The Development
of Modern Epidemiology

The Development of Modern Epidemiology: Personal Reports From Those Who Were There

Edited by

Walter W. Holland

Emeritus Professor of Public Health Medicine
and Visiting Professor of London School
of Economics and Political Science,
University of London, UK

Jørn Olsen

President of the International Epidemiology Association;
Professor and Chair, Department of Epidemiology,
School of Public Health, UCLA,
Los Angeles, USA

and

Charles du V. Florey

Emeritus Professor of Epidemiology and Public Health,
University of Dundee, UK

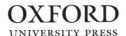

OXFORD
UNIVERSITY PRESS

OXFORD
UNIVERSITY PRESS

Great Clarendon Street, Oxford OX2 6DP

Oxford University Press is a department of the University of Oxford.
It furthers the University's objective of excellence in research, scholarship,
and education by publishing worldwide in

Oxford New York

Auckland Cape Town Dar es Salaam Hong Kong Karachi
Kuala Lumpur Madrid Melbourne Mexico City Nairobi
New Delhi Shanghai Taipei Toronto

With offices in

Argentina Austria Brazil Chile Czech Republic France Greece
Guatemala Hungary Italy Japan Poland Portugal Singapore
South Korea Switzerland Thailand Turkey Ukraine Vietnam

Oxford is a registered trade mark of Oxford University Press
in the UK and in certain other countries

Published in the United States
by Oxford University Press Inc., New York

A catalogue record for this title is available from the British Library

Library of Congress Cataloging in Publication Data

(Data available)

Typeset by Cepha Imaging Private Ltd., Bangalore, India
Printed in Great Britain
on acid-free paper by Biddles Ltd., King's Lynn

ISBN 978–0–19–856954–1 (Hbk.)

10 9 8 7 6 5 4 3 2 1

Whilst every effort has been made to ensure that the contents of this book are as complete, accurate and up-to-date as possible at the date of writing, Oxford University Press is not able to give any guarantee or assurance that such is the case. Readers are urged to take appropriately qualified medical advice in all cases. The information in this book is intended to be useful to the general reader, but should not be used as a means of self-diagnosis or for the prescription of medication.

Preface

This book collects the experiences of eminent scientists who have been responsible for the amazing advances that have been made in our ability to prevent the conditions that afflict humankind, by improving the health services, reducing occupational and environmental hazards, and in developing the methods that we can apply to these problems. The foundation of the International Epidemiological Association (IEA) by Pemberton and Willard 50 years ago was a landmark event. Their genius in identifying the need to provide a forum for those involved in epidemiology globally attracted many of the already well known epidemiologists as well as those who were to play a major role in the development of the subject. This book brings together contributions from many of those who have played a crucial role in this endeavour to celebrate the 50th anniversary of the IEA, though contributors were not selected because of their IEA membership. It is both an account of past achievements and the lessons learnt by those involved and a critical analysis which can serve as guidance for the future.

Professor Walter W. Holland

Acknowledgements

We are extremely greatful to Mrs Champa Heidbrink for her unfailing helpfulness and co-ordinating abilities. Without Dr Nic Williams and her colleagues at Oxford University Press this work would not have been so well produced.

Contents

Section 3: **Applications and role of epidemiology in related domains**

Section 4: **Methodology**

Section 5: **Regions and countries**

Contributors

Kunio Aoki
Professor Emeritus of Nagoya University,
Japan;
Honorary Member of the International
Epidemiological Association

Haroutune K. Armenian
Professor of Epidemiology,
Bloomberg School of Public Health,
Johns Hopkins University,
Baltimore, MD, USA;
President,
American University of Armenia,
Oakland, CA, USA

Arpo Aromaa
Professor and Director of Department,
Department of Health and Functional Capacity,
The National Public Health Institute,
Helsinki, Finland

Elizabeth Barrett-Connor
Professor and Chief,
Division of Epidemiology,
Department of Family and Preventive
Medicine, School of Medicine,
University of California,
San Diego, CA, USA

Robert Beaglehole
Director, Chronic Diseases and
Health Promotion, Noncommunicable
Diseases and Mental Health,
World Health Organization, Geneva,
Switzerland

Henry Blackburn
Mayo Professor Emeritus, Division of
Epidemiology and Community Health,
School of Public Health, University of
Minnesota, Minneapolis, MN, USA

Francisco Bolúmar
Catedrático de Medicina, Preventiva y
Salud Pública, Universidad Miguel
Hernandez, Elche, Spain;
Departamento de Ciencias Sanitarias y
Médico-Sociales Universidad de Alcala,
Madrid, Spain

Gérard Bréart
Professor of Public Health,
Université Pierre et Marie Curie,
Paris, France;
Director, Unité de Recherches en Santé
Périnatale et Santé des Femmes,
INSERM, France

Lester Breslow
Professor Emeritus and former Dean,
School of Public Health,
University of California,
Los Angeles, CA, USA

George W. Comstock
Professor of Epidemiology Emeritus,
Johns Hopkins Bloomberg School
of Public Health;
Director Emeritus,
George W. Comstock Center for Public
Health Research and Prevention,
Baltimore, MD, USA

Andrew G. Dean
Information Systems,
HIV/AIDS Clinic, La Romana,
Dominican Republic

Roger Detels
Professor of Epidemiology and Infectious
Diseases, Department of Epidemiology,
School of Public Health,
University of California,
Los Angeles, CA, USA

Richard Doll (1912–2005)
Honorary Consultant,
Clinical Trial Service Unit and Epidemiology
Study Unit (CTSU), University of Oxford, UK

Charles du V. Florey
Emeritus Professor of Epidemiology
and Public Health,
University of Dundee, UK

Eduardo L. Franco
James McGill Professor
Department of Epidemiology and
Biostatistics and Department of Oncology,
McGill University,
Montreal, Canada

Julio Frenk
Ministry of Health, Mexico

Rebecca Fuhrer
Professor and Chair,
Department of Epidemiology,
Biostatistics and Occupational Health,
McGill University, Montreal, Canada

Octavio Gómez-Dantes
Director General for Performance Evaluation,
Ministry of Health, Mexico

Malcolm Harrington
Emeritus Professor of Occupational Medicine,
University of Birmingham, UK

Richard Heller
Emeritus Professor of the Universities
of Manchester, UK, and Newcastle,
Australia

Basil S. Hetzel
Former Foundation Professor of Social and
Preventive Medicine, Monash University,
Melbourne, Australia; Former Executive
Director and Chairman, International Council
for Control of Iodine Deficiency Disorders,
Adelaide, Australia;
Emeritus Professor of Medicine,
University of Adelaide, Australia

Walter W. Holland
Emeritus Professor of Public Health and
Visiting Professor of London School of
Economics and Political Science,
University of London, UK

Manolis Kogevinas
Professor and Co-Director,
Centre for Research in Environmental
Epidemiology (CREAL), Municipal Institute
of Medical Research (IMIM), Barcelona,
Spain; Department of Social Medicine,
Medical School, University of Crete,
Heraklion, Greece

Rafael Lozano
Director General for Health Information,
Ministry of Health, Mexico

Adetokunbo O. Lucas
Adjunct Professor,
Harvard School of Public Health,
Harvard University, Cambridge, MA, USA

Wieslaw Magdzik
Emeritus Professor of Epidemiology,
National Institute of Hygiene,
Warsaw, Poland

Salaheddin M. Mahmud
Department of Community Health Sciences,
University of Manitoba,
Winnipeg, Canada

Ahmed Mandil
Professor and Dean,
College of Health Sciences,
University of Sharjah,
United Arab Emirates

Colin Mathers
Department of Measurement and
Health Information, Evidence and
Information for Policy Cluster,
World Health Organization Headquarters,
Geneva, Switzerland

Franco Merletti
Unit of Cancer Epidemiology and Centre
for Oncologic Prevention,
University of Turin, Italy

Olli S. Miettinen
Professor,
Department of Epidemiology
and Biostatistics, and Department of
Medicine, McGill University,
Montreal, Canada

Alfredo Morabia
Professor of Epidemiology,
Center for the Biology of Natural Systems,
School of Earth and Environmental Sciences,
Queens College, City University of
New York, NY, USA

Richard H. Morrow
Professor of International Health,
Johns Hopkins University Bloomberg School
of Public Health,
Baltimore, MD, USA

William J. Moss
Associate Professor of Epidemiology,
Johns Hopkins University Bloomburg
School of Public Health,
Baltimore, MD, USA

Landon Myer
Senior Lecturer,
School of Public Health and Family Medicine,
University of Cape Town, South Africa; and
Department of Epidemiology, Mailman
School of Public Health,
Columbia University, New York, NY, USA

Kenrad Nelson
Department of Epidemiology,
Johns Hopkins University Bloomberg
School of Public Health,
Baltimore, MD, USA

Jørn Olsen
President of the International Epidemiological
Association

John Pemberton
Emeritus Professor of Social and Preventive
Medicine, the Queens University of Belfast,
1958–1976

Ian Prior
Director,
Epidemiology Unit, Wellington Hospital
and Wellington School of Medicine,
New Zealand

Lee Robins
Emeritus Professor of Psychiatry,
Department of Psychiatry,
Washington University, St Louis, MO, USA

Claude Rumeau-Rouquette
Former Director of Research at Institut
National de la Santé et de la Recherche
Médicale (INSERM)

Rodolfo Saracci
Director of Research in Epidemiology,
National Research Council, Pisa, Italy;
Adjunct Professor,
University of Aarhus, Denmark;
Former president, 1996–1999,
International Epidemiological Association

Itsuzo Shigematsu
Consultant Emeritus of Radiation Effects
Research Foundation; Honorary Member of
the International Epidemiological Association

Chitr Sitthi-amorn
The College of Public Health and
the Institute of Health Research,
Chulalongkorn University, Thailand

Tom Sorahan
Professor of Occupational Epidemiology,
University of Birmingham, UK

Frank E. Speizer
Edward H. Kass Professor of Medicine,
Harvard Medical School;
Professor of Environmental Science,
Harvard School of Public Health;
Channing Laboratory, Brigham and
Women's Hospital, Boston, MA, USA

Mervyn W. Susser
Gertrude H. Sergievsky Professor Emeritus
of Epidemiology; Special Lecturer
in the Mailman School of
Public Health, Columbia University,
New York, NY, USA

Ira B. Tager
Professor of Epidemiology,
Division of Epidemiology,
School of Public Health,
University of California, Berkeley, CA, USA

Benedetto Terracini
Former Professor of Cancer Epidemiology,
Unit of Cancer Epidemiology,
University of Turin, Italy

Mohamed H. Wahdan
Assistant Regional Director—Poliomyelitis
Eradication, World Health Organization,
Regional Office for the Eastern Mediterranean
Region (WHO/EMRO), Cairo, Eygpt

Kerr L. White
Former President International
Epidemiological Association; Founding Chair,
Department of Health Care Organization,
the Johns Hopkins University,
Baltimore, MD, USA;
former Deputy Director for Health Sciences,
the Rockefeller Foundation,
New York, NY, USA

Warren Winkelstein Jr
Professor of Epidemiology Emeritus,
Division of Epidemiology,
School of Public Health,
University of California,
Berkeley, CA, USA

Miroslaw J. Wysocki
Professor of Epidemiology,
Deputy Director,
National Institute of Hygiene,
Warsaw, Poland

Yu Shun-Zhang
Professor,
Institue of Preventive Medicine,
Fudan University, Shanghai, China

Jan E. Zejda
Professor and Prorector (Research) and Head,
Department of Epidemiology, Medical
University of Silesia Katowice, Poland

Section 1

History and setting the scene

Introduction

Walter W. Holland, Charles Florey, and Jørn Olsen

The establishment in 1956 of the International Epidemiological Association (IEA) by John Pemberton and Harold Willard was a landmark in the internationalization of epidemiology. It created a group of individuals who were passionate about its development. They wanted to 'spread the gospel'. This book is intended to illustrate how the subject has developed in the past 50 years by providing personal stories from prominent leaders of the discipline. The majority of the authors illustrate their commitment to the improvement of not only knowledge but also the social conditions and health of the population. We asked each of the contributors to describe how and why they came to the subject. The major drivers in almost all instances were the example of their mentors, the recognition that there was a need to have a wider perspective than the treatment of individual patients if one wished to influence health, a social conscience, and, of course, luck, opportunity, and being in the right place at the right time. We also asked them to describe the obstacles they met when they started doing research. Some mention problems relating to the publication of findings that were unwanted by people in power, but it is surprising that only a few talk about internal conflicts within health research. Maybe these problems are only emerging now, when epidemiology is a serious competitor for a much larger proportion of research funds than 50 years ago.

Pemberton and Willard's contributions cannot be overestimated. Their original intention of a club to promote the dissemination of knowledge and improve the teaching of the subject has been achieved. Their contributions illustrate how the existence of the IEA helped create the necessary conditions for establishment of the academic discipline in most regions and countries, and how the knowledge, methods, and philosophy have been disseminated.

It is remarkable how over the years epidemiology has become a respected subject in medicine, rather than simply a fringe discipline. The chapters on individual diseases illustrate how epidemiological findings have contributed to the knowledge on specific diseases but also how such knowledge has enabled major advances in preventing some diseases from occurring and eliminating others.

We have not attempted to be comprehensive in the choice of subjects—for example there is no chapter on the eradication of smallpox. This story of the work of D. A. Henderson and his colleagues is well known; instead we chose to include a chapter by another IEA stalwart, Basil Hetzel, on the eradication of iodine deficiency disorders, a rather less well known example of how a disease can be eradicated.

The book has been organized to illustrate a number of themes. The first section sets the scene, and gives an historical account of concepts and ideas and portrays the current importance of the subject to the World Health Organization (WHO) and to global health issues.

The second section is intended to illustrate the advances and contributions to epidemiological knowledge in a number of specific disease areas, for example cancer, cardiovascular diseases, malaria, and tuberculosis. Again, this is not intended to be comprehensive but to illustrate in a few conditions how epidemiology has progressed and how it has developed in its concepts and contributed to the developments in health improvement and health policy in both communicable and non-communicable disease. Chapter 10 on perinatal epidemiology illustrates particularly well the development of knowledge and the contribution that good epidemiology can make to improvement in maternal and child health and how epidemiological science helps in the formulation of health policy. It also demonstrates the dangers of reliance on central direction in modern heterogeneous populations. Armenian's chapter on non-biological disorders (Chapter 11) is of paramount importance at this time in illustrating how epidemiology can be used in coping with war and disasters, what actions can and should be taken, but also in questioning the ways in which the findings are used.

Detels comments in Chapter 12 on why new infectious diseases have emerged as important health issues, what we know about them, and how they may be tackled. HIV is probably only one of the warning signals of other emerging diseases that relate to global trade, travel, and social injustice. There may be opportunities to contain these diseases at a very early stage if we have sufficient advanced monitoring systems and enough competence to act. If these opportunities are missed the health consequences may be devastating, as they were and are for HIV/AIDS. Comstock, in Chapter 13 on tuberculosis, provides a model of how epidemiology tackles an issue and the advances that have occurred as a result of sound research worldwide in the control of one of the world's scourges. He illustrates the need for proper diagnosis to trace the natural history and thus to be able to prevent and treat the condition. He also shows how modern genetic studies can and will be used in disease control. Morrow and Moss's chapter on malaria (Chapter 14), as well as providing a brief historical account, demonstrates that thorough basic research is required if one wishes to develop appropriate methods of treatment and control—a lesson often disregarded by some of us who consider that only applied research is required in the health field. Their emphasis on the need to teach mothers about the prevention of malaria is a salutary example of the multidisciplinary nature of epidemiology.

The chapters by Blackburn on cardiovascular disease (Chapter 7) and Speizer and Tager on respiratory disease (Chapter 8), two of the commonest 'chronic' diseases, illustrate the development of epidemiological methods and their application to these conditions. Both also illustrate the importance of serendipity in charismatic researchers in identifying suitable, testable hypotheses—success in both these conditions in identifying methods of prevention and then applications has led to a marked diminution in both the prevalence and incidence of these diseases in some countries.

Section three illustrates the application of epidemiology in cognate domains. Breslow and Detels in Chapter 15 have chosen four major public health areas—smallpox, kuru, injuries, and health behaviours—in which the contributions of epidemiological findings have been crucial in improving health. Kerr White, in Chapter 16 on health services research (HSR), illustrates the importance of sound epidemiology to the improvement and development of medical care and health services starting with the contributions of Florence Nightingale in the middle of nineteenth century, which contributed both to improvement in the care of soldiers in a war, but also to the design of hospitals and the measurement of performance in peacetime. In all countries there is an inexorable growth in demand for health services. Thus there is need to develop evidence for improving the effectiveness and efficiency of both health service and health practice. Kerr White wonders why epidemiology is often neglected in the investigation and design of policies, services, and practices. His chapter ends on an optimistic note for the future interaction between epidemiology and health services research. There is no doubt that his optimism is justified in the acceptance of the application of research methods—but the application of findings in the development of prevention, cure, rehabilitation, and caring in the health services must be viewed more cautiously. It is true that the development of services concerned with the prevention of disease is almost always based on sound epidemiological evidence. But in the developed world the situation is more problematic. Immunization policies, based on sound research, are often threatened by the power of fringe groups seizing on aberrant, or even false, findings, as in the case of MMR immunization. In spite of outstanding research in the world's wealthiest country, the USA, showing the benefits of medical services, services for the poor are neglected. In the UK, even though proper evidence is required for the treatment of individual patients, health policy is often formulated without evidence of effectiveness or efficiency but on the prejudices or beliefs of ministers and their advisers. Thus although epidemiology has become recognized and accepted in investigations of the causes of disease and their treatment and prevention by the health professions it has not yet attained the necessary authority of use in the design of health policy or services by intelligent laypeople in positions of power.

Chapter 17 on occupational and environmental epidemiology provides a thorough account of how registers can be and are being used in the identification and surveillance of occupational/environmental factors in the development of disease and how risks are identified. With the demise of heavy industries such as coal mining or steel production in many developed countries concern with occupational risk has unfortunately diminished—although there is still a paramount need to be concerned with workplace hazards, such as from the manufacture of chemical agents and drugs or other modern high-tech products. Occupational conditions in such enterprises as offices or hospitals may have important health consequences, too often neglected. The identification of such hazards is often far more difficult, as the effects are more subtle and take longer to develop than those of 'older' industries. The chapter also emphasizes the methodological issues in occupational epidemiology. The authors' prediction of the future is not rosy in view of the mobility of populations, the restrictions posed by data/information protection, the interference of the media and legislative processes, and the demise of trade union power with a concomitant increase in entrepreneurial power. The importance of these issues, particularly in the developing world, should not be underestimated. We need to make modern and powerful research methods available for health personnel who are in charge of workers' health in countries which become recipients of dangerous work conditions/practices that are no longer acceptable in more affluent countries.

Susser and Myer's chapter on social epidemiology (Chapter 18) outlines the different ways in which this subject has developed in the USA compared with the UK and other countries. In the USA the subject was not developed to the same extent in the 1960s as in the UK, and the major drivers for methodological and subject interests were in psychiatry. By contrast, the underlying feature of UK concern was inequality. One of the editors (W.H.) was advised when the title of his department was being considered that the term 'social medicine' had to be linked to 'clinical epidemiology' if he wanted to retain his links with colleagues in the USA. More recently Susser and Myer outline that the major drivers in the USA have been concerned with psychological factors and stress, and the studies have been largely descriptive with few examples of interventions. The contrast with the UK, and the effect of the 1980 Black Report (*Inequalities in health. Report of a research working party*, DHSS, London) are emphasized. It is of interest that individuals of South African origin and experience (John Cassell, Mervyn Susser) have had such a powerful influence on the development of this aspect of epidemiology in both the USA and the UK.

Several chapters illustrate that differences in opinion on whether epidemiology should focus upon proximal determinants of disease or more distant drivers of poor health are not new. These opinions have political roots as well as roots in whether epidemiology should link with demography or molecular epidemiology. Should epidemiologists develop their hypotheses on determinants of disease by studying disease patterns over time and between different populations, or should they follow recent developments in modern biology? At present, some of the advantages of epidemiology seems to have been forgotten. Theories are developed without consideration of whether these theories make any sense at the macro level. Does disease in the population follow a pattern that is at least compatible with the hypothesis? Or is it only a matter of biological plausibility? A similar dilemma exists for the clinical epidemiologist. Should there be an interest in the population of patients or should one try to use epidemiological methods to study the mechanism of treatment effects? Without doubt several approaches are needed; in some instances one uses epidemiology to study biological phenomena, in others one uses biology to facilitate epidemiology, as illustrated by Hetzel, and the problem is to find a proper balance.

In Chapter 19 Hetzel illustrates two remarkable epidemiological developments. His chapter on nutrition outlines how epidemiological observations followed by laboratory investigations and a randomized controlled trial have led to the elimination of iodine deficiency disorder, a major health scourge in many parts of the world. This is a superb example of how powerful a tool epidemiology can be, but also of the importance of cooperation with the basic sciences. His second example, of the investigation of diet in the aetiology of heart disease, demonstrates the complexity of the subject—similar findings were shown in the USA and Australia, but the findings could not be demonstrated in the UK.

Section four is largely concerned with methodological developments in which Miettinen (Chapter 20) has played an important role. There have been enormous strides in the statistical methods used in epidemiology. To some extent, concerns about experimental design or the choice of population to study, observer variability, response rates and methods of measurement in the testing of specific hypotheses have been replaced by intricate, sophisticated statistical methods, made possible by computers, particularly small PCs. For some 'old stagers' the change from concern with biology to reliance on mathematics has not necessarily been welcomed. The elegance of some of the older studies, for example those of Donald Reid on air pollution, is no longer common. Reid's work on air pollution in England was parsimonious in its use of resources. By comparing sickness absence in postal deliverymen, who worked outdoors, with that of individuals working in the same area of London and recruited from the same population with similar rates of pay but who worked indoors sorting the mail, he showed that cold temperatures and air pollution were associated with more frequent episodes of bronchitis. Nowadays far larger population groups, and far more variables, are investigated, and confirm these findings. This change has influenced recruitment to epidemiology: whereas in the past the majority of epidemiologists were medically qualified and the approach to investigations was led by biology, now mathematically trained graduates with social or environmental qualifications are common, or biologists only trained in laboratory methods, particularly in the USA and the UK.

Part of this change in methodology has been influenced by the availability of much more data on health and populations, as outlined in Chapter 22 by Kogevinas. Large-scale repeated national surveys on health, behaviour, environment, and economic issues are now available and easily accessible. Many health services also collect large amounts of administrative data, which often include diagnostic information. This means that it is often much cheaper to use available information and data sets to answer epidemiological problems than to devise the collection of data from specific population groups. Kogevinas does, however, emphasize some of the problems with these large data sets, which have usually not been collected to answer a specific question.

Nelson, in Chapter 21, illustrates the developments that have taken place in the investigation of outbreaks of infectious disease. He illustrates the advances that have occurred as a result of the use of molecular tests and of the development of surveillance now possible with the use of computers. Much modern technology has yet to be implemented on a large scale and at a more rapid rate. It has to be linked to population monitoring both humans and animals worldwide, as illustrated by the current epidemic of bird flu. His chapter complements Chapter 13 on tuberculosis by Comstock. We need to ensure that, as with many of the other chapters, this enthusiasm and the excitement of epidemiology is portrayed in our educational programmes on infectious and non-communicable disease epidemiology. Each has much to learn from the other. Both are equally important if we are concerned with health improvement.

Clinical epidemiology has been a term widely used, particularly in North America, Australia, and the Far East. In Chapter 23, Heller, a major proponent of the use of this label, gives a very balanced account and emphasizes that the clinician is now able to understand that epidemiology enables the application of a scientific approach to clinical medicine. He suggests that its major methodological themes have been statistics and implementation. Clinical epidemiology has served as an excellent bridge between clinicians and epidemiologists and has helped to involve health economists in epidemiology. 'Interaction is the key to clinical epidemiology', as Heller outlines: unless one is concerned with large numbers of patients, one cannot study the natural history of diseases nor can one understand the performance of a diagnostic test—unless one knows about group probability. Paradoxically, he suggests, public health, at least in the UK, now neglects epidemiology and has become too closely linked to political imperatives with neglect of sound epidemiological findings or the need for evidence. An example given is the universal introduction of 'health trainers', a middle-class fad which has not been shown to be effective in reducing morbidity or mortality.

Section five looks at the development of the subject and the concerns of individual countries or regions. Each shows the concerns and changes that have occurred. In some instances accounts of specific health hazards and their investigation and control are given.

These chapters are fascinating. In the description of development in the Americas (Chapter 24), the rise in the application of computers to the analysis of data is chronicled. Of particular interest is the development of Epi Info, a widely used program, particularly for the surveillance of infectious disease. This chapter describes the increasing use of statistical and mathematical methods to improve the analysis and interpretation of epidemiological data. However, the authors caution investigators on the need to know their data properly before using these highly sophisticated methods.

Chapter 25 demonstrates the important role played by the WHO, IARC, and the EU in fostering education, training, and cooperation in epidemiology in Europe. But it also emphasizes the problems faced. The possibilities for improving the health of the population in Europe have not and are not being exploited in an optimal way. Unfortunately the concentration on wealth creation and the illusory glamour of developing new technologies, for example molecular biology, permeates international bodies as much as it does national governments.

Lucas (Chapter 26) in his fascinating account of trends in Africa emphasizes the role that classical 'shoe-leather' epidemiology and cartography has played in the increase in our knowledge of tropical disease and thus the control of these conditions.

One of the best and most characteristic accounts of how individuals are attracted to epidemiology is given by Prior and Beaglehole in Chapter 27. They emphasize the importance of family background and their forebears concern with social justice and 'environmental' issues such as cannibalism. But this is not enough—it needs to be linked to academic curiosity as well as scientific rigour. The work that they initiated in South Sea Islanders demonstrates the importance of community participation and involvement and how this can and should be linked to medical care and the development of health policy. Their chapter also emphasizes the role of mentoring in the recruitment and retention of future epidemiologists.

An excellent account of obstacles to epidemiology and the difficulty of coping with disease outbreaks with political implications is given by Wahdan and Mandil (Chapter 28). This illustrates that epidemiology needs an official 'code of conduct' to prevent the suppression and manipulation of research findings. In 1969 a cholera outbreak in Egypt with more than 80,000 cases was renamed 'summer diarrhoea', while the occurrence of an outbreak of bubonic plague at this time was hidden. The lack of adequate statistics until the beginning of this century has meant that information on poliomyelitis and typhoid in Egypt has been lacking. The lessons we can learn from this for global control, eradication, and surveillance are important. Both Wahdan and Mandil demonstrate the importance of the support of the WHO in disease control in developing countries and the need for coordination and cooperation. The results in the control of meningitis and hepatitis B in the region are a clear example. They emphasize the role of education in changing the attitudes of both doctors and other health policy-makers.

Chapter 29, by Yu Shun-Zhang from China, reinforces these messages and illustrates the enormous progress that has been made in the control of infectious diseases through the application of sound epidemiological principles. This chapter also provides a warning of the simultaneous increase in chronic disease as a health problem, even before the problems of communicable disease have been tackled.

Sitthi-Amorn's contribution (Chapter 30) complements these chapters both by outlining the history of epidemiology in his country but also by his discussion of the 'politics' of studies of 'modern' diseases such as HIV/AIDS and SARS and their control.

Aoki and Shigematsu show in Chapter 31 how epidemiology has developed over the years in Japan. It should be noted that, as elsewhere, one of the main drivers to the growth in importance of epidemiology and its involvement in health policy was partly the investigation of a number of major environmental disasters, such as cadmium and mercury poisoning, and the need to follow up the survivors of the atom bombs in Hiroshima and Nagasaki to better understand the long-term effects of radiation exposure. Japan also showed the way in the exploitation of disease registers—and now demonstrates the ability to investigate the cause of rare diseases through nationally coordinated studies.

In Chapter 32 Frenk and his colleagues from Mexico describe the major changes in health which have occurred in Central America, and link these to both the frequency of individual groups of diseases and changes in fertility. From the perspective of a Minister of Health it is emphasized that epidemiology is the key to changes in health policy.

Barrett-Connor and Winkelstein in their consideration of developments in North America (Chapter 33) suggest that one of the most important reasons for the growth in importance in funding of epidemiology in the USA after the Second World War was concern with germ warfare (later biological warfare) and the Cold War. They illustrate the importance of Goldberger's work on the identification of the causes of pellagra and its control, the analysis and determination of cause and effect in lung cancer and smoking, and the epidemiology of cervical cancer as major stimuli in the development of epidemiology in the USA.

Wysocki and Magdzik (Chapter 34), while demonstrating the improvement in health in Poland (and Eastern Europe) due to the control of communicable disease, also show that in the past 40 years there have been major advances in the study of chronic respiratory diseases, cancer, and diabetes which have led to better methods of control. They illustrate the emergence of studies in children and environmental hazards to illustrate how epidemiological research has attempted to develop methods for the prevention and control of chronic disease.

In Chapter 36 Saracci, Terracini, and Merletti, describe events in Italy over the past 50 years. Starting with the strong basis of genetics and the social movement of the 1960s, epidemiology began to gain a foothold in academic institutions. A major impetus for use of the subject was the need to investigate a number of environmental disasters, such as Seveso. The creation of the Associazione Italiano di Epidemiologia (Italian Association of Epidemiologists) provided a firm foundation for the subject and it has prospered greatly since then.

Bolúmar, in his description of the development of epidemiology in Spain (Chapter 37), emphasizes the past, as well as the present. The association of pellagra with diet was made in

Valencia in 1790 and a Spanish book of 1803 is claimed to have been the first to have used epidemiology in its title. The import effect of the political and social environment on teaching, practice, and research in epidemiology is illustrated. The progress made in the early years of the twentieth century was halted, and disputed, by the Civil War and its aftermath. Only since the fall of the Franco regime has epidemiology been able to progress. The link to the service of public health is emphasized in Bolúmar's description of epidemiological developments. As with Italy, the creation of a national association has ensured that there is a firm foundation for the subject.

Conclusion

The accounts of developments in individual disease areas, countries, and methods provide a fascinating picture and how much we have developed. Obviously there are differences, but the underlying themes amongst those who have contributed have been their social concerns, their intellectual curiosity, and their intentions to improve health.

The problems we face today have been present right from the start. Should we focus our attention on the causes of diseases or ill-health; upstream or downstream in the river of causation? Should we get our research ideas from studying disease patterns in human populations or follow new trends in molecular biology, or both? We divide the subject by the type of population studied; healthy or sick (as in clinical epidemiology), by the exposures of interest (as in social epidemiology or genetic epidemiology), or by the disease under study (as in epidemiology of infectious diseases or cancer). What binds all this together is a common set of methods developed to make inferences based on data from populations. Development of this set of methods may come from new ways of assessing the data we use, from a deeper understanding of the concepts we apply, or from understanding more about the sources of bias that are present when complex systems are being studied.

Whereas the subject has been accepted by clinicians and used by them in the development of medical science, treatment, and prevention, this has not necessarily been so with health policy-makers. There have been many advances in concepts and methods; most striking, however, has been the re-emergence of infectious disease which has again encouraged a greater link to laboratory research. With the increasing predominance of statistics and modelling some consider that there has been an unfortunate decline in biologically driven research, with a concomitant decline in the involvement of medically qualified scientists. It would also appear that whereas the earlier investigators were largely driven by their wish to improve health, more recent entrants have a greater interest in methodology rather than application. Epidemiology would be best served if a dynamic balance is maintained between the two perspectives.

This book certainly illustrates the enormous contributions epidemiology has made in the past 50 or more years, both in methods and as well as applications to health improvements. The IEA can be proud to have fostered this activity and provides an excellent foundation for the future advancement of the discipline.

2

Setting the scene (largely from the UK point of view)

John Pemberton

The epidemiology of infectious disease

When I became a medical student in London in 1930 'epidemiology' meant the study of epidemics of infectious disease. It was included in the course of lectures on public health given by the local medical officer of health. He described the common infectious diseases, vaccination against smallpox, and the laws relating to the control of the physical environment. Many students found the subject uninteresting. We saw very few cases of infectious disease in our teaching hospitals and did not realize how common they were in the community. We certainly did not appreciate the enormous successes that had been achieved in their control by the great public health movement started in the nineteenth century and the devoted work of many medical officers of health. Most of the patients we saw in our teaching hospital were suffering from non-communicable conditions. The social aspects of these illnesses were hardly ever considered and their epidemiology was unknown territory.

Social medicine and clinical medicine

In the 1930s general physicians were aware of specific occupational diseases such as lead poisoning and the nutritional deficiency diseases such as rickets and scurvy. Few recognized the more general relationships of occupation or nutrition to health, although the Registrar General's report *Occupational mortality* published in 1938 which related death rates from many diseases to occupational class clearly showed a connection between heath and income (The Stationery Office 1938). The nutrition surveys organized by John Boyd Orr in the 1930s, in one of which I was privileged to take part, demonstrated that a large proportion of the population was not getting enough to eat for growth and health (Orr 1936).

It was my work with Boyd Orr, which involved the clinical examination of about 4000 children, many from very poor homes, in sixteen centres in Great Britain, combined with my socialist convictions that led me to decide to spend my professional life in social medicine and epidemiology.

One of the few clinicians who, at that time, recognized the importance of social conditions in the causation of disease was James Spence, the first professor of child health in the UK. He reported that the children he saw from the professional classes were heavier, taller, and had higher haemoglobin values than the children from poor homes (Spence and Charles 1934).

Social medicine and politics

In 1930 a small group of UK doctors who were socialists founded the Socialist Medical Association (SMA), headed by a consultant surgeon from the Middlesex Hospital, Somerville Hastings. A main aim of the SMA was:

> To work for a socialised medical service, both preventive and curative, free and open to all, to secure the highest standards of health for the British people.
>
> Stewart (1999)

The SMA became affiliated to the Labour Party and provided some of the basic ideas underlying the National Health Service created by the Labour Government in 1948. Some of the early members of the SMA were attracted to the concepts of social medicine because they believed that poverty was an important cause of ill-health and that some solutions to health problems required political action. Several of the early members of the SMA later became heads of university departments and research units in social medicine and epidemiology, including Maurice Backett, Richard Doll, and myself.

War and the advancement of social medicine

The coming of war in 1939 caused a great disruption of the health services and led to new ideas about the financing and administration of these, which were embodied in the historic Beveridge Report of 1942. The report included the assumption that there would be a National Health Service after the war, which would be universal in coverage and free at the time of use (The Stationery Office 1942).

The registration of the whole population with a general practitioner which followed when the National Health Service was established in 1948 helped to make possible some large-scale epidemiological and health service studies which came later. In 1942 the Chief Medical Officer, Wilson Jameson, in an article entitled 'War and the advancement of social medicine' referred to the creation of a national nutrition policy which owed a lot to Boyd Orr's research and also helped towards the introduction of social medicine into medical education (Jameson 1942).

Social medicine accepted as part of the training of a doctor

In 1943 the Royal College of Physicians of London published a report which recommended 'That every medical school, should establish a Department of Preventive and Social Medicine' and that the social medicine course should replace the traditional course in public health and should be closely associated with students' clinical work (Royal College of Physicians of London 1943). The report was not very clear about what social medicine was and still restricted the term 'epidemiology' to infectious diseases, but it did give the stamp of approval of a highly respected medical institution to the inclusion of the subject in the medical course.

The appointment by the University of Oxford in 1943 of a distinguished Professor of Medicine, John Ryle, to the first Chair of Social Medicine in the UK confirmed the acceptance of social medicine as an important subject in the training of a doctor. Edinburgh and Birmingham universities soon followed Oxford by creating academic departments of social medicine and ultimately nearly all the UK universities followed suit. The university departments that were being created at the end of the 1940s and in the 1950s were starting research as well as designing and introducing social medicine teaching programmes like that at Sheffield (Hobson and Pemberton 1950). Much of the research started by these new departments consisted of medical–social surveys of specific population group such as old people living at home (Hobson and Pemberton 1955).

Their aim was to describe the health of these groups, and to identify the causes of ill-health. The pioneering medical–social survey of Sheldon on 'Some aspects of old age' (Sheldon 1948) compelled the attention of the medical profession to this age group and led to the recognition of geriatrics as a medical speciality.

So far I have concentrated on what was called 'social medicine' in the UK in the period from the early 1930s to the early 1950s.

The social aspects of a patient's illness were increasingly considered in the practice of clinical medicine. Those working in the new university departments of social medicine were beginning to realize that this led to comparisons of groups of people exposed to different social conditions such as diet, housing, and occupation. There was an increasing awareness that epidemiological methods were required to investigate these differences, especially in the field of non-communicable disease. University departments and research units of social medicine were beginning to embark upon epidemiological research.

Remarkably, J. N. Morris had started as early as 1942 to carry out epidemiological research on non-communicable disease, namely juvenile rheumatism and peptic ulcer (Morris 1942, 1944).

The London School of Hygiene and Tropical Medicine

In addition to the university departments of social medicine which were being set up following Oxford's example in 1942 an important centre of epidemiology, the London School of Hygiene and Tropical Medicine (LSHTM), of London University, began to undertake research on the epidemiology of non-communicable disease.

After the end of Second World War a group of doctors came to the LSHTM to take the course leading to the Diploma in Public Health or to take up research posts. Bradford Hill who had followed Greenwood as Professor of Epidemiology had a considerable influence on this group of young doctors which included A. L. (Archie) Cochrane, Richard Doll, J. N. (Jerry) Morris, and Richard Schilling, all of whom later made important contributions to the epidemiology of non-communicable disease.

The Medical Research Council (MRC) made an important contribution by creating the Pneumoconiosis Research Unit (PRU) in 1945, directed by Charles Fletcher, and the Social Medicine Research Unit under J. N. Morris in 1948 at the London Hospital Medical School. Members of the PRU made significant contributions to the development of epidemiology, including the creation of instruments to measure pulmonary function and providing a definition of chronic bronchitis which made it possible to carry out accurate surveys of chronic respiratory disease.

The stage was now set for a big development in epidemiology in which the International Epidemiological Association was to play a significant role.

The origins and contribution to epidemiology of the International Epidemiological Association

For those of us who wished to make a career in social medicine there were few jobs available; perhaps a lectureship or research fellowship in a university department or a MRC research unit or a similar job at the LSHTM, but little else. We had a passionate belief in the importance of social medicine but were not sure what the subject included, how we should teach it, what research would be appropriate, and whether it would be possible to make a career in it.

Some of us decided to try and get a grant to visit the USA to see what was going on there.

I received valuable advice from Professor Robert Cruickshank, Professor of Bacteriology at St Mary's in the USA. He later became the first chairman and wise adviser of the international group we were to set up.

My visit to the USA was almost prevented when the New York immigration officer read my introductory letter from the MRC which said that it was my 'intention to study the teaching of social medicine in the USA'. He almost exploded and shouted out 'We don't want any of that filth here'. It was the end of the McCarthy period.

In the New York Hospital I met a young doctor, Harold Willard, who was doing a study on what happened to patients after they left hospital. He had been shocked by some of his findings.

We both worked in departments of clinical medicine and had been encouraged by our chiefs to pursue our interest in social medicine. We knew a few others with similar interests, some of whom were already working in the small number of centres where social medicine was being developed. In 1954 we decided to get in touch with them with a view to forming a corresponding club to find out what was going on in the field. We found 29 other enthusiasts, mainly in the UK and USA, and started to circulate a six-monthly bulletin containing information about what was going on in their centres. We called ourselves 'The International Corresponding Club' (ICC).

The object of the ICC was:

> To facilitate the communication between physicians working for the most part in university departments of social and preventive medicine or in research institutes devoted to these aspects of medicine, throughout the world.

This was to be achieved by the publication of the bulletin twice a year and by members endeavouring to ensure a friendly welcome for visiting colleagues. Many friendships were made in this way and later helped to create a warm atmosphere at our international meetings.

We found however that the bulletin and occasional personal contact were not enough to keep in touch with all that was now going on in the growing field of social medicine, so we decided to organize an international meeting on a small scale. The Ciba Foundation provided a meeting place and accommodation in London and a meeting was held on two days at the end of June 1956. Twenty of the correspondents attended and nine invited visitors.

We were very choosy about whom we invited to become members of the ICC. We did not invite any heads of departments nor medical officers of health, unless they had carried out relevant research. We thought the former would cramp our style and that the latter group might swamp us. Later when some of our members became heads of departments we dropped that rule but not the other. The wisdom of this was illustrated later when I wrote to the only contact I had in the USSR and asked him if he could recommend an epidemiologist to join us and he replied 'Yes of course. We have 20,000 epidemiologists in the USSR'. Meaning of course medical officers concerned with the control of infectious disease.

Scientific papers were given at the London meeting including one by J. N. Morris on 'Epidemiology as a research tool' in which he referred to several examples of research on the epidemiology of non-communicable disease. Richard Doll gave a paper on 'Prospective and retrospective studies'. One session at the London Meeting was devoted to 'international aspects' and Professor A. Querido of Amsterdam invited the ICC to hold a small international meeting in The Netherlands in 1957. At another session of the London meeting it was decided to found 'The Society for Social Medicine' for the UK and Ireland.

The international meeting took place at Noordwijk in The Netherlands on 1–6 September 1957. Fifty-eight doctors from 44 university departments in 20 countries attended and the papers given were published as a book in 1958. The great majority were on the epidemiology of non-communicable disease with a few on health services research (Pemberton and Willard 1958). It was clear that the epidemiological aspects of social medicine had become the major interest of members of the ICC and that its application to research on non-communicable disease was its exciting growing point. Morris's book, *Uses of epidemiology*, published in the same year as the Noordwijk meeting provided a valuable account of the methods of, and successes achieved in, the epidemiology of non-communicable disease up to that time (Morris 1957). The first Executive Committee of the ICC (which later became the International Epidemiological Association or IEA), was elected at the end of the Noordwijk meeting and consisted of:

Robert Cruickshank (UK), Chairman

Lester Breslow (USA)

Branko Cvjetanovic (Yugoslavia)

Charles Fletcher (UK)

A. Querido (The Netherlands)

Jack Weir (USA)

John Pemberton (UK) and Harold Willard (USA), joint editors of the bulletin.

The second international meeting was held at the Universidad delle Valle in Cali, Colombia, in 1959 when the present title of the International Epidemiological Association (IEA) was adopted.

The third international meeting was held 2 years later at Korcula, Yugoslavia and after that meetings took place every three years.

Considerable interest in the foundation of the IEA was shown by some leading clinicians and professors of medicine such as George Pickering (Cambridge), Melville Arnott (Birmingham), Jack Ustvedt (Oslo), and Gunnar Biörck (Stockholm), who came to and contributed to the early meetings. This interest was aroused because epidemiological research on non-communicable disease was throwing new light on the causation and prevention of the diseases in which they were most interested, such as heart disease and cancer. Their support was very encouraging and helped to increase the influence of the IEA. The membership continued to grow in an increasing number of countries, encouraged by the organization of seminars, workshops, and regional meetings in various parts of the world at the request, and with the cooperation of, local epidemiologists.

More detailed histories of the IEA have been published elsewhere (Anon 1977, 1984; Pemberton 2005) and on the IEA website. The archives are held in the Wellcome Institute for the History of Medicine in London.

Probably the most important contribution of the IEA to epidemiology was the encouragement it gave to those who were carrying out epidemiological research, especially in the field of non-communicable disease; in the words of its first chairman, Robert Cruickshank, it helped 'to spread the gospel of epidemiology' throughout the world.

The *International Journal of Epidemiology*

An important decision was taken by the IEA in 1971. This was to found an international journal of epidemiology. Walter Holland agreed to become the first editor and he established its fine reputation as the IEA's official journal. The journal has flourished under successive editors. It now covers every aspect of epidemiology and publishes contributions from epidemiologists from all over the world. It has played a seminal role in the development of modern epidemiology.

Health services research and randomized controlled clinical trials

Two important by-products of modern epidemiology have developed in the last half century; health services research (HSR) (see Chapter 16) and randomized controlled clinical trials (RCT). Both have led to more efficient and effective treatments, and members of the IEA have made many important contributions to these disciplines. A. L. (Archie) Cochrane, a founder member of the IEA, did a great deal to develop them in his slender monograph, published in 1972, entitled *Effectiveness and efficiency. Random reflections on health services* (Cochrane 1971).

The future

The biggest contribution that epidemiology has made to the health of populations has been to discover a good many of the causes of disease and to indicate how these conditions could be prevented. In the field of non-communicable disease the demonstration by Doll and Hill of the causal relationship between tobacco smoking and lung cancer has been perhaps the greatest achievement (Doll and Hill 1952). Many more studies of this type and quality are needed. The success of HSR and RCTs in making medical treatment more efficient and more effective are of great importance but have contributed little to our knowledge of the causes and prevention of disease.

It is important that the movement of epidemiologists into these fields does not reduce the numbers available to work on causation and prevention because there are still huge problems in both communicable and non-communicable disease which might be better understood as a result of epidemiological research. Among these conditions, and excluding the great global problems of infections and malnutrition, are chronic arthritic disease, obesity, diabetes, depression, addictions, and violent and accidental deaths.

The epidemiological approach might also be used more often and more effectively in the study of serious social problems such as crime, dysfunctional families, and educational failure.

Poverty is a major general cause of disease and premature death. Modern epidemiology, as described in this book, if applied to deprived populations in order to define the specific causes of ill-health associated with poverty, could make an immense contribution to the health of nations.

References

Anon (1977). History of the International Epidemiological Association 1954–77. *International Journal of Epidemiology*, **6**, 304–24.

Anon (1984). The history of the International Epidemiological Association brought up to date. *International Journal of Epidemiology*, **13**, 139–41.

Cochrane AL (1971). Effectiveness and efficiency. Random reflections on health services. Nuffield Provincial Hospitals Trust, London.

Doll R and Hill AB (1952). A study of the aetiology of cancer of the lung. *British Medical Journal*, **2**, 1272–86.

Hobson W and Pemberton J (1950). Teaching of social medicine in the University of Sheffield. *Lancet*, **2**, 323–4.

Hobson W and Pemberton J (1955). *The health of the elderly at home*. Butterworth, London.

Jameson W (1942). War and the advancement of social medicine. *British Medical Journal*, **2**, 475–80.

Morris JN (1942). Epidemiology of juvenile rheumatism. *Lancet*, **1**, 59–62.

Morris JN (1944). Epidemiology of peptic ulcer. *Lancet*, **2**, 841–5.

Morris JN (1957). *Uses of epidemiology*. E and S Livingstone, London.

Orr JB (1936). *Food health and income*. Macmillan, London.

Pemberton J (2005). Commentary on the article by Lester Breslow on the origins and development of the IEA (with photograph of founders). *International Journal of Epidemiology*, **34**, 729–31.

Pemberton J and Willard H (ed.) (1958). *Recent studies in epidemiology*. Blackwell, Oxford.

Royal College of Physicians of London (1943). *Social and Preventive Medicine Committee, interim report*. Royal College of Physicians of London, London.

Sheldon JH (1948). Some aspects of old age. *Lancet*, **1**, 59–62.

Spence JA and Charles JC (1934). Investigation into the health and nutrition of the children of Newcastle upon Tyne between the ages of one and five. City and Council of Newcastle upon Tyne.

Stewart J (1999). The battle of health. A political history of the Socialist Medical Association, 1930–51. Ashgate, Aldershot.

The Stationery Office (1938). The Registrar-General's decennial supplement 1931 Part 2a occupational mortality. HMSO, London.

The Stationary Office (1942). *Report on social insurance and allied services* [Beveridge Report], Cmnd 6404. HMSO, London.

3

Epidemiological methods and concepts in the nineteenth century and their influences on the twentieth century

Alfredo Morabia

Personal experiences

After graduation from medical school in 1978, I specialized in internal medicine and was considering sub-specializing in occupational medicine. In 1982, I went to Milan, Italy, where I discovered that a generation of young doctors trained in the 1960s and 1970s had gone into occupational medicine. For many, if not most, this was their way to defend the workers and support their political movements. I obtained some funding from Switzerland to study the emerging Italian system of prevention in the workplace (Morabia 1984). I interviewed dozens of doctors and health inspectors and accompanied them to industrial plants almost daily for a year. They had extraordinarily broad inspection expertise and showed me how they attempted, often with the help of trade unions, to reduce deleterious exposures in very diverse occupational settings such as the metallurgical/mechanical, chemical, iron and steel, or tyre and rubber industries, just to name a few. It was fascinating. This is when I first heard of epidemiology. Some of my interviewees were so passionate when they referred to epidemiology that, by curiosity, I bought the Italian translation of Michael Alderson's (1978) *Introduction to epidemiology*. I read it like a novel, a very joyful experience. I was completely seduced by the mode of reasoning. It struck me like a thunderbolt that an epidemiologist was what I wanted to be. Back in Switzerland in 1984, I successfully applied for a training grant from the Swiss National Research Foundation. The grant covered tuition and living expenses for 3 years. I went to The Johns Hopkins University School of Hygiene and there obtained one of, if not the first, 'Swiss' PhDs in epidemiology. I still remember listening to Leon Gordis teaching *Epidemiology 1* in September 1986 and feeling that if paradise existed it was there. In the summer of 1990, I returned to Geneva to lead a newly created Unit (and later Division) of Clinical Epidemiology, another first in Switzerland, and that is where I have been until February 2007 when I moved to New York.

Epidemiology belongs to the nineteenth-century disciplines, such as sociology, economy, and evolutionary biology, which had in common the study of populations rather than individuals. The first epidemiologists of the nineteenth century were guided by their research intuition in the absence of formal theory. In public health and in hospital medicine, it progressively appeared that the combination of population thinking with an experimental approach consisting of comparing subgroups of people was an efficient way to solve some key aetiological and therapeutic problems. This combination of population thinking and group comparison became the methodological hallmark of epidemiology. Nineteenth-century epidemiologists carried out some of the most famous investigations in the history of our discipline. These include the work of Snow, Farr, Louis, Semmelweis, etc. But the validity of their findings was not immediately recognized. Their experimental approach faced obvious difficulties in design, measurement, and interpretation. Observational 'researches' were always threatened by the identification of spurious associations in the presence of multiple potential causes, which we refer to today as confounding. The threat of confounding generated scepticism towards the epidemiological approach in medicine and public health, especially in the last quarter of the nineteenth century. The formalization of modes to prevent confounding 'fallacies', has been one of the main tasks and achievements of the early twentieth-century epidemiologists. They improved the study designs and invented and/or implemented new techniques such as randomization of treatment, stratification or restriction of the study population, and statistical standardization, which allowed them to prevent or control for confounding. In laying the theoretical foundations for rigorous observational research, Weinberg, Lane-Claypon, Goldberger/ Sydenstricker, Greenwood, Frost, young Bradford Hill, amongst others, created the necessary conditions for the rapid expansion of epidemiology after the Second World War.

Populations and science

There are many ways to describe the importance of epidemiology in the nineteenth century. One can focus on its contribution to medicine and public health. This is a very ambitious approach, which actually overlaps the history of medicine and public health. The approach that I choose here, however, describes the emergence of what I believe (and have argued elsewhere; Morabia 2004) has historically been, the specific contribution of epidemiology to science; that is, the progressive constitution of a coherent ensemble of methods and concepts, aimed at assessing health determinants and based on two principles—population thinking and group comparisons.

To the best of my knowledge, before the eighteenth century there was no research based on population thinking or group comparisons and could therefore be no materialization of epidemiology. We could expect historians to dig out new examples of precursors of epidemiology but it is unlikely that these examples will substantially precede the date of the first textbook of probability by Huygens in 1657 (Hacking 1975).

Until the nineteenth century, the examples of researches that carry the attributes of epidemiological research, such as the work of John Graunt or James Lind, are rare. Johann Peter Frank (1745–1821) was, as Henry Sigerist has put it, 'one of the most outstanding figures of the great public health movement that took place in the second half of the eighteenth century' (Frank 1941). He was convinced that misery was the main cause of human diseases and epidemics and proposed abolishing serfdom as a way of alleviating the burden of disease on populations. But this essentially remains an elaborate 'clinical' description of the living conditions of his contemporaries. Events are not quantified. There is no attempt to formally compare rich and poor, or subgroups of the populations. This is not specifically epidemiological.

An additional argument in favour of considering epidemiology as a nineteenth-century discipline is that its emergence is not an isolated event. Several new scientific disciplines appear in the nineteenth century which have the common characteristic of studying populations. And epidemiology is one of them.

Thomas Malthus (1766–1834), considered as the founder of demography, wrote 'An essay on the principle of population' (1798). His theory relating population growth to societal collapse has been very influential because of either its supporters or its detractors. His main argument was that the number of people was growing faster than food production. Thus, when the lot of people exceeds the available food supply, societies collapse.

Malthus inspired Charles Darwin (1809–82), who explained in his autobiography that it was after having read 'for amusement' in October 1838 Malthus' book on population that the question of how selection could be applied to organisms living in a state of nature [as opposed to artificial selection] became clear to him. He proposed that when societies were about to collapse because of the insufficient resources described by Malthus, the crisis would preserve variations within species that better suited the new environment and destroy the unfavourable variants. Hence, new species would be formed or become more prevalent. The theory of selection, on which Darwin worked in the following years, can only be understood in terms of populations. Populations with certain traits replace populations with different traits. The dialectical materialism developed by Karl Marx (1818–83) according to which the struggle between opposed classes within societies explains the historical changes of societal structures can also only be understood in terms of population thinking. Classes are population groups. They appear, fight, and disappear. Marx was critical of Malthus, but knew his work well.

Some consider Adolphe Quetelet (1796–1874) as a demographer, others as a statistician, and still others as a sociologist. Quetelet observed that when one represented graphically the frequency of values of some human characteristics, such as height, these values tended to cluster around a central parameter, which was the mean value. The most common values were concentrated around the mean. Values distant from the mean were rare. Overall, distributions had the shape of a bell, as in the normal law described by Laplace some years before. That the normal curve accurately described biological (e.g. height) or social phenomena was an astounding surprise. It implied that it was possible to find order and meaning in thousands of observations which looked a priori independent from each other. Quetelet analyzed data on the height and thorax circumferences of Scottish soldiers, which had been collected to plan the production of military equipment. Both characteristics were normally distributed. Quetelet believed that the mean value was the normal value and that the variation around the mean stemmed from measurement errors. As strange as it may sound today, Quetelet was convinced that a similar distribution would be obtained if one had measured many times the thorax of the same soldiers instead of having measured the thorax of thousands of soldiers. For Quetelet, the existence of regular distributions centred by means reflected a divine intention to create an 'average man'. One of the greatest contributions of Quetelet to population thinking was to suggest that characteristics of homogeneous groups tended to be normally distributed because every distance from the mean could be attributed to chance (Stigler 1990).

The cases of Malthus, Darwin, Marx, and Quetelet are not exhaustive of the impact of population thinking on the social and human sciences of the nineteenth century. The population phenomenon also reached medicine (Tröhler 2000) and would give birth to sociology, anthropology, etc.

To get the complete picture we have to remember that after the French Revolution and during the whole nineteenth century, populations acquired a central role in the political arena and in the transformation of most European and North American societies into parliamentary democracies.

Some of the new, non-medical disciplines, such as sociology or political economics, were interested in identifying indicators of health status at the population level. In his classical description of the conditions of the working class in England, Friedrich Engels (1820–95), Marx's close friend and colleague, gave a vivid but squalid description of the ignominious working environment, diet, and living constraints imposed upon labourers by industrialization. This led him to ask: 'How is it possible, under such conditions, for the lower class to be healthy and long lived?' His approach to answering the question was quite eloquent: 'Let us see', wrote Engels, 'how the facts stand' (Engels 1845). Well, the facts were epidemiological data comparing health outcomes across socio-economic subgroups. Indeed, Engels cites the deposition of a physician, Dr P. H. Holland in Manchester, who investigated Chorlton-on-Medlock, a suburb of Manchester, under official commission. It reads:

> The Report on the Sanitary Condition of the Working-Class contains information which attests the same fact. In Liverpool, in 1840, the average longevity of the upper classes, gentry, professional men, etc., was thirty-five years; that of the business men and better-placed handicraftsmen, twenty-two years; and that of the operatives, day-labourers, and serviceable class in general, but fifteen years. The Parliamentary reports contain a mass of similar facts.
>
> Engels (1845)

Pre-formal epidemiology

Epidemiology is one of the new scientific disciplines that emerged in the nineteenth century that dealt with populations, but specifically from a medical and public health perspective. That epidemiology is closely related to population thinking to address (public) health determinants, is clearly expressed in the writing of its most brilliant contributors, e.g. William Augustus Guy: 'Does the numerical method admit of application to individual cases? It must be conceded by the most strenuous advocate of this method, that such application is limited' (Guy 1839).

Pierre Charles Alexandre Louis: 'For the appreciation of treatment, the necessity of numerous facts is peculiarly apparent, for though a hundred cases would be valuable evidence in favor of any one system of cure, it is only by comparison with others that its real efficacy can be decided' (Louis 1843) (cited in *The Lancet* 1834–5, 2, 296).

And John Snow: 'To ascertain the cause of cholera, we must consider it not only in individual cases but also in its more general character as an epidemic' (Snow 1849).

What differentiates the related disciplines of demography, biology, sociology, and political economy, from epidemiology? All these disciplines rely on population thinking and even use population data to discuss the potential determinants of health states. Some, such as sociology, follow a path that is so closely related to that of epidemiology, that it sometimes becomes difficult to distinguish an epidemiologist from a sociologist. Neither discipline uses exactly the same analytical methods but they share many concepts and even study designs. Consider the case of the Frenchman Louis-René Villermé (1782–1863). Even though he was not a socialist, Villermé produced the French equivalent to Engels' description of the condition of the English working class. He used vital statistics to describe health inequalities. This piece on longevity is very similar to that cited earlier by Engels:

> The excessive mortality among families of workers employed in the cotton spinning and weaving mills in Mulhouse mainly affects the younger age groups. In fact, one-half of the children born to the class of manufacturers, businessmen, and factory managers reach the age of 29, whereas one-half of the children of weavers and factory workers in the spinning mills will die, as hard as it may seem to believe, before the age of 2.
>
> Villermé (1839); also in Pan American Health Organization (1988)

But in contrast to Engels, Villermé conducted his own investigations. His 'Tableau de l'état physique et moral des ouvriers employés dans les manufactures de coton, de laine et de soie' (Villermé 1839) was the result of a patient investigation. Moreover, Villermé performed quantified group comparisons. In order to provide evidence, which he defined as 'observations which would remove all doubts', of the poorer health conditions of the working class compared to other classes, he used data from military recruitment:

> Unfortunately no one has yet compiled and described. This is what led me to undertake research in this respect. However, the time available only enabled me to carry out this work for the city of Amiens. My results show that the men aged 20 to 21 who were most often found unfit to serve in the army by reason of their size, constitution, or health, often came from the poorer classes, one could even say from the factory working class. In order to find 100 men fit for military service, 193 men have to be drafted in the more comfortable classes and up to 343 have to be drafted in the poorer classes.
>
> Villermé (1839); also in Pan American Health Organization (1988)

Villermé was even quite creative in his presentation of vital statistics. At home ('à *domicile*') mortality rates in 1817–21 were 16.1 per thousand in the first and richer arrondissement and 23.3 per thousand in the 12th and poorer arrondissement of Paris. Taking the inverse of these rates, 1/16.1 and 1/23.3 Villermé presented the numbers of inhabitants for one death, which were, respectively, 62 and 43.

Whether Villermé qualifies as an epidemiologist or a sociologist is a matter of opinion. I prefer to characterize him as a sociologist because he was primarily concerned with the socio-economic aspects of poverty and because of the nature of the details that he collected and described in his survey. Villermé made minute observations of the life of workers in the textile industry. He collected first-hand description of the way workers had their meal, occupied their leisure time, behaved in the workplace, etc. The primary purpose of his investigations was to describe economic and hygienic conditions, which could be improved by the State. He convinced that diseases were caused by the miasma of filth and was not seeking to identify new health determinants.

Thus, the boundaries between epidemiology and other population thinking disciplines are not clear-cut in the nineteenth century. These disciplines are related because they have common ancestors. They are all somewhat connected to the important theoretical activity in statistics, peaking in the work of Laplace, Poisson, and Bernouilli (Stigler 1990). Pre-formal epidemiologists, demographers, political economists, etc. may not have consulted the work of these statisticians but they must have been aware of their ideas and of the trend of new ideas in society.

The emergence of group comparisons

The combination of group comparison and population thinking will provide a powerful tool to identify relevant determinants of population health. The development and refinement of the methods and concepts needed to implement group comparisons will lead to the emergence of the scientific discipline we today call epidemiology.

The first reported usage of group comparison dates back from the eighteenth century. Group comparisons were performed by physicians such as James Lind (1753) or the English proponents of quantified medicine that is, the use of mass observations collected on patients as an additional source of knowledge for medical practice beyond the teaching of the great clinicians (Tröhler 2000). But the real emergence of scientific work that can be considered as epidemiology dates back from the nineteenth century. Even the philosophical bases for group comparison can be traced to J. S. Mill, that is, the mid-nineteenth century (Mill 1881).

Pre-formal epidemiologists performed the first exposed/non-exposed or affected/non-affected group comparisons. John Snow's 1854 'Grand Experiment' compared the mortality from cholera of households exposed to polluted water and households that were not. But another investigation during the same epidemic around the Broad Street pump compared frequencies of exposure to the water pump in people affected versus those not affected by cholera (Paneth et al. 2004). Pierre Louis described his work on the use of bleeding in the treatment of pneumonia in terms of exposed/unexposed comparison, but he also used affected/unaffected comparisons in other circumstances, as when for example to assess the potential hereditary origin of emphysema, a chronic lung disease leading to respiratory insufficiency, he wrote that of 28 patients with emphysema, '18 had their mother or father affected by that same disease' while 'of 50 individuals free of emphysema, only three had affected relatives' (Louis 1837).

The conjunction of population thinking and group comparisons was necessary for the emergence of a new discipline, epidemiology. Progress into the understanding of the causes of infectious diseases only became apparent when public health data were ordered and analyzed according to the principles of group comparisons.

I present here some classic examples of group comparisons performed in the nineteenth century.

Pierre Charles Alexandre Louis

In the aftermath of the French Revolution, François Joseph Victor Broussais (1772–1838), an influential Parisian physician, predicated that fevers were manifestations of organ inflammation and that bloodletting and leeches were efficient to treat them all. Pierre Charles Alexandre Louis (1787–1872), another French physician, doubted the validity of Broussais' theory. Louis reports the following analysis of the large collection of case descriptions which he had accrued during years of intensive clinical activity and autopsy in the Parisian Hospital La Charité (Louis 1835). He found in his clinical records a total of 77 patients who were comparable because they had a well-characterized form of pneumonia (Morabia and Rochat 2001) and were in perfect health when the first symptoms of the disease appeared. Twenty-seven of them had died. For each patient he computed the duration of illness from disease onset to death or recovery. Louis compared the duration of disease and the frequency of death in relation to the time interval at which the patient was first bled during the course of the disease. Louis grouped those first bled during days 1 to 4 of the disease (early bloodletting) and those bled for the first time during days 5 to 9 after the onset of disease (late bloodletting). The two groups of patients were of comparable age. Louis wrote that he had carefully checked that the severity of the disease was on average similar in both groups. Mortality was 44% in the patients bled during the first 4 days of disease compared to 25% among those bled later. These results ruled out the strong protective effect of early bleeding claimed by Broussais.

John Snow

Most epidemiologists are familiar with John Snow's investigations of the 1854 epidemic of cholera in London and of the now famous outbreak around the Broad Street pump (Snow 1855).

In 1852, one of the major water suppliers of London, the Lambeth Water Company, in accordance with an Act of Parliament, changed its source of Thames water. Its pumps were moved from near Hungerford Bridge, where the water was certainly soiled by sewage, to a place well outside London, beyond the influence of the tide and therefore out of reach of the London sewage. In contrast, another water supplier, the Southwark and Vauxhall Company, continued to draw its water from Battersea Fields, a seriously polluted area.

William Farr had noticed that the weekly mortality from cholera in the districts partly supplied by the Lambeth Water Company (61 per 100,000 inhabitants) was lower than that for those districts entirely supplied by the Southwark and Vauxhall Company (94 per 100,000). Note that the rate (between 0.5 to 1 per 10,000 inhabitants per week) and the ratio (94/61= 1.5) imply that these were relatively rare events with a weak association. When cholera returned to London in July 1854, John Snow himself started the fieldwork that was needed to determine the exact effect of the water supply on the progress of the epidemic (Snow 1855).

The most cited paragraph of the second edition of '*On the mode of communication of cholera*' stresses the novel idea behind group comparisons that Snow had striven to achieve:

> The experiment, too, was on the grandest scale. No fewer than three hundred thousand people of both sexes, of every age and occupation, and of every rank and station, from gentlefolks down to the very poor, were divided into two groups without their choice, and, in most cases, without their knowledge; one group being supplied with water containing the sewage of London, and, amongst it, whatever might have come from the cholera patients, the other group having water quite free from such impurity.
>
> Snow (1855)

During the first 7 weeks of the epidemics there were 1361 deaths from cholera in the districts supplied by the two companies: 1263 (315 per 10,000 households) occurred in those supplied by

Southwark and Vauxhall versus 98 (37 per 10,000 households) in those supplied by Lambeth. The ratio (315/37) was 8.5. Sceptics could still argue that the association was caused by a third variable, such as poverty or elevation above sea level. But Snow also compared the mortality from cholera of the houses supplied by the same company in 1849 and 1854, that is, before and after the Lambeth Water Company had moved its pumps to cleaner areas. Mortality had remained constant for the Southwark and Vauxhall patrons but was four times lower for those of the Lambeth Water Company. Thus, the experiment offered a double perspective on group comparisons: concurrent differences in mortality, and 'before and after' changes in exposure comparisons.

Ludwig Panum

The role of the group comparison is really to compare what is observed in the exposed group to what would be expected had the exposed group not been exposed. In order to show the magnitude of the epidemic of measles on the Faeroe Islands in 1846, the Danish physiologist Peter Ludwig Panum (1820–85) did not have such an unexposed group. He therefore compared the age-specific number of deaths from measles during the epidemic, that is, for the first 8 months of 1846, with the average number of annual deaths from 1835 to 1845, that is, the 10 years that had preceded the epidemic. The latter provided the expected frequency in the absence of an epidemic and served as a comparison group. For example, there had been 50 deaths under the age of 1 in 1846 versus '18 1/11th' in 1835–45, a ratio of observed versus expected of 2.8. Panum wrote that:

> Number of times mortality in first two-thirds of 1846 was greater than the usual in an ordinary whole year: about 2 9/11.

> Pan American Health Organization (1988)

Ignaz Philipp Semmelweis

Ignaz Philipp Semmelweis (1818–65), a Hungarian physician teaching medicine in Vienna, observed that the mortality from puerperal fever was two to four times higher among women delivered by physicians compared with women delivered by midwives. In 1846, mortality had been about 11.4% in medical deliveries ('First clinic') versus 2.7% in midwife deliveries ('Second clinic') (Carter 1983). Semmelweis speculated that these differences were caused by the fact that examining physicians went from pathological dissections and consequent contact with dead bodies, to deliveries without thorough cleansing their hands between the two activities. At the end of May 1847 Semmelweis introduced the practice of washing the hands with a solution of chlorinated lime before the examination of lying-in women. Subsequently, the mortality from puerperal fever stabilized around 2% or less for both midwives and physicians (Carter 1983). The contaminated hands of physicians were the culprit.

William Farr

In his report on the mortality of Cornish miners, 1860–62, William Farr (1807–83), responsible for the collection of vital statistics in England and Wales, compared annual mortality rates from pulmonary diseases observed for metal miners with those for 'males exclusive of metal miners' within 10-year age categories:

> . . . assuming as before that the rate of mortality among the males exclusive of miners is represented at each period of life by 100, then that among the miners would be represented by 114 between the ages of 15 and 25 years, by 108 between 25 and 35, by 186 between 35 and 45, by 455 between 45 and 55,

by 834 between 55 and 65, and by 430 between 65 and 75 years. It is therefore evident that pulmonary diseases are the chief cause of the excess mortality among the Cornish miners.

Pan American Health Organization (1988)

This comparison showed that within in each category, miners had a higher mortality from pulmonary diseases than males who were not miners.

Adolphe Vorderman

Christiaan Eijkman (1858–1930), a Dutch physician and Nobel laureate, identified in Java a potential 'natural experiment' to test his firmly established hypothesis that beriberi was caused by a diet based on polished rice. Beriberi was a disease of fatigue, involving weight loss, muscle weakness, loss of feeling and eventually death in up to 80% of the cases. In the local idiom, the word 'beri' means weak, and doubling the term intensifies its meaning. Between May and September 1896, Adolphe Vorderman (1857–1902), supervisor of the Civil Health Department of Java, compared the occurrence of beriberi among the 280,000 inmates of 100 Javan prisons. According to local customs, prisoners were fed polished rice, half-polished rice, or a mixture of both. Beriberi was found in 2.7% of the prisons feeding half-polished rice (corresponding to 1 in 10,000 prisoners), in 46.1% of the prisons preparing a mixture of polished and half-polished rice (1 in 416 prisoners), and in 70.6% of the prisons serving exclusively polished rice (1 in 39 prisoners) (Allchin 2000; Carpenter 2000). On the other hand, beriberi was not associated with hygienic conditions of the prisons such as the age of the building, the permeability of the floor, ventilation, or population density. The deficiency of thiamine (vitamin B_1) in polished rice was later established as the cause of beriberi.

Population thinking

As seen above, most population thinking in nineteenth-century epidemiology is very primitive. People essentially relied on ratio (e.g. the ratio of cholera deaths over number of households in Snow's work) or proportions. The exception was William Farr, who established a clear conceptual difference between risks and rates (Farr 1838). Risk and rates are so fundamental to epidemiological thinking that they were already used by Graunt, but without being formally identified as such. Graunt used an equivalent of risk to assess the impact of plague on the London population, and the equivalent of a rate to describe the fluctuation of risk across time which he considered as evidence that plague is due to environmental rather than endogenous factors (Morabia 2004).

Farr, in contrast, showed that the 'force of mortality' (i.e. the mortality rate) had a different meaning than the mortality risk. The first indicated how fast a disease took its burden while the latter reflected the burden of disease itself. Compared to tuberculosis, cholera had a higher mortality rate and a lower mortality risk. Tuberculosis therefore appeared less frightful than cholera because it killed the sick at a slower pace.

The obstacle of confounding

It is striking that the balance between success and failure of pre-formal epidemiology is more positive when we look at it in retrospect than it was for the nineteenth-century community: Snow was right, Semmelweis was right, Louis was right, and so on. Still, their contemporaries did not trust their findings and conclusions. If we add up the preventable deaths of young parturients, the worldwide recurrence of cholera after 1854, the pneumonitis patients killed by bloodletting, etc., scores of lives have been lost because of this unwarranted scepticism.

The medical community was more prone to accept the conclusions of unsupported theories or uncontrolled experiments than the results of pre-formal epidemiology. Consider the case of Broussais, whose theory had been debunked by Louis. His theory on inflammation being the universal cause of fevers was purely speculative. It was attractive because it appealed to a convenient 'one theory fits all' post-revolutionary sensibility. Millions of leeches were imported; millions of patients were bled uselessly and probably died because of it. Consider too, the treatment of cholera in the mid-nineteenth century. Bleeding was prescribed against all common sense to patients who were massively losing fluids through diarrhoea and vomiting. Think also of the tragedy of puerperal fever, which killed at given moments one in every three young women entering a hospital ward for delivery. That the problem was in the hospital and not in the women, or in the doctor's ward but not in the midwives clinic, was obvious to the population. The rich delivered at home and the poor, fearful of being handled by doctors, begged the midwives to preside. But doctors themselves were unbelievably blind to the wisdom of the masses.

Few scientists practiced group comparison and population thinking but it proved to be a powerful approach. The combination revealed the conventional knowledge of today, in terms of hygienic protocol and standard procedures. Pump clean water, wash hands, don't bleed patients with pneumonia.

Still, the findings were met with scepticism. One reason is, I believe, that epidemiological findings did not discover the mechanisms through which the identified 'cause' produced disease. Indeed, epidemiology thrived in these situations where mechanisms were unknown and which were therefore out of reach of the laboratory sciences. Another reason is that probabilistic findings could not be reproduced for each individual patient. They by their very essence work on average. The mechanism being unknown, many singular cases, in confinement from one another outwardly seemed to contradict the theory.

However, the main motive for the lack of recognition of pre-formal epidemiology has to do with what we refer to today as *confounding*. People simply did not believe that the compared groups were comparable and therefore found a wealth of reasons for which non-comparability between groups could explain the observed differences.

William Farr in November 1853 argued that:

> To measure the effect of bad or good water supply, it is requisite to find two classes of inhabitants living at the same level [elevation], moving in equal space, enjoying an equal share of the mean of subsistence, engaged in the same pursuits, but differing in this respect, – that one drinks water from Battersea [supposedly polluted water], the other from Kew .... But of such experimenta crucis the circumstances of London do not admit ....

> (cited by Vinten-Johansen *et al* 2003, p. 260)

The critic asked for a comparison between two groups equally exposed to 'miasma', the most popular cause of cholera in nineteenth-century public health circles, believing that the association with water was confounded by poverty. A similar type of argument was raised against Semmelweis's findings. Critics argued that delivery rooms were not adequately ventilated, among other things.

I propose that pre-formal epidemiologists lacked the tools to convincingly rule out confounding, because there is no absolute proof of its absence in observational studies. Endless debates can arise if the opposed groups have different models of causation in mind. Snow was a contagionist, and this belief guided his theory and interpretation of the experiment. Similarly, Farr believed in miasma as the cause of cholera and would see poverty as a primary determinant.

The characteristic of this first phase of epidemiology, is the absence of theory. Scientists used population thinking and group comparisons, spontaneously, as a commonsense approach. People such as Lind, Snow, and Farr invented their way into epidemiological research and therefore set the basis for the future development and formalization of methods and concepts. I have proposed to call them 'pre-formal' precisely because there is no formal theory backing their practice.

Without a theory of group comparison, it was not possible to build a theory of confounding. Finding a solution to this inherent menace of all observational group comparison will be one of the main methodological concerns of epidemiologists in the following phase.

Influence of nineteenth-century epidemiology on early modern epidemiology

Early modern epidemiology characterizes the development phase in which some epidemiological concepts and methods become assembled for the first time into a theory of population thinking and group comparisons.

Early modern epidemiologists essentially built on their nineteenth-century predecessors and started to formalize some of their empirical developments. During this second phase, epidemiological methods and concepts acquired some theoretical foundations. These were somewhat less commonsensical than that proposed in the previous phase but nevertheless remained quite simple. A major theoretical contribution to this phase consisted in identifying sources of fallacious interpretations of group comparisons 'affected by a multiplicity of causes', and in proposing solutions to minimize them. Indeed, confounding was initially conceptualized as a 'fallacy'.

The confounding fallacy

The Cambridge statistician G. Udny Yule (1871–1951) first formally described some 'fallacies that may be caused by the mixing of records'. He used the hypothetical example of an attribute that was not transmitted by fathers to their sons or mothers to their daughters but that showed 'considerable apparent inheritance' when the data of fathers, sons, mothers, and daughters were analyzed together (Yule 1903).

For Yule, the reason for the fallacy was that the parental attribute was more common in fathers than in mothers and the childhood attribute was more common in sons than in daughters. Thus, gender was associated with having the attribute in children and with having the attribute in parents.

Major Greenwood (1880–1947), 32 years after Yule's publication, produced an almost identical demonstration of the fallacy in his 1935 textbook *Epidemics and crowd diseases* (Greenwood 1935). The example used by Greenwood referred to an immunization experiment. Group 1 had a higher mortality but more individuals in Group 2 had been inoculated. Inoculation had no effect in Groups 1 and 2 taken separately but, when mixing Groups 1 and 2, inoculation became spuriously effective.

Two years after Greenwood's text, Austin Bradford Hill also (1897–1991) presented an almost identical demonstration of Yule's fallacy in his 1939 textbook *Principles of medical statistics*. In Hill's example, more men than women were treated and women died more than men. The treatment had no effect in neither men nor women, but appeared to reduce mortality when the male and female data were combined.

Thus, in the early 1900s a formal theory of confounding appeared all of a sudden in three publications, including the two earliest textbooks of epidemiology. The authors of these publications, Yule, Greenwood, and Hill, did not refer to each other (even though Hill worked in Greenwood's department) but clearly confounding was a matter of concern for that generation of researchers.

Early analyses of confounding

One of the first analytical adjustments for confounding was performed by Joseph Goldberger (1874–1929) and Edgar Sydenstricker (1881–1936). Goldberger and Sydenstricker studied the causes of pellagra, sometimes called the disease of the four Ds—dermatitis, diarrhoea, dementia, and death. By 1912, the state of South Carolina alone reported 30,000 cases and a case fatality rate of 40%, but the disease was hardly confined to Southern states. The US Congress requested an investigation, which Goldberger and Sydenstricker carried out in the spring of 1916 in South Carolina. They selected seven representative cotton-mill villages, enumerated their populations, and sampled 750 households, comprising 4160 people, who were exclusively Whites of Anglo-Saxon origin.

A statistical adjustment was made for age when analyzing the relation between pellagra incidence and income. Pellagra occurred 16 times more frequently within the poorest households (adjusted risk 41 per 1000) when compared with households that were economically better off (adjusted risk 2.5 per 1000). The authors explained that they standardized the pellagra risks for age because age was associated with both income and pellagra incidence. Age-adjusted and crude rates were practically identical. (Goldberger *et al.* 1920).

The total population (all incomes) served as the standard population. They noted that the agreement between the crude and the adjusted risks ruled out the possibility that 'differences in the sex and age distribution in the different income classes might give rise to' the inverse association of income and pellagra (Goldberger *et al.* 1920). They appropriately pooled the data of males and females: the gender-specific rates across income categories were substantially different but the relative risks of income and pellagra incidence were similar in men and women.

Cohort analysis

Wade Hampton Frost (1880–1938), the first Professor and Chairman in the Department of Epidemiology and Public Health Administration at The School of Hygiene and Public Health of the Johns Hopkins University in Baltimore, addressed another manifestation of confounding. In a posthumous paper (Frost 1939), he described the fallacy that may occur when naively interpreting cross-sectional changes in death rates with age (Comstock 2004; Doll 2004).

Mortality rates from tuberculosis in Massachusetts peaked at ages 0 to 4, were lowest at ages 5 to 9, and then rose across age groups. This apparent age effect was difficult to explain. Was it that a lower exposure to *Mycobacterium tuberculosis* during infancy resulted in more severe infections in adults? Frost showed that when death rates were computed within a categorical birth 'cohort' (e.g. people born between 1871 and 1880) rates tended to steadily decline after age 20. Similar observations across several cohorts allowed Frost to conclude that the inexplicable variations of mortality rates with age occurring in the cross-sectional analysis was due to a third factor, exposure to tuberculosis, which was associated both with age and with mortality. In the cross-sectional analysis, each age group represented a different birth cohort. Stratifying by birth cohort produced groups that were homogeneous with respect to exposure to tuberculosis and thus revealed the true association of age and mortality.

Alternative allocation of treatment

Random allocation of treatment was another answer proposed by epidemiologists to solve group non-comparability. In the trial of the Medical Research Council on the serum treatment of lobar pneumonia (Therapeutic Trial Committee of the Medical Research Council 1934), patients admitted to Aberdeen, London, and Edinburgh hospitals for pneumonia received, by design and according to the order of admission, either a serum treatment or the conventional treatment, which served as a control. Hill had advocated alternate allocation of treatment as a way of balancing in the compared groups the distribution of characteristics associated with both exposure and outcome (Hill 1939). With large numbers it was reasonable to expect that they would be equally, or nearly equally, represented in all groups (Hill 1939).

Conclusions

Early epidemiologists clearly established confounding as a problem of non-comparability for factors related to both exposure and outcome. In collaboration with statisticians, they proposed tools (i.e. stratification, adjustment, matching, and random allocation of treatment) to deal with confounding in a variety of situations. These early solutions to the confounding problem released the grip of criticism of non-comparability and set the stage for the rapid growth of epidemiology after the Second World War. When Fisher invoked confounding against the smoking–lung cancer association (Stolley 1991), epidemiologists were prepared to address the criticism, drawing from the experience of their predecessors and similar conceptual developments that had occurred in sociology (Vandenbroucke 2004).

References

Alderson M (1978). Introduction to epidemiology [Introduzione all'Epidemiologia]. *Epidemiologia e Prevenzione*, **5–6**, 1–116.

Allchin D (2000). *Of rice and men.* http://www1.umn.edu/ships/modules/eijkman1.htm (posted 15 October 2000; accessed 21 September 2006).

Carpenter KJ (2000). *Beriberi, white rice, and vitamin B: a disease, a cause and a cure.* University of California Press, Berkeley.

Carter KC (1983). *Ignaz Semmelweis. The etiology, concept and prophylaxis of childbed fever.* University of Wisconsin Press, Madison.

Comstock GW (2004). Cohort analysis: W.H. Frost's contributions to the epidemiology of tuberculosis and chronic disease. In *History of epidemiological methods and concepts* (ed. A Morabia), pp. 223–31. Birkhäuser, Basel.

Doll R (2004). Cohort studies: history of the method. In *History of epidemiological methods and concepts* (ed. A Morabia), pp. 243–74. Birkhäuser, Basel.

Engels F (1845). *The condition of the working class in England,* p. 117. Reprinted 1987. Penguin Classics, London.

Farr W (2004). 'On prognosis' by William Farr (British Medical Almanack 1838; Supplement 199–216) Part 1 (pages 199–208). In *History of epidemiological methods and concepts* (ed. A Morabia), pp. 159–78. Birkhäuser, Basel.

Frank J (1941). The people's misery: mother of diseases (1790). Introduction and translation by HE Sigerist. *Bulletin of the History of Medicine,* **9**, 81–100.

Frost WH (1939). The age selection of mortality from tuberculosis in successive decades. *American Journal of Hygiene,* **30**, 91–6.

Goldberger J, Wheeler GA, and Sydenstricker E (1920). A study of the relation of family income and other economic factors to pellagra incidence in seven cotton-mill villages of South Carolina in 1916. *Public Health Representative,* **35**, 2673–714.

Greenwood M (1935). *Epidemics and crowd diseases: introduction to the study of epidemiology.* Ayer Company Publishers, Inc., North Stratford, NH.

Guy W (1839). On the value of the numerical method as applied to science, but especially to physiology and. medicine. *Journal of the American Statistical Association,* **2**, 25–47.

Hacking I (1975). *The emergence of probability.* Cambridge University Press, Cambridge.

Hill AB (1939). *Principles of medical statistics,* pp. 5–6. The Lancet Ltd, London.

Lind J (1753). *A treatise of scurvy.* Reprinted 1953. University Press, Edinburgh.

Louis PCA (1835). *Recherches sur les effets de la saignée dans quelques maladies inflammatoires et sur l'action de l'émétique et des vésicatoires dans la pneumonie.* Librairie de l'Académie royale de médecine, Paris.

Louis PCA (1837). Recherche sur l'emphysème des poumons. *Mémoires de la Société Médicale d'Observation,* 160–257.

Louis PCA (1843). *Recherches anatomiques, pathologiques et thérapeutiques sur la phthisie.* Deuxième édition considérablement augmentée. J.-B. Baillière, Paris.

Mill JS (1881) A system of logic, 8th edn. In *Philosophy of scientific method* (ed. E Nagel), pp. 3–356. Hafner Publishing Co., New York.

Morabia A (1984). *The Italian system of primary prevention in the workplace. Theoretical model and applications.* University of Geneva, Cahier Ecotra No 5, Geneva. (In French.)

Morabia A (2004). Epidemiology: an epistemological perspective. In *History of epidemiological methods and concepts* (ed. A Morabia), pp. 1–126. Birkhäuser, Basel.

Morabia A and Rochat T (2001). Reproducibility of Louis' definition of pneumonia. *Lancet*, **358**, 1188.

Pan American Health Organization (1988). *The challenge of epidemiology. Issues and selected readings.* PAHO, Washington, DC.

Paneth N, Susser E, and Susser M (2004). Origins and early development of the case-control study. In *History of epidemiological methods and concepts* (ed. A Morabia), pp. 291–312. Birkhäuser, Basel.

Snow J (1849). On the pathology and modes of communication of cholera. *London Medical Gazette*, **44**, 745–52.

Snow J (1855). *On the mode of communication of cholera*, 2nd edn. Churchill, London.

Stigler S (1990). *The history of statistics: the measurement of uncertainty before 1900*, p. 205. Belknap Press, Boston.

Stolley PD (1991). When genius errs: R.A. Fisher and the lung cancer controversy. *American Journal of Epidemiology*, **133**, 416–25.

Therapeutic Trial Committee of the Medical Research Council (1934). The serum treatment of lobar pneumonia. *Lancet*, **1**, 290–5.

Tröhler U (2000). *To improve the evidence of medicine: the 18th century British origins of a critical approach.* Royal College of Physicians, Edinburgh.

Vandenbroucke JP (2004). The history of confounding. In *History of epidemiological methods and concepts* (ed. A Morabia), pp. 313–26. Birkhäuser, Basel.

Villermé L (1839). De la santé des ouvriers employés dans les fabrications de soie, de coton et de laine. *Annales d'hygiène publique et de médecine légale*, **21**, 338–420.

Vinten-Johansen P, Brody H, Paneth N, Rachman S, Rip MR (2003). *Cholera, Chloroform and the Science of Medicine: A Life of John Snow.* Oxford University Press, Oxford.

Yule GU (1903) Notes on the theory of association of attributes in statistics. *Biometrika*, **2**, 121–34.

4

Epidemiological concepts pre-1950 and their relation to work in the second half of the century

Rodolfo Saracci

Personal experiences

I enrolled in the medical school at the University of Pavia more than half a century ago, after some hesitation between medicine and physics. Like nearly all medical students, I was envisaging a future in clinical medicine, most likely as an internist. In the 6 years of the school curriculum 'epidemiology' meant some 40 pages on health statistics and 100 or so on the descriptive aspects of infectious diseases, with no numbers. During the summer holiday of the fourth year I came across, entirely by chance, an announcement offering a scientifically and financially attractive fellowship to students in biology or medicine wishing to prepare an experimental dissertation at the Institute of Genetics. I applied, I was accepted, and I spent 2 and 1/2 years on a project in immunogenetics within an environment which left an indelible imprint in terms of research spirit, methodology, and a quantitative approach to biological phenomena. I had there my first introduction to statistics in biology. This turned out to be an asset when, in 1961, I moved, after completing my MD dissertation (and buying a small car, the now mythical 'Fiat 500', thanks to the fellowship savings), to the Department of Clinical Medicine at the University of Pisa. Colleagues soon started to ask for statistical help when trying to interpret the data from their clinical studies: I began to plead for proper planning, rather than only late stage chi-square tests, of these studies and to strengthen my own competence—particularly in the clinical trial field—I decided to spend a year abroad. I had read the just published book *Sequential medical trials* by Peter Armitage (1964): I contacted him and was advised to join the MRC Statistical Research Unit in London directed by (at that time) Dr Richard Doll. While working (1965) on the analysis of a clinical trial on acute leukaemia I discovered that the largest portion of the unit's activity was devoted to a kind of investigation about which I had not had the slightest idea: the epidemiology and aetiology in humans of the very diseases I was interested in as an internist. Epidemiology became my field of research, teaching, and expertise.

The rise of the epidemiology of non-communicable diseases

I had arrived at epidemiology as a second level choice, via genetics and clinical medicine. Whatever the specifics, via microbiology, pathology, or clinical specialities, this was a common path, at least until the late 1960s, for physicians, who represented the dominant participants in the field, the other important but numerically smaller component being statisticians.

A major change in the very objects of epidemiological research had intervened in the decade of the Second World War (1939–45). Communicable diseases underwent a sharp and sustained fall. In a southern Europe country, Italy, the crude mortality rate per 100,000 (both sexes combined) fell from above 1300 in the last pre-war year (1939) to about 1000 ten years later, essentially due to advances in control of infectious and respiratory causes, mainly tuberculosis: cancers and

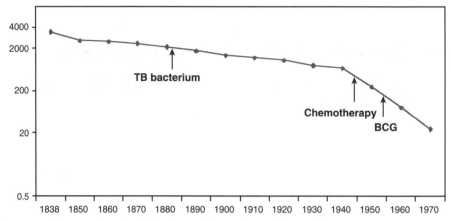

Fig. 4.1 Respiratory tuberculosis: death rates for England and Wales (x-axis, year; y-axis, log annual death rate per million). (Reproduced with permission and modification from McKeown T (1976). *The role of medicine*. The Nuffield Provincial Hospitals Trust, London.)

cardiovascular diseases already ranked as the leading causes of death, although rates were substantially lower than, for instance, in UK or USA. A similar trend occurred throughout most European countries. The graph of mortality for respiratory tuberculosis in England and Wales (McKeown 1976), when plotted on a logarithmic, rather than arithmetic, scale, shows clearly that the secular rate of decline, essentially due to improvements in hygiene and nutrition, underwent a brisk acceleration thanks to the discovery of antibiotics such as streptomycin active against the TB mycobacterium (Fig. 4.1). As a consequence, non-communicable diseases emerged as the most prominent and largely intractable problems in health, prompting research on their aetiology, control, and treatment. Even a very short overview of the three most investigated class of non-communicable diseases—cancers, cardiovascular, and respiratory diseases—can show how the research approach developed its own conceptual and technical tools, partly similar and partly in contrast to those prevailing until then in the study of communicable diseases.

In the area of cancer the need for accurate figures of incidence, rather than only mortality, had already become apparent, as it had been decades before for infectious diseases, although in the latter case the control of sources of infection was the original rationale for notification. In Europe the first cancer registry started to operate in Denmark in 1942, preceded in the United States by the Connecticut register in 1940. By 1965 Clemmesen had published, largely out of 25 years' experience with his registry, a monumental work (Clemmesen 1965) which still makes valuable reading. In the introduction he pointed out that 'it may be significant to notice some distinction between malignant neoplasms and the infectious diseases from which we have borrowed various of our terms and gradually – erroneously – also some notions'. He went on, stressing in particular the large 'multiplicity of causes' of each cancer making the part played by any one agent far less dominant than an infective agent in bacterial epidemiology; and, related to this, he sceptically questioned as a 'caricature' of the human situation the isolation of single agents for tests in animal experiments. Some of the most remarkable discoveries of epidemiology soon arose in the cancer area. In 1952 three case–control studies, two from the USA (Levin *et al.* 1950; Wynder and Graham 1950) and one from Britain (Doll and Hill 1950), were published almost concurrently, clearly showing the association—probably causal in nature—between tobacco smoking and lung cancer.

One of the three studies, by Doll and Hill (1950), was the forerunner of a series of investigations, based on a cohort of British doctors who have been followed up for 50 years, the first report being published in 1964 (Doll and Hill 1964) and the most recent in 2004 (Doll *et al.* 2004). The associations, repeatedly found in numerous observational studies, between tobacco smoking and respiratory cancers as well as with other chronic conditions, in particular several cardiovascular and respiratory ones, focused attention on the all-pervasive problem of how to ascertain with reasonable confidence the causal nature of an association, even in absence of experimental confirmation in animal models. Criteria were proposed for this purpose, substantially departing from the received wisdom in the area of infectious disease, which required instead some experimental confirmation: I will return to this important dissonance between old and new epidemiology.

The epidemiology of cardiovascular disease had in common with cancer epidemiology an attention to the wide variation of rates between geographical areas, pointing to likely environmental determinants: but from this starting point it took a different line of development. In cancer epidemiology the relatively clear-cut pathological (histological) case confirmation made population based registries a viable possibility: the wide variations in cancer incidence rates, pointing to the role of the environment (broadly defined), and the total lack of pathophysiological indicators of cancer growth before it emerges clinically channelled the epidemiological investigations towards environmental exposures, for which the case–control design represented a suitable instrument. Questionnaires were developed to inquire about past exposures, in the general, local, and personal environment, in cases and controls; hence to the present day cancer epidemiology has seen, side by side with a limited number of important cohort studies, a vast proliferation of case–control investigations on virtually all cancer sites. In the cardiovascular domain the case definitions of conditions like myocardial infarction and stroke have been based on syndromic and functional criteria rather than on pathological confirmation, and even the relevant defining lesions are debatable: as a consequence population based registries have become a much less common instrument here, and are usually limited in time and extension (World Health Organization 1976) compared with the cancer field. Physiological variables such as blood pressure or blood cholesterol were suspected to affect clinical endpoints like myocardial infarction and stroke; the case–control design is unsuitable for investigating these, as their values would most likely have been affected by the very occurrence of the endpoint. Hence the epidemiology of cardiovascular disease has provided little room for registries and no room for case–control studies, but has developed cohort studies in selected populations. These studies have focused either on interindividual differences within a cohort, like the prototype Framingham study (Dawber *et al.* 1963), or on between-cohort (populations) differences, like the 'Seven countries' studies (Keys 1970). Keys, the initiator and principal investigator of this study, attended the first UN Food and Agriculture Organization nutrition conference in 1950 in Rome (Keys 1995). Only nutritional deficiencies were discussed, and when he ventured a question on diet and the new (in the USA) coronary heart disease epidemic he was told that, for instance, coronary heart disease 'was no problem in Naples'. Keys decided to go to Naples and find out for himself: anecdotal evidence confirmed that indeed coronary heart disease appeared to be rare except 'among the small class of rich people whose diet differed from that of the general population—they ate meat every day instead of every week or two'. And the serum cholesterol level turned out to be very low, except among members of the Rotary Club. This was the initial spark of what developed into a now classic long-term prospective study in seven countries with markedly different dietary habits. Interestingly, and in line with the combination of epidemiology with experimental study common in the infectious diseases domain, Keys also conducted a series of controlled experiments (in US mental hospital subjects) showing the effect of diets on serum cholesterol. He died a centenarian in 2003, after spending his long retirement in Campania, southern Italy, where he had the first intuition of the health benefits of the Mediterranean diet.

Respiratory diseases of the chronic type, at that time a mixed bag of conditions lending to considerable variability in classification by different clinicians, presented diagnostic issues and study options closer to those for cardiovascular disease than for cancer: but first of all they very clearly posed the basic problem of characterizing in an unambiguous way what 'disease' was going to be studied epidemiologically, avoiding the vagaries of the clinical diagnoses. The Medical Research Council's questionnaire on chronic bronchitis (Medical Research Council 1960) represented in this sense a pioneering work. It allowed an accurate identification of the condition for studies of natural history and aetiology and ushered in an approach which was later extended to encompass lung function tests, and even more generally to other syndromes.

If non-communicable diseases became the main focus for the growth of epidemiology, it was through communicable diseases that rigorous procedures for the evaluation of interventions made their way into the field. Two landmark randomized trials were the British study of streptomycin in pulmonary tuberculosis (Medical Research Council 1948) and the big field trial of the Salk vaccine against poliomyelitis in the United States (Francis *et al.* 1955).

Methodological developments and syntheses

The expanding field of the epidemiology of non-communicable disease was the first beneficiary of the considerable advances that had been made in the first half of the twentieth century in theoretical and applied statistics for data analysis as geared to study design. Developments specific to epidemiological problems soon took place. A prominent example, at the crossroads between the different types of studies, is the work of Cornfield. In a seminal 1951 paper (Cornfield 1951) he showed that the odds ratio computable from the results of a a case–control study would correctly estimate the relative risk that would be obtainable from a cohort study in the same population, provided that one makes the assumption that the incidence rate of the disease is low (the 'rare disease' assumption, which does not need to be a hindrance as a disease can be 'rendered rare' by sampling cases and the corresponding controls within suitably short time intervals). A decade later, when working on the risk of coronary heart disease, he showed (Cornfield 1962) that the risk could be simultaneously related to a number of different factors by using logistic regression. In the 1960s this kind of application, which was practically prohibitive for manual calculations when more than two or three independent variables were involved, became routinely feasible and its real worth testable thanks to the advent of electronic computers.

If papers mark the dates of the appearance of original advances, reference books (a status that after the Second World War could in practice be reached only by books written in or translated into English) offer a comprehensive cross-section of the methodological knowledge available at different points in time. *Epidemiologic methods* by MacMahon, Pugh, and Ipsen was published in 1960 and represented the first attempt to assemble within a coherent frame the methods of epidemiology, with a clear emphasis on non-communicable disease. It deals with the issues of study design, conduct, and interpretation, with only essentials on statistical procedures. Methodological progress blossomed in the 1960s and 1970s, critically scrutinizing existing procedures of population sampling, measuring events, and analysing data, which were still based mostly on empirical grounds ('they worked'). Solid conceptual and formal foundations were provided for them—thanks to the work of authors such as Miettinen (1985)—enabling a basis on which to build methods capable of tackling more complex study designs and data analyses.

Concurrently with the methodological boom the need for orderly summary compilations became apparent. The most lasting and successful (until present day) proved to be the twin volumes by

Breslow and Day, on case–control (1978) and cohort studies (1985), which dealt with statistical methods in cancer epidemiology studies, and which are in fact suitable for studies of most non-communicable diseases as well. While they give a detailed illustration of each method, these books present a unifying synthesis (not a compilation) of them, based on the fundamental equivalence of the case–control and cohort approaches. Between the publication of the first and the second of these twin volumes the book *Epidemiologic research* by Kleinbaum, Kupper, and Morgenstern appeared in 1982, didactically organized and with substantial parts on statistics: the axis of synthesis was the chronology of issues that arise during the investigation of a disease, from the formulation of a hypothesis and event measures to the interpretation of results. In 1986 the adjective 'modern' made its way for the first time into a compact book of methodology (*Modern epidemiology* by Rothman (1986)): the second edition by Rothman and Greenland (1998) was much extended both in the statistical sections and in a series of sections dealing with nutritional epidemiology, genetic epidemiology, and other speciality areas, and represents the most comprehensive presentation of methods currently available. An even more basic and elegant unification of methods, on the basis of the statistical likelihood principle, was later introduced by Clayton and Hills in their *Statistical models in epidemiology* (1993). Of the three methodological constituents of any epidemiological study, i.e. exposure measurement, health condition measurement, study design and analysis, the latter two had been the subject of texts throughout the 1960s, 1970s, and beyond: it was, however, not until 1992 that the first book, by Armstrong, White, and Saracci, was published specifically devoted to the principles of exposure measurement in epidemiology.

Epidemiology, old and new

Old and new are relative terms: clearly in the first decades of the period 1950–2000 non-communicable disease was the new component and communicable disease the old one, the latter being already well established before the Second World War. A number of differences emerged between the two areas.

In the first place the often separate development of both strands simply translated in each the non-specific and general secular trend in science towards increasing specialization, inherent in the increasing volume and complexity of knowledge: this necessarily accentuated the divergences while obscuring the common elements between streams of epidemiological research.

A second but specific difference had to do with the different stages of evolution of the two areas of epidemiology—aetiological knowledge about non-communicable diseases being roughly where knowledge of the communicable diseases had been some 80 or 100 years previously. Once the communicable nature of a disease was just generically suspected an entire technological armamentarium was already at hand, or could be perfected *ad hoc*, to identify the agent, or otherwise to exclude the infectious nature of the disease: in the case of AIDS it took only 3 years between recognition of the syndrome in 1981 and identification of the virus responsible (HIV) in 1983–84 (Shaw 1992). In the area of non-communicable disease one was instead starting at the stage of circumscribing, out of a multitude of heterogeneous factors, those likely to be causal, before proceeding to firmly isolate the culprits. When Hill and Doll (1950) started their case–control study on lung cancer, which appeared to show a striking increase in the immediate post-Second World War period, they encompassed in their questionnaire a range of environmental factors; indeed their attention had been primarily attracted by the possible role of atmospheric pollution which badly affected London in those days. As it turned out, tobacco smoking emerged among the other factors as being strongly associated with lung cancer.

The criteria, or better guidelines, elaborated in the mid-1960s to establish with reasonable confidence the causal nature of associations between an environmental agent, such as tobacco smoking, and a disease, mark one of the relevant differences between old and new epidemiology. One set of guidelines was presented, for the specific issue of tobacco, in the milestone report 'Smoking and health' of the US Surgeon General in 1964 (US Department of Health, Education and Walfare 1964). A closely related set of nine elements of evidence more widely applicable to environmental agents was elaborated by Hill in 1965 and became popularly known as the 'Hill guidelines' to infer causality in general in epidemiology (Hill 1965). Up to that time the criteria for establishing causality were those that Koch had spelled out in 1882 for infectious agents (Fredericks and Relman 1996): they prescribed that the agent should be recovered from all cases of disease, that it should not be recovered in other conditions, and that it should reproduce the disease in suitable animal systems. Although already not satisfied by definitely infectious pathogens (cholera) during Koch's lifetime, and subsequently modified, for instance for viruses, the Koch's criteria represented a revered canon of reference: and in any case reproducibility in animals has constantly remained, to the present day, a favourite requirement in the domain of infectious disease. This was, however, a stumbling block against recognizing tobacco smoking as a causal factor because 'Few attempts have been made to produce bronchogenic carcinoma in experimental animals with tobacco extracts, smoke, or smoke condensate. With one possible exception, none has been successful' (US Department of Health, Education and Welfare 1964). Confronted with overwhelming epidemiological evidence in humans and the absence of reproducible evidence in animals the authors of 'Smoking and health' sensibly rallied, as Hill did in his more general guidelines, on positing only the weaker requirement of biological 'plausibility', which indeed was available for tobacco, as tar extracts had been shown to be carcinogenic in skin painting experiments in mice. However, the fact that the Hill guidelines soon became a general reference had the unfortunate consequence that the relevance of (re)producing disease in animal experiments, fundamental in physiology, pathology, pharmacology, and toxicology, often ended by being eclipsed in the study of non-communicable diseases, as if different kinds of biology were bizarrely underlying the old and the new epidemiology. This was not without important practical consequences, as witnessed by the continuing controversies surrounding the regulation of toxic agents in the environment based on clear evidence of pathogenicity in animal species but in the absence of adequate human data—a circumstance of which carcinogens provide prominent examples (International Agency for Research on Cancer 1972–2004).

A third differential development between the old and new epidemiologies stemmed from two parallel sources: (1) the research on unambiguous, accurate operational definitions of normal and pathological conditions (such as chronic bronchitis or angina pectoris) for epidemiological purposes, which critically scrutinized the properties of physical, instrumental, and laboratory techniques as used in clinical medicine; (2) the early randomized trials of treatments, whose methodology spread from the area of communicable disease to the testing of the growing number of drugs, such as corticoids or psychoactive drugs, that were probably effective in non-communicable conditions in humans. Investigations in these two areas converged in the birth of a general approach that went beyond epidemiological research back into the clinical world, developing a culture and methodology of evaluation of all kind of interventions—preventive, diagnostic, therapeutic, and rehabilitative—used in clinical practice or public health. Morris's book *Uses of epidemiology* (Morris 1957, 1964) provided early suggestions of such developments; Holland's series on screening in *The Lancet* (Holland 1974) represents a fully fledged and specific example of the approach; and Cochrane's *Effectiveness and efficiency* its systematic message book (Cochrane 1972). It ushered in and articulated over the years what has become known as 'evidence-based medicine', the core of clinical epidemiology; namely, research carried using the tools of epidemiology in populations of patients.

Notwithstanding all these differences there is not, at a conceptual level, any fundamental difference between old communicable disease and new non-communicable disease epidemiology: both share a common population-based approach employing such key concepts as probability and unbiased comparisons. Moreover, many methods are (or would be if researchers would communicate better) adaptable from one sector to another. Still, when it comes to the actual historical unfolding, the homogeneous field of epidemiological concepts and methods materializes into differentiated streams of research, not seldom proceeding in quasi-isolation one from the other. This becomes strikingly manifest if not only research and knowledge *per se* are considered but also the institutional aspect, namely the people, institutions, and resources devoted to such research. In continental Europe, where I have been carrying on my work, the institutional split between old and new epidemiology was particularly marked at the beginning of the 1950–2000 period, slowing down the development of both sectors. It has persisted with only a gradual reduction for several decades and had not totally disappeared even at the end of the century, particularly in Eastern Europe.

Current epidemiology: modern or post-modern?

Is the new 'old' at the end of the 1950–2000 period? One could be tempted to say 'yes' on the account of the remarkable revival of the epidemiology of infectious disease. Virtually all major findings (in terms of health impact) acquired so far in the aetiology of non-communicable disease had already been firmly or almost firmly established by the end of the 1970s (Holland *et al.* 1985). Major epidemiological findings in the 1980s and 1990s concerned diseases which have been found to have an infectious aetiology, like cancer of the liver (International Agency for Research on Cancer 1994a) and stomach (International Agency for Research on Cancer 1994b). In fact what has happened is a confluence of the methodologies of old and new epidemiology; for instance, observational cohort studies of AIDS patients have not only allowed us to demonstrate the efficacy of the tri-therapies but have come to represent 'epidemiological laboratories' from which valuable lessons can be drawn for the search and investigation of non-infectious pathogens (Samet and Munoz 1998). A second powerful stimulus to the confluence of methodologies has been the increased use of biological markers of exposure, early pre-clinical lesions, and of susceptibility, which has expanded in non-communicable disease epidemiology since the 1980s, followed by the massive irruption of genetic biomarkers in both old and new epidemiology in the 1990s. Past differences were vanishing by the end of the century and it may be premature to say whether the new difference emerging between the 'newest' epidemiology, based on laboratory and biomarkers, particularly genetic, and the more 'traditional' one based on questionnaire data, measurements in the environment (personal, local, or general), and physiological tests will become sufficiently established to acquire the same historical status that justified the distinction between new and old epidemiology after the Second World War.

What about 'modern' epidemiology? The term essentially denotes epidemiology as developed on rigorous methodological foundations in all substantive areas in the first decades of the period 1950–2000, and vigorously continued afterwards. By the same token it consecrates methodology as a distinctive primary trait. In this sense it can be said that 'epidemiology is needed everywhere' in medicine and public health. This all pervasive, actual or forthcoming, presence of epidemiology could not be obtained without a cost. The cost is that an always-needed tool also becomes an all-purpose tool, with no sharp priorities.

At the turn of the century this cost may have already started to materialize for current epidemiology, particularly because the dominant ideology in society profoundly differs from the one which provided the seeds and the greatest thrust to the development of modern epidemiology. In the period of roughly 1945–1975 the ideology reflected the impulse of post-war reconstruction and economic expansion and a dominant, if not universal, sense of solidarity stemming directly from the harsh wartime experiences shared by men and women of all social standing. This climate favoured epidemiology in at least two ways. First the concept of health as the right of everybody gained wide acceptance for the first time, and for this purpose epidemiology, with its focus on populations rather than individuals and prevention rather than late disease events, presented as a suitable instrument to be developed and financially supported. Second epidemiologists could reasonably and comfortably assume that the results of their studies would be translated by decision-makers into benefits for the whole population, as witnessed, for instance, by the establishment in many countries of systems of universal health insurance. In the neoliberal climate prevailing at the turn of the century the assumption of an unobstructed continuity between epidemiological results and their translation into benefits for all sections of society appears to be no longer warranted, as an economically based (or often so alleged) political barrier may be raised to impede or distort this transfer at any stage.

To ensure that these pervasive obstacles are overcome and the results of research are effectively transferred into benefits for all demands an active involvement which may take variable forms, from assistance to full participation in decision-making, from social critique to advocacy initiatives. Whatever the form, it is an engagement of an essentially political inspiration which many epidemiologists see well beyond their all-absorbing commitment to research, notably in a period in which rapid advances in genomics, proteomics, metabolomics, and developmental biology open multiple new avenues to epidemiological intelligence. To the extent that this attitude prevails, current epidemiology may be described as 'post-modern'. Post-modernism (Lyotard 1992) shies away from any utopian project, including the one of universal human betterment born with the Enlightenment: for good and bad, current epidemiology is doing much the same.

References

Armitage P (1964). *Sequential medical trials*. Blackwell, London.

Armstrong B, White E, and Saracci R (1992). *Principles of exposure measurement in epidemiology*. Oxford University Press, Oxford.

Breslow NE and Day NE (1980). *Statistical methods in cancer research. Volume 1—The analysis of case-control studies*. International Agency for Research on Cancer, Lyon.

Breslow NE and Day NE (1987). Statistical methods in cancer research. Volume 2—The design and analysis of cohort studies. International Agency for Research on Cancer, Lyon.

Clayton D and Hills M (1993). *Statistical models in epidemiology*. Oxford University Press, Oxford.

Clemmesen J (1965). *Statistical studies in malignant neoplasms*. Munskgaard, Copenhagen.

Cochrane AL (1972). *Effectiveness and efficiency*. The Nuffield Provincial Hospitals Trust, London.

Cornfield J (1951). A method for estimating comparative rates from clinical data. Applications to cancer of the lung, breast and cervix. *Journal of the National Cancer Institute*, **11**, 1269–75.

Cornfield J (1962). Joint dependence of the risk of coronary heart disease on serum cholesterol and systolic blood pressure. A discriminant function analysis. *Federation Proceedings*, **21**, 58–61.

Dawber TR, Kannel WB, and Lyell LP (1963). An approach to longitudinal studies in a community: the Framingham study. *Annals of the New York Academy of Sciences*, **107**, 539–56.

Doll R and Hill BA (1950). Smoking and carcinoma of the lung: preliminary report. *British Medical Journal*, **II**, 739–48.

Doll R and Hill BA (1964). Mortality in relation to smoking: ten years' observations of British doctors. *British Medical Journal*, **I**, 1399–1410, 1460–7.

Doll R, Peto R, Boreham J, and Sutherland I (2004). Mortality in relation to smoking: 50 years' observation of male British doctors. *British Medical Journal*, **328**, 1519–28.

Francis T, Korns RF, Voight RB, et al. (1955). An evaluation of the 1954 poliomyelitis vaccine trials—summary report. *American Journal of Public Health*, **5**, 1–63.

Fredericks DN and Relman DA (1996). Sequence-based identification of microbial pathogens: a reconsideration of Koch's postulates. *Clinical Microbiology Reviews*, **9**, 18–33.

Hill BA (1965). The environment and disease. Association or causation? *Proceedings of the Royal Society of Medicine*, **58**, 295–300.

Holland WW (1974). Screening for disease. Taking stock. *Lancet*, **II**, 1494–7.

Holland WW, Detels R, and Knox G (1985) (ed.). *Oxford textbook of public health*, 1st edn, Vol. 4. Oxford University Press, Oxford.

International Agency for Research on Cancer (1994a). *Hepatitis viruses*. IARC Monographs on the Evaluation of Carcinogenic Risks to Humans, Vol. 59. International Agency for Research on Cancer Lyon.

International Agency for Research on Cancer (1994b). Schistosomes, liver flukes and *Helicobacter pylori*. *IARC Monographs on the Evaluation of the Carcinogenic Risks to Humans*, Vol. 61. International Agency for Research on Cancer, Lyon.

International Agency for Research on Cancer (1995). Human papilloma viruses, *IARC Monographs on the Evaluation of the Carcinogenic Risks to Humans*, Vol. 64. International Agency for Research on Cancer, Lyon.

International Agency for Research on Cancer (1972–2006). *IARC Monographs on the Evaluation of the Carcinogenic Risks to Humans*, Vols 1–86. International Agency of Research on Cancer, Lyon.

Keys A (1970). *Coronary heart disease in seven countries*, American Heart Association Monograph no 29. AHA, New York.

Keys A (1995). Mediterranean diet and public health: personal reflections. *American Journal of Clinical Nutrition*, **61**, S1321–S1323.

Kleinbaum DG, Kupper LL, and Morgenstern H (1982). *Epidemiologic research*. Lifetime Learning Publications, Belmont, CA.

Levin ML, Goldstein H, and Gerhardt PR (1950). Cancer and tobacco smoking: a preliminary report. *Journal of the American Medical Association*, **143**, 336–8.

Lyotard JF (1992). *The postmodern condition: a report on knowledge*. Manchester University Press, Manchester.

MacMahon B, Pugh TF, and Ipsen J (1960). *Epidemiologic methods*. Little, Brown and Co., Boston.

Miettinen O (1985). *Theoretical epidemiology*. Wiley, New York.

McKeown T (1976). *The role of medicine*. The Nuffield Provincial Hospitals Trust, London.

Medical Research Council (1948). Streptomycin treatment of pulmonary tuberculosis. *British Medical Journal*, **II**, 769–82.

Medical Research Council (1960). Standardized questionnaire on respiratory symptoms. *British Medical Journal*, **II**, 1665–8.

Morris JN (1957). *Uses of epidemiology*, 1st edn. Livingstone Ltd, Edinburgh.

Morris JN (1964). *Uses of epidemiology*, 2nd edn. Livingstone Ltd, Edinburgh.

Rothman KJ (1986). *Modern epidemiology*, 1st edn. Little, Brown and Co, Boston.

Rothman KJ and Greenland S (1998). *Modern epidemiology*, 2nd edn. Lippincott-Raven, Philadelphia.

Samet JM and Munoz A (1998). Prospective: cohort studies. *Epidemiology Review*, **20**, 135–6.

Shaw GM (1992). Biology of human immunodeficiency viruses. In *Cecil textbook of medicine*, 19th edn (ed. JB Wyngaarden, LH Smith, and JC Bennett), pp. 1913–18. WB Saunders, Philadelphia.

US Department of Health, Education and Welfare (1964). *Smoking and health—report of the Advisory Committee to the Surgeon General of the Public Health Service*. US Department of Health, Education and Welfare, Public Health Service, Washington, DC.

World Health Organization (1976). *Myocardial infarction community registers*, Public Health in Europe no 5. WHO, Copenhagen.

Wynder EL and Graham EA (1950). Tobacco smoking as a possible etiologic factor in bronchiogenic carcinoma: a study of six hundred and eighty-four proved cases. *Journal of the American Medical Association*, **143**, 329–36.

5

Epidemiology and world health

Colin Mathers

Personal experiences

I originally trained as a physicist at the University of Sydney in Australia during the 1970s. One of my professors was Bob May, then a theoretical physicist, who went on to play a major role in the development of chaos theory and the application of mathematical modelling techniques in population ecology and infectious disease epidemiology (May and Anderson 1991). In Australia, as in many other countries, a significant citizens' movement against nuclear power developed in the latter half of the 1970s, with a focus in Australia on the prevention of uranium mining in Australia's Northern Territory. I became involved, with a small group of physicists at the university, in the public debate, on one occasion sharing a public platform with a junior opposition parliamentarian, Paul Keating, later to become Prime Minister of Australia.

Some work in assessing the impact on population health of nuclear power and other forms of energy generation led to an interest in epidemiology and the application of statistical and mathematical techniques to questions around population health. On completion of my doctorate in theoretical physics at the end of the 1970s, I took a job with the newly established National Perinatal Statistics Unit and contributed to the development of a national monitoring system for congenital malformations. During this time, I also undertook epidemiology and demography course work for a masters degree in public health.

In 1986, I joined a newly created statutory authority, the Australian Institute of Health (AIH), created by the Australian government to address the need for national information and comparable state-level information to support health policy-making. My first major project was to develop a national database and report on hospital costs, use, and efficiency. Over the next 13 years, I was fortunate to be able to take a leading role in the development of new national activities and reports across a wide range of population health and health system issues.

In this chapter, I examine major developments in summarizing population health over the last 30 years, and focus particularly on developments in global descriptive epidemiology, on the global burden of disease approach to summarizing population health, and on the issues and controversies surrounding these developments. Reliable and comparable information about levels and trends in population health, about the main causes of loss of health in populations, and how these are changing, is a critical input for debates about international and national health policies and priorities.

Summarizing the health of populations

The regular assessment of levels of population health is a key component of the public policy process. It enables analysis of variations in levels of health across and within populations and changes in levels of health over time for populations and by age and sex—to show whether levels of health are improving. With accelerating ageing of populations during the second half of the twentieth century came increasing recognition that it was important to assess not only mortality but also morbidity and disability at the population level. In particular, there was considerable interest in the question of whether populations were becoming more or less healthy as life expectancies increased: an issue referred to as compression or expansion of morbidity (Fries 1980).

The concept of combining data on the health or disability status of populations with mortality data in a life table to generate estimates of expected years of life in various health states was first proposed in the 1960s (Sanders 1964; Sullivan 1966) and disability-free life expectancy (DFLE) was calculated for a number of countries during the 1970s and 1980s. A Network for Health Expectancy and the Disability Process, known by its French acronym of REVES, was established in 1989 largely due to the energy and enthusiasm of Jean-Marie Robine of the French Institute for Health and Medical Research (INSERM). REVES has focused much of its efforts on the harmonization of calculation methods and identification of the conditions necessary for the comparison of estimates of health expectancy, both across populations and over time (Robine *et al.* 2003).

In 1990, I accidentally stumbled across a short paper by Jean-Marie Robine on the calculation of DFLE, and as I had all the requisite data to hand, completed the first calculations of DLFE for Australia that same day. I attended the next REVES meeting in Leiden in 1991 and over the following years contributed to the development of methods and calculations for health expectancies globally (Mathers 2002; Robine *et al.* 2003). During the 1990s, there was a dramatic increase in the number of health expectancy calculations carried out, almost all using the Sullivan method.

As a summary measure of the average level of health in a population, health expectancies have two advantages over other summary measures:

◆ the concept of an equivalent 'healthy' life expectancy is relatively easy to explain to a non-technical audience, and

◆ health expectancies are measured in units (expected years of life) that are meaningful to and within the common experience of non-technical audiences (unlike other indicators such as mortality rates or incidence rates).

In its early meetings the REVES network identified that the main challenge in the international use of health expectancies was the use of different questions, response scales, and concepts (impairment, disability, handicap, quality of life, etc) in nationally representative surveys. For a long time this was thought to be the most important problem in the development of summary measures of population health, and REVES and international agencies devoted much attention to the development of standard concepts, methods, and instruments.

In the 1990s, a number of cross-national surveys became available that used a common instrument and consistent sampling methods. One example was the European Community Household Panel survey conducted in 13 countries in 1994. It became apparent from these surveys that standardized instruments did not solve the problems of comparability across countries. These problems relate much more fundamentally to unmeasured differences in expectations and norms for health, since the meaning that different populations attach to the labels used for each of the response categories in self-reported questions can vary greatly.

Consider a self-reported survey question that asks respondents whether they have difficulty walking up stairs. For such a question the response categories are labelled 'no difficulty', 'mild difficulty', 'moderate difficulty', 'severe difficulty', and 'extreme/cannot do'. The identical response of 'mild difficulty' in walking up stairs could indeed map to different levels of mobility in different populations. The survey results would be reliable and valid within each population but the results cannot be compared across populations without adjustment. In fact, self-report survey data on difficulty in carrying out activities of daily living (ADL) typically show difficulty prevalences five to ten times higher in developed countries compared with developing countries.

Global burden of disease

While health expectancies provide a potentially useful summary measure of the overall levels of population health, combining mortality risks and morbidity or disability information, they do not lend themselves readily to causal decomposition. As with life expectancy, all causes contribute to the resulting summary indicator and it is only possible to decompose the contributions of specific diseases and injuries through counterfactual analyses in which causes are deleted one by one and the resulting increases in the indicator calculated. Such cause-deleted increments in life expectancy or healthy life expectancy are not additive, and this significantly limits their utility as a tool for communicating the impact of different causes on population health.

For this reason, I experimented in 1992 with generalizing the concept of potential years of life lost to include lost good health, and applied this to the calculation of lost years of healthy life due to cancers in Australia. Unknown to me at the time, Chris Murray at Harvard University and Alan Lopez at the World Health Organization (WHO) were developing and applying a similar indicator, the disability adjusted life year or (DALY), to the estimation of the burden of disease for all regions of the world. At the same time, they were carrying out the most ambitious meta-synthesis of population health and mortality information ever attempted (Murray and Lopez 1996a,b). The Global Burden of Disease (GBD) study was commissioned by the World Bank to provide a comprehensive assessment of disease burden in 1990 from over 100 diseases and injuries, and from 10 selected risk factors, for the world as a whole and eight regions. These assessments were combined with regional estimates of the cost-effectiveness of health interventions to recommend essential packages of intervention for countries at different stages of development (World Bank 1993).

The motivations for interest in an alternative summary measure of population health of this type was essentially twofold: (1) the need to decompose the summary measure by disease and injury (and risk factor) causes in order to address the needs of policy-makers for information on the causes of loss of health, and (2) the need for a measure that was comparable across population groups, a need which, it had become clear, health expectancies based on self-report information could not meet.

The disability-adjusted life year (DALY)

The DALY is a summary measure which combines time lost through premature death and time lived in states of less than optimal health, loosely referred to as 'disability'. The DALY is a generalization of the well known potential years of life lost (PYLL) measure to include lost good health. One DALY can be thought of as one lost year of 'healthy' life, and the measured disease burden is the gap between a population's health status and that of a normative reference population. DALYs for a specific cause are calculated as the sum of the years of life lost due to premature mortality (YLL) from that cause and the years of healthy life lost due to disability (YLD) for incident cases of the health condition.

The YLL are essentially calculated as the number of cause-specific deaths multiplied by a loss function specifying the years lost as a function of the age at which death occurs. The loss function chosen by Murray and Lopez did not use an arbitrary age cut-off such as 70 years, but instead specified it in terms of the life expectancies at various ages in global standard life tables, with life expectancy at birth fixed at 82.5 years for females and 80.0 years for males. The loss function was specified to be the same for all deaths of a given age and sex, irrespective of other characteristics such as socio-economic status or relevant current local life expectancies.

Because YLL measures the incident stream of lost years of life due to deaths, an incidence perspective is also taken for the calculation of YLD. To estimate YLD for a particular cause during a particular time period, the number of incident cases in that period is multiplied by the average duration of the disease and a weight factor that reflects the severity of the disease on a scale from 0 (perfect health) to 1 (dead). The health state weights formalize and quantify social preferences for different states of health, and thus allow time (years of healthy life) to be used as the common currency for combining non-fatal health states and years of life lost due to mortality. DALYs can thus also be thought of as a particular form of the more general concept of 'quality-adjusted life years' or QALYs, widely used in economic evaluations for health interventions.

Health economists have developed a number of choice-based methods to measure preferences for health states, although there is considerable heterogeneity in the conceptualization of what the preferences relate to, ranging from health, through quality of life and wellbeing, to utility. (Salomon and Murray 2004). The original GBD study used two forms of the person trade-off method and asked participants in weighting exercises to make a composite judgement about the severity distribution of the condition and the preference for time spent in each severity level (Murray 1996). This was largely necessitated by the lack of population information on the severity distribution of most conditions at the global and regional levels. The participants were not representative of general populations, but were by and large public health professionals involved in a WHO meeting with representation from all regions, and in training workshops held in several different regions.

In developing the DALY indicator Murray (1996) argued that two additional value choices should be made explicit in the formulation of the summary measure, namely:

♦ Is a year of healthy life gained now worth more to society than a year of healthy life gained in 20 years' time? In other words, should time discounting be applied to the stream of incident lost healthy years represented by the DALY?

♦ Are lost years of healthy life valued more at some ages than others? Is a year of life at young adult ages valued more than in old age or infancy? In other words, should unequal age weights be applied to years of healthy life lost at different ages?

He chose to apply a 3% time discount rate to the years of life lost in the future to estimate the net present value of years of life lost in calculating DALYs. Time discounting was included for consistency with the measurement of health outcomes in cost-effectiveness analyses; to prevent giving excessive weight to deaths at younger ages; and to address the disease eradication and research paradox. Assuming that investment in research or disease eradication has a non-zero chance of succeeding, then without discounting, all current expenditure should be shifted to such investment because the future stream of benefits is infinite.

Murray also incorporated non-uniform age weights that gave less weight to years lived at younger and older ages. This was based on human capital arguments and on a number of studies that suggest the existence of a broad social preference to value a year lived by a young adult more highly than a year lived by a young child or an older person (Murray 1996). The particular age weights used in the GBD study result in greater weight being given to all deaths below the age of 39 compared with deaths at older ages.

Burden of disease analysis

A key feature of the GBD approach to descriptive epidemiology was to include assessments of all causes of disease and injury burden, even in the face of limited or missing data, to produce a comprehensive and unbiased, if uncertain, overview of the importance of specific diseases and risk factors in causing loss of health. Two key tools in dealing with limited or missing data were to carefully screen sources of health data for plausibility and completeness, drawing on expert opinion and on cross-population comparisons; and to explicitly ensure the internal consistency of estimates of incidence, prevalence, case fatality, and mortality for each specific cause of disease.

Estimating prevalence and incidence is usually much harder than estimating mortality. Data collection, when done, is often limited in terms of both time and geographical area, and problems of case definition abound. Not surprisingly, data are frequently incomplete, and when available, their validity may be in doubt. In particular, given differences in the way the data for incidence, prevalence, and mortality are collected, it is almost inevitable that observations are internally inconsistent. For example, when a cohort study misses more incident cases than deaths, the observed incidence will be too small to account for the observed mortality.

To address such issues, the GBD exploited two kinds of knowledge:

- Disease characteristics, such as remission, case fatality rates, and duration, may be relatively constant across countries and known from studies in some populations, from clinical studies, or from expert knowledge.

- Because the various epidemiological variables are causally linked by a disease process, a disease model that explicitly describes these causal pathways allows us to infer missing data if existing data are sufficient to do so. Supplementing observed data with expert knowledge on other aspects of the disease process may help to overcome a lack of data.

A software tool called DISMOD was developed for the GBD study to help model the incidence and duration parameters needed for calculations of YLD from available data, to incorporate expert knowledge, and to check the consistency of different epidemiological estimates and ensure that the estimates used were internally consistent. Figure 5.1 shows the underlying model used by DISMOD.

Impact of the original GBD study

The GBD study had a very large impact on the global public health community, but was also controversial. For the first time, the comparative importance of over 100 diseases and injuries, and 10 major risk factors, for global and regional health status was assessed using a common metric which simultaneously accounted for both premature mortality and the prevalence, duration, and severity of the non-fatal consequences of disease and injury. As a result, mental health

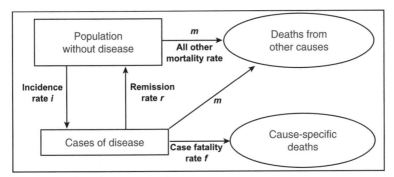

Fig. 5.1 The basic disease model underlying DISMOD. Reproduced from Mathers *et al.* (2006a). Sensitivity and uncertainty analyses for burden of disease and risk factor estimates. In *Global Burden of Disease and Injury Series*, Vol. 2. Harvard School of Public Health, Cambridge, MA on behalf of the WHO.

conditions and injuries, for which non-fatal outcomes are of particular significance, were identified as being among the leading causes of disease/injury burden in both high- and low-income countries, with clear implications for policy, particularly prevention.

The leading causes of disease burden in 1990 were childhood diseases (lower respiratory diseases, diarrhoeal diseases, and perinatal causes such as birth asphyxia, birth traumas, and low birth weight), in part because of the greater weight given to deaths at younger ages by the DALY. To the surprise of many, depression ranked fourth globally, ahead of ischaemic heart disease, cerebrovascular disease, tuberculosis, and measles. Road traffic accidents also ranked in the top 10 causes of DALYs worldwide. In terms of broad disease categories, non-communicable diseases, including mental disorders, were estimated to have caused 41% of the global burden of disease, only slightly less than communicable, maternal, perinatal, and nutritional conditions combined (44%), with 15% due to injuries. The GBD study identified in very clear terms that non-communicable diseases caused a very substantial disease burden in developing as well as developed countries.

In addition, the GBD study attempted to quantify the attributable mortality and burden for 10 major risk factors, and to project mortality and burden forward for 30 years.. Almost 16% of the entire global burden of disease and injury for 1990 was attributed to malnutrition, another 7% to poor water and sanitation, 3.5% each to unsafe sex and alcohol, and between 1% and 3% from risks such as tobacco, occupational exposures, hypertension, and physical inactivity.

Much of the comment and criticism of the original GBD study has focused on the construction of DALYs (Anand and Hanson 1997; Williams 1999), particularly the social choices incorporated in it, and relatively little around the uncertainty in the basic descriptive epidemiology, especially in Africa, which is likely to be far more consequential for setting health priorities (Cooper *et al.* 1998). Some critics have argued against the use of age weights that give lower value to years of life lived in early childhood and older ages and some recent national and international burden of disease studies have used time discounting but not age weights (Jamison *et al.* 2006b; Mathers *et al.* 1999). Murray and others have responded to the criticisms of the value choices made for the original GBD study (Murray and Acharya 1997; Murray and Lopez 2000).

A second criticism has been that burden of disease analysis may result in incorrect policy decisions because priorities for health action might be set solely on the basis of the magnitude of burden of disease. Some health economists have taken this concern to such an extreme that they have argued that one should never measure the size of a problem but only the marginal cost-effectiveness of interventions, i.e. the health that can be gained for a given expenditure (Mooney *et al.* 1997).

However, neither Murray nor anyone else involved with the burden of disease work has ever claimed that size of problem should be used to set priorities. In fact, the original GBD study, and the later round of GBD work at WHO, discussed further below, have both been accompanied by a substantial effort in cost-effectiveness analysis, and an explicit recognition that health priority setting requires not only information on the size and causes of health problems, but on the cost-effectiveness of interventions and on other information relating to equity and social values.

A third area of criticism has related to the methods used to elicit the disability weights with claims that the person trade-off method used in the GBD is unethical, in that it involves hypothetical scenarios trading off saving the lives of people in full health versus saving the lives of people with specified health conditions (Arnesen and Nord 1999). Subsequent work on eliciting health state valuations has moved away from reliance on the person trade-off method. Additionally, the DALY results are generally much more sensitive to the data and assumptions on the severity distributions and durations of the disabling sequelae of diseases and injuries than to variations or uncertainty in disability weights (Mathers *et al.* 2006b).

Perhaps the most persistent criticisms have come from disability lobby groups and from some health analysts and policy-makers, largely in the developed countries, who have seen the quantification of disease burden in terms of disease and injury causes as a retreat to 'the medical model of health' and the inclusion of disability in the DALY as implying that people with disability are less valued than people in full health. I return to these issues later.

National burden of disease

The methods and findings of the original GBD study have spawned numerous national disease burden exercises of varying quality and ambition. The earliest comprehensive studies were for Mexico and Mauritius (Lozano *et al*. 1995; Vos *et al*. 1995). A Dutch study in the mid-1990s devoted considerable effort to the estimation of disability weights using improved methods and a lay group as well as several groups of health professionals (Stouthard *et al*. 1997). I carried out the first Australian national burden of disease study during 1997 to 1999 in collaboration with Theo Vos (Mathers *et al*. 1999), who also carried out a parallel study for one state in Australia involving district level analyses and projections (Public Health Division 1999). Theo Vos had been the principal investigator on the Mauritius burden of disease study and his experience and knowledge of the disease models and assumptions used in the GBD study were invaluable in enabling the completion of the Australian studies in 2 years with a relatively small combined team of around six people.

The Australian burden of disease studies have had a considerable impact on public health policy in Australia. Apart from helping to raise the profile of low-mortality conditions such as mental health, musculoskeletal disorders, sensory disorders, and dementia, the burden of disease studies have increased policy-makers' attention to interventions aimed at risk factors. Additionally, they have been used as a starting point for economic analyses of public health interventions and priorities and for an influential report on returns on investment in public health. In Victoria, the regional analyses have had a major effect in focusing policy-makers' attention on geographical and social inequalities in health and in regional health service provision, funding, and priorities.

During the last 5 years, comprehensive national burden of disease studies have also been carried out in countries such as Brazil, Malaysia, Turkey, South Africa, Zimbabwe, Thailand, and the USA, and studies are under way in Canada and several other countries. The results of these studies have been widely used by government and non-governmental agencies alike to argue for more strategic allocation of health resources to disease prevention and control programmes that are likely to yield the greatest gains in population health. Some of these studies have also led to substantially more data on the descriptive epidemiology of diseases and injuries, as well as to improvements in analytical methods.

Measuring the health of populations at global, regional, and national levels

When Dr Gro Harlem Brundtland took office as Director-General of WHO in July 1998, she also brought Chris Murray to the WHO to provide a stronger focus on evidence for health policy, not only in terms of better evidence on population health and its determinants, but on cost-effectiveness of interventions and on the performance of health systems. I came to the WHO at the beginning of 2000 to work with Chris Murray and Alan Lopez on the global burden of disease analyses and on the development of summary measures of population health for comparing levels of health of WHO member states, a key outcome measure for health systems. From 2002 to 2005, I had management responsibility for the work on summary measures of population health, updating of the GBD analyses and the annual updating of estimates of incidence, prevalence, mortality, and burden for a comprehensive set of disease and injury causes.

My first task at the WHO was to work on the estimation of healthy life expectancy for 191 WHO member states, a key output measure in the health system performance assessment published in the World Health Report 2000 (WHO 2000). This report ranked countries on healthy life expectancy, a measure of level of health, as well as on other important inputs and goals of health systems, and also ranked countries on their overall health system performance. The report generated considerable media attention, great controversy among WHO member states, and heated debates in academic and expert forums and journals. In response to this controversy, technical and regional consultations were undertaken, new forms of survey data collection were implemented, and a scientific peer review group was established to review the framework and methods for future analysis (Murray and Evans 2003). It is beyond the scope of this chapter to examine the controversies around the health system performance work except as they relate to the measurement and summarizing of levels of population health and causes of loss of health.

Healthy life expectancy

The WHO reported for the first time on the average levels of population health for its 191 member states using a health expectancy measure in the World Health Report 2000 (WHO 2000). Healthy life expectancy (HALE) is a form of health expectancy that, like the DALY, applies disability weights to health states to compute the equivalent number of years of life expected to be lived in full health. The first HALE calculations attempted to use existing health survey data together with imputed national-level data from the GBD study. The difficulties in comparing self-reported health data across populations, discussed above, severely limited the information input from population-representative surveys. To address this problem, as well as to improve the availability of country-level empirical data, the WHO embarked on an ambitious multicountry survey study (MCSS) in 2000–2001 involving 63 surveys in 55 countries. These surveys also included a health state valuation module involving multiple valuation methods to address criticisms of the original GBD valuation methods, including the reliance on experts rather than population-based respondents).

The measurement and valuation of the health states of survey respondents was conceptualized in terms of a set of six core domains: pain, affect, cognition, mobility, self-care, and usual activities (including household- and work-related activities). To address the fundamental comparability issues of respondents' use of response categories, the surveys included anchoring vignettes and some measured tests on selected domains that were intended to calibrate the description that respondents provided of their own health. Statistical methods have been developed for correcting biases in self-reported health using such calibration data (King *et al.* 2003).

Estimates of healthy life expectancy for the year 2000 were published in the World Health Report 2001 using improved methods and incorporating cross-population comparable survey data for 55 countries from the MCSS. Figure 5.2 shows average HALE at birth for 192 countries in 2002 as published in the World Health Report 2004. These are plotted against income per capita (GDP measured in international dollars using purchasing power parity conversion rates) on a logarithmic scale. The error bars show estimated 95% uncertainty ranges for HALE at birth.

Some commentators have argued that the data demands and complexity of the calculations make healthy life expectancy impractical for use as a summary measure of population health. Although the concept of healthy life expectancy is relatively simple to understand, health encompasses multiple domains and mortality risks, and with the additional requirement to ensure comparability of estimates across countries, any acceptable methods used to compute healthy life expectancy will inevitably be complex and highly data demanding. The HALE estimates published by the WHO based on GBD analyses and the multicountry survey study results have much

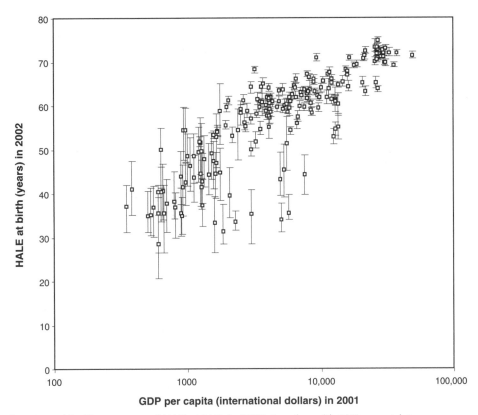

Fig. 5.2 Healthy life expectancy (HALE) at birth in 2002, together with 95% uncertainty ranges, versus gross domestic product (GDP) per capita for 2001 in international dollars, for 192 WHO member states. Reproduced with permission from the WHO.

wider uncertainty ranges compared to the life expectancy estimates, and further work is needed both on statistical methods for ensuring cross-population comparability and on data collection.

New assessments of the global burden of disease

Between 1998 and 2004, WHO undertook a new assessment of the global burden of disease for the years 2000 to 2002, with annual assessments published in Annex Tables to the World Health Reports. These new assessments were based on an extensive analysis of mortality data for all regions of the world together with systematic reviews of epidemiological studies and population health surveys. These revisions drew on a wide range of data sources, and incorporated a range of methodological improvements. Additionally, a major and expanded research programme was undertaken to quantify the global and regional attributable mortality and burden for 26 major risk factors (Ezzati *et al.* 2003).

The recent revisions of the GBD have been documented in detail, with information on data sources and methods as well as uncertainty and sensitivity analyses, in a book published as part of the Disease Control Priorities Project, along with the second edition of *Disease control priorities in developing countries* (Jamison *et al.* 2006a; Lopez *et al.* 2006). The Disease Control Priorities Project is a joint project of the World Bank, WHO, and the National Institutes of Health, funded by the Gates Foundation.

The basic units of analysis for the first GBD study were the eight World Bank regions defined for the 1993 World Development Report. The heterogeneity of these large regions limited their value for comparative epidemiological assessments. For the new GBD assessments, a more refined approach was followed. Mortality estimates by disease and injury cause, age, and sex were first developed for each of the 192 WHO member states using different methods for countries with different sources of information on mortality. Epidemiological estimates for incidence, prevalence, and YLD were first developed for 17 groupings of countries, and then imputed to country populations using available country-level information and methods to ensure consistency with the country-specific mortality estimates. The resulting country-level estimates have been made available at a summarized level, and also facilitate the production of regional estimates for any desired regional groupings of countries.

Perhaps the major methodological progress since the original GBD study was with respect to risk-factor quantification. Although the 1990 study estimated the attributable mortality and burden for 10 risk factors, there were serious concerns about the comparability of the estimates. There was little consistency across disparate risk factors, particularly with regard to the definition of 'hazardous' exposure, the strength of evidence on causality, and the availability of epidemiological research on exposure and outcomes. Moreover, exposures were treated as dichotomous following traditional epidemiological approaches to risk quantification, with exposure defined according to some, often arbitrary, threshold value. For the GBD 2000–2002 study, a new framework for risk factor quantification was defined which calculated attributable fractions of disease due to a risk factor based on a comparison of disease burden expected under the current estimated distribution of exposure, with that expected if a counterfactual distribution of exposure had applied, and also took into account excess risk across the entire range for continuous exposures such as cholesterol, blood pressure, and body mass index burden, that would be expected under different population distributions of exposure (Murray and Lopez 1999). The counterfactual distribution was defined for each risk factor as the theoretically achievable population distribution of exposure that would lead to the lowest minimum levels of disease burden. The case of tobacco use is particularly clear: the theoretical minimum distribution would be 100% of the population being life-long non-smokers. For body mass index, it would be a population distribution of body mass index normally distributed with mean and standard deviation of 21 and 1 kg/m^2 respectively (Ezzati *et al.* 2003).

What do the GBD studies tell us about world health?

While changes in the availability of data and revisions in methods and disease models make it difficult to compare the results of the original 1990 GBD study with the new assessments, it is possible to draw some conclusions on broad trends in global health. There have been impressive improvements in global health in the twentieth century: for example, life expectancy at birth has increased from a global average of 46 years in 1950 to 65 years in 2000. However, huge disparities across countries remain, with life expectancy at birth ranging from over 80 years in the most developed countries to just over 40 years in the most disadvantaged countries. In almost all countries women have longer life expectancy than men, with the notable exception of countries in the eastern Mediterranean region and North Africa.

Life expectancy increased during the 1990s for most regions of the world, with the notable exception of Africa and the former Soviet countries of Eastern Europe. In the latter case, male and female life expectancies at birth declined by 3.2 years and 2.7 years, respectively, over the 10-year period between 1990 and 2000. In sub-Saharan Africa, life expectancies for countries most affected by the HIV/AIDS epidemic declined by 10 to 20 years. In Botswana, for example, life expectancy decreased from nearly 65 years in 1985–90 to just over 40 years in 2002. In the absence of AIDS it would have been expected to rise to 66 years by 2005. HIV/AIDS is now the leading cause of death in sub-Saharan Africa, with more women infected than men.

The epidemiological transition in low- and middle-income countries has resulted in a 20% reduction since 1990 in the per capita disease burden due to communicable, maternal, perinatal, and nutritional conditions. Without the HIV/AIDS epidemic, this reduction would have been substantially greater, at 30% over the last 11 years. Several of the 'traditional' infectious diseases, such as tuberculosis and malaria have not declined, in part because of weak public health services and the increased numbers of people with immune systems weakened by HIV/AIDS.

The extent of the global inequalities in health is illustrated by the large variations in child mortality rates (under 5 years of age). The risk of dying under the age of 5 ranges from 17% in sub-Saharan Africa to 0.7% in high-income countries in 2001. If all countries had the Japanese rates, the lowest in the world, there would be only 1 million child deaths each year, instead of the current 10 million deaths. Low- and middle-income countries account for 99% of global deaths in children under the age of 5 years; 85% of these are in the low-income countries and can be attributed to just five preventable conditions—pneumonia, diarrhoeal diseases, malaria, measles, and malnutrition.

The per capita disease burden in Eastern European and Central Asian countries has increased by nearly 40% from 1990 to 2001, so that this region now has worse health than all other regions of the world apart from South Asia and sub-Saharan Africa. The unexpected increase in disease burden, and concomitant reductions in life expectancy, in countries of this region, appear to be related to identifiable factors including alcohol abuse, suicide, and violence which are seemingly associated with societies facing social and economic disintegration. The rapidity of these declines has dramatically changed our perceptions of the time frames possible for substantial change in chronic disease burden, and the potential for such adverse health trends to occur elsewhere.

The main findings of the GBD study for the year 2001 are summarized in Tables 5.1 and 5.2 for low- and middle-income countries, for high-income countries, and for the world. The high-income countries include the countries of Western Europe, North America, Australia, New Zealand,

Table 5.1 Deaths by cause: low- and middle-income countries, high-income countries[a] and world, 2001

	Low- and middle-income	High-income	World	
Total deaths (thousands)	48,351	7891	56,242	
Death rate per 1000 population	9.3	8.5	9.1	
Age-standardized death rate per 1000[b]	11.4	5.0	10.0	
Leading global disease and injury causes	Number (thousands)			% of total
1 Ischaemic heart disease	5699	1364	7063	12.6
2 Cerebrovascular disease	4608	781	5390	9.6
3 Lower respiratory infections	3408	345	3753	6.7
4 Chronic obstructive pulmonary disease	2378	297	2676	4.8
5 HIV/AIDS	2552	22	2574	4.6

Continued

Table 5.1 (continued) Deaths by cause: low- and middle-income countries, high-income countries[a] and world, 2001

		Low- and middle-income	High-income	World	
6	Perinatal conditions[c]	2489	32	2522	4.5
7	Diarrhoeal diseases	1777	6	1783	3.2
8	Tuberculosis	1590	16	1606	2.9
9	Trachea, bronchus and lung cancer	771	456	1227	2.2
10	Malaria	1207		1208	2.1
11	Road traffic accidents	1069	121	1189	2.1
12	Diabetes mellitus	757	202	960	1.7
13	Hypertensive heart disease	760	129	889	1.6
14	Self-inflicted injuries (suicide)	749	126	875	1.6
15	Stomach cancers	696	146	842	1.5
16	Cirrhosis of the liver	654	118	771	1.4
17	Measles	762	1	763	1.4
18	Nephritis and nephrosis	552	111	663	1.2
19	Colon and rectum cancers	357	257	614	1.1
20	Liver cancer	505	102	607	1.1
Selected global risk factors[d]		Attributable number (thousands)			% of total
1	High blood pressure	6223	1392	7615	13.5
2	Smoking	3340	1462	4802	8.5
3	High cholesterol	3038	842	3880	6.9
4	Childhood underweight	3630		3630	6.5
5	Unsafe sex	2819	32	2851	5.1
6	Low fruit and vegetable intake	2308	333	2641	4.7
7	Overweight and obesity	1747	614	2361	4.2
8	Physical inactivity	1559	376	1935	3.4
9	Alcohol use	1869	24	1893	3.4
10	Indoor smoke from household use of solid fuels	1791		1791	3.2
11	Unsafe water, sanitation, and hygiene	1563	4	1567	2.8
12	Zinc deficiency	849		849	1.5
13	Urban air pollution	735	76	811	1.4
14	Vitamin A deficiency	800		800	1.4
15	Iron-deficiency anaemia	613	8	621	1.1
16	Contaminated injections in health-care setting	407	4	412	0.7
17	Illicit drug use	189	37	226	0.4

Table 5.1 (continued) Deaths by cause: low- and middle-income countries, high-income countries[a] and world, 2001

		Low- and middle-income	High-income	World	
18	Non-use and use of ineffective methods of contraception	162		162	0.3
19	Child sexual abuse	65	6	71	0.1
	All risk factors together	22,014	3473	25,488	45.3

Adapted from: Lopez AD, Mathers CD, Ezzati M, Murray CJL, and Jamison DT (2006). *Global burden of disease and risk factors, Disease Control Priorities Project*. Oxford University Press, Oxford.

[a] Countries grouped according to gross national income per capita.

[b] Age-standardized using the WHO world standard population.

[c] Includes 'Causes arising in the perinatal period' as defined in the International Classification of Diseases, and does not include all causes of deaths occurring in the perinatal period.

[d] Note that deaths attributable to individual risk factors cannot be added due to multicausality.

Table 5.2 DALYs[a] by cause: low- and middle-income countries, high-income countries[b] and world, 2001 (adapted from Lopez *et al.* 2006)

		Low- and middle-income	High-income	World	
Total DALYs (thousands)		1,386,709	149,161	1,535,871	
DALYs per 1000 population		265.7	160.6	249.8	
Age-standardized DALYs per 1000[c]		281.7	128.2	256.5	
Leading global disease and injury causes		Number (thousands)			% of total
1	Perinatal conditions[d]	89,068	1408	90,477	5.9
2	Lower respiratory infections	83,606	2314	85,920	5.6
3	Ischaemic heart disease	71,882	12,390	84,273	5.5
4	Cerebrovascular disease	62,669	9354	72,024	4.7
5	HIV/AIDS	70,796	665	71,461	4.7
6	Diarrhoeal diseases	58,697	444	59,141	3.9
7	Unipolar major depression	43,427	8408	51,835	3.4
8	Malaria	39,961	9	39,970	2.6
9	Chronic obstructive pulmonary disease	33,453	5282	38,736	2.5
10	Tuberculosis	35,874	219	36,093	2.3
11	Road traffic accidents	32,017	3045	35,063	2.3
12	Hearing loss, adult onset	24,607	5387	29,994	2.0
13	Cataracts	28,150	493	28,643	1.9
14	Congenital anomalies	23,533	1420	24,952	1.6

Continued

Table 5.2 (continued) DALYs[a] by cause: low- and middle-income countries, high-income countries[b] and world, 2001 (adapted from Lopez *et al.* 2006)

		Low- and middle-income	High-income	World	
15	Measles	23,091	23	23,113	1.5
16	Self-inflicted injuries	17,674	2581	20,255	1.3
17	Diabetes mellitus	15,804	4192	19,997	1.3
18	Violence	18,132	765	18,897	1.2
19	Osteoarthritis	13,666	3786	17,452	1.1
20	Alzheimer and other dementias	9640	7468	17,108	1.1
Selected global risk factors[e]		Attributable number (thousands)			% of total
1	Childhood underweight	120,579	67	120,647	7.9
2	High blood pressure	78,063	13,887	91,950	6.0
3	Unsafe sex	80,270	909	81,179	5.3
4	Smoking	54,019	18,900	72,919	4.7
5	Alcohol use	49,449	6580	56,029	3.6
6	High cholesterol	42,815	9431	52,246	3.4
7	Unsafe water, sanitation, and hygiene	51,622	289	51,911	3.4
8	Overweight and obesity	31,515	10,733	42,248	2.8
9	Indoor smoke from household use of solid fuels	41,731	2	41,734	2.7
10	Low fruit and vegetable intake	32,836	3982	36,819	2.4
11	Zinc deficiency	27,631	5	27,636	1.8
12	Physical inactivity	22,679	4732	27,411	1.8
13	Iron-deficiency anaemia	23,933	789	24,722	1.6
14	Vitamin A deficiency	24,686	1	24,686	1.6
15	Illicit drug use	7890	2024	9914	0.6
16	Urban air pollution	8707	664	9371	0.6
17	Contaminated injections in health-care setting	8974	76	9050	0.6
18	Non-use and use of ineffective methods of contraception	7411	23	7434	0.5
19	Child sexual abuse	5381	699	6079	0.4
	All risk factors together	500,066	51,092	551,158	35.9

[a]DALYs calculated with 3% time discounting but without age weighting.

[b]Countries grouped according to gross national income per capita.

[c]Age-standardized using the WHO world standard population.

[d]Includes 'Causes arising in the perinatal period' as defined in the International Classification of Diseases, and does not include all causes occurring in the perinatal period.

[e]Note that DALYs attributable to individual risk factors cannot be added due to multicausality.

Japan, the Republic of Korea, and Singapore. These tables clearly illustrate the 'double burden' of disease faced by low- and middle-income countries. Countries that are still struggling with epidemics of old and new infectious disease must now also deal with the emerging epidemics of chronic non-communicable disease such as heart disease, stroke, diabetes, and cancer.

Rapid demographic changes, particularly in poorer regions of the world, will lead to an ageing population and an increase in the burden of non-communicable diseases in the absence of preventive action. However, it is difficult for poorer countries and international health agencies to focus on medium-term preventive strategies in the face of more immediate communicable disease problems, particularly in sub-Saharan Africa. The 'double burden' of disease is being superseded by the 'triple burden'. To the unfinished agendas of communicable and non-communicable disease prevention and control, are being added new health threats associated with globalization such as those posed by avian flu and global warming.

Figure 5.3 illustrates the regional variations in disease burden in 2001. Group I conditions (communicable, maternal, perinatal, and nutritional disorders) account for 70% of the burden of disease in sub-Saharan Africa and 44% of the burden in South Asia. In other low- and middle-income countries, group I conditions account for around one-quarter of the disease burden. The total disease burden in the countries of Europe and Central Asia is now higher than for other developing regions of the world apart from South Asia and sub-Saharan Africa. Sensory disorders, principally hearing and sight loss, contribute significantly to disability in all regions of the world.

In Latin America and Caribbean countries, Europe and Central Asian countries, and the Middle East and North Africa, more than 30% of the entire disease burden among male adults aged 15–44 is attributable to injuries, including road traffic accidents, violence, and self-inflicted injuries. Additionally, deaths from injury are noticeably higher for women in some parts of Asia and the Middle East and North Africa, in part due to high levels of suicide and violence.

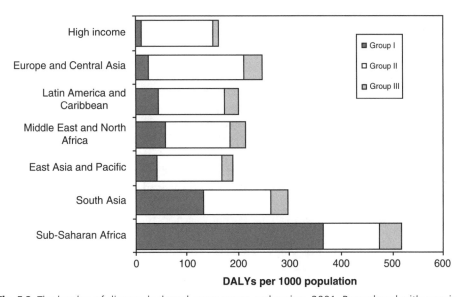

Fig. 5.3 The burden of disease, by broad cause group and region, 2001. Reproduced with permission from Lopez AD, Mathers CD, Ezzati M, Murray CJL, and Jamison DT (2006). *Global burden of disease and risk factors*. Oxford University Press, Oxford.

As Tables 5.1 and 5.2 suggest, the world is also experiencing a 'risk factor' transition. Already in low- and middle-income countries, the 10 leading risk factors include underweight, unsafe sex, unsafe water and sanitation, and indoor air pollution but also include risk factors for chronic disease that have traditionally been thought of as conditions of affluence: tobacco, suboptimal blood pressure, alcohol, cholesterol, overweight, and low fruit and vegetable intake. An analysis of the joint effects of the 19 risk factors listed in Tables 5.1 and 5.2 suggest that almost half of global mortality can be attributed to these risk exposures, and just over one-third of the disease and injury burden. In addition, just five risk factors—unsafe sexual practices, alcohol use, indoor air pollution, occupational exposures, and tobacco use—account for around 20% of the world's disease burden.

Issues and controversies

The burden of disease methodology and the DALY remain controversial in the international and national health policy arena and in the epidemiological research community. Critics of the GBD approach fall into two main groups. First, are a group of critics concerned with the extrapolation of population health estimates where data are limited, uncertain, or missing. Second, are a group of critics concerned about a number of issues in the way that the DALY summarizes fatal and non-fatal health outcomes. These two groups of issues are largely separate. The first relates to any attempts to synthesize partial and fragmentary data to provide a comprehensive picture of the burden of disease that does not leave blanks in the tables for some causes or populations (which will be interpreted as 'no problem'). The second relates more to social value choices and concepts of health and the degree to which these can be applied universally.

The GBD analyses have been criticized for making estimates of mortality and burden of disease for regions with limited, incomplete, and uncertain data, and have even been characterized by some critics as having at best only tenuous links to empirical evidence. Murray and colleagues have argued that health planning based on uncertain assessments of the available evidence, that attempt to synthesize it while ensuring consistency and adjustment to known biases, will almost always be more informed than planning based on ideology, and that there will be practically no cases where we are totally ignorant about an issue to the point where there is no alternative to ideology (Murray *et al.* 2003).

Some epidemiologists would argue that there is a fundamental difference between an estimate based on a review of all the available evidence plus the application of plausible methods and 'proper' measurements required for research studies. There is a tendency in descriptive epidemiology to refuse to make estimates where data are sparse, uncertain, or based on studies that do not reach certain methodological standards. In contrast, disciplines such as demography and economics more often aim to make the best possible estimates from the available data, using a range of techniques depending on the type and quality of evidence. It is also important to note that the quantities of interest in the GBD analyses are unbiased population-level estimates of the complete incidence, prevalence, and mortality for clearly defined causes of disease and injury, and the derived summary measures.

For example, the WHO and many national statistical agencies routinely make available data on the statistic 'Deaths detected by the civil registration system'. However, policy-makers are interested in different statistics, namely the age- and sex-specific mortality risk due to a specified disease, and a related quantity, the realized numbers of deaths occurring due to that risk. As many civil registration systems detect only a fraction of total deaths, and even in systems with complete registration there may be biases and limitations in the identification and coding of cause of death, the quantity 'Deaths in the population due cause x' is distinctly different from 'Deaths detected by the civil registration system and coded to cause x'.

In general, the death notification data sets provide input to the production of the best unbiased estimates of population-level mortality risks and numbers of deaths. Thus, there is not a conflict between the use of 'data' and 'estimates', rather that the two quantities of interest are different. Decision-makers, and even many technical groups, do not have the skills, relevant background knowledge, or resources to themselves convert the input data sets to information on the quantities of interest at the population level. On the other hand, the GBD approach to the estimation of population-level quantities of interest requires the use of judgement on the quality and completeness of data sets, and the adjustment of estimates to take into account the identified biases. Such procedures are sometimes beyond the comfort zones of national and international analysts, particularly in regions of the world without a strong culture of challenging official information and confronting different data sources.

The revisions of the GBD for the years 2000–2002 drew on a wider set of information on population health and mortality than the original GBD study. In excess of 770 country-years of death registration data from over 100 countries in all regions of the world were used together with over 3000 additional sources of information on levels of child and adult mortality and on specific causes of death to estimate global and regional patterns of mortality. Together with the more than 8700 data sources used for the estimation of YLD, the GBD 2001 has incorporated information from over 10,000 data sets relating to population health and mortality. This represents the largest synthesis of global information on population health carried out to date. To address criticisms about lack of transparency in some areas of the GBD analyses, substantial effort was also put into documenting cause-specific analyses and the overall analytical approach (Mathers *et al.* 2006a).

Despite the criticisms that the GBD study is inadequately empirically based, particularly in Africa, it is notable that fully one-third of the more than 10,000 data sources used by the GBD 2001 relate to sub-Saharan African populations, albeit with serious limitations in the information available on mortality. The fact that estimates are possible does not obviate the need to put higher priority on addressing the serious lack of information on levels of adult mortality and causes of death in some regions of the world, particularly Africa.

DALYs have received a great deal of criticism from disability advocates. Some of this criticism relates to ethical issues, such as the claim that DALYs devalue the life of disabled people or that cost-effectiveness analysis imposes an implicit utilitarianism on assessing social preferences. A more fundamental criticism is that the conceptualization of disability found in DALYs confounds the ideas of 'health' and 'disability'. Many disability advocates in high-income countries, justifiably concerned about stigma and social and environmental barriers to full participation in society by people with disabilities, have taken a position that the causes of disability lie in the interaction of the person and the environment, and that people with disabilities are no less healthy than anyone else. In response to these critics, the conceptual basis for the measurement of health and the valuation of health states has been further developed and clarified (Salomon *et al.* 2003).

It is probably unfortunate that the term 'disability' was used in the original GBD study since there is so little consensus on the meaning of this term. As used by the GBD and in the DALY it is essentially a synonym for health states of less than full health. The DALY is actually attempting to quantify loss of health, and the disability weights should thus reflect social preferences for health states. Thus disability weights reflect the general population preference for health states, or judgements about the 'healthfulness' of defined states, not any judgements about quality of life or a person's worth.

To be more precise, the disability weights are intended to quantify the functional status of individuals in terms of capacities (as defined in the WHO International Classification of Functioning) in a set of core domains of health such as mobility, affect, pain, cognition, etc. Where some disability advocates argue that a person with one leg is as healthy as a person with two legs, and the only problem is possibly the lack of good prostheses and a facilitating environment, I would argue that all societies do want their health systems to prevent impairments such as loss of legs in populations and do perceive the loss of a leg as a loss of functioning and health. There is thus a need for a health measure that quantifies those aspects of health that people value and are collectively willing to put social priority on preventing or treating the loss of.

Conclusions

I remain convinced of the importance of generating unbiased and cross-population comparable evidence on levels of population health and causes of the loss of health. Cross-population comparability creates possibilities for investigating broad determinants of population health at national and cross-national level. The generation of unbiased evidence on population health requires a comprehensive framework that addresses all causes, not just those that happen to be priorities for some institutions or sectional interests, that includes all ages, and that includes non-fatal health outcomes, not just mortality. In both international and national health policy arenas, with many actors and sectional interests, such evidence is valued by some and but threatening to others.

Global health policy and priority setting in health will be much better served if international health agencies such as the WHO and partners establish and implement a concerted effort to improve data collection and synthesis, and hence our knowledge, about the true extent of the disease burden worldwide. Even efforts that substantially reduce uncertainty will be a major advance towards this goal. With increasing pressure on resources for health in all countries, priority setting in the health sector will depend more and more on comprehensive, comparative information about the impact of diseases, injuries, and risk factors on population health.

In the last 2 years, the WHO has shifted its focus from the production of evidence to support health policy to technical support and capacity building at country level. Recently, the Gates Foundation has funded a $50 million initiative, the Health Metrics Network, currently hosted by the WHO, to address gaps in country health information and to build capacity in health information systems at national and local levels. The Health Metrics Network is funding health information system capacity-building projects in low-income countries, as well as providing technical advice and support.

Murray and colleagues have recently argued for an independent agency outside the WHO to take on the role of the production of unbiased and objective information on population health (Murray *et al.* 2004). They argued that the WHO has an inherent conflict of interest in relation to the production of unbiased and objective information on population health, since often the very WHO departments undertaking such syntheses are also the departments whose performance in implementing global health policy and interventions is being judged on the basis of such information. Additionally, they argued, as a political organization whose policies are determined to a large extent by member states, the WHO is under continual pressure to accept and rely on data supplied by member states, data that are often biased and inaccurate.

In 2005, Larry Ellison, head of the Oracle corporation, agreed to provide $115 million initial funding for the establishment of an independent organization headed by Chris Murray, the Ellison Institute, for the generation of credible, comparable, and comprehensive information on population health and its determinants, on health resources and interventions, and on the effectiveness of health systems. Ellison later changed his mind, and Murray is currently seeking other sources of funding for a new round of global burden of disease work. Murray and several colleagues have also won the Gates Grand Challenge 13 to develop new and improved methods for the measurement and monitoring of population health.

There remain a large number of remaining methodological and empirical challenges for better global and national estimates of disease burden. Academic research groups could be valuable partners for existing global health agencies such as the WHO, UNICEF and the World Bank, in improving the measurement and policy use of information on population health, and on priorities for funding interventions to improve health. It remains to be seen whether genuine collaborative efforts will occur, and whether the differing interests of the parties can be transcended in the interests of global health improvement.

Acknowledgements

I wish to acknowledge the many WHO staff and external collaborators who have contributed to the global burden of disease revisions for 2000–2002 and to the work on summary measures of population health. The author alone is responsible for the views expressed in this publication, which do not necessarily reflect the opinion of the World Health Organization or of its member states.

References

Anand S and Hanson K (1997). Disability-adjusted life years: a critical review. *Journal of Health Economics*, **16**, 685–702.

Arnesen T and Nord E (1999). The value of DALY life: problems with ethics and validity of disability adjusted life years. *British Medical Journal*, **319**, 1423–5.

Cooper RS, Osotimehin B, Kaufman JS, and Forrester T (1998). Disease burden in sub-Saharan Africa: what should we conclude in the absence of data?. *Lancet*, **351**, 208–10.

Ezzati M, Lopez A, Rodgers A, and Murray CJL (2003). Comparative quantification of health risks: global and regional burden of disease attributable to several major risk factors. WHO, Geneva.

Fries J (1980). Aging, natural death, and the compression of morbidity. *New England Journal of Medicine*, **303**, 130–5.

Jamison DTJ, Breman G, Measham AR, *et al.* (2006a). *Disease control priorities in developing countries*, 2nd edn. Oxford University Press, Oxford.

Jamison DTJ, Breman G, Measham AR, *et al.* (2006b). *Disease control priorities in developing countries*, 2nd edn. Oxford University Press, New York.

King G, Murray CJL, Salomon JA, and Tandon A (2003). Enhancing the validity and cross-cultural comparability of measurement in survey research. *American Political Science Review*, **93**, 567–83.

Lopez AD, Mathers CD, Ezzati M, Murray CJL, and Jamison DT (2006). *Global burden of disease and risk factors, Disease Control Priorities Project*. Oxford University Press, Oxford.

Lozano R, Murray CJL, Frenk J, and Bobadilla J (1995). Burden of disease assessment and health system reform: results of a study in Mexico. *Journal for International Development*, **7**, 555–64.

Mathers CD (2002). Health expectancies: an overview and critical appraisal. In *Summary measures of population health: concepts, ethics, measurement and applications* (ed. CJL Murray, JA Salomon, CD Mathers, and AD Lopez). WHO, Geneva. pp. 171–204.

Mathers CD, Vos T, and Stevenson C (1999). *The burden of disease and injury in Australia*. Australian Institute of Health and Welfare, Canberra.

Mathers CD, Lopez AD, and Murray CJL (2006a). The burden of disease and mortality by condition: data, methods and results for 2001. In *Global burden of disease and risk factors* (ed. AD Lopez, CD Mathers, M Ezzati, CJL Murray, and DT Jamison). Oxford University Press, Oxford, pp. 45–240.

Mathers CD, Salomon JA, Ezzati M, Begg S, and Lopez AD (2006b). Sensitivity and uncertainty analyses for burden of disease and risk factor estimates. In *Global burden of disease and risk factors* (ed. AD Lopez, CD Mathers, M Ezzati, CJL Murray, and DT Jamison). Oxford University Press, Oxford, pp. 399–426.

May RM and Anderson RM (1991). *Infectious diseases of humans.* Oxford University Press, Oxford.

Mooney G, Irwig L, and Leeder S (1997). Priority setting in healthcare unburdening from the burden of disease. *Australian and New Zealand Journal of Public Health,* **21,** 680–1.

Murray CJL (1996). Rethinking DALYs. In *The global burden of disease* (ed. CJL Murray and AD Lopez), Global Burden of Disease and Injury Series, Vol. 1. Harvard School of Public Health, Cambridge, MA, pp. 1–98.

Murray CJL and Acharya AK (1997). Understanding DALYs. *Journal of Health Economics,* **16,** 703–30.

Murray CJL and Evans DA (2003). *Health systems performance assessment: debates, methods and empiricism.* WHO, Geneva.

Murray CJL and Lopez AD (ed.) (1996a). *Global health statistics: a compendium of incidence, prevalence and mortality estimates for over 200 conditions,* Global Burden of Disease and Injury Series, Vol. 2. Harvard School of Public Health, Cambridge, MA.

Murray CJL and Lopez AD (ed.) (1996b). *The global burden of disease: a comprehensive assessment of mortality and disability from diseases, injuries and risk factors in 1990 and projected to 2020,* Global Burden of Disease and Injury Series, Vol. 1. Harvard School of Public Health, Cambridge, MA, pp. 715–26.

Murray CJL and Lopez AD (1999). On the comparable quantification of health risks: lessons from the global burden of disease study. *Epidemiology,* **10,** 594–605.

Murray CJL and Lopez AD (2000). Progress and directions in refining the global burden of disease approach: a response to Williams. *Health Economics,* **9,** 69–82.

Murray CJL, Mathers CD, and Salomon JA (2003). Towards evidence-based public health. In *Health systems performance assessment: debates, methods and empiricism* (ed. CJL Murray and D Evans). WHO, Geneva,

Murray CJ, Lopez AD, and Wibulpolprasert S (2004). Monitoring global health: time for new solutions. *British Medical Journal,* **329,** 1096–100.

Public Health Division (1999). *Victorian burden of disease study: morbidity.* Victorian Government Department of Human Services, Melbourne.

Robine JM, Jagger C, Mathers CD, Crimmins EM, and Suzman RM (2003). *Determining health expectancies.* John Wiley & Sons, Chichester.

Salomon JA and Murray CJL (2004). A multi-method approach to estimating health state valuations. *Health Economics,* **13,** 281–90.

Salomon J, Mathers CD, Chatterji S, Sadana R, Ustun TB, and Murray CJL (2003). Quantifying individual levels of health: definitions, concepts and measurement issues. In *Health systems performance assessment: debate, methods and empiricism* (ed. CJL Murray and D Evans). WHO, Geneva, pp. 301–18.

Sanders BS (1964). Measuring community health levels. *American Journal of Public Health,* **54,** 1063–70.

Stouthard M, Essink-Bot M, Bonsel G, Barendregt J, and Kramers P (1997). *Disability weights for diseases in the Netherlands.* Department of Public Health, Erasmus University, Rotterdam.

Sullivan DF (1966). *Conceptual problems in developing an index of health.* National Center for Health Statistics, Rockville, MD (available at: http://www.cdc.gov/nchs/data/series/sr_02/sr02_017.pdf).

Vos T, Tobias M, Gareeboo H, Roussety F, Huttley S, and Murray CJL (1995). *Mauritius health sector reform. National Burden of Disease Study, final report of consultancy.* Ministry of Health and Ministry of Economic Planning and Development, Mauritius.

Williams A (1999). Calculating the global burden of disease: time for a strategic reappraisal. *Health Economics,* **8,** 1–8.

World Bank (1993). *World Development Report 1993. Investing in health.* Oxford University Press, New York.

World Health Organization (2000). *The World Health Report 2000. Health systems: improving performance.* WHO, Geneva.

Section 2

Specific disease areas of concern

6

Development of the epidemiology of cancer

Richard Doll

Editors' note

This chapter was commissioned from Richard Doll, a founder member of the IEA, and the world's leading cancer epidemiologist. Richard agreed to write the chapter—but stated that this would be his last piece of work. Unfortunately he became ill soon after. Nonetheless he completed this chapter, while in hospital, just before his death in July 2005. It provides a fascinating account of the contributions and advances of knowledge in the past 50 or more years. It has been edited with a very light touch in order to emphasize his style and contributions.

Personal experiences

When I qualified in medicine in 1937 I had it in mind to be a neurosurgeon, but war intervened. When I came out of the army it was too late start on such prolonged training and I aimed at being a general physician. There was, however, no national health service and it meant ingratiating yourself with senior physicians at some general teaching or specialist hospital—a process that didn't attract me. I had always been interested in the use of numerical methods in medicine and had written what must have been one of the earliest articles on the use of the χ^2 test in the St Thomas' Hospital Gazette while still a student. I leapt at the opportunity suggested by a friend at MRC headquarters to act as a research assistant to Dr (subsequently Sir) Avery Jones, a leading gastroenterologist at the Central Middlesex Hospital. Avery wanted to carry out a study of the different prevalences of peptic ulcers in men and women with different work patterns, involving regular or irregular meals. In the course of the work I took the short course in medical statistics at the London School of Hygiene under Professor (also subsequently Sir) Austin Bradford Hill. He, it appears, was impressed with my work with Avery Jones, in that I had succeeded in getting interviews with 98% of the workers we wished to study, and he offered me the job in his unit to carry out a study to discover the reason for the dramatic increase in the mortality attributable to cancer of the lung, something the MRC had asked him to investigate. There was no looking back, I had found my niche in life and quickly became a committed epidemiologist, to my lasting satisfaction.

Epidemiology has contributed more than any other branch of science to our knowledge of the causes of cancer. Mortality rates and a few isolated epidemiological studies were reported before the Second World War; but it was only after the war ended that such studies began to transform our knowledge of how different types of cancer were caused and how they could be prevented. I consider below the development of the subject in relation to cancer under three headings: descriptive epidemiology, case–control studies, and cohort studies.

Descriptive epidemiology

The first reports linking specific cancers to specific occupations are more properly ascribed to clinical acumen than to epidemiology, as they were qualitative in nature and made no quantitative comparison: notably Ramazzini's (1743) account of the frequency of cancer of the breast in nuns, Pott's (1775) of the association between cancer of the scrotum and employment as a chimneysweep when a boy, and Sommering's (1795) of the association between pipe smoking and cancer of the lip. Similar reports subsequently linked many skin cancers to occupational exposure to coal tar and some cancers of the tongue and mouth, as well as cancer of the lip, to the smoking of pipes.

Credit for the first formal use of epidemiological methods should probably go to Rigoni Stern (1842) in Padua, when he provided estimates of the mortality from cancer among women in Verona, and concluded from the separate study of married and unmarried women that breast and uterine cancers were complementary to one another. The latter was particularly uncommon among nuns, in whom the ratio of breast to uterine cancers was 9:1 while it was 0.5:1 for women who were married.

Subsequent studies were for long limited to accounts of clinical and pathological series of causes expressed as a proportion of all cancers or, for example, of all hospital admissions or all autopsies. The findings were often difficult to assess, depending, as they necessarily did, on the frequency of conditions other than the cancer under special study. They have, however, sometimes been the only type of epidemiological information obtainable in areas where the provision of medical services is scarce and they have, at times, provided valuable information about the type of cancer occurring in underdeveloped countries, as, for example, Cook and Burkett's (1971) data for variation of the frequency of some 30 types of cancers admitted to hospitals throughout sub-Saharan Africa. These draw attention to some remarkable variations which inspired regional differences in aetiological factors.

Mortality data

Meanwhile a major advance was made when, in 1900, representatives of a group of countries considered the recommendation by the International Statistical Institute to adopt a classification of the causes of death, which had been drawn up by Jacques Bertillon, head of statistics in the city of Paris (Moriyama 1993). Different lists had been used previously in different countries. In England one had been adopted by William Farr for use in the First Annual Report of the Registrar General of Births and Marriages in 1837, which was useful enough to permit comparison of the mortality from asthma in young people for over a century (Speizer and Doll 1968); but it ceased to be adequate with the passage of time and did not compete with Bertillon's. The latter had been extended to include 161 conditions and could be abbreviated to include only 99 or 44. In the event, the 1900 conference, which had been convoked by the French government, modified Bertillon's list and accepted a classification in 179 groups, which could be abbreviated to only 35. The lists, it was agreed, should come into use on 1 January 1901 and revisions should be undertaken approximately every 10 years under the auspice of the French government. This arrangement continued until 1948, when responsibility for the sixth and subsequent revisions was accepted by the World Health Organization, which had taken over responsibility for global health from the health section of the League of Nations.

With causes of death recorded in a standard way and agreement reached at the initial conference on how to deal with deaths where several causes were mentioned on the death certificate, comparisons could be made of the rates observed in different countries, standardized for sex and age, and, with the passage of time, of rates observed at different periods. It was these last data that brought to the fore the enormous increase in the occurrence of cancer of the lung in the first half of the twentieth century that led eventually to the analytical studies that enabled the disease to be related to the smoking of cigarettes.

Comparisons between different communities have been less dramatically productive, but they quickly showed that the mortality from all types of cancer that were at all common anywhere varied much more than could be attributed to differences in the efficacy of treatment or in genetic constitution, and they have given rise to many testable hypotheses about cancer causation. In 1965, for example, it was found that among 38 communities the mortality from cancer of the oesophagus in men varied 12 times, cancer of the stomach nine times, and cancer of the colon five times (Doll 1965). Much greater differences have, of course, been observed in special studies, including, most notably, a remarkable study of rural China (Chen *et al.* 1990). Conditions throughout China are very heterogeneous and Chen and colleagues sought to utilize this by comparing the mortality from seven different types of cancer in 65 counties selected so as to maximize the differences observed in the nationwide study of mortality in 1973–75. Twenty-five households were chosen within each of four communities in two villages in each county, and blood and urine samples were obtained from adults together with personal dietary and other lifestyle histories. Altogether 285 biochemical and other characteristics were defined for each county and made available for correlation with the mortality from each of the seven types of cancer. The study was repeated 10 years later (Chen *et al.* 2005) so that it should now be possible to decide which features are consistently most characteristic of each county and so provide more informative data for correlation with each of the seven cancers.

Incidence data

Mortality, however, is of little epidemiological value when fatality rates are low and can be misleading when the efficacy of treatment varies and it is of limited value in just those circumstances where comparisons are of particular interest, namely those of risks in the developed and underdeveloped worlds. For such purposes there is no substitute for incidence.

Practical steps to record incidence on a routine basis began in Connecticut in the United States, at the instigation of a group of physicians in New Haven who persuaded the state government to establish a registry that recorded the occurrence of all cases of cancer in the state (Eisenberg 1966; Griswold *et al.* 1953). Retrospective examination of hospital records enabled figures to be provided by sex and age annually from 1935 on. Eight years later, in 1943 during the Second World War, the first registry to record the incidence of cancer in a whole country was established in Denmark (Clemmesen 1955) which served a population about 70 times greater than that of Connecticut. Three years later another was started in Miyagi prefecture Japan (Segi 1966). Several others followed, including a few special registries set up temporarily for research purposes in places where routine registration would have been impractical and, in 1964, the geographical pathology committee of the International Union against Cancer recommended that data from all the known registries, both national and local, that had recorded their data in an adequate way should be brought together and set out in a form that facilitated comparisons. A book containing these data was published with the title of *Cancer incidence in five continents* under the auspices of the International Union against Cancer (1966). Responsibility for bringing together the data was subsequently taken over by the International Agency for Research on Cancer which has published a series of volumes every few years under the same title. The 2002 volume was published in conjunction with the International Association of Cancer Registries and records data for up to 50 types of cancer in 215 populations in 55 countries (International Agency for Research on Cancer, International Association of Cancer Registries 2002). Taken altogether the contents of this volume provide a mine of information for correlation studies over time and between many varied cultures with different dietary, behavioural, and environmental characteristics.

Case–control studies

The earliest example I have found of a case–control study that is up to modern standards was by Lane-Claypon (1926). She studied 508 women with breast cancer and 508 without the disease admitted to nine hospitals in London and Glasgow. Women were asked about their marital status, their childbearing and breastfeeding practices, their family history of cancer, menstrual patterns, and disorders of the breast, including trauma. The women with breast cancer had been married for a shorter period and were less likely to have had children than the comparison group—and Major Greenwood assisted with the analyses, developing 'a multiple regression equation, for establishing the number of children in terms of age at marriage and duration of marriage'. They concluded that the low parity of women with breast cancer could not be accounted for by their later age at marriage. Another early example was the study by Stocks and Karn (1933) of the characteristics of people with or without cancer. The study which embraced 462 patients with cancer and 435 men and women of approximately the same ages without the disease, recorded answers to questions about the individuals' home-life, habits, temperament, diet, and medical history and is memorable, in retrospect, for the findings that the cancer patients, in general, ate less wholemeal bread and fewer vegetables than the controls. The two groups were, however, recruited to the study in such varied ways that it is impossible to assess how representative they were of the population that the authors wished to study or what biases might have influenced them.

Similar criticisms apply to a lesser extent to two studies of lung cancer that were reported in Germany shortly before or during the war (Müller 1939; Schairer and Schöniger 1943) and to another carried out in The Netherlands a few years later (Wassink 1948). The technique, however, was rapidly coming into general use and five such studies of lung cancer were reported in 1950, four in the USA and one in the UK. All recorded a higher proportion of smokers in the cancer patients than in the controls and in one the authors felt able to conclude from the results (I quote) 'that cigarette smoking is an important cause of cancer of the lung' (Doll and Hill 1950). Patients had been notified to the investigators by the hospitals to which the patients had been admitted 'on suspicion of having lung cancer', as requested formally by the Secretary of the Medical Research Council, along with other patients suspected of having cancers of the stomach or large bowel. Controls, in contrast, were selected by specially trained interviewers from other patients with other diseases (other than cancers of the upper respiratory and digestive tracts) who were in the same ward, in the same hospital, or (in a few instances when the patients were admitted to specialized hospitals) in other specialized hospitals serving the same area. To reach their conclusion the authors showed, first, the extreme unlikelihood that the results could be due to chance ($P < 10^{-7}$) they then tested for bias, eliminating respectively selection bias and recall bias by comparing the findings in the selected controls with those in the patients independently notified as having gastric or large bowel cancer and by comparing the findings in the patients notified with a suspected diagnosis of lung cancer, who subsequently proved, after interview, to have or not to have the disease. Confounding was more difficult to exclude, but it could be excluded by twin studies for the rather unappealing suggestion made by Fisher (1958) that some genetic factor caused people both to smoke and to have susceptibility to the disease. Lastly the authors sought positive evidence in favour of causality as an explanation for the observed association from the internal and external evidence, as subsequently summarized by Hill (1965) as 'guidelines' to causality.

These papers, published in 1950, marked a turning point in the epidemiological study of cancer, and indeed of many other non-infectious diseases. With minor modifications the method of investigation and the method of interpreting the findings became the standard initial approach for investigating the causes of different types of cancer throughout the world.

Cohort studies

Equally important, if not more so, than case–control studies are the cohort studies that are now used routinely to measure occupational hazards and to confirm relationships revealed or suggested by other methods. The history of the methods has been described elsewhere by Doll (2001a,b), unfortunately omitting reference to Lane-Claypon's (1916) splendid but neglected study of the growth of infants fed different types of milk, which was probably the first example of the use of the method. Shortly after it was applied to demonstrate an occupational hazard of cancer of the nasal sinuses and lungs in nickel refiners by Bradford Hill; he did not publish his account in detail, as the work was privately commissioned by the relevant industry. Subsequently, however, he described the findings in his book on statistical methods to illustrate the fact that you might not need repetition in other studies to draw a conclusion about causality if the hazard was large enough and the internal relationship was specific for a particular subgroup of the population (in his case a thousand-fold increase in the risk of nasal cancer in the specific group of process workers).

The first detailed account of the application of the method was given in a report of a study of men employed in the manufacture of coal-gas which demonstrated an approximate doubling of the risk of lung cancer in men who had been specifically employed in the retort houses where the exposure to the products of heated coal would have been highest. The study was undertaken because gas-workers were known to be specially liable to develop cancer of the skin and bladder (Henry *et al.* 1931) and Kennaway and Kennaway (1947) had noted that, in an analysis of male deaths attributed to cancer of the lung in England and Wales during the period 1921–38, seven out of the 56 occupations studied were different groups of gas-workers and that in each case the number observed was greater that the number expected from the experience of the whole, although the number of exposed men could be estimated only approximately. The study is also of some interest as reflecting the different attitudes of a private and nationalized industry. The medical officer of the gas company concerned (Dr R. E. W. Fisher) (see Doll *et al.* 1965) had been encourage to assist in the study but, before the report was published, the industry had been nationalized and Dr Fisher was not allowed to put his name to it.

Very many similar studies have been carried out since then, some on an immense scale. In the majority the greatest problem has been to quantify the extent to which individual workers were exposed to the suspected carcinogens and hence to provide a dose–response relationship that would permit estimates to be made of the effect of exposure to small amounts of the carcinogen in other situations. Examples include exposure to white (chrysotile) asbestos (Peto *et al.* 1985) and above all the massive study of the risk of a wide range of cancers from exposure to the explosion of the atomic bombs at Hiroshima and Nagasaki undertaken jointly by the American and Japanese at the Radiation Effects Research Institute.

The origin of this study is of particular interest, for when concern was raised about the long-term impact of the Hiroshima and Nagasaki explosions the Atomic Board Casualty Commission organized regular clinical examination of a relatively small selected group. Conclusive evidence that ionizing radiation increased the risk of leukaemia, cataracts, and mental retardation in children most heavily exposed *in utero* was rapidly obtained by a variety of methods, but by 1954 the plan for repeated clinical examination was foundering in the face of negative findings and declining participation and a cohort study was initiated to determine specific mortality rates in a group of some 100,000 people (subsequently increased to about 120,000) selected from nearly three times that number known to have been resident in the two towns at the time of the national census on October 1950 and whose history of exposure was known. This became the basis for the Life Span Study which is still continuing and—in conjunction with the evidence from the local cancer registry—has provided the principal evidence on which our current knowledge of the long-term effects of ionizing radiation is based. At first designed specifically to quantify the risk of cancer, it has now begun to show that moderate doses may also have some relatively minor effect on the risks of vascular and possibly some other diseases as well. For many years now the results of this study have provided data for the estimate of risks from different levels of exposure to ionizing radiation that are used routinely for the protection of radiation workers, patients exposed for medical purposes, and the public (see Chapter 31).

References

Chen J, Campbell TC, Li J, and Peto R (1990). *Diet, life-style, and mortality in China: a study of the characteristics of 65 Chinese counties.* Oxford University Press, Oxford.

Chen J, Liv B, Wenham P, *et al.* (2005). *Geographic study of mortality, biochemistry, diet and lifestyle in rural China* (text updated 26 January 2006). Website of Clinical Trials Service Unit, Oxford. Results and Reports. Chinese Ecology Study. www.ctsu.ox.ac.uk.

Clemmesen J (1955). The Danish Cancer Registry, under the National Anti-Cancer League. *Danish Medical Bulletin*, 2, 124.

Cook PJ and Burkett DP (1971). Cancer in Africa. *British Medical Bulletin*, 27, 14–20.

Doll R (1965). *Worldwide distribution of gastrointestinal cancer*, National Cancer Institute Monograph No 25. National Cancer Institute, Bethesda, MD.

Doll R (2001a). Cohort studies: history of the method—I. Prospective cohort studies. *Soziale Präventivmedizin*, 46, 75–86.

Doll R (2001b). Cohort studies: history of the method—II. Retrospective cohort studies. *Soziale Präventivmedizin*, 46, 152–60.

Doll R and Hill AB (1950). Smoking and carcinoma of the lung. Preliminary Report. *British Medical Journal*, 228, 1451–5.

Doll R, Fisher REW, Gammon EJ, *et al.* (1965). Mortality of gas workers with special reference to cancers of the lung and bladder, chronic bronchitis and pneumoconiosis. *British Journal of Industrial Medicine*, 22, 1–12.

Eisenberg H (1966). USA, Connecticut. In *Cancer incidence in five continents* (ed. R Doll, P Payne, and J Waterhouse) pp. 97–100. Springer-Verlag, Berlin.

Fisher RA (1958). Cigarettes, cancer and statistics. *Centennial Review*, 2, 151–66.

Griswold MH, Wilder CS, Cutler SJ, and Pollack ES (1953). *Cancer in Connecticut, 1935–1950.* Connecticut State Department of Health, Hartford, CT.

Henry SA, Kennaway NM, and Kennaway EL (1931). The incidence of cancer in the bladder and prostate in certain occupations. *Journal of Hygiene*, 31, 125–37.

Hill AB (1965). The environment and disease: association and causation. *Proceedings of the Royal Society of Medicine*, 58, 295–300.

International Agency for Research on Cancer, International Association for Cancer Registries (2002). *Cancer incidence in five continents*, Vol. 8 (ed. DM Parkin, SL Whelan, F Ferlay, L Teppo, and DB Thomas). International Agency for Research on Cancer, Lyon.

International Union Against Cancer (1966). *Cancer incidence in five continents*, UICC Technical Report (ed. R Doll, P Payne, and J Waterhouse). Springer-Verlag, Berlin.

Kennaway NM and Kennaway EL (1947). A further study of the incidence of the lung and larynx. *British Journal of Cancer*, 1, 260–98.

Lane-Claypon JE (1916). *Milk and its hygienic relations.* Longmans, Green & Co., New York.

Lane-Claypon JE (1926). *Reports on public health and medical subjects*, No 32. The Stationery Office, London.

Moriyama IM (1993). *Historical Development of Cause of Death Statistics.* International Institute for Vital Registration and Statistics, Bethseda.

Müller FH (1939). Tabakmissbrauch und Lungencarcinom. *Krebsforschung,* **49**, 52–85.

Peto J, Doll R, Hermon C, Binns W, Clayton R, and Goffe T (1985). Relationship of mortality to measures of environmental asbestos pollution in an asbestos textile factory. *The Annals of Occupational Hygiene,* **29**, 305–55.

Pott P (1775). *Chirurgical observations relative to the cataract, polypus of the nose, the cancer of the scrotum, the different kinds of ruptures and the mortification of the toes and feet.* Hawes, Clarke & Collins, London.

Ramazzini B (1743). *De morbis artificum. Diatriba.* J Corona, Venice.

Schairer E and Schöniger E (1943). Lungenkrebs und Tabakverbrauch. *Krebsforschung,* **54**, 261–9.

Segi M (1966) Japan, Miyagi. In *Cancer incidence in five continents* (ed. R Doll, P Payne, and J Waterhouse), pp. 10–119. Springer-Verlag, Berlin.

Sommering (1795). *De morbis vasorum absorbentium corporis humani.* Varrentsapp and Wenner, Frankfurt am Main.

Speizer F and Doll R (1968). A century of asthma deaths in young people. *British Medical Journal,* **3**, 245–6.

Rigoni Stern D (1842). Fatti statistici relativi alle malattie cancerose. *Gioru Prog Patol Terep,* **2**, 507–17.

Stocks P and Karn M (1933). A co-operative study of the habits, home life, dietary and family histories of 450 cancer patients and of an equal number of control patients. *Annals of Eugenics,* **5**, 237.

Wassink WS (1948). Ontstaans voorwanden voor longkranken. *Nederlands Tijdschrift voor Geneeskunde,* **92**, 3732–47.

7

Cardiovascular disease epidemiology

Henry Blackburn

Personal experiences

I arrived at cardiovascular disease (CVD) epidemiology from an early interest in electrocardiography as a medical student under George Burch at Tulane in the late 1940s. Later, I did a Masters thesis at Minnesota with Ernst Simonson and Otto Schmitt on the 'spatially corrected' QRS interval. It was pedestrian research but good training in careful measurement, repeat variability, defining the 'normal', simple statistical analysis, and practical aspects of survey methods.

This thesis work, carried out in the intensely searching atmosphere of physiologist Ancel Keys' Laboratory of Physiological Hygiene, came at a romantic time in the early history of CVD epidemiology, when Keys had become a 'medical Marco Polo'. From travels about the world with Paul Dudley White, the international 'dean of cardiology', he would return to Minnesota with bountiful news and hypotheses about cultural differences in the frequency of heart attacks. The Holy Grail lay, he suspected, in the diet and 'mode of life' of populations living varieties of traditional lifestyles.

Several things in Keys' vision rang true from my experience. In the summer of 1949 in eastern Cuba I had discovered the severe limitations of medicine to cope with mass diseases due mainly to poverty and ignorance. These were matters for public health and the political economy, quite beyond the meagre efforts of medical missionaries.

That first view of the sociocultural origins of common diseases was confirmed while I was serving as public health officer for the US Displaced Persons Program in the camps of Austria and Germany from 1950 to 1953. From these exposures I was primed, when the opportunity arose, for a career in public health and for a 'population view' of epidemic cardiovascular diseases.

Ancel Keys' 1956 invitation to become a research associate in 'The Lab' and project officer for the cross-cultural Seven Countries Study of cardiovascular diseases, offered an international career exploring a major phenomenon of public health and involving my early interests and experience. It was too attractive to refuse, despite its paltry stipend.

Keys' direct challenge to me—to render the clinical components of cardiac diagnosis sufficiently unambiguous, quantitative, valid, and reliable for comparative field surveys of CVD—I found feasible and even 'right down my alley'. It led to early signature publications: 'The electrocardiogram in population studies' (the Minnesota Code), and, with Geoffrey Rose, the WHO manual, *Cardiovascular survey methods*.

The same day as Keys' invitation, I received the offer of a junior faculty position in the medical school. I soon learned from its annoyed chief of medicine that my signing on with Ancel Keys and 'those weird people doing those crazy things under Gate 27 of the football stadium', would almost certainly exclude me from the academic elite of internal medicine!

So be it. Interesting and important things, including the birth of cardiovascular disease epidemiology, were under way at Minnesota and abroad.

Introduction

Recognition of epidemic heart attack in the mid-twentieth century, with attempts by pioneers to explain and reduce its burden, provides lessons and drama unparalleled in chronic disease epidemiology. At that historic moment, several streams of knowledge and circumstance converged to provoke formal epidemiological study:

- Cardiovascular experts were making advances in cardiac diagnosis and in the understanding of atherosclerosis and hypertension, two processes fundamental to the cardiovascular disease (CVD) epidemic.

- Observers of trends in CVD deaths before, during, and just after the Second World War proposed arguments that these trends were real and that the abrupt decline in CVD deaths in Europe was due to wartime changes in nutrition.

- Others, returning from travels, brought back tales about large differences in the frequency of heart attack, along with hypotheses about the cultural origins of those differences.

A few pioneers in the trenches, mainly experts in cardiovascular fields and most without epidemiological training, integrated evidence from these several sources. They posed critical questions about the possible causes of CVD and undertook studies in populations, creating a new field in what would become the broader epidemiology of non-communicable diseases.

The creation was no 'Big Bang', but it did occur abruptly—around 1948—and the universe expanded rapidly. Independent beginnings in several centres internationally coincided with a deliberate effort by the US Public Health Service in which the Framingham Heart Study was initiated (Dawber 1980; Oppenheimer 2005). This designated 'moment of creation', 1948, saw the start of formal prospective epidemiological research into possible causes of CVD among healthy cohorts, beginning in Minnesota and in Framingham.

That early period also saw the founding of bodies critically supportive of this 'new' kind of research: the World Health Organization (WHO), the US National Heart Institute (NHI), and the American Heart Association (AHA), which had just reorganized into a public agency. Coincident with these activities were new directions in research and training at the London School of Hygiene and Tropical Medicine and soon thereafter in numerous centres worldwide (Morris 1957).

Origins: pre-1948

A small coterie of CVD experts recognized heart attack as epidemic among several industrialized countries in the years just before and after the Second World War, predominantly among men from upper economic classes and in their prime years. Heart attack was even popularly called 'executive disease'. A few leaders turned their curiosity about the causes of the epidemic to the community and culture from which the many cases derived.

The state of medical ignorance and cautious attitudes about the possible environmental influences on CVD *circa* 1948 can hardly be appreciated today. Hypertension was known to have a direct relation to heart failure and to stroke but its connection with heart attack was not clear, and at any rate there was little to be done about it. Vascular diseases generally were relegated to 'an inevitable consequence of aging'. The importance of 'cholesterol', long known as a main component of arterial plaque and a cause of experimental dietary atherosclerosis, was for many years 'pooh-poohed', along with habitual diet, as 'a simplistic causal view of something as complex as atherosclerosis' (Jeremy Swan, personal communication, early 1970s). Smoking and obesity were merely distasteful; physical activity was dangerous and unfashionable; 'stress' and heredity were fundamental but inescapable.

'Be wise. Reduce your weight', was about as far as preventive practice went in the late 1940s. Research was informal, clinical, and privately funded. And public health recommendations to avoid risk were nowhere to be seen.

Pathology

The initiative of Ignatowski and Anitschkow, pathologists in the Russian Imperial Medical Institute, led to the modern understanding of atherosclerosis as the anlage of epidemic CVD. In the early twentieth century, they hypothesized that a 'rich' diet was responsible for accelerated aging and atherosclerosis. In those flourishing days for experimental pathology, they fed human diets to rabbits, producing fatty arterial lesions resembling those of human disease. Anitschkow determined that dietary lipids and cholesterol, rather than protein as Ignatowski postulated, were the arterial pathogen. His classic review of experimental atherosclerosis, in Cowdry's popular text of the 1930s, anticipated virtually every issue about atherogenesis explored since that time, including regression of atheroma (Anitschkow 1933).

Anitschkow's findings and syntheses were widely disseminated, stimulating much clinical-pathological study and causal ideation (McGill 1968).

Diagnosis

At the turn of the twentieth century, Wilhelm Einthoven of Leiden developed the string galvanometer electrocardiograph, which vastly facilitated cardiological diagnosis, particularly after its clinical application by the British investigator, Thomas Lewis (Einthoven 1903). Paul White came to study with Lewis in the 1920s and, with others, brought the apparatus and the art of electrocardiology back to the USA.

Some years later, Herrick's description of myocardial infarction with survival is generally given priority in Western medicine for establishing the syndrome of clinical and electrocardiographic manifestations (Herrick 1912; White 1948). The electrocardiogram became the major diagnostic tool in early clinical and epidemiological studies of coronary heart disease.

Stroke, on the other hand, was properly diagnosed much earlier, though it was only with development of brain imaging in the 1970s that its origins were successfully differentiated, during life, as thrombotic, embolic, or haemorrhagic.

Wartime mortality fluctuations

The rise of CVD mortality during the first half of the twentieth century was recognized early by a few experts internationally, including Joseph Mountin of the US Public Health Service, who, as we shall learn, initiated the Framingham Heart Study. The trend, however, was long attributed by the medical establishment to artefact—to improved diagnosis in an aging population.

In 1950 Haqvin Malmros of Sweden published an influential report about spectacular wartime changes in CVD deaths in Scandinavia (Malmros 1950). He had made the important assumption that diagnostic custom and medical care changed little in his neutral country during the Second World War; therefore, the dramatic downward trend in reported CVD mortality in the war years was probably real. If real, it was probably due to wartime privations, among which Malmros (an internist trained in nutrition and biochemistry) postulated the role of decreased dietary fat consumption.

Others in Europe found a similar wartime picture, including reduced arterial pathology at autopsy. Their independent reports, indicating an abrupt sociocultural–environmental impact on CVD death rates and on the fundamental arterial disease itself, heightened awareness of the coronary epidemic and pointed both to its mutability and its possible causes.

An informal romantic period

As early as 1916, Cornelis De Langen, a young Dutch physician sent to teach medicine in Indonesia, was struck by the contrast among colonial Dutch and the native Javanese in the frequency of angina pectoris, gall bladder disease, and post-operative thrombotic events, all of which he came to regard in the light of different lifestyles, diet, and blood cholesterol levels. He systematically made the seminal clinical and laboratory observations and then, to confirm them, went to a population of Javanese ship stewards living in a Dutch environment. From this, he proceeded to dietary experiments in which reversal of Dutch and Javanese habitual eating patterns produced profound changes in serum cholesterol levels (De Langen 1916).

De Langen's work is historically significant in the development of CVD epidemiology not only for its priority, scope, and use of several methodologies, but because its legacy can be traced in a direct line to the Dutch colleagues with whom he corresponded regularly: Isidore Snapper and Juda Groen. They, in turn, studied other contrasting populations and communicated their findings widely, influentially, and in English.

For example, De Langen's colleague and successor as house officer in Groningen was Isidore Snapper, who in the late 1930s became Rockefeller Professor in the Peking Union Medical School. There, Snapper undertook systematic study of ECG manifestations of coronary disease in populations and reported on their rarity in northern China. In 1941, in a book well-known to historians, *Chinese lessons to Western medicine*, he suggested that 'poor' working Chinese were protected from vascular disease by their mainly vegetarian diet, citing De Langen for priority in this view (Snapper 1941).

Juda Groen, student and colleague of both De Langen and Snapper, documented other dietary 'natural experiments'. He found, for example, lower blood cholesterol levels in vegetarian Trappists than in Benedictine monks and, at the Hadassah University Hospital in Israel, found lower vascular disease rates in Yemenite than in European immigrants to Israel (Groen *et al*. 1962; Kallner and Groen 1966).

The teachings and writings of this 'Dutch dynasty' touched the imagination of several pioneers of formal CVD epidemiology, particularly that of Ancel Keys, who had read both Snapper and De Langen when he met Groen in Amsterdam in 1952 and worked with him on a WHO expert committee in 1955 (Aneel Keys, personal communication 1955).

An early synthesis

Thus, Ancel Keys of Minnesota was well aware of this wartime mortality experience and of the early Dutch accounts. At mid-century, he and Paul Dudley White of Boston, based on their international eminence in nutrition and clinical cardiology, respectively, were invited around the world to witness contrasts in the prevalence of coronary cases and in diet and culture. Their early formulations about the influence of lifestyle on these differences led them to undertake and encourage others to take up formal epidemiological investigations. White and Keys promulgated an international strategy for CVD prevention, helped found and lead the new professions of CVD epidemiology and preventive cardiology, and effectively escorted these fields into the mainstream of international cardiology (Keys and White 1956).

The early era: 1948–72

Formal epidemiological research in cardiovascular diseases took several forms, beginning in 1948. Prospective study among defined cohorts, a 'new' strategy, focused on traits for individual risk within affluent, high-prevalence populations of the industrial world. Clearly, this summary chapter cannot give proper attribution to the many international investigations initiated early or late. Unquestionably, however, the prototype and icon of these was the Framingham Heart Study, discussed below (Dawber *et al*. 1951). Early studies, with similar design and intent to Framingham, spread rapidly across the USA and worldwide, as identified in Table 7.1.

Table 7.1 Early prospective (cohort) studies: 1948–72[a]

Alameda County Study	Honolulu Heart Study
Albany Civil Servants Study	Ikawa-Akita Study
Belgian Bank Study	Israel Ischemic Heart Disease Study
Bogalusa Heart Study	Lipid Research Centers Population Study
British Physicians Study	London Transport and Postal Workers Studies
Busselton Heart Study	Los Angeles Civil Servants Study
California Longshoreman Study	Malmö Study of Men Born in 1914
Charleston Heart Study	Minnesota Business and Professional Men Study
Chicago Heart Association Detection Project in Industry	
	NIHONSAN Study
Chicago Peoples Gas Company Study	Noichi-Kochi Study
Chicago Western Electric Study	Olmsted County Study
Community Syndrome of Hypertension, Atherosclerosis Study	Paisely-Renfrew Study
	Paris Prospective Study
Cooperative Lipoprotein Study	Puerto Rico Cardiovascular Disease Study
Dupont Company Study	Seal Beach Study
Evans County Heart Study	Seven Countries Study
Finnish Social Insurance Institution Study	Stockholm Study
FINRISK Study	Tecumseh Community Health Study
Framingham Heart Study	United Airlines Study
Glostrup Study	US Railway Study
Göteborg Study of Men Born in 1913	Western Collaborative Group Study
Göteborg Primary Prevention Cohort Study	Whitehall I Study
Harvard Alumni Study	Yao-Osaka Study
Helsinki Policemen Study	Yugoslavia Cardiovascular Disease Study
Hisayama Study	

[a]Initiated by 1972.

A different model, cross-cultural comparisons, was presaged by Epstein's study among New York City Italian and Jewish garment workers (Epstein and Boas 1955). But the icon of such formal studies is the Seven Countries Study, which began in the mid-1950s and is ongoing today. It also looked at individual risk prospectively within cohorts but focused main questions on the relationships between population-wide characteristics and CVD rates among cultures, in this case populations contrasting in habitual diet. It combined the goals of cohort studies with the older strategy of 'geographic pathology' (Keys 1970, 1980; McGill 1968).

Surveillance of CVD mortality was carried out in the early era, as it had been during the origins of CVD epidemiology, but trends in vital statistics on deaths continued to be treated as suspect by the medical community and were rarely examined systematically.

Experiment, also an early epidemiological thrust, was explained by Frederick Epstein in his Ancel Keys Lecture: '. . .a point is reached in the course of observational studies when it becomes

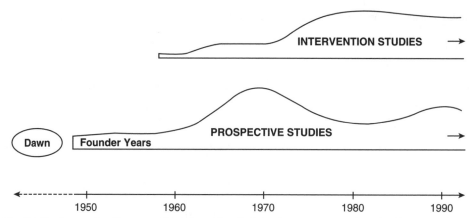

Fig. 7.1 Cardiovascular disease epidemiology historical development. Reproduced with permission from Epstein FH (1996). Cardiovascular disease epidemiology. A journey from the past into the future. Based on the 1993 Ancel Keys Lecture. *Circulation*, **93**, 1755–64. With permission from Lippincott Williams & Wilkins.

imperative to test whether predisposing factors not only predict clinical disease but whether their reduction causes a decline in the risk of disease' (Epstein 1996). In Fig. 7.1 from that presentation he depicted the time sequence of overlapping research strategies in CVD epidemiology, which coincides closely with the chronology conceived here.

Early trials of the effect of lowering of risk factors among randomized individuals or populations are listed in Table 7.2. Later and more definitive preventive trials are dealt with in appropriate detail elsewhere (Labarthe 1998; Black 2001; Steinberg 2005).

The core questions and the radiating arms of formal CVD epidemiology took form in the design, conduct, and analysis of these early studies that addressed the main candidate risk factors: blood pressure, diet, blood cholesterol, body mass, physical activity, and cigarette smoking. Such a broad new initiative required methods that were largely unfamiliar to the pioneer researchers. Soon, however, they learned and adopted elements of a common method and sound protocol (see Methods below).

The first formal cohort studies

A summary chapter cannot deal exhaustively with the myriad prospective studies that exploded from 1948 onward. Only a couple of these are discussed here because of their obvious priority in time or their role as prototypical of the genre.

The Minnesota Business and Professional Men's Study

The Minnesota Business and Professional Men's Study by physiologists Ancel Keys, Henry Taylor, and colleagues at the University of Minnesota examined 500 men in great physiological detail, annually from autumn 1947 to 1963, and followed them to 1983 (Keys *et al.* 1963). Though its epidemiological concept and prospective design provided a historical precedent for formal CVD studies, its resources and sample size were inadequate to produce predictive information until long after 'risk factors' were well laid out in larger cohort studies. The early Minnesota study, nevertheless, posed the appropriate questions about lifestyle risk factors; it defined 'norms', refined survey methods, and provided a stimulus and preparation for the Seven Countries Study and others that followed internationally.

Table 7.2 Early clinical trials in CVD risk factor reduction 1948–72[a]

Anti-Coronary Club Trial	Oslo Trial on Treatment of Mild Hypertension
Bierenbaum St. Vincent's Hospital Study	Oslo Study of Diet and Anti-smoking Advice
Chicago Coronary Prevention Evaluation Program	Physical Activity and CHD Pilot Trial
Coronary Drug Project	Program on Surgical Control of Hyperlipidemias (POSCH)
Finnish Mental Hospital Study	Scottish Society of Physicians Clofibrate Trial
Göteborg Multifactorial Primary Prevention Trial	MRC Low Fat Diet Trial
Hypertension Detection and Follow-up Program (HDFP)	MRC Soya Bean Oil Trial
Lipid Research (LRC) Coronary Primary Prevention Trial	Stanford Three-community Project
Lyon Mediterranean Diet Trial	Stockholm Prevention Trial with Clofibrate and Niacin
Morrison Diet-Heart Study	University Group Diabetes Program (UGDP)
Multiple Risk Factor Intervention Trial (MRFIT)	USPHS Hospitals Collaborative Trial in Mild Hypertension
Multifactorial CVD Prevention Trial in Helsinki Businessmen	VA Cooperative Trials of Hypertension
National Diet-Heart Pilot Trial	VA Domiciliary Diet Trial
North Karelia Project	WHO Cooperative (Clofibrate) Trial
	WHO Collaborative MRF Trial

[a]Initiated by 1972.

Of greater historical interest is how the Minnesota study was conceived in the first place. In 1948, Keys, who was a physiologist and nutritional scientist, had just completed a classic study of experimental starvation. In it, he had been struck by the rapid modifiability of heretofore-considered 'constitutional' characteristics such as body type, blood pressure, blood cholesterol, and vascular responses. Meanwhile, he had become curious about the phenomenon of epidemic heart attack, apparently from Minnesota newspaper reports of the day (Keys 1999). We know from an action photograph taken in 1946 that Keys had plotted a hypothetical projection toward intersection of the rising slope of heart deaths and the falling slope of other deaths in the city of Minneapolis. This antedated by two decades published discussions of 'the epidemiological transition' (Ancel Keys Photographic Archive, University of Minnesota).

Keys recounts in his memoirs:

> As news of the war and its aftermath receded from the newspapers, I was struck by the frequency of reports of executive men dropping dead, victims of what seemed to be a new plague, an increase in the frequency of coronary heart disease.... The cause... was unknown. I thought that we could record the characteristics of a large number of executives when they were apparently healthy, and then follow their status over the years, during which time some of them would develop coronary heart disease. By comparing the records of the afflicted men with those of the group that stayed healthy, we could discover which characteristics were related to the tendency to develop the [arterial] deposits.
>
> Keys (1999)

The Framingham Study

The Framingham Study was initiated by Joseph Mountin, Assistant Surgeon General, head of the Division of Chronic Diseases of the US Public Health Service (USPHS), and, according to his contemporaries, an 'architect of modern public health' (Mountin 1956; Oppenheimer 2005). The special public health orientation and competence of Mountin and the original designers of that study set it apart from many others that sprang up around the world in the early 1950s.

Invited to Massachusetts by Harvard's David Rutstein, the proposed USPHS–community study set up shop in 1948 in Framingham, MA, a small, independent township near Boston, and, soon after, its management was incorporated into the National Heart Institute (NHI). There the study was redesigned by the NHI chief of biometrics, Felix Moore, and the first medical director, Gilson Meadors, who made estimates of the sample size required for a definitive study having the likelihood of establishing, in a 5- to 10-year period, the relationship of given characteristics to the risk of heart attack.

The original goals of the study were submitted to Bert R. Boone, Heart Disease Section, USPHS, in a letter of 19 July 1947, attributable to Meadors: 'This project is designed to study the expression of coronary artery disease in a "normal" or unselected population and to determine the factors predisposing to the development of the disease through clinical and laboratory examination and long-term follow-up of such a group'. In fact, the Framingham manual of operation listed 28 hypotheses specific to these possible characteristics of risk.

The same memorandum opined that there is no 'perfect sample' of a population and it went on to provide a further insight: 'It is of less importance to have such a [perfect] sample than to record rather accurately the characterization of the group studied'. Other pioneers who recruited the first CVD cohorts shared the view that bias of selection is diminished and generalization strengthened by large numbers, careful measurement, and long-term observation.

Early in-house opposition to epidemiological studies at the National Institutes of Health (NIH), by clinical and bench scientists, was overcome, in considerable part, by arguments of the Heart Institute's chief advisor and Advisory Council executive, the Boston cardiologist Paul Dudley White. Then, in 1950, a vigorous young internist in the USPHS hospital division, Roy Dawber, was appointed Framingham director and brought his practical ideas and management skills to the study. He set the tone of clinical relevance that Framingham has maintained over the decades (Dawber 1980).

Framingham and others of the original US cohort studies published an early monograph on the predictive power for heart and blood vessel diseases of blood pressure, blood cholesterol level, and cigarette smoking habit (Multiple authors 1957). A subsequent publication established Framingham investigators' priority in use of the term 'risk factor' (Kannel *et al.* 1961). These investigators went on to elaborate many of the central concepts and practical tools now employed in the identification of personal cardiovascular risk.

In the late 1960s, Framingham underwent a major crisis when powerful interests wedded to bench and clinical research at NIH, along with Nixon administration budget cuts, removed support for most of Framingham's staff. Roy Dawber and Bill Kannel, under official threats, valorously resurrected and then maintained the study in an arrangement between the National Heart, Lung, and Blood Institute (NHLBI) and Boston University that still thrives today.

The congruent findings from Framingham and other early analytical epidemiological studies worldwide (listed in Table 7.1) sparked a revolution in understanding of the risk of heart attack and stroke among 'healthy' populations. The findings of these pioneer studies, taken together, produced the 'risk factor paradigm', a concept of predictive factors along the causal pathways of CVD. This, in turn, provided an international framework for ongoing research questions on causation and for a generation of professional activity in CVD prevention. This risk idea and its quantitative evidence continue to provide the base for the academic discipline of CVD epidemiology, the specific indications for interventions on individual risk, and the stimulus for ongoing research and public policy in CVD prevention.

The Seven Countries Study

In the 1950s, a different epidemiological approach to understanding the causes of CVD focused on comparisons among whole populations across a wide spectrum of diet or lifestyle in efforts to define the mass, as well as the individual, characteristics related to high or low population risk. The Seven Countries Study tested specific hypotheses among largely rural, traditional populations contrasting greatly in habitual diet. It was carried out by Ancel Keys and international colleagues in a collaboration starting in the late 1950s and ongoing today (Keys 1970, 1980; Kromhout *et al.* 2002). Major differences in CVD risk were found among samples of working middle-aged men followed for 30 years in 14 areas of seven countries, with the lowest rates in Japan and the Greek islands and the highest in the United States and Finland.

The Seven Countries Study provided the first credible data about major population differences in CHD and stroke rates. It also confirmed large variations in death rates from all causes. It found that a habitual diet of less than 10% calories from saturated fatty acids, with its associated lower blood cholesterol values, was apparently a necessary factor in lower population rates of CVD, whereas other risk factors failed to 'explain' the geographical differences. Within Seven Countries populations having different mortality, however, the 'traditional' CVD risk factors of diet, serum cholesterol, blood pressure, and cigarette smoking were universally predictive of an individual's risk, albeit with culturally different 'slopes' or force of the relationship (Keys *et al.* 1972; Kromhout *et al.* 2002).

The Seven Countries Study provided new and strong evidence for a policy of risk reduction at the population level. And it infected with the epidemiological method and mystique the medical and public health 'virgin forest' in each of its seven countries.

The spread of CVD epidemiology

Historical analysis remains to be made about how much of the rapid spread of CVD epidemiology in the 1950s was directly infective from the early foci in Framingham and Minnesota and how much was independent 'spontaneous generation'. Studies began early throughout North America and in the United Kingdom and Scandinavia and a little later in Japan. The London School of Hygiene and Tropical Medicine (LSHTM) was the nidus of early UK efforts as well as of much international enterprise in CVD epidemiology, based in the philosophy, research, and active teaching programme of Bradford Hill. He and his colleagues (see below) comprised a powerful academic centre of chronic diseases epidemiology, research, and training.

Of the many prospective, analytical studies initiated internationally in the early decades of CVD epidemiology (see Table 7.1), several became centres of ongoing academic activity and public health import. As relevant historically is whether the spread of CVD epidemiology was superfluous to the original investigations, whether 'merely' confirmatory or importantly contributory to the validation, strength, and generalizability of epidemiological method and the risk factor concept, or was the main value of its spread simply the alerting of professionals to their population's particular risk, with the knowledge they would need for regional preventive strategies? These issues beg historical analysis.

The evolution of risk factors

Ideas and evidence central to the evolution of the risk factor concept came mainly from (originally) non-epidemiologist investigators having particular interests or training in subject areas of CVD. Those include diet and nutrition, blood lipids and lipoproteins, blood pressure and 'hypertensive disease', obesity, metabolism, and diabetes, physical inactivity and fitness, respiratory disease and tobacco use, and various facets of the social, ethnic, psychological, and behavioural picture intuited to affect CVD risk. Rapid advances in understanding in this early period came from the ability of some of these investigators to move comfortably between the clinic, the laboratory, and populations in the field, or to collaborate effectively across disciplines (Gofman *et al.* 1950; Keys and White 1956; Morris 1957).

Therein lies much of the rich content as well as the *Sturm und Drang* of CVD epidemiology, which, again unfortunately, defies reduction for this summary chapter. For insights into the active to and fro among disciplines in the investigation of specific risk characteristics in CVD pathogenesis and prevention, I recommend a few recent reviews: physical activity, Leon (1997); lipids, Steinberg (2005); all risk factors, Labarthe (1998) and Stamler (2005).

Method, design, analysis, and computation

The naïvety of pioneer investigators about epidemiological methods led to increased communication among them, then to improved methodology. A certain collegiality emanated from early conferences on survey methods, study design, and work-in-progress. These were held by the WHO in Geneva from 1955 onward, at Beaconsfield in 1957, Princeton in 1959, at annual AHA meetings starting in Chicago in 1960, early on and at regular intervals at the LSHTM, and in expert groups of the International Society of Cardiology (ISC).

Essential to the comparisons of early CVD prevalence surveys and the prospective studies that followed were pioneer contributions made to standard, validated survey methods, including symptom questionnaires, blood pressure and other physical measurements, the electrocardiogram, blood lipid and other chemical measures, and diagnostic criteria. Diagnoses made in prior surveys and recorded in death certificates were poorly repeatable and of uncertain validity. By contrast, new field methods were rigorously and systematically developed, often collaboratively among the WHO, the LSHTM and St Thomas's and Guy's Hospital in London, the Laboratory of Physiological Hygiene in Minnesota, and committees of the AHA and the ISC (Holland 1962; Rose and Blackburn 1968).

In the early 1960s, those caught up in the new field of CVD epidemiology were suddenly able to put aside their cumbersome mechanical calculators and start sorting punched cards to get their row and column sums, summed squares, and products. But no sooner had researchers become comfortable with cross-classifications and chi-square statistical tests of differences, two variables at a time, than electronic computers burst upon the scene, rapidly expanding the horizons of computation and inference. Computer facilitation of data storage and management, of computation of correlations and regressions, along with the capacity for handling multiple variables simultaneously, was technically akin to its contemporary phenomenon of blasting off into space!

Electronic computers made possible one of the major contributions of modern epidemiology, that is, analysis of the effect of multiple variables while adjusting for their interactions. For example, the multiple logistic regression was first implemented in CVD epidemiology by Jerry Cornfield (Truett *et al.* 1967), soon followed by Cox's proportional hazards ratios and life table regression (Cox 1972).

Bradford Hill is given the credit for assimilating epidemiological–statistical methods from the past and developing new methods for improving the design of observational studies, for the design and analysis of randomized clinical trials, and for compiling the now-classic considerations for causal inference from statistical correlations in observational studies. His pioneering study of a cohort of British physicians and their smoking habits made a dramatic impact on design in epidemiology as well as on knowledge about the use of tobacco in relation to CVD and lung cancer (Doll and Hill 1954). Hill also trained many pioneers in chronic diseases epidemiology.

Jerry Morris's study of London Transport workers similarly provided innovations in the design and early understanding of the limitations of occupational studies for causal research in CVD epidemiology as well as early evidence about the role of habitual physical activity as a risk factor (Morris *et al.* 1953).

Automated chemistry vastly improved the reliability and efficiency of survey measurements as did the role of the WHO, the NIH, and Centers for Disease Control (CDC) in providing laboratory standards, testing, and manuals for survey methods.

The central role of the evolution of design and analysis in the development of modern epidemiology is, however, beyond the scope of this summary (see Conceptual evolution below).

Institutions and support agencies

Governmental support agencies, WHO, and heart foundations internationally were crucial to the rapid and effective progress in CVD epidemiology and prevention research. Each organization had particular ways of operating, funding assets, strengths, and institutional 'personalities'. Mainly they were complementary in roles of advice, design, funding, coordination, and direction.

The WHO

The efforts of the WHO in CVD prevention research and programmes were fostered from the outset by an international community of its supporters and consultants. The WHO responded by assembling experts in prevention research and policy and by establishing, in 1957, a CVD section at its Geneva headquarters and an operational European office in Copenhagen.

The first WHO CVD director, Zdenek Fejfar, organized timely expert reports and manuals on epidemiological methods, study design, and procedure, defining major CVD problems and enlisting expert solutions. In 1964, he commissioned *Cardiovascular survey methods*, initially a collaboration of the LHSTM and the University of Minnesota, now in its third edition, which provides detailed formularies, criteria, and a bare-bones standard strategy for surveys (Rose and Blackburn 1968; Luepker *et al.* 2004).

The WHO also initiated and coordinated major pioneering collaborative studies: the first cholesterol-lowering trial (the Clofibrate Trial) in the 1960s, and the European Multiple Risk Factor Intervention Trial in Industry in the 1970s, each among the earliest experimental interventions on risk; the Myocardial Infarction Registers organized by the Copenhagen office in the 1970s, and more recently, the MONICA Project, among the few research-oriented approaches to CVD surveillance, which provided systematic analysis of international disease trends.

The UK Medical Research Council (MRC)

The MRC was formed in 1913 as the Medical Research Committee and incorporated as the Medical Research Council by Royal Charter in 1920. In the 1950s, in parallel with the British National Health Plan, the MRC undertook to stimulate and fund research in chronic diseases. Several early units had a strong epidemiological and social medicine focus, one a Statistical Research Unit at the LSHTM under Bradford Hill with Richard Doll, another a Social Medicine Research Unit under Jeremy Morris at the London Hospital Medical School, and finally an Epidemiological Research Unit under Archie Cochrane at Cardiff, with Ian Higgins and William Miall. All had more or less orientation toward cardio-respiratory problems and pioneered in CVD surveys, prospective studies, and trials among civil servants and in the population of the Rhondda Fach (Higgins *et al.* 1963).

MRC units developed in other parts of the UK and Commonwealth, including Scotland and Jamaica, studying local vagaries of CVD and conducting trials, including the treatment of mild hypertension.

US National Institutes of Health (NIH)

The NHI opened as a new institute of the NIH in 1948, with a mission to support extramural research in CVD. From the outset it established a balanced strategy of support for clinical, laboratory, and epidemiological research and soon took jurisdiction over the Framingham Heart Study. James Watt, an epidemiologist and early institute director, strengthened the policy and organizational base of the population approach to research at the Heart Institute, at WHO, and internationally (personal communication James Watt to Zdenek Fejfar, 1959).

The eventual NHLBI became an international engine of epidemiological and prevention-related research, in which it has led its sister institutes and the larger community. As pointed out below, while it led the field, it wrestled with the expansion of costly population studies and trials and became more directive of them under the guise of 'fiscal responsibility'.

Heart foundations

In the early twentieth century, public health-oriented cardiologists within the New York Heart Association influenced its restructure into the AHA. The leaders of the AHA, in turn, championed its conversion into a public agency in 1948. The broad community views and initiatives of these leaders, particularly Felix Moore and Oglesby Paul, eventually led, in 1964, to formation of a Scientific Council on Epidemiology and Prevention having active programmes in research communication, methodology, and training. It became the parent body and philosophical home of CVD epidemiology in North America.

Guided by Paul Dudley White and Ancel Keys, the ISC, a consortium of regional professional societies, began research programmes and formal training in CVD epidemiology in the 1950s and 1960s. These leaders co-opted the cardiology elite into conferences on design and methods; they organized international seminars on CVD prevention; and they moulded the ISC into scientific councils with research and training missions. The ISC, joined by national heart foundations to become the International Society and Federation of Cardiology, was further reformed as the World Heart Federation in the 1990s and continues to support international seminars in CVD epidemiology. Several of its component regional foundations, such as the European Society of Cardiology, have organized active working groups to forward research and training in CVD epidemiology and prevention.

Academia and CVD epidemiology

Formal training programmes in observational CVD epidemiology and clinical trial design and analysis were among early and influential academic developments in the epidemiology of non-communicable diseases. The LSHTM pioneered in this development in the mid-1960s, initiating short courses, led by Donald Reid and Geoffrey Rose, which attracted an international audience.

The ISC research committee organized the first international Ten-day Seminar in CVD Epidemiology in 1968, which was led by Geoffrey Rose, Richard Remington, Jerry and Rose Stamler, and later by Darwin Labarthe, Dag Thelle, and K. T. Khaw. It is on-going almost 40 years later. With its regional counterpart at Lake Tahoe in the USA and other language-specific regional seminars, this seminar has exposed hundreds of younger CVD investigators from many countries to rigorous exercises in literature criticism and study design. Seminarians gain a new view of population strategies and preventive practice and, as alumni, form an international core of academicians and practitioners who foment epidemiological research and forward prevention policy and practice.

Many schools of public health and medical faculties maintain active research programmes, and graduate and post-doctoral training and degree programmes with majors in CVD epidemiology, which serve as models of training in epidemiological research for other chronic diseases.

Numerous texts and reviews in CVD epidemiology and in preventive cardiology have wide readership.

The modern era: 1972–present

Formal prevention policy and trials of the 1970s

The early 1970s marked a dramatic period of transition in CVD epidemiology; that is, between the period producing the evidence that formed the risk factor concept and the launching of the prevention policy and broad action implicit in the risk paradigm.

In particular, there was an uncomfortable interim in the USA while the National Diet–Heart Pilot Trial underwent a succession of evaluations after its results were published in 1968, accompanied by strong recommendations for a definitive diet–heart trial (National Diet–Heart Study Research Group 1968). It was finally and irrevocably deemed infeasible as a blinded, single-factor, diet–heart trial by an NIH task force led by E. H. Ahrens, Jr. This was based purportedly on practical issues of staffing and cost rather than on the scientific validity of its design or the public health import of diet in CVD. (Another appropriate and fascinating subject for historians would be the decisions, manipulations, and consequences surrounding that NIH decision.)

Frustration among the prevention research community during that period came from the inability to elicit any clear governmental policy on CVD prevention, either in research or programme, when the Lalonde Report had come out in Canada and when the AHA, the WHO, and other non-governmental agencies had called vigorously for a broad public policy and programme in CVD prevention. The medical establishments and governments of the USA and Europe seemed to drag their feet, unprepared either to accept the congruent evidence supporting prevention and to back lifestyle changes for the public or, its logical alternative, to authorize further preventive trials of risk factor modification.

In response, a band of pioneers in prevention mobilized efforts to stimulate the needed grand plan for research and policy, resulting in the following actions internationally:

- The Report on Preventive Trials in Coronary Heart Disease, from the ISC Conference in Makarska in 1968, recommended specific single and multiple risk factor trials of primary and secondary CVD prevention. The meeting and report were directly influential in subsequent policy decisions at the NIH, WHO, and internationally.

- Pioneer epidemiological researchers, Richard Remington, Jeremiah Stamler, and Henry Taylor, with a band of expert collaborators, submitted a proposal to NIH in 1969, dubbed 'Jumbo' because of its immense size, for a primary prevention trial to lower multiple risk factor levels, as the more powerful and efficient approach to 'prove' the feasibility of CVD prevention. ('Jumbo' was rejected, but helped stimulate a policy response. Requests for proposals for such a trial, and others, were finally issued from NIH in 1972.)

- The WHO sponsored several initiatives in 1970–71 on individual and industry-based multiple risk factor trials of both primary and secondary prevention.

- The US Joint Commission on Heart Disease Resources published its seminal report of recommendations for major research and broad social strategies of CVD prevention (Inter-Society Commission for Heart Disease Resources 1970). (No prevention policy recommendations before or since have been nearly as comprehensive.)

- The 1971 report of the National Heart and Lung Institute (NHLI) Task Force on Arteriosclerosis, in conjunction with the Joint Commission Report and clamour from the scientific community, led Theodore Cooper, the NHLI director, to propose major national policy for CVD prevention in 1972 (National Heart and Lung Institute 1971).

'A giant leap for mankind'?

These activities all converged in a new and international wave of research policy and action that at the time was considered a great step forward for CVD epidemiology and prevention. Some, however, found that the new direction toward experimental 'proof' was redundant to the clear findings of observational epidemiology, which, in turn, were congruent with clinical and laboratory evidence about the causes of CVD. Many of the subsequent generation of preventive trials proved to be academic and costly and a diversion from the socially oriented research and health promotion programmes that many CVD epidemiologists thought justified by the evidence. But the die was cast.

Gigantic trials, both explanatory and pragmatic, were undertaken in many places in the next decades (too extensive to document here) to modify single and combined risk characteristics in simultaneous efforts to prove causation and test the feasibility and safety of secondary and primary prevention of CVD (Blackburn *et al.* in preparation). They occupied the resources and energies of much of the cardiovascular research community worldwide. These ponderous, multi-centre, 'government issue' approaches were in many respects inimical to investigator initiative, coherence, and efficacy; their eventual outcomes were sometimes ambiguous. But they were essential, in the tenor of the times, to enlist the medical establishment in prevention. They became 'the only show in town' for academic CVD epidemiology; almost everyone 'got on board'.

The Lipid Research Centers (LRC) Primary Prevention Trial, part of a vast NHLBI–LRC empire internationally, at long last 'proved' the effectiveness of lipid lowering as a prevention strategy to reduce coronary risk (Lipid Research Clinics Program 1984). The Hypertension Detection and Follow-up Program, carried out in the same period, 'proved' the beneficent effects of a 'community approach' to hypertension control, while parallel British and Australian hypertension trials found drugs better than placebos (Black 2001).

On the other hand, these 'successful' 1970s trials substantially determined the overwhelmingly medical–pharmaceutical orientation, or 'medicalization', of subsequent CVD prevention policy and programmes in much of the industrial world.

A population strategy of CVD prevention emerges

As the risk factor paradigm from CVD epidemiology became more generally accepted, leaders and institutions moved forward with new prevention strategies. Policy-makers sought to integrate the traditional medical approach—to lower risk in the high-risk individual—with a complementary and more powerful population-wide health promotion strategy. This idea grew through several iterations until elaborated most clearly by Geoffrey Rose and colleagues in a WHO Expert Report on the population strategy of CHD prevention (World Health Organization Expert Committee on the Prevention of Coronary Heart Disease 1982) and in Rose's post-retirement classic, *The strategy of preventive medicine* (Rose 1992).

Another fundamental preventive strategy was formulated in 1978 by Toma Strasser at WHO, who proposed the term 'primordial prevention' to denote prevention of the epidemic occurrence of elevated CVD risk factors themselves—an alternative to detection and treatment once they are present. This was seen as a possible means for 'preserving entire risk-factor-free societies', thereby averting expansion of CVD as a global health problem (Strasser 1978).

Frederick Epstein, in particular, extended this idea, based on evidence that stopping smoking, modifying eating patterns, controlling hypertension, and improving physical activity and weight control, would profoundly reduce the age-specific rates of many common causes of mortality, including some cancers (Epstein 1994). This broader concept was stimulated further by evidence from several sources: the low-CVD-risk societies found in the Seven Countries Study, which often had lower all-causes mortality as well (Menotti *et al.* 1987), and Stamler's findings on the small but impressive very-low-risk segment of American cohorts (Stamler *et al.* 1993). Epstein proposed that this concept be explored with health promotion in whole populations as well as in youth, gender, and ethnic subgroups threatened but not yet at high CVD risk (Epstein 1996). (Epidemiological interest in recent years has extended toward prediction of all-causes deaths and longevity, to analysis of trends in risk and disease rates and their possible explanation, and to the impact of prevention on the population age pyramid. It is appropriate, therefore, to continue to ask what, indeed, are the ultimate aims of 'prevention'?)

Global health policy for CVD prevention gained support from Omran's 'theory of epidemio-logic transition' (Omran 1971), which forecast mounting proportions of deaths from CVD in all regions of the world due to rising burdens of 'man-made and degenerative diseases'. Policy devel-opment continues to the present day, building on accumulated knowledge and experience, expressed in landmark reports such as 'International action on cardiovascular disease: a platform for success based on international cardiovascular disease (CVD) declarations' (International Heart Health Society 2005), and in a number of specific national plans.

'The decline' (in CVD mortality rates)

It was in this period of the 1970s that the decline in age-specific mortality rates for coronary heart disease, having first been observed in the 1960s in California, was belatedly recognized throughout Western industrial society. This remarkable course correction in a raging non-communicable disease epidemic has become a major impetus to international research and policy for CVD prevention, leading to international conferences on 'the decline' and to the evolu-tion of systematic surveillance research and strategies of disease monitoring (Gillum *et al.* 1984; The ARIC Investigators 1989; Tunstall-Pedoe 2003).

These programmes have documented the decline in CVD mortality rates in many countries and the equally dramatic rise in others such as the Eastern Block in Europe and in the developing world. They have established clearly that population strategies of risk detection and health pro-motion, and innovations in medical and surgical cardiac care, have each contributed substan-tially to the decline in CVD mortality rates. Again, the limits of space prevent elaboration of the specific improvements in public health and in cardiac care that are documented to have reduced mortality and improved survival rates from CVD.

The challenge to epidemiology has been to explain the trends, that is, to link preventive pro-grammes or trends in mass health behaviours such as eating and smoking patterns, and levels of specific risk factors, to the trends in incidence and mortality rates. Research on CVD surveil-lance, with modelling of risk change effects, has entered the evolution of methods for modern epidemiology. These, in turn, are significantly led by work in CVD epidemiology.

'Circular epidemiology' and community studies of the 1980s

The first generation of preventive trials was followed by a period of elaboration of the risk factor paradigm that some called 'circular epidemiology', going 'round and round' on the same old issues (Kuller 1999). In an effort to move beyond repetitive cohort studies and trials, at least two other major directions were taken in the 1980s: in a few centres in the USA, Europe, and South Africa, large-scale, 'quasi-experimental' public health trials or community demonstrations of CVD health promotion strategies were approved after extensive peer review (Winkleby *et al.* 1997). In parallel, formal surveillance programmes were established to document and attempt to explain the dramatic international trends in CVD death rates that had begun in the 1960s (Gillum *et al.* 1984; Tunstall-Pedoe 2003).

Many of these preventive and epidemiological undertakings, too, were large and expensive, and again, some had ambiguous results. For example, the designs and interventions of the public health trials in California, Minnesota, and Rhode Island were insufficiently powerful to demonstrate significant short-term treatment effects over and above the dynamic trends on-going in health behaviour that were lowering risk levels throughout the industrial West in the 1980s (Winkleby *et al.* 1997). Few in the medical establishment accepted the community trial findings in Finland and the USA for what they really were: strong documented evidence for a profound change in health behaviour and CVD risk at ground level, irrespective of any true experimental effect.

An unintended consequence of the two decades of large and expensive CVD population studies and trials was mobilization of a powerful bench and clinical elite against what they termed 'those huge, costly, everlasting, epidemiological projects', along with calls for their rapid 'sunset' (personal communications to the NHLBI Advisory Council, multiple authors, 1988–92). It may be that the prevention research community has not fully recovered from the fallout of this sometimes rancorous rally against funding for CVD epidemiology in the late 1980s and early 1990s.

A millennial pause in the 1990s

At the moment in history when age-specific CVD mortality rates were in maximal decline in much of the West, and when the potential for prevention was clearly an open, if not guaranteed, opportunity, a reversal of fortunes in CVD epidemiological and prevention research developed, both in policy and programme. An opinion vigorously registered by the head of the 1991 NHLBI Task Force on Research in Atherosclerosis characterized attitudes of the clinical and bench scientific establishment at that juncture. He remarked to the effect that: 'Epidemiology made its contribution in the '60s and '70s. Now there are more interesting and important things to do' (personal communication, Daniel Steinberg, *circa* 1992).

That 1991 Task Force report was the first in the series of these influential milestones in US national research policy that failed to describe continued needs for epidemiological study or to maintain the balance among research disciplines in NHLBI programmes and policies, a policy highly productive over the prior decades. This departure represented a deliberate and qualitative change in national research policy for atherosclerotic–hypertensive cardiovascular diseases.

My Ancel Keys Lecture of 1991 summarized the unrest pervading the CVD epidemiology community in response to that official rejection of research balance as well as to NIH budget straits and the 'sunset' mentality of shutting down existing research. It also addressed increasing and discriminatory NHLBI restrictions on, and control of, epidemiological studies and trials. And it cited a general regression in energy, funding, and status of population research implicit in the national focus on individual, medical, and high-tech approaches to cardiological care and prevention (Blackburn 1992).

Subsequent calls for action by the epidemiological community caused the director of the NHLBI to assemble in 1992 an *ad hoc* 'Task Force on Research in Epidemiology and Prevention of Cardiovascular Diseases', a ploy that calmed the waters but avoided the basic issues of institute policy inimical to epidemiological research (National Heart, Lung, and Blood Institute 1994). Millennial unrest in the US academic community of CVD epidemiology was further diverted when Clinton and then Bush administration proposals were carried out to 'double the NIH budget in 5 years'. More people, in the USA, for a little while, got a larger 'piece of the pie'.

Internationally, where most countries never 'had it good' in the first place from strong government policy or funding on prevention, the picture of CVD epidemiology and prevention research has remained more or less static.

Progress, nevertheless

I should not exaggerate. Many positive elements are noted from the 1990s and since the millennium. CVD mortality rates have continued to decline in many countries, though at a slower rate. (Exceptionally, they have climbed steeply in eastern Europe, India, and southern Africa.) Epidemiological evidence has accumulated that CVD risk factor modification substantially reduces the risk of many non-CVD illnesses including some cancers; that is, it reduces total mortality. And the interchange among epidemiology, clinical, and bench science has become more natural and productive.

Epidemiology also made substantial specific contributions to a revived interest in the role of inflammation in atherosclerosis and thrombosis. Epidemiology and trials extended knowledge of the effects of diet independent of lipids and they led to effective use of prevention strategies in those at highest risk, such as patients with diabetes and renal disease. New interpretations of observational evidence increased the appropriate use of absolute over relative risk in efficacious prevention strategies. And epidemiology produced evidence about social inequities in risk, coming up with serious projections for CVD epidemics in the developing world.

Meanwhile, in the 1990s, the mature academic field of CVD epidemiology was having internal perturbations, including self-criticism of its 'circular' pursuits: study of 'the same old', or slightly refined, add-on risk factor analyses. Searching for the 'new', researchers faced the magnetic attraction, both intellectual and economic, of priorities in the gene–environment questions of individual CVD risk, finding direction in these mechanisms rather than in those of societal risk. Such a direction appeared to flourish within a social milieu preoccupied with medical–pharmacological approaches to individual and even population-wide risk, amidst a wider culture in which 'personal responsibility' for health trumped social obligation.

Post-millennial trends for the 2000s

CVD epidemiology remains a vigorous discipline of non-communicable disease epidemiology. The high quality and number of abstracts and publications submitted to the major scientific assemblies and journals concerned with CVD is evidence of progress. The youthful composition of those assemblies and of the regional and international Ten-day Seminars in CVD Epidemiology also is a positive sign. Observational epidemiology maintains fairly stable governmental review and absolute funding levels, despite rigid new policy rules and 'programme priorities'. A few centres remain productive with cohort studies addressing poorly understood issues of socio-economic class and CVD risk. Clinical trials, with a few happy exceptions such as the DASH study of diet and blood pressure, no longer mainly test hygienic or public health interventions but rather are drug-related and increasingly supported by industry.

Innovative epidemiological strategies abound, such as postal surveys and trials, with long-term follow-up among massive numbers of responsive professional men and women; nested case–control studies within older survey and cohort populations; international multicentre and cross-cultural surveys and clinical trials; meta-analyses of worldwide cohort and trial data; systematic international and regional surveillance studies; and an occasional group-randomized trial of health promotion.

Faculty positions and graduate and post-doctoral training programmes in CVD epidemiology remain stable, their collaborations increasing with genetics, physiology, metabolism, clinical trials, and 'clinical research'. Many branches of medicine, even surgery, now proudly proclaim the goal of prevention. Thus, the picture is far from bleak, though research funding for CVD epidemiology and prevention is far from plentiful. It remains perennially incommensurate with the disease burden.

The conceptual evolution in CVD epidemiology

Concepts have evolved steadily in CVD epidemiology, along with new evidence, methods, and professional training. Problems of design and analysis central to the whole field of epidemiology are increasingly recognized and dealt with as analysts (and their computers) acquire greater sophistication. 'Over lightly' the following conceptual issues evolve:

◆ Bias and confounding continue to be the main livelihood of epidemiological theorists and methodologists.

◆ Regression–dilution bias, the great weakener of epidemiological evidence, is systematically corrected.

◆ The funnel-shaped relation between precision, significance, and sample size is explored.

◆ Meta-analysis has left the realm of the investigator and moved to world centres that aggressively acquire and reanalyse everyone else's data.

◆ The old intellectual hierarchy of case–control versus cohort study versus randomized trial is challenged when their risk estimates are found increasingly similar as study design and methods improve.

◆ The provenance and training of epidemiologists shifts such that knowledge of the biology and mechanisms of disease phenomena can no longer be assumed. (And its absence is found disadvantageous to good study design and interpretation.)

◆ Clinical–laboratory–epidemiological cross-fertilization and collaboration increases.

◆ Separate and complementary roles of individual and ecological correlations are appreciated.

◆ Low CVD risk is found among entire populations and in low-risk segments of high-incidence populations, confirming and strengthening the risk paradigm.

◆ Criteria are honed for enhanced causal inference from observational evidence.

◆ The generalizability is increasingly questioned of experimental 'proof' from the 'platinum meter' of clinical trials (always carried out in select populations).

◆ The ultimate role of epidemiology is appreciated: to establish real-world implications of small-world evidence, and so on!

Leitmotifs in CVD epidemiology

The medical establishment has traditionally been slow to accept epidemiological evidence on diet and culture among the basic causes of atherosclerosis and CVD. The more favourable interpretation of this incomprehension is the 'necessary' medical focus on care rather than prevention and on the individual rather than the collectivity. In any case, recommendations for diet and lifestyle change in the general population, even when based on congruent evidence, have been unsupported by traditional medicine without 'conclusive proof' from human experiment, proof that is often infeasible, costly, or unethical to attain.

Such attitudes are, at best, an ongoing symbolic challenge to epidemiology, but they are also a significant impediment to reasoned public policy based on the best available evidence at any given time.

Another leitmotif in the development of modern epidemiology is its struggle for recognition as an essential basic science as well as a utilitarian applied science. Epidemiology continues to fight for intellectual and administrative equity within institutions and their policies. Among the three medical research disciplines 'We are number 3. Thus, we try harder!'

Clearly, such issues at the heart of modern epidemiology justify more thoughtful treatment and historical analysis than this summary presentation allows.

Epilogue

CVD epidemiology in the new millennium has evolved into a productive and mature discipline paralleled by rich findings from clinical and laboratory researches and, *pari passu*, a decline of CVD mortality rates in many places.

Historically, the field is unique in its origins and in its contributions to the concepts, evidence, and methods of modern epidemiology. But while epidemiology has helped establish the promise of population-wide prevention and has led medical science and public health to the brink of its accomplishment, actual research and programmes for effective population control of the CVD epidemic have languished.

Molecular biology, which for a time has dominated CVD research, enhances the understanding of mechanisms of disease and ultimately is expected to improve medical practice. On the other hand, the relevance of studies in gene and gene–environment associations to the mass causes and prevention of epidemic CVD is under question. Left to future judgement is the wisdom of a deliberate shift of intellectual focus, energy, and national policies away from the challenge of population-wide primary prevention and toward high-tech medical strategies and the biogenetics of personal risk and 'resurrection'.

Today's challenges for CVD epidemiology include the effects of 'incomplete prevention'. In that current state, the decline in mortality rates slows (at least, in the USA), while improved survival along with stable incidence rates tends to expand the CVD burden among aging affluent populations. Further progress in prevention at the population level requires priority for research into risk inequities and prevention strategies among youth, the elderly, women, and minorities, and into the looming threat of epidemic CVD in developing countries. There, high rates of tobacco use and of hypertension wait ominously for the projected upward shift in the distributions of risk factors related to diet and physical activity.

The history of CVD epidemiology strongly suggests, nevertheless, a continuing opportunity, achievable through scientific research and its fruits, for another global epidemiological transition—to longer, healthier, and different lives.

Acknowledgements

The collaboration is gratefully acknowledged of Darwin Labarthe, MD, Kalevi Pyörälä MD, and Research Assistants in the Minnesota Program on the History of Science and Medicine: Karen Ross and Suzanne Fischer (Program Head: John Eyler PhD). Support is acknowledged from the Division of EPICH and the Dean's Office of the School of Public Health, University of Minnesota, from the American Heart Association Council on Epidemiology and Prevention, the National Library of Medicine, NIH grant no 1G13 LM008214, and from the Frederick Epstein Foundation and Doris Epstein of Zurich.

References

Anitschkow N (1933). Experimental atherosclerosis in animals. In *Atherosclerosis: a survey of the problem* (ed. E Cowdry), pp. 271–322. Macmillan, New York.

Black H (2001). *Clinical trials in hypertension*. Marcel Dekker, New York.

Blackburn H (1992). Ancel Keys Lecture. The three beauties. Bench, clinical, and population research. *Circulation*, **86**, 1323–31.

Blackburn H, Labarthe D, and Pyörälä K (in preparation). *Prevention of heart attack and stroke. A history of cardiovascular disease epidemiology*. Oxford University Press, Oxford.

Cox D (1972). Regression models and life tables. *Journal of the Royal Statistical Society Series B*, **34**, 187–220.

Dawber TR (1980). *The Framingham Study: the epidemiology of atherosclerotic disease.* Harvard University Press, Cambridge, MA.

Dawber TR, Meadors GF, and Moore FE (1951). Epidemiological approaches to heart disease: the Framingham Study. *American Journal of Public Health*, **41**, 279–86.

De Langen CD (1916). Cholesterine-stofwisseling en rassenpathologie. *Geneeskundig Tijdschrift voor Nederlansch-Indie*, **56**, 1–34.

Doll R and Hill AB (1954). The mortality of doctors in relation to their smoking habits. A preliminary report. *British Medical Journal*, **1**, 1451–5.

Einthoven W (1903). Die galvanometrische Registrierung des menschlichen Elektrokardiogramms, zugleich eine Beurteilung der Anwendung des Capillar-Elektrometers in der Physiologie. *Pflügers Archiv für die gesamte Physiologie des Menschen und der Tiere*, **99**, 472–80.

Epstein FH (1994). Will measures to prevent coronary heart disease protect against other chronic disorders? In *Lessons for science from the seven countries study* (ed. H Toshima, Y Koga, H Blackburn, and A Keys), pp. 179–93. Springer, New York.

Epstein FH (1996). Cardiovascular disease epidemiology. A journey from the past into the future. Based on the 1993 Ancel Keys Lecture. *Circulation*, **93**, 1755–64.

Epstein FH and Boas EP (1955). The prevalence of manifest atherosclerosis among randomly chosen Italian and Jewish garment workers. A preliminary report. *Journal of Gerontology*, **10**, 331–7.

Gillum RF, Hannan PJ, Prineas RJ, *et al.* (1984). Coronary heart disease mortality trends in Minnesota 1960–1980: the Minnesota Heart Survey. *American Journal of Public Health*, **74**, 360–2.

Gofman JW, Lindgren F, Elliott H, *et al.* (1950). The role of lipids and lipoproteins in atherosclerosis. *Science*, **3**, 166–71, 186.

Groen JJ, Tjiong BK, Koster M, Willebrands AF, Verdonck G, and Pierloot M (1962). The influence of nutrition and ways of life on blood cholesterol and the prevalence of hypertension and coronary heart disease among Trappist and Benedictine monks. *The American Journal of Clinical Nutrition*, **10**, 456–70.

Herrick J (1912). Clinical features of sudden obstruction of the coronary arteries. *Journal of the American Medical Association*, **59**, 2015–20.

Higgins I, Cochrane A, and Thomas A (1963). Epidemiological studies of coronary disease. *British Journal of Preventive and Social Medicine*, **17**, 153–65.

Holland WW (1962). The reduction of observer variability in the measurement of blood pressure. In *Epidemiology. Reports on research and teaching* (ed. J Pemberton). Oxford University Press, London. pp. 271–81.

International Heart Health Society (2005). *International action on cardiovascular disease: a platform for success based on international cardiovascular disease (CVD) declarations.* International Heart Health Society (available at http://www.internationalhearthealth.org/Publications/Synthesis%20Document.pdf).

Inter-Society Commission for Heart Disease Resources (1970). Primary prevention of the atherosclerotic diseases. Report of Inter-Society Commission for Heart Disease Resources. *Circulation*, **42**, A55–A95.

Kallner G and Groen JJ (1966). Mortality and hospitalization in relation to coronary and cerebral vascular disease in Israel. *Journal of Atherosclerosis Research*, **6**, 419–29.

Kannel WB, Dawber T, Kagan A, Revotskie N, and Stokes J (1961). Factors of risk in the development of coronary heart disease—six-year follow-up experience. The Framingham Study. *Annals of Internal Medicine*, **55**, 33–50.

Keys A (ed) (1970). Coronary heart disease in seven countries. *Circulation*, **41**, I1–I211.

Keys A (ed) (1980). *Seven countries: a multivariate analysis of death and coronary heart disease.* Harvard University Press, Cambridge, MA.

Keys A (1999). *Adventures of a medical scientist. Sixty years of research in thirteen countries.* Crown Printing, St Petersburg.

Keys A and White PD (ed.) (1956). *Cardiovascular epidemiology: selected papers from the Second World Congress of Cardiology and Twenty-seventh Annual Scientific Sessions of the American Heart Association.* Hoeber-Harper, New York.

Keys A, Aravanis C, Blackburn H, *et al.* (1972). Probability of middle-aged men developing coronary heart disease in five years. *Circulation*, **45**, 815.

Keys A, Taylor HL, Blackburn H, Brozek J, Anderson JT, and Simonson E (1963). Coronary heart disease among Minnesota business and professional men followed 15 years. *Circulation*, **28**, 381–95.

Kromhout D, Menotti A, and Blackburn H (2002). *Prevention of coronary heart disease. Diet, lifestyle, and risk factors in the Seven Countries Study*. Kluwer Academic Publishers, New York.

Kuller L (1999). Circular epidemiology. *American Journal of Epidemiology*, **50**, 897–903.

Labarthe DR (1998). *Epidemiology and prevention of cardiovascular diseases: a global challenge*. Aspen Publishers, Inc., Gaithersburg, MD.

Leon AS (ed) (1997). *Physical Activity and Cardiovascular Health. A National Consensus*. Human Kinetics, Champaign, IL.

Lipid Research Clinics Program (1984). The Lipid Research Clinics Coronary Primary Prevention Trial Program. I. Reduction in incidence of coronary heart disease. *Journal of the American Medical Association*, **251**, 351–64.

Luepker R, Evans A, McKeigue P, and Reddy K (2004). *Cardiovascular survey methods*, 3rd edn. WHO, Geneva.

Malmros H (1950). The relation of nutrition to health. A statistical study of the effect of the war-time on arteriosclerosis, cardiosclerosis, tuberculosis and diabetes. *Acta Medica Scandinavica Supplementum*, **246**, 137–53.

McGill H (1968). *The geographic pathology of atherosclerosis*. Williams and Wilkins Co., Baltimore.

Menotti A, Mariotti S, Seccareccia F, and Giampaoli S (1987). The 25-year estimated probability of death from some specific causes as a function of twelve risk factors in middle-aged men. *European Journal of Epidemiology*, **4**, 60–7.

Morris JN (1957). *Uses of epidemiology*. Livingstone, Edinburgh.

Morris JN, Heady JA, Raffle PAB, Roberts CG, and Parks JW (1953). Coronary heart disease and physical activity of work. *Lancet*, **2**, 1053–7.

Mountin JW (1956). *Selected Papers of Joseph W. Mountin, M.D.* Joseph W. Mountin Memorial Committee.

Multiple authors (1957). Measuring the risk of coronary heart disease in adult population groups (part II). *American Journal of Public Health*, **47**, 1–63.

National Diet–Heart Study Research Group (1968). *The national diet-heart study final report*, AHA Monograph No 18. American Heart Association, Inc., New York.

National Heart and Lung Institute Task Force on Arteriosclerosis (1971). *Arteriosclerosis: a report*. National Institutes of Health, Bethesda, MD.

National Heart, Lung, and Blood Institute (1994) *Report of the Task Force on Research in Epidemiology and Prevention of Cardiovascular Diseases*. National Institutes of Health, Bethesda, MD.

Omran AR (1971). The epidemiologic transition: a theory of the epidemiology of population change. *Millbank Memorial Fund Quarterly*, **49**, 509–38.

Oppenheimer GM (2005). Becoming the Framingham Study 1947–1950. *American Journal of Public Health*, **95**, 602–10.

Rose G (1992). *The strategy of preventive medicine*. Oxford University Press, Oxford.

Rose GA and Blackburn H (1968). *Cardiovascular survey methods*. WHO, Geneva.

Snapper I (1941). *Chinese lessons to Western medicine*. Interscience Publishers, Inc., New York.

Stamler J, Dyer AR, Shekelle RB, Neaton J, and Stamler R (1993). Relationship of baseline major factors to coronary and all-cause mortality and to longevity: findings from long-term follow-up of Chicago cohorts. *Cardiology*, **82**, 191–222.

Stamler J (2005). Established major coronary risk factors: historical overview. In *Coronary heart disease epidemiology from aetiology to public health* (ed. M Marmot and P Elliott). Oxford University Press, Oxford, pp. 18–31.

Steinberg D (2005). The pathogenesis of atherosclerosis. An interpretative history of the cholesterol controversy: part II: the early evidence linking hypercholesterolemia to coronary disease in humans. *Journal of Lipid Research*, **46**, 179–90.

Strasser T (1978). Reflection on cardiovascular diseases. *Interdisciplinary Science Reviews*, **3**, 225–30.

The ARIC Investigators (1989). The Atherosclerosis Risk in Communities (ARIC) Study: design and objectives. *American Journal of Epidemiology*, **129**, 687–702.

Truett J, Cornfield J, and Kannel W (1967). A multivariate analysis of the risk of coronary heart disease in Framingham. *Journal of Chronic Diseases*, **20**, 511–24.

Tunstall-Pedoe H (ed.) (2003). *MONICA. Monograph and multimedia sourcebook*. WHO, Geneva.

White PD (1948). *Heart disease*. Macmillan Company, New York.

Winkleby M, Feldman H, and Murray D (1997). Joint analysis of three U.S. community intervention trials for reduction of cardiovascular disease risk. *Journal of Clinical Epidemiology*, **50**, 645–58.

World Health Organization Expert Committee on the Prevention of Coronary Heart Disease (1982). *Prevention of coronary heart disease*. WHO, Geneva.

8

Chronic respiratory disease epidemiology

Frank E. Speizer and Ira B. Tager

Personal experiences

In 1958, through a special education programme sponsored by the California State Department of Public Health designed to introduce medical students to public health research, Frank Speizer had the opportunity of being introduced to three brilliant public health researchers. These three individuals, two of whom became deans of schools of public health (Raual 'Stoney' Stallones, University of Texas; Lester Breslow, University of California at Los Angeles) and the third, John Goldsmith, who became a major force in public health in Israel and one of the founders of the International Environmental Epidemiology Association, converted a medical student interested in a summer job in Los Angeles for personal reasons into a lifelong investigator in population-based research by demonstrating how clinical medicine, physiology, statistics, and preventive medicine could be combined into a satisfying and productive career.

Following medical school, Dr Speizer took a fellowship in respiratory physiology at the Harvard School of Public Health. This was a unique opportunity to conduct applied research that tested the physiological responses from exposure to SO_2 in both dogs and humans, and, at the same time, to participate in the design and execution of a study of responses of free-living subjects to environmental levels of ambient pollutants.

After spending three additional years in clinical training, Dr Speizer spent 2 years working with Sir Richard Doll in London, when Sir Richard was the Director of the MRC Statistical Research Unit. During this period Dr Speizer identified and reported on the excess risk of mortality from asthma in young people and had the opportunity to work with Charles Fletcher who was exploring the natural history and risk factors for chronic bronchitis and emphysema. This work was continued by Dr Speizer over the next 30 years and was the basis for the development of the first training programme in the USA on chronic respiratory disease epidemiology, in which Dr Ira Tager was the first trainee.

Ira Tager, initially working with Drs Speizer and Ed Kass at the Channing Laboratory, combined his interest in infectious diseases and chronic respiratory disease to explore risk factors for the development of chronic obstructive pulmonary disease (COPD) in both adults and children. He soon realized that his real interest had less to do with the infectious diseases component and more to do with the lung itself and the effect of the environmental exposures on lung function. In concert with the mentoring he got from Dr Speizer, Dr Tager acquired the knowledge about pulmonary mechanics that he needed for his work. This effort was aided by the generosity of Dr Roland Ingram and Professor Jere Mead.

As a result of some serendipitous observations, his early work focused on the effects of exposure to second-hand smoke (SHS), both *in utero* and after birth, on the development of lung function and airways reactivity in children, and the direct effects of smoking on lung function in young adults. Dr Tager, along with Dr Speizer were among the first to identify the 'plateau phase' in the natural history of the development of lung function and the fact that a major effect of cigarette smoking was to reduce or eliminate this plateau phase—thereby initiating the increased decline in lung function observed in smokers as a group.

In 1995, Dr Tager initiated a major research effort related the effects of air pollution on the development of lung function in children and adolescents. This work has built on the model of the effects of SHS and has already shown similarities with respect to effects on small airways.

The modern era of the study of the epidemiology of chronic obstructive pulmonary disease (COPD), although originally defined in the early part of the nineteenth century (Badham, 1808) did not blossom until the middle of the twentieth century. Before that time clinicians generally believed that much of the symptomatology associated with the disease represented a 'normal' state. Collis (1923) reported the common view that:

> The trite observation that familiarity breeds contempt is essentially true with regard to the outlook on chronic bronchitis: those afflicted are inclined to accept the complaint as inevitable, as something troublesome, but not serious. Those called upon to treat it do not find it sufficiently interesting to study closely. At hospital it tends to be disregarded with an out-patient mixture yet. . .records in England and Wales show that when mortality and morbidity are taken together, bronchitis is the most important of all diseases and further. . .it is at the same time a most preventable disease.

The formal beginning of population-based approaches to chronic respiratory disease had its origin in a combination of social, political, and (although not expressed in such terms) economic philosophies of a uniquely qualified group of physicians and mathematicians in the late 1930s. Prior to that time, epidemiological research was dominated by explorations of approaches to control infectious diseases (Winslow 1952). Clean water, insect control, and other efforts to control vectors of common infectious diseases were the primary foci.

In the early part of the twentieth century, particularly in Great Britain, coal was the major source of energy, and much of that coal was mined in South Wales. By the mid 1930s, it was recognized that radiographic evidence of silicosis was associated with chronic pulmonary disease. At that time in Great Britain silicosis was a compensatable disease. However, what was also recognized was that most of the coal mining in South Wales was not associated with exposure to high quartz content; and, although miners and their local physicians recognized some form of respiratory disease, it was not diagnosed as silicosis and, therefore, it was not compensatable. Moreover, it was not related to tuberculosis, the occurrence of which was known to be associated with coal mining. This resulted in a somewhat dissatisfied work force. Because of concern about the importance of the work force (with an impending war) and concern about the health and welfare of that work force, the government asked the Medical Research Council (MRC) to establish a research group to determine the magnitude of the problem. The MRC brought together a remarkable group of investigators that established the research foundation of modern chronic respiratory disease epidemiology and became the resource for the leaders in the development of chronic respiratory disease epidemiology research for the remainder of the twentieth century. Initially this group was called the MRC Pneumoconiosis Research Unit and, subsequently, a second unit, the MRC Epidemiology Unit, was formed. The concept and importance of large-scale population-based surveys with exceptionally high response percentages (Archie Cochrane); the role of standardized diagnostic clinical approaches (Charles Fletcher); the use of physiological measures of lung function (Phillip Hugh-Jones), the importance of application of statistical methods to evaluate observed associations (Peter Oldham), and the measurement of exposure (John Gilson) all had their beginnings in these units—particularly as related to chronic respiratory diseases. Through their efforts, coal workers' pneumoconiosis, with the presence of progressive massive fibrosis, became a compensatable disease not only in Great Britain but throughout the developed world. (For a full account of the development of these units see Wellcome Witnesses to Twentieth Century Medicine (2002).)

Within this context, the stage was set for consideration of the wider impact of chronic respiratory diseases, which went beyond the occupational setting. A further stimulus for this larger view came in 1952 when London experienced an episode of stagnant air pollution associated with coal combustion contaminants that resulted in an estimated 4000 extra deaths over a 2-week period (Ministry of Health 1954). Most of the deaths were in people with pre-existing respiratory or cardiovascular diseases. Remarkably, Firket (1931) in reporting on a similar episode of pollution occurring in the Meuse Valley in Belgium, suggested that if a similar event were to occur in London that approximately 3000 excess deaths could be predicted. Reanalysis of this episode in the late 1990s suggested that the excess mortality may have been as high as 12,000 deaths (Bell and Davis 2001). Other documented episodes had previously been recorded in the USA Donora, PA (Schrenk 1949) and subsequently by others (Holland 1979). The London episode stimulated a broad concern and led to the recognition of the importance of the health burden associated with chronic respiratory diseases and alerted researchers to the need for a set of standardized and valid criteria with which to identify these diseases. Subsequently, efforts to reduce pollution in London through smoke abatement programmes by control of the use of soft coal have resulted in less frequent pollution episodes and to episodes with far less excess mortality. The importance of this 1952 episode for the understanding of effects of the environment on the occurrence of chronic respiratory disease is testified to by the many investigations over the past 25 years that have looked back at the mortality consequences of the event and its role as a stimulus to 'air pollution epidemiology'.

South Wales was not the only place in which developments in chronic respiratory disease epidemiology research were taking place. In 1947, Tiffeneau and Pinelli reported on the usefulness of a measure of pulmonary function in exercise to define functional status. Although this is recognized as the beginning of the modern use of pulmonary function testing, Hutchinson (1846) first described the vital capacity and demonstrated that it could be used as screening tool to predict mortality. However, much of the mortality at that time was due to consumption (tuberculosis). In 1951 Ed Gaensler, a surgeon in the USA, developed a timing device that allowed the vital capacity to be subdivided, and subsequently Brian Gandevia and Phillip Hugh-Jones (1957), in a report of the Thoracic Society of the United Kingdom, defined the terminology currently used to describe the components of pulmonary function.

Because of the difficulties in making uniform clinical diagnoses of chronic respiratory diseases and the clinical confusion brought about by the British use of the term chronic bronchitis and the American use of emphysema to describe what would appear to have been the same disease, in 1959, a Ciba Guest Symposium (1959) was held in an attempt to identify a uniform set of definitions for chronic respiratory disease (see Table 8.1). Although the effort brought together a distinguished group of experts, and the definitions appeared to be clinically useful, they suffered from not being defined for epidemiological purposes. Subsequently, the Medical Research Council (1960) published a standardized respiratory questionnaire that has been used widely, and,

Table 8.1 Definitions of chronic obstructive respiratory diseases

Disease	Definition	Comment
Chronic bronchitis	Chronic expectoration	Questionnaire definition
Asthma	Reversible airways obstruction	Physiological definition
Emphysema	Distal air space enlargement	Pathological definition
Chronic obstructive lung disease (COLD)	Irreversible air flow obstruction due to bronchitis or emphysema	Combination of above criteria

Source: Ciba Guest Symposium (1959). Terminology, definitions, and classification of chronic pulmonary emphysema and related conditions. *Thorax*, **14**, 286–99.

brought to the forefront of the field the concept of standardized data collection that has been essential for the comparison of results across different populations and across time within the same populations (Holland and Reid 1965; Peto *et al.* 1983; Higgins *et al.* 1984). Although modified on several occasions (Medical Research Council 1960; Ferris 1978), and most currently in its incarnation as the ATS-DLD questionnaire (O'Conner and the ATS Working Group 2006), many of the original questions related to cough, phlegm, and breathlessness have remained unchanged for almost 50 years—a testimony to the care that went into the design and, in the case of phlegm, real validation of these questions (Samet 1978).

As standardized surveys began to be conducted in the late 1950s, what became apparent was the overwhelming impact of cigarette smoking on the risk of chronic respiratory disease. Levin *et al.* (1950), Wynder and Graham (1950), and Doll and Hill (1950) had already reported in case–control studies the role of smoking in lung cancer. However, at that time most of the evidence about chronic respiratory diseases, other than cancer and tuberculosis, was obtained from retrospective assessments of patients seen at hospitals. For the purpose of convenience for the remainder of this chapter we will use the term COPD to describe what would otherwise be called simple chronic bronchitis or chronic mucus hypersecretions, obstructive bronchitis, emphysema, or chronic obstructive pulmonary disease. Some investigators have also included asthma in this definition. These studies led to speculations about the origins of and risk factors for COPD. Orie *et al.* (1961) suggested what was later termed by Fletcher (1970) the 'Dutch hypothesis', that COPD and asthma had common origins in that the intrinsic make-up of individuals resulted in different responses to common environmental exposures (e.g. air pollution and or cigarette smoking). This was in contrast to the hypothesis offered by Fletcher (the 'British hypothesis') that suggested that the infectious nature of acute respiratory illnesses resulted in recurrent bronchitis and subsequent development of obstructive airways disease (Fig. 8.1). Pathological correlates of each of the stages of disease could be identified (Hogg *et al.* 1968).

Although reduction in environmental exposures would play a major role in the management of these diseases, from the standpoint of explaining the origins of COPD and identifying research and clinical strategies, distinguishing between these hypotheses became important. If the British hypothesis were true, one should be able to interfere with the infectious nature of the recurrent bronchitis and thus block the development of obstructive airways disease and/or mitigate the exacerbations that characterized the disease. In contrast, if the Dutch hypothesis were true,

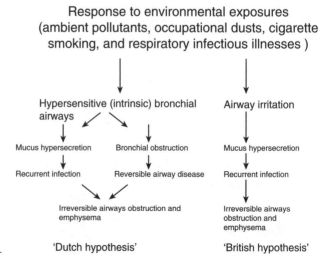

Fig. 8.1 Comparison of the 'Dutch' and 'British' hypotheses.

it became more important to identify the characteristics of those who were susceptible to the development of hyper-responsive airways and to identify methods to block such reactions. The retrospective nature of most of the data that led to these hypotheses and the need for longitudinal data to test them was an important impetus that has stimulated much of the work in the field of chronic respiratory disease epidemiology over the last 30 years.

One of the first studies that began to look prospectively at risk factors for COPD was designed by Charles Fletcher and was stimulated by the visionary ideas of Sir Richard Doll (Fletcher *et al.* 1976). In 1958, Fletcher suggested that a prospective assessment of a population of healthy working men evaluated with standardized questionnaires and repeated pulmonary function testing along with sputum assessments could be used to test the British hypothesis. The difficulty at that time was the fear that the volume of data generated over the relatively short period of 8 years of repeated testing would be impossible to handle by available analytical techniques. At that time, Doll suggested that by the time the data were ready to be analysed there would be 'machines' available that could handle the data effectively and economically. It also was Doll's vision that the developing expertise of computer-oriented biostatisticians would make such efforts feasible. This vision was fulfilled by the mid-1960s with the development of the Atlas computer at the University of London and through the ongoing collaboration of Doll's MRC Statistical Research Unit and investigators such as Richard Peto.

At the same time, in the United States, Ben Burrows at the University of Chicago, after meeting Charles Fletcher, established a cohort of diseased patients and assessed prospectively the characteristics of their disease (Burrows and Earle 1969). In addition, Ben Ferris, in Boston, after a visit with John Gilson in MRC Pneumoconiosis Unit in South Wales, brought the concept of standardized population-based respiratory disease surveys to his studies in Berlin, NH, where he used the MRC Standardized Respiratory Disease Questionnaire along with pulmonary function testing in cross-sectional assessments of the associations between smoking, occupational, and environmental exposures and chronic respiratory disease morbidity (Anderson and Ferris 1962). It was also at about this time that the Framingham Study (a community-based study of 6000 residents of a small Massachusetts town) began to include regular assessments of pulmonary function as part of its repeated clinical assessments.

To test the 'Dutch hypothesis', there needed to be developed reliable, standardized tests of airway reactivity that could be used in community settings. Much of the effort in the 1960s was directed toward the establishment of protocols for such tests, and it was not until much later that these tests became used in population-based surveys.

In the 1970s, through initiatives established by the National Institutes of Health in the USA, studies were designed to follow population-based samples prospectively across time to test the importance of a number of risk factors for the establishment of COPD. Similar investigations were begun in Europe. These efforts established what came to be called by some as the recurrent wave design in which cohorts of subjects were followed for upwards of 15–20 years with repeated assessments for the development of COPD as defined by standardized questionnaires or change in pulmonary function. The idea behind these studies was that through studying a wide spectrum of overlapping age groups, investigators could piece together the natural history of the development of COPD. Along the way specific hypotheses were used to test prospectively the impact of putative risk factors. Within the first group of studies a revival of interest in the familial patterns of COPD, exclusive of asthma, and the application of methods of population genetics to the subject was initiated (Tager *et al.* 1977; Lewitter *et al.* 1984).

Over the past 25–30 years several aspects of the British and Dutch hypotheses have been elucidated and, to some extent, parts of each hypothesis have been supported Airway hyper-responsiveness has been associated with decreased growth (Redline *et al.* 1989) and accelerated decline in lung function (Rijcken *et al.* 1995). Mucus hypersecretion also has been associated with increased declines in lung function, even after adjustment for smoking history (Sherman *et al.* 1992), and mucus hypersecretion, independent of lung function and smoking, has been associated with increased mortality, in part associated with infection (Annesi and Kauffmann 1986; Prescott *et al.* 1995). Clearly, cigarette smoking plays a major role in the development of COPD. However, although most active smokers will have respiratory symptoms, only about 15–20% actually progress to develop irreversible obstructive pulmonary disease, i.e. clinically recognizable consequences of airway obstruction and/or mucus hypersecretion (see above). Moreover, cigarette smoking decreases the maximum level of growth of lung function (Wang *et al.* 2004) and accelerates the age at which decline in lung function begins (Tager *et al.* 1988). In children, *in utero* and passive exposure to tobacco smoke products is associated with reduced airway size and increased airway reactivity (Hanrahan *et al.* 1992). Children who live in smoking households have lower lung capacity and lower lung function later in life (Cunningham *et al.* 1994), and second-hand exposure in adult life also appears to be associated with decreased lung function (Kauffmann *et al.* 1983). Furthermore, children tend to track in the growth of their pulmonary function, and thus, those with early life exposures and lower lung function tend not to reach their predicted maximum level of function. Once maximum level of pulmonary function is obtained, smokers tend to lose function from that level at a faster rate than non-smokers. Among smokers there are subgroups who are destined to become patients with COPD, and this group makes up about a quarter of all smokers who lose pulmonary function the fastest. Of interest, if one restricts the loss to this lower quartile of the population the rate of loss of lung function in these relatively healthy (or at least uncomplaining subgroups) is on average equivalent to the rate of loss recorded in patients initially seen by physicians because of respiratory complaints (Fig. 8.2).

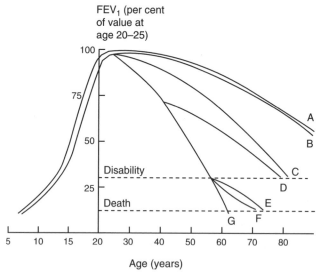

Fig. 8.2 Theoretical curves representing varying rates of changed in FEV by age. Curve A represents normal decline in FEV_1. Curve B shows less than optimal development of normal lung function. Often, the disability-related decline continues as a variable-rate curve (C). Curve D shows the effect of smoking cessation; also seen in disabled individuals (curve E). Curve F is a disability-related decline continuing at a variable rate. Curve G represents the accelerating decline in FEV_1 with cigarette smoking and continuing rapid decline until death as a consequence of respiratory failure. Reproduced with permission from Bumgarner JR and Speizer FE (1991). Chronic obstructive pulmonary disease. *In Disease control priorities in developing countries* (ed. DT Jamison, WH Mosley, AR Measham, and JL Bobadilla), p. 596. World Bank/Oxford University Press, New York/Oxford.)

Much of the epidemiological research in the last 15 years, not counting the various clinical trials of both therapeutic agents and efforts at smoking cessation, has been directed to identifying the characteristics of these subgroups at risk before clinical disease is apparent. Data obtained from laboratory studies of both humans and animals have suggested mechanisms of injury that could be tested in population samples. For example, the recent editorial by Nadel (2005) comments on the role of clearance, mucin production, epidermal growth factors, and receptors, and Shapiro (2003) discusses how matrix metalloprotease inhibitors may play a role in COPD. With the completion of the Human Genome Project in 1999, and the more recent development of the Human Haplotype Genome Map, the opportunities to carry out population-based genetic studies in phenotypically well-characterized human samples of sufficient size to assess risk for particular mechanisms of injury suggest a paradigm shift in epidemiological research in respiratory disease. As the technology is further developed, first with family studies of putative genetic markers of injury pathways and subsequently through the application of whole-genome scans, one can anticipate further discovery of risk profiles of gene–environment interactions that will have both risk predictive as well as potentially therapeutic value. Much of the potential in this area is summarized in the recent efforts of an international collaborative group to bring the fields of respiratory medicine, epidemiology, and genetics together (Silverman *et al.* 2005.) To carry out such studies will require the continued collaborations of a large number of scientific disciplines: because of the obvious importance of smoking (which unfortunately will not go away) and the well-characterized effect of smoking on chronic respiratory diseases, the respiratory epidemiologist of the twenty-first century must be trained and prepared to work in these areas.

References

Anderson DO and Ferris BG Jr (1962). Role of tobacco smoking in the causation of chronic respiratory disease. *New England Journal of Medicine*, **267**, 787–94.

Annesi I and Kauffmann F (1986). Is respiratory mucus hypersecretion really an innocent disorder? *American Review of Respiratory Disease*, **134**, 688–93.

Badham C (1808). *Observations on the inflammatory affections of the mucous membrane of the bronchie.* Callow, London.

Bell ML and Davis DL (2001). Reassessment of the lethal London Fog of 1952: Novel indicators of acute and chronic consequences of acute exposure to air pollution. *Environmental Health Perspectives*, **109**, S389–S395.

Burrows B and Earle RH (1969). Course and prognosis of chronic obstructive lung disease. *New England Journal of Medicine*, **280**, 398–404.

Ciba Guest Symposium (1959). Terminology, definitions, and classification of chronic pulmonary emphysema and related conditions. *Thorax*, **14**, 286–99.

Collis EL (1923). The general and occupational prevalence of bronchitis and its relation to other respiratory diseases. *Journal of Industrial Hygiene and Toxicology*, **5**, 264–76.

Cunningham J, Dockery DW, and Speizer FE (1994). Maternal smoking during pregnancy as a predictor of lung function in children. *American Journal of Epidemiology*, **139**, 1139–52.

Doll R and Hill AB (1950). A study of the aetiology of carcinoma of the lung. *British Medical Journal*, **2**, 740–48.

Ferris BG (1978). Epidemiology standardization project. *American Review of Respiratory Disease*, **118** (Suppl.).

Firket J (1931). Sur les causes des accidents survenus dans la vallée de la Meuse, lors des brouillards de décembre 1930. *Bulletin Academie Royale Medicine Belgique*, **11**, 683–741.

Fletcher CM (1970). Summary of the session on epidemiology of chronic non-specific lung disease (CNSLD). In *Bronchitis III Proceedings of the Third International Symposium on Bronchitis at Groningen, the Netherlands* (ed. NGM Orie, R Van Der Lende, C Charles, and A Thomas), p.138. Royal Van Gorcum, Assen, The Netherlands.

Fletcher CM, Peto R, Tinker CM, and Speizer FE (1976). *The natural history of chronic bronchitis: An eight year follow-up study of working men in London.* Oxford University Press, Oxford.

Gaensler EA (1951). An instrument for dynamic vital capacity measurements. *Science,* 114, 114.

Gandevia B and Hugh-Jones P (1957). Terminology for measurements of ventilatory capacity. *Thorax,* 12, 290–3.

Hanrahan JP, Tager IB, Segal MR, *et al.* (1992). The effect of maternal smoking during pregnancy on early infant lung function. *American Review of Respiratory Disease,* 145, 1129–35.

Higgins MW, Keller JB, Landis JR, *et al.* (1984). Risk of chronic obstructive pulmonary disease: collaborative assessment of the validity of the Tecumseh Index of Risk. *American Review of Respiratory Disease,* 130, 380–5.

Hogg JC, Macklem PT, and Thurlbeck WM (1968). Site and nature of airways obstruction in chronic obstructive lung disease. *New England Journal of Medicine,* 278, 1355–60.

Holland WW (1979). Health effects of particulate pollution: reappraising the evidence. *American Journal of Epidemiology,* 110, 527.

Holland WW and Reid DD (1965). The urban factor in chronic bronchitis. *Lancet,* 1, 445–8.

Hutchinson J (1846). On the capacity of the lungs, and on the respiratory functions, with a view of establishing a precise and easy method of detecting disease by the spirometer. *Medico-Chirurgical Transactions,* 29, 137–252.

Kauffmann F, Tessier JF, and Oriol P (1983). Adult passive smoking in the home environment: a risk factor for chronic airflow limitation. *American Journal of Epidemiology,* 117, 269–80.

Levin ML, Goldstein H, and Gerhardt PR (1950). Cancer and tobacco smoking. A preliminary report. *Journal of the American Medical Association,* 143, 329–36.

Lewitter FI, Tager IB, Tishler PV, Speizer FE, and McGue M (1984). Genetic and environmental determinants of level of pulmonary function. *American Journal of Epidemiology,* 120, 518–30.

Medical Research Council (1960). Standardized questionnaire on respiratory symptoms. *British Medical Journal,* 2, 1665.

Ministry of Health (1954). *Mortality and morbidity during the London fog of December 1952.* Her Majesty's Stationery Office, London.

Nadel JA (2005). Role of the airway epithelium in defense against inhaled invaders. *COPD,* 3, 285–7.

O'Conner G (2006). ATS-DLD revised respiratory questionnaire project 2006 (personal communication).

Orie NGM, Sluiter HJ, Vries K, DeTameling GJ, and Witkop J (1961). The host factor in bronchitis. In *Bronchitis, an International Symposium* (ed. NGM Orie and HJ Sluiter). Royal Van Gorcum, Assen, The Netherlands. pp.43–59.

Peto R, Speizer FE, Cochrane AL, *et al.* (1983). The relevance in adults of airflow obstruction, but not of mucus hypersecretion, to mortality from chronic lung disease: Results from 20 years of prospective observation. *American Review of Respiratory Disease,* 128, 491–500.

Prescott E, Lange P, and Vestbo J (1995). Chronic mucus hypersecretion in COPD and death from pulmonary infection. *European Respiratory Journal,* 8, 1333–8.

Redline S, Tager IB, Segal MR, Gold D, Speizer FE, and Weiss ST (1989). The relationship between longitudinal change in pulmonary function and nonspecific airway responsiveness in children and young adults. *American Review of Respiratory Disease,* 140, 179–84.

Rijcken B, Schouten J, Xu X, Rosner B, and Weiss S (1995). Airway responsiveness to histamine associated with accelerated decline in FEV_1. *American Journal of Respiratory and Critical Care Medicine,* 151, 1377–82.

Samet JM (1978). A historical and epidemiologic perspective on respiratory symptom questionnaires. *American Journal of Epidemiology,* 108, 435–46.

Schrenk HH, Hermann H, Clayton GD, and Gafater WM (1949). *Air pollution in Donora, PA,* Public Health Bulletin 306. Government Printing Office, Washington, DC.

Shapiro SD (2003). Proteolysis in the lung. *European Respiratory Journal,* 22, S30–S32.

Sherman CB, Xu X Speizer FE, Ferris BG Jr, Weiss ST, and Dockery DW (1992). Longitudinal lung function decline in subjects with respiratory symptoms. *American Review of Respiratory Disease*, **146**, 855–9.

Silverman EK, Shapiro SD, Oomas DA, and Weiss ST (2005). *Respiratory genetics*. Hodder Arnold, London.

Speizer FE and Tager IB (1979). Epidemiology of chronic mucus hypersecretion and obstructive airways disease. *Epidemiologic Reviews*, **1**, 124–42.

Tager I, Tishler PV, Rosner B, Speizer FE, and Litt M (1979). Studies of the familial aggregation of chronic bronchitis and obstructive airways disease. *International Journal of Epidemiology*, **7**, 55–62.

Tager IB, Segal MR, Speizer FE, and Weiss ST (1988). The natural history of forced expiratory volumes: effect of cigarette smoking and respiratory symptoms. *American Review of Respiratory Disease*, **138**, 837–49.

Tiffeneau R and Pinelli A (1947). Air circulant et air captive dans l'exploration de la function vertilatirse pulmonaire. *Paris Medicine*, **37**, 624–8.

Wang X, Mensinga TT, Schouten JP, Rijcken B, and Weiss ST (2004). Determinants of maximally attained level of pulmonary function. *American Journal of Respiratory and Critical Care Medicine*, **169**, 941–9.

Wellcome Witnesses to Twentieth Century Medicine (2002). *Population-based research in South Wales. The MRC Pneumoconiosis Research Unit and the MRC Epidemiology Unit*, Wellcome Witnesses to Twentieth Century Medicine Vol. 13 (available at http://www.ucl.ac.uk/histmed/publications/wellcome-witnesses/witness13.html).

Winslow C-EA, Smillie WG, Doull A, and Gordon JE (ed.) (1952). *The history of American epidemiology*. CV Mosby Co., St Louis.

Wynder EL and Graham EA (1950). Tobacco smoking as a possible etiologic factor in bronchogenic carcinoma. *Journal of the American Medical Association*, **143**, 329–36.

9

The epidemiological study of mental disorders since the beginning of the twentieth century

Rebecca Fuhrer and Lee Robins

Personal experiences

The authors began their respective careers in psychiatric epidemiology at different points in its evolution during the second half of the twentieth century. The contributions and accomplishments of one of them (L.R.) greatly influenced the other (R.F.)

Lee Robins received her PhD in sociology from Harvard University and began her research career by designing an interview study of attitudes toward birth control. She had learned how to conduct such studies while working in the US Government's Division of Program Surveys, which later moved to the University of Michigan as the Center for Behavioral Science. Next, in the Department of Psychiatry at Washington University, she followed into their forties children who had attended one of the first child guidance clinics in the United States. She selected from public school records of that era a control group who had grown up in the same neighbourhoods as the clinic patients. She found the two samples equally locatable and equally agreeable to be interviewed about their childhoods and their current mental health. Clinic-referred antisocial boys had as adults an excess of antisocial personality and psychoses. Because the juvenile court, which the clinic served, might somehow have selected for referral youngsters particularly likely to develop adult mental disorders, she repeated her study in young black men selected from St Louis public school records of the 1930s, a truly epidemiological sample. Not only did it confirm the earlier findings, but it provided the first study of heroin use in a general population. That in turn led to an invitation to lead a study of drug use after return to the United States by soldiers exposed to heroin in Vietnam. She next attempted to explain why white older men have more suicides than do black men. She did a comparison of disability in in-patients and then in men on pensions. She found that white pensioners were more unhappy about their retirements and less happy with how they are treated by their families. They were also less religious than the black men, and therefore less anxious about disapproval by God if they committed suicide. Her next project aimed at translating the 'department interview', a list of symptoms with unwritten but carefully followed traditions for combining them into major psychiatric diagnoses, into a fully structured interview scored by computer. The comparability of its results when used by trained lay interviewers to the results of the department interview given by psychiatrists had just been established when an interview to be used in the Epidemiologic Catchment Area (ECA) study was sought by the National Institute of Mental Health. The Diagnostic Interview Schedule was selected, and Lee Robins became one of the principal investigators for that large epidemiological study. She is a member of the WHO scientific advisory board for the Composite International Diagnostic Interview (CIDI).

Rebecca Fuhrer trained in psychology (CUNY, Brooklyn College) and then in medical information science at the University of California, San Francisco (UCSF). As a research assistant in psychiatric research at the Langley Porter Neuropsychiatric Institute, UCSF, in the 1970s she queried the selection of study subjects to explore the nature of psychopathology. It seemed that the volunteer nature of some, and the 'patient' origins of the others, did not provide any representation of the population at large. Furthermore, diagnostic practices seemed to vary by practitioner, which meant fuzzy patients groups that were less than homogeneous. Fuhrer's original intention was develop expert medical decision support systems. She realized that medical decision-making could only be as effective as the knowledge base about pathology, its signs and symptoms, its course, and risk factors. This redirection encouraged her to move towards research that would augment the knowledge base, i.e. epidemiology. Although Fuhrer started conducting psychiatric epidemiological research in 1982 when she moved to France and joined INSERM (Institut National de la Santé et de la Recherche Médicale), the former experiences had left their mark. The ECA studies had just started to publish their findings in 1984. French psychiatric epidemiology at that time was primarily based on hospitalized patients and grounded in the use of administrative data with limited clinical validity and reliability. French psychiatry was only just starting to develop an empirically based perspective. Inspired by the British studies of mental disorders in general practice patients, a large scale study of 367 GPs and over 5000 patients was undertaken to study depression and its treatment. Subsequently, she became involved in a large-scale community-based study of cognitive aging and the role of depression in this declining process. Following a move to the UK, Fuhrer continued to study depression and its social determinants in an occupational cohort of British civil servants. She is currently working to strengthen and further develop psychiatric epidemiology at McGill University, Montreal, Canada.

Psychiatric epidemiology at the present time is much like epidemiology in the rest of medicine. It attempts to count the prevalence and incidence of a disease or group of related diseases, in this case all specific mental disorders in the population, whether treated or untreated, and to estimate each disorder's burden in terms of morbidity and mortality. Furthermore, it seeks to identify risk and protective factors, so that prevention and treatment strategies can be designed. Indeed, psychiatric epidemiology, or the epidemiology of mental disorders, has had great visibility in the past 25 years and research findings have led the World Health Organization (WHO) to claim that one mental disorder, depression, alone accounts for more disability and loss of years of active and productive life than does any physical illness.

1901–60

Early epidemiology primarily studied causes of death. Although those affected by mental disorder do have a shortened life expectancy from suicide, homicide, complications of alcohol, tobacco, and other drug addictions, and during the first half of the twentieth century, from complications of institutionalization, such as poor diet and infection, the specific cause of death is not often a mental disorder *per se*. Interestingly, statistics of insanity were collected from the mid to late nineteenth century, mostly reporting on the inhabitants of asylums that were created for the pauper insane. Although the statistics collected were primarily limited to the asylums, suicide statistics were one exception. The use of epidemiological approaches to shed light on mental disorders not necessitating hospitalization is a modern phenomenon. More recently, the motivation for an epidemiology of mental disorders has roots in different types of questions and hypotheses in contrast to the statistics of insanity or causes of death or, later on, morbidity, and has been carried out by social scientists in addition to psychiatrists.

A review of the epidemiological literature shows that psychiatric epidemiology has not been part of mainstream epidemiology, which might be explained in part by the state and development of psychiatry itself, including issues of psychiatric nomenclature. In the first three-quarters of the twentieth century, psychiatry's official manuals suffered from a lack of careful clinical descriptions of the symptoms and course of disorders, and rules for deciding on whether a patient qualified for a diagnosis, as illustrated by the Diagnostic and Statistical Manual (DSM) editions I and II (American Psychiatric Association 1952 and 1968) and the International Classification of Diseases (ICD) (World Health Organization 1957) editions prior to ICD-8

(World Health Organization 1968). In the early 1960s, the mental health programme of the WHO became actively engaged in aiming to improve the diagnosis and classification of mental disorders. Based on consultations with a wide range of experts from different disciplines, from various schools of psychiatry, and from all parts of the world, numerous proposals were made to improve the classification of mental disorders, and the 1970s saw further growth of interest in improving classification in many countries. Over time, these diagnostic descriptions and guidelines moved further away from theoretical implications.

All the while, in clinical practice, there was doubt, particularly in the United States and France, that psychiatric diagnosis was meaningful because, under the influence of Freud, many psychiatrists and social scientists thought that all psychiatric disorders shared common causes. Therefore, the particular pattern of symptoms was important only as a symbolic disclosure of the traumas of childhood that accounted for them.

Another heritage from Freud's writings was the conviction on the part of social scientists that the general population would be likely to be in denial about, to minimize, or to have forgotten ('repressed') their mental symptoms. Thus, it was the clinician or interviewer's job to help the subject express and recall them. This view resulted in early studies that asked about symptoms without inquiring about their severity and duration, or the impairment they caused. Such interviews did not eliminate transient feelings and concerns that are the common problems of everyday life. Nor did they inquire about age of onset or history of remissions to learn whether the course fitted clinically defined descriptions. The interviews were based on experience with psychiatric patients, with little or insufficient knowledge about the occurrence of these symptoms in the general population. As one might expect, these methods led the early studies to report very high proportions of the populations as having mental disorders, leading to what was often jocular treatment in the public media.

Many of the issues raised were inherent to the field of psychiatric epidemiology regardless of the country in which the study was conducted. To a large extent, the developments described are based on the US experience; the last half century has been not very different in other countries. Michael Shepherd at the Institute of Psychiatry in London trained several generations of epidemiological psychiatrists and left his imprint on rigorous modern methods applied to the epidemiology of mental disorders, with emphasis on the disorders most frequent in primary care. He founded the journal *Psychological Medicine* as a forum for methodological and substantive articles, and remained its editor for over 20 years until he retired (Williams *et al.* 1989).

While the evolution of the field was also similar in France in some ways, the timeline and turning points were also culture bound. The use of psychological testing had been part of clinical culture specific to Hôpital Sainte Anne in Paris under the influence of Jean Delay, and then Pierre Pichot, starting in the late 1940s. Their work on diagnosis and measurement was exemplary for that time, but limited to the world of biological psychiatry and the treatment of the severe mental disorders in the hospitals and asylums. These schools were seriously engaged in developing treatments and they applied scientific rigour in order to arrive at homogeneous groups of patients. Although services for outpatients and community-based pathology were organized into catchment areas as early as the 1960s, the epidemiological study of these areas did not seem to be a priority. Statistics on causes of hospitalization were routinely collected and analysed with a quasi-actuarial approach, but studies of general population samples or of persons registered with general practices were virtually unheard of prior to the 1980s. This was the beginning of a new wave, and followed in the footsteps of the ECA community-based samples in the USA and the UK studies in general practice.

In the USA, the earliest method for determining mental health problems, in non-patient populations, was developed for purposes for which diagnosis was irrelevant. This was a result of the observation that during the selection of draftees for the US military in the Second World War there were extremely variable rates of rejection by draft boards for psychiatric causes. It was believed that these differences were much more likely to be explained by the different beliefs and methods of the doctors evaluating the men than by variation in mental health in different areas of residence. To solve this problem, Shirley Star (a psychologist) (Star 1950) was asked to create a standardized interview for doctors to use. Not a psychiatrist herself, she used the items in the Minnesota Multiphasic Personality Inventory (MMPI) (Hathaway 1951), without the scoring system that transformed the answers into dimensional scores related to diagnosis, but not into diagnoses. Ironically, Star's interview never served its original purpose—selecting draftees—because the war ended before it was completed.

The early interviews used in epidemiological studies in the USA and Canada were based on Star's interview, assessing 'mental health' or 'mental disorder' without specifying a diagnosis e.g. the Home Interview Survey (HIS) (Langner 1962) used in the Midtown Manhattan Study (Srole *et al.* 1962) and the Health Opinion Survey (HOS) (MacMillan 1957) used in the Stirling County study (Leighton *et al.* 1963).

Not only did these early studies fail to make specific psychiatric diagnoses, they always counted as psychiatric those symptoms which are common in both psychiatric and physical diseases, such as fatigue, lack of appetite, weakness, and insomnia, without eliminating those that might well have been explained by a concomitant physical illness. A similar disregard for diagnosis was common in the UK, where a commonly used epidemiological instrument was the General Health Questionnaire (GHQ) (Goldberg 1972), which collected symptoms chiefly of depression and anxiety, and counted them to decide whether a respondent was positive or negative for unspecified mental disorder. Epidemiological studies that did pay attention to diagnosis (e.g. Hollingshead and Redlich 1958) relied on psychiatrists' records, without checking the validity of that diagnosis. Not until H. Warren Dunham's (1965) study of schizophrenia was there attention by epidemiologists to correcting hospital diagnoses.

Unlike their English-speaking counterparts, Scandinavians and Germans conducted psychiatric epidemiological studies in confined areas—an island or a county or city or a small country—where the researchers were often the local psychiatrists personally familiar with the clinical history of those who had received treatment. The researchers were also the interviewers. The subjects to be interviewed were often not a sample, but rather every resident of a small area (e.g. Fremming 1951; Essen-Moller 1956; Hagnell 1966; Helgason 1964). These studies did not use standardized questions. Rather, the psychiatrist typically carried a list of topics to be addressed, and made a diagnosis on the spot. By contrast, Helgason's work was exemplary in that he brought his observations to a group of five psychiatrists who had been his mentors during his residency, and this group worked on achieving diagnostic consensus. While Helgason was a psychiatrist himself, he did the study while in training as a resident, and felt the need for his seniors' agreement with his judgement. Interestingly, Helgason's father was the only psychiatrist in Iceland and had treated all the 'cases'.

Even though the diagnoses made in these early European studies may have been more accurate than studies being conducted in the USA or Great Britain during this time, there were too few study subjects due to the small geographical areas of the target population to provide reliable data on any but the more common disorders.

Modern psychiatric epidemiology, attempting to assess many disorders including the relatively rare ones, required large samples. Large samples, collected over a short period to avoid the effects of historical change, are simply not achievable if the interviewers have to be psychiatrists. They did and do not have the time, there are not enough of them, and their services are prohibitively expensive. There is also the problem of the reliability of the psychiatrists' diagnoses, the problem that prompted the construction of standardized questions by Shirley Star (Star 1950). Finally, there is the problem that the psychiatrists in these early studies had much more detailed information about subjects who had been in treatment than about subjects never treated. Reliable prevalence estimates require equal levels of inquiry and data about all subjects (Lapouse 1967).

Following up epidemiological samples over time is not essential to measuring the prevalence of psychiatric disorders, but it is the ideal way of estimating incidence—the frequency with which new cases appear in a defined time period. Follow-ups also reduce the length of recall requested of the subject. Some of the early studies tried only to assess current symptoms. Although not always planned in advance, several of the studies in both North America and Europe followed up their samples after a number of years to learn about the incidence of new cases and the remission of cases identified originally. This allowed the exploration of risk and protective factors that determined who became psychiatrically ill and who among the ill recovered.

Improving diagnosis and counting the prevalence of a broad spectrum of disorders

By the mid-1970s a number of events converged to convince the US National Institute of Mental Health (NIMH) and the WHO's Division of Mental Health that something had to be done to obtain more and better information about the prevalence of mental disorders. The lack of adequate information became painfully obvious when the NIMH was endeavouring to gather data for the President's Commission on Mental Health (Carter 1978). The Commission's goal was to determine how many people had psychiatric disorders and how many of those affected were in appropriate treatment and how many were not. It was glaringly clear that the numbers were just not available; nor was there any agreement on how to obtain those numbers. There was, moreover, growing consensus that the breadth of mental disorders went far beyond the severe psychiatric diseases that were treated in psychiatric hospitals.

In the same period, i.e. the mid to late 1970s, NIMH funded a study on the course of depressive illnesses, and appointed both Eli Robins at Washington University and Robert Spitzer at Columbia University to the small group of psychiatrists leading that study (Spitzer *et al.* 1978). The Washington University Department of Psychiatry was unique in this period for its lack of interest in psychoanalysis and its view that psychiatric disorders should be studied and treated in the same way that medicine approached physical disorders. For researchers at Washington University diagnosis was a prime interest. In the years leading up to the NIMH study, the Department of Psychiatry had developed criteria to identify and study 14 of the most common psychiatric disorders. The criteria included a minimum number of symptoms, a method for excluding symptoms caused by physical illness, minimum criteria for severity, clinical significance, and course as described by ages of onset, remissions, and relapses. Dr Spitzer, with a long-standing interest in computer scoring of diagnoses, was persuaded that these criteria should be used in the depression study. This was the start of a paradigm shift in the study, diagnosis, and understanding of mental illness that extended beyond the Washington University Department of Psychiatry.

The remarkable next event was that Dr Spitzer was asked by the American Psychiatric Association to lead the production of the third edition of the DSM (DSM-III American Psychiatric Association 1980), and he decided to follow Washington University's pattern for systematic diagnosis in that volume, abandoning the aetiological emphasis common to DSM-II (American Psychiatric Association 1968) and psychoanalysis. This dropping of an aetiological emphasis was an important shift in philosophy for psychiatry, which lacked objective methods of confirming diagnoses with blood cultures, x-rays, and biopsies that verify the presence and cause of many physical disorders.

In those days, the Washington University Psychiatry Department was doing clinical research using what was called the 'department interview'. In appearance, it looked much like the interview forms used in Scandinavian epidemiological studies—a mere list of topics that the clinician was to cover. However, the department had also developed a tradition of how to ask about each topic and how to evaluate the responses. While not written down at that time, these traditional elements were explained to young psychiatrists and were observable on videotapes made for training.

One of the authors (L.R.) and a group of other department members were interested in using 500 department interviews from a clinical study of outpatients to see whether the interview could be shortened without changing the diagnostic outcome. When symptoms were found to be necessary, fully specified questions were written for them. However, there was no way to validate the shortened version without writing a full version, with identical questions plus questions to cover rejected symptoms so that a fair test of the screening instrument could be made. Computer programs were written to score the responses in the way traditionally done. Tests were conducted to demonstrate that the fully specified version was valid and reliable. Validity was evaluated by agreement between diagnoses when the instrument was given by a lay interviewer and scored by computer, and when it was given by a clinician. Reliability was evaluated by the level of agreement between two lay interviewers conducting independent interviews. Shortly after this work that established the validity and reliability of the instrument (Robins *et al.* 1981), NIMH began searching for an instrument to use in a large epidemiological study.

The large epidemiological survey of psychiatric disorders was planned and intended to provide the information needed to fulfil the objectives of the President's Commission, and so the Epidemiological Catchment Area (ECA) Study was born (Robins and Regier 1991). It was also used to ascertain a count of cases diagnosed according to the soon to be published DSM-III rules, while additionally providing an investigation of the use of treatment services by those who had a positive score. The interview composed by Lee Robins' group was selected as the model for that study and revised to match DSM-III. Drs Spitzer and Endicott collaborated in its revision to create the Diagnostic Interview Schedule (DIS-III). This was not a difficult task because the DSM-III had in large part been based on the research diagnostic criteria, which had grown out of the Spitzer, Endicott, and Eli Robins' modifications of the department interview.

Because NIMH had sponsored the DIS, it was selected for a host of other studies, in part because the principal investigators felt that using it improved their chances of getting a grant and also for reasons of comparability. It was also translated into many languages for use in numerous countries. Researchers came to St Louis, MI (home to Washington University) for training and then set up training centres in their own countries. Under the auspices of the WHO, the DIS evolved into the Composite International Diagnostic Interview (CIDI) (Robins *et al.* 1988). The CIDI maintained many of the features of the DIS but allowed for arriving at both DSM and ICD diagnoses. Large-scale studies were undertaken in parallel in many countries using this instrument, including most recently in the WHO World Mental Health surveys of over 60,000 community-based adults in 14 countries (World Health Organization 2004).

It seems clear that the DIS marked a major turning point in the field of mental health epidemiology. Studies were now able to be standardized by using the same questions and scored by the same computer algorithms. As a result, studies conducted in different settings could be compared, allowing researchers to identify different patterns of psychiatric disorders in different cultures, and to determine whether risk factors and treatment provision differed. Because the questions covered the whole lifetime, it was possible to see whether recovery was more rapid and more complete in some settings than in others.

With more thorough and accurate modes of study, researchers in mental health epidemiology were able to ascertain far more detailed results than ever before. While fruitful and informative, these results were also very sobering, highlighting that psychiatric disorders were very common and that there were not nearly enough psychiatrists, psychologists, and social workers to treat them all. Additionally, many of the affected did not want treatment, either because they had already had it without great success, because they thought they could handle their psychiatric problems on their own, or because they had little expectation of treatment success. Moreover, many of the current patients did not meet full criteria for a disorder, but nonetheless wanted help. Given all this, it was painfully obvious that the Presidential Commission's original view that treatment could be and should be available to everyone with a psychiatric illness was overly idealistic.

Identifying the target population

Whereas earlier epidemiological studies used small geographically defined samples, the new epidemiology of psychiatric disorders challenged the appropriateness of this approach for estimating prevalence and incidence in order to identify service needs. Survey methodology was brought to bear on selecting appropriate samples of the target populations, large enough to ensure sufficient numbers of cases and cases in treatment. One large and interesting study was the WHO Collaborative Study of schizophrenia that was conducted in 12 countries and provided strong support that incidence of the first-contact episode was similar across different cultures, but that prognosis appeared to be better in less industrialized cultures. This study had as its focus the determinants of outcome, and used a facilities-based approach for sampling given the rarity (1%) of the disorder (Jablensky *et al.* 1992). The typical case–control study approach used in other areas of epidemiology was barely used in psychiatric epidemiology. This could be explained by various factors that are inherent to the case–control design and the very nature of psychiatric pathology, particularly the differentiation of mild cases from the normal experiences of everyday life. Another reason, however, was that much of psychiatric epidemiology for the latter quarter of the twentieth century was oriented to the identification of unmet health-care needs, and the case–control method does not provide these data.

Prevalence and annual incidence studies can contribute to estimating service needs, but are far more problematic for identifying risk and protective factors. Prospective studies of birth cohorts are demonstrating that many adult-onset disorders actually are manifest in childhood or adolescence, but go unrecognized or not identified as reflecting psychopathology amenable to intervention. This means that, ideally, studies of aetiology or vulnerability should start as early as possible, preferably at or even before birth, and the UK birth cohort studies are examples. Other studies in different countries have modelled themselves on these influential studies. But with few exceptions, most of the birth cohorts were assessing a diversity of factors and diseases, and could not monopolize the time needed to evaluate psychopathology across the lifecourse. Without relevant study findings, prevention strategies are compromised and unlikely to succeed.

The challenge for identifying the target population in the study of psychiatric disorders is linked to the strong potential for selection bias. By sampling only within community-based households, some subgroups at high risk of mental disorders were ineligible for study inclusion. Most surveys sample households, choosing one resident from each. This design misses small, but important, subgroups at high risk of mental disorder: the homeless and those in prisons.

Some mental illnesses can interfere with social trajectories, thereby overlooking and excluding the subjects from identification and study participation. Mental illnesses that begin in childhood, adolescence, and young adulthood (such as schizophrenia or early onset depression), often interfere with family formation or make families exceptionally fragile and can also interfere with steady employment. Consequently, those affected with mental illness who do not have families willing and able to support them may become homeless or hospitalized.

Mental illnesses that start with substance abuse have a tendency to involve illegal behaviours such as public drunkenness or possession of illicit drugs, leading to incarceration, as do the impulsive or aggressive behaviours symptomatic of mania, antisocial personality disorder, psychosis, and drug intoxication.

Because of the association of mental illness with homelessness, incarceration, and hospitalization, epidemiological methods limited to samples living in households underestimate both the proportion of the population affected and the average severity of their disorders. The ECA did sample penal and psychiatric institutions, but not the homeless. Since then, studies of the homeless have been conducted (North *et al.* 1996) demonstrating very high rates of psychopathology in these populations and likewise for studies for prison populations (Teplin 1990).

While long-term hospitalization has become uncommon in recent years, it still occurs, particularly for people judged not to be guilty of a crime by reason of insanity, for those too difficult to manage at home because of diseases such as dementia, or for patients without family to assume care when they are ready for release.

The scope of psychiatric epidemiological studies

Most epidemiological studies are designed around one disease or a group of related diseases, or exposures. No epidemiological study has covered every psychiatric diagnosis listed in the official manuals. In the first place, there are simply too many disorders to allow evaluating them all in a single interview. Also, there are disorders that have to be omitted because the diagnostic manuals do not list their criteria in sufficient detail to guide their translation into a set of structured questions. For example, in recent studies, investigators have chosen to omit disorders that previous epidemiological studies have found to be rare, such as anorexia nervosa and somatization disorder. One important study has artificially made the common disorder dementia rare by setting its sample's upper age limit below the age at which dementias become common (Kessler *et al.* 1994). Some common and well-described disorders have been dropped or made optional because they are thought to be 'sensitive', including antisocial personality, dependence on 'hard' drugs (Kessler *et al.* 1994), and sexual and gender identity disorders (ECA). Dropping 'sensitive' disorders has occurred either because the institutional review boards or government agencies (Office of Management and Budget (OMB)) have prohibited their inclusion or the investigators' fear that the questions needed to evaluate them would upset respondents or discomfit interviewers. In some studies of current disorders, interviews have avoided disorders the symptoms of which include current risk of violence or child neglect. Learning about them would violate confidentiality because the study would be obliged to report the respondent to the authorities.

This incomplete coverage of disorders in mental health epidemiological studies means that estimates of the total burden of mental disorder obtained by these studies is not a meaningful number in itself, nor is the comparison of this total across studies informative. Its only legitimate use is within a single study, where the proportion with any covered disorder can be compared across genders, age cohorts, historical eras, etc. This is because all subsamples of that study had been evaluated for the same disorders.

A measure rarely used in other areas of epidemiology is the notion of 'lifetime prevalence', i.e. the prevalence of a specific disorder over the lifetime. This has been assessed retrospectively, and so recall bias, selection bias, and healthy survivors can influence the results obtained by underestimating the true extent of pathology.

Multiple diagnoses and comorbidity

The issue of multiple diagnoses has long concerned psychiatry. All editions of the DSM have had exclusion rules in which some diagnoses for which enough positive symptoms are present to qualify are excluded if the symptoms occur only in the presence of another disorder assumed to explain them. For example, DSM-IV notes that positive symptoms of generalized anxiety do not qualify if the anxiety and worry are only about symptoms of other disorders for which the person also qualifies or if they occur only during post-traumatic stress disorder; similarly, pathological gambling is not diagnosed if it occurs only during an episode of mania. In the absence of such specified exceptions, multiple diagnoses are allowed. In the original DSM (1952), drug addiction could be a secondary diagnosis when the patient had another underlying disorder (although, oddly, alcohol addiction could not.) DSM-II (1968) allowed multiple diagnoses but urged parsimony, with the first diagnosis being either the one most in need of immediate treatment, the more serious one, or the underlying one. The third (1980) and fourth editions (1994) became more encouraging of multiple diagnoses: '. . . multiple diagnoses should be made when necessary to describe the current condition'. Although one diagnosis is selected as the 'principal diagnosis', i.e. the one chiefly responsible for coming to clinical attention, completeness is urged instead of parsimony.

Because epidemiological studies assess people not in treatment as well as those seeking care, the reason for coming to treatment cannot be used to decide which of multiple diagnoses is the principal one. Nor is that the best way to decide priority of diagnoses even for those in treatment, since symptoms of a less important disorder may be used to persuade a reluctant patient of the need for treatment.

In epidemiological studies, one cannot limit consideration of multiple diagnoses to the picture at the time of interview, as is frequently done in clinical practice. Because specific disorders are relatively rare in general populations, epidemiological studies typically try to maximize the opportunity to identify cases and their risk factors by asking whether a disorder occurred at any time in the respondent's lifetime. To do so, they ask when the first symptom occurred and when the most recent symptom ended. If there are multiple disorders, these questions allow investigators to decide which disorder began first and which disorders continued even when the disorder with which it had co-occurred remitted. Although a subject's recollections of their first and last symptoms may not be completely accurate, these questions provide important clues to two important issues: the frequency of concurrent disorders and the possibility that an earlier disorder may be a risk factor for a later one.

Epidemiological studies have shown that having more than one diagnosis is the norm for those with any psychiatric diagnosis (Robins and Regier 1991). This observation is unsettling to clinicians who have traditionally made only one diagnosis per patient. Indeed, it does raise questions about the validity of the current diagnostic system. If a disorder almost never appears except when comorbid with another disorder, it might better be considered a subtype of that comorbid disorder rather than an independent diagnosis. Or, it may indicate excessive specificity in the diagnostic system: for example, if a typical drug abuser takes a variety of drugs, and substitutes one for another when supplies are scarce, the user may not be a reliable informant about drugs on which he or she is dependent.

What is the current status of epidemiological studies of mental disorders?

Although we have not addressed the genetic epidemiology of psychiatric disorders, this has been ongoing as part of the nature versus nurture debate. Despite many efforts to identify the gene for pathologies such as schizophrenia and manic depressive disorder, each great discovery disappeared after attempts to replicate the findings. As the technology of genetics evolves and as the diagnostic nomenclature improves, genetic causes may be identified. But the focus more recently is not on genes versus environment, but rather on the gene–environment interaction. The methodology to study gene–environment interaction is developing and should help to disentangle the contribution of each in the presence of the other.

The goal of most of the studies carried out so far has been to assess the prevalence of disorders as described in the standard nomenclature, their risk factors and correlates, and the disabilities they account for. However, these findings from epidemiological studies that obtain the lifecourse of disorders can also be used to critique and improve the standard nomenclature. Combining the data about signs and symptoms and how they cluster together and how they evolve can contribute to defining and refining diagnostic categories and improving the validity of psychiatric diagnoses (Robins 2004).

How much have we learned and how much do we know about the epidemiology of mental disorders? We can certainly conclude that we have learned about the burden of these disorders in the community. They are far more frequent than many people, professionals included, would have thought. Also, many people remain untreated and yet recover from individual episodes, with and without subsequent relapse. The implications for the person and his/her family and community are quite different when the disorder is one of the more common ones or one of the more severe forms of pathology.

We did not discuss the epidemiological history of pediatric psychopathology during the same time period. On reason is that many of the methodological issues were not different and similarly the objectives of studies were similar to investigations in adult samples. Another reason is the fact that this would have significantly lengthened the chapter. However, it remains important to cite the early studies by Michel Rutter and colleagues that provided first estimates of psychopathology in children and adolescents (Rutter 1976). These studies were in limited geographic areas (Isle of Wight) and inner London, and used relatively standardized interviews administered by psychiatrists. The findings were important, and the studies and their instruments influenced several decades of epidemiological research on pathology in children and youth.

We have chosen to focus on the methodological developments in the last 60 years as this is where the greatest progress has taken place. As a result, we believe we know more about health service needs and we understand that differences in incidence between countries are not as great as originally thought, but the differences are more pronounced for the prevalence rates. We need better data on how to provide effective and needed treatment and preventive services, and how to fund these costly initiatives. The cost and burden to society of not addressing these needs is nonetheless more expensive, and thus must be confronted. These are the challenges for the next generation of psychiatric epidemiologists.

References

American Psychiatric Association (1968). *Diagnostic and statistical manual of mental disorders*, 3rd edn (DSM-II). American Psychiatric Association, Washington, DC.

American Psychiatric Association (1980). *Diagnostic and statistical manual of mental disorders*, 3rd edn (DSM-III). American Psychiatric Association, Washington, DC.

American Psychiatric Association (1994). *Diagnostic and statistical manual of mental disorders*, 3rd edn (DSM-IV). American Psychiatric Association, Washington, DC.American Psychiatric Association, Committee on Nomenclature and Statistics (1952). *Diagnostic and statistical manual: mental disorders*. American Psychiatric Association Mental Hospital Service, Washington, DC.

Dunham W (1965). *Community and schizophrenia: an epidemiological analysis*. Wayne State University Press, Detroit.

Essen-Möller E, Larsson H, Uddenberg CE, and White G (1956). Individual traits and morbidity in Swedish rural populations. *Acta Psychiatrica et Neurologica Scandinavica*, Suppl. 100, 1–160.

Fremming K (1951). The expectation of mental infirmity in a sample of the Danish population, based on a biographical investigation of 5,500 persons born in the years 1883–1887. *Occasional Papers on Eugenics*, No 7. Eugenic Society, London.

Goldberg DP (1972). *The detection of psychiatric illness by questionnaire.* Oxford University Press, London.

Hagnell O (1966). *A prospective study of the incidence of mental disorder.* Norstedts Svenska Bosorlaget, Stockholm.

Hathaway SR (1951). *The Minnesota Multiphasic Personality Inventory.* Psychological Corp., New York.

Helgason T (1964). Epidemiology of mental disorders in Iceland. *Acta Psychiatrica Scandinavica,* **40**(Supp. 173), 1–258.

Hollingshead AB and Redlich FC (1958). *Social class and mental illness: a community survey.* John Wiley & Sons, New York.

Jablensky A, Sartorius N, Ernberg G, *et al.* (1992). Schizophrenia: manifestations, incidence and course in different cultures. A World Health Organization ten-country study. *Psychological Medicine Monograph,* **20**, S1–S97.

Kessler RC, McGonagle KA, Zhao S, *et al.* (1994). Lifetime and 12-month prevalence of DSM-III-R psychiatric disorders in the United States. Results from the National Comorbidity Survey. *Archives of General Psychiatry,* **51**, 8–19.

Langner TS (1962). A twenty-two item screening score of psychiatric symptoms indicating impairment. *Journal of Health and Human Behavior,* **3**, 269–76.

Lapouse R (1967). Problems in studying the prevalence of psychiatric disorder. *American Journal of Public Health,* **57**, 947–54.

Leighton DC, Harding JS, Macklin DB, Hughes CC, and Leighton AH (1963). Psychiatric findings of the Stirling County Study. *American Journal of Psychiatry,* **110**, 1021–6.

MacMillan AM (1957). The Health Opinion Survey: technique for estimating prevalence of psychoneurotic and related types of disorder in communities. *Psychological Report,* **3**(Monograph Suppl. 7), 325–39.

North CS, Smith EM, Pollio DE, Spitznagel EL (1996). Are the mentally ill homeless a distinct homeless subgroup? *Annals of Clinical Psychiatry,* **8**, 117–28.

Robins LN (2004). Using survey results to improve the validity of the standard psychiatry nomenclature. *Archives of General Psychiatry,* **61**, 1188–94.

Robins LN and Regier DA, eds. (1991). *Psychiatric disorders in America: the Epidemiological Catchment Area Study.* The Free Press, New York.

Robins LN, Helzer JE, Croughan J, Ratcliff KS (1981). National Institute of Mental Health Diagnostic Interview Schedule. Its history, characteristics, and validity. *Archives of General Psychiatry,* **38**, 381–9.

Robins LN, Wing J, Wittchen HU, *et al.* (1988). The Composite International Diagnostic Interview: an epidemiological instrument suitable for use in conjunction with different diagnostic systems and in different cultures. *Archives of General Psychiatry,* **45**, 1069–77.

Spitzer RL, Endicott J, and Robins E (1978). Research diagnostic criteria: rationale and reliability. *Archives of General Psychiatry,* **35**, 773–82.

Srole L, Langner ST, Michael MK, and Rennie TAC (1962). *Mental health in the metropolis: the Midtown Manhattan Study,* Vol. 1. McGraw-Hill, New York.

Star SA (1950). The screening of psychoneurotics in the army: technical development of tests. In *Measurement and prediction,* Vol. IV (ed. SA Stouffer, L Guttman, EA Suchman, PF Lazarsfeld, SA Star, and JA Clausen), pp. 486–567. Princeton University Press, Princeton.

Teplin LA (1990). The prevalence of severe mental disorder among male urban jail detainees: comparison with the Epidemiologic Catchment Area Program. *American Journal of Public Health,* **80**, 663–9.

Williams P, Wilkinson G, and Rawnsley K (ed.) (1999). *The scope of epidemiological psychiatry.* Routledge, London.

World Health Organization (1957, 1968). *International classification of diseases, injuries and causes of death.* WHO, Geneva.

World Health Organization World Mental Health Survey Consortium (2004). Prevalence, severity, and unmet need for treatment of mental disorders in the World Health Organization World Mental Health Surveys. *Journal of the American Medical Association,* **291**, 2581–9.

10

Perinatal epidemiology

Claude Rumeau-Rouquette and Gérard Bréart

Personal experiences

Claude Rumeau-Rouquette: In the early 1950s, epidemiology, in French medical schools covered only contagious diseases; statistics and survey methods were barely mentioned. I learnt about techniques for surveys and statistical tests in my social psychology class, which played a decisive role in the direction of my career.

When I finished medical school, in 1954, I joined the team of Daniel Schwartz, a young engineer. He had conducted research into the biology of the tobacco plant. He was then appointed to organize an investigation of the role of smoking in the aetiology of bronchial cancers, under the aegis of the Institut National d'Hygiène (INH) and the Cancer Institute (Institute Gustave Roussy (IGR)). The results were conclusive, and we extended our research to other cancers and other risk factors. I thus began studies of the aetiology and prognosis of breast and cervical cancers in 1956.

By 1962, Schwartz's team, which had initially included four people, had grown considerably. The INH allowed us to start a laboratory at IGR. It was time to explore new fields of research. The thalidomide tragedy led me to turn, in 1963, towards the domain of reproduction and perinatology.

Gérard Bréart: In the late 1960s, when I finished medical school, I was interested in epidemiological research. In1969, I decided to join the laboratory directed by Professor Daniel Schwartz and I began to work in the team of Claude Rumeau-Rouquette.

In 1970, the perinatal actions programme adopted by the government gave the opportunity to develop scientific evaluation of prevention and care. So, I participated with the team in charge of the national perinatal surveys in 1972, 1976, and 1981. At the same time, I increased the collaboration of our laboratory with maternity units, introducing the practice of randomized controlled trails to evaluate the prevention of preterm deliveries, intra-uterine growth retardation, and other neonatal anomalies.

In the 1980s, I extended my field research to the epidemiology of osteoporosis and, when I succeeded Claude Rumeau-Rouquette as director of our laboratory, our research covered the perinatal period, handicaps, and health of the mother as women at work, violence, and aging problems.

Now, as professor of epidemiology and adviser to the ministry of health I participate in the new developments of research in public health.

Major obstacles to undertaking epidemiological research on the perinatal period in 1963

Before discussing these obstacles, it must be stressed that they were much smaller than those encountered 10 years earlier. That is, the early epidemiological research in which we were involved, in 1954, had faced two major obstacles: the substantial lag of France behind other countries in the field of medical statistics and the decline in the teaching of public health. By 1963, several favourable changes had occurred, but obstacles still remained.

Several favourable changes

At this time the teaching of statistical methods was increasing. Daniel Schwartz had established courses in medical statistics (Schwartz 1963) outside medical schools, and these were attracting increasing numbers of students. Courses in epidemiology began to follow the same path (Rouquette and Schwartz 1970).

The rapid development of medical research within the INH had enabled our small team to attract young medical doctors and mathematicians. By 1962, 25 people worked together in Unit 21, one of the earliest INH laboratories. Our research, originally limited to oncology, turned towards cardiology and then reproduction. Benefiting from the experience of our English colleagues, we moved from aetiological surveys to randomized trials (Schwartz *et al.* 1960).

In 1963, public health research received a boost from the new executive director of INH, Eugène Aujaleu, who had previously had an important position at the Ministry of Health. Under his direction, INH became INSERM (Institut National de la Santé et de la Recherche Médicale). A new division was formed specializing in public health research with the aim of improving information and research for public health activities.

Major obstacles

Despite this progress, our specialization in reproductive research faced several obstacles. The first was internal—the weakness of the research team. The second was related to the very unequal development of obstetrics and paediatrics.

A tiny team

In 1963, only five people were involved in my team. The INH and the Ministry of Health, aware of the important questions raised by thalidomide, allocated us a budget large enough to recruit physicians and statisticians.

Another weakness was lack of experience. Our knowledge of statistics and epidemiology had certainly advanced in 10 years, but we knew nothing about human reproduction except what I had learned in the medical school, which was very little.

In spite of these conditions, we planned a prospective survey intended to cover 18,000 pregnancies to study the aetiology of congenital malformations. Some will be astonished at our rashness—and at that of our superiors, who trusted us. During this pioneering period, such adventures happened to others too, and surprisingly often they succeeded.

Unequal development of medicine

Paediatrics in France had progressed considerably. From the 1930s, Robert Debré and his students had conducted active clinical research on childhood diseases, especially those transmitted genetically. This momentum continued after the Second World War and, in the early 1960s, Jérôme Lejeune discovered—at the same time as Down—trisomy 21 and its consequences. During the same period, young paediatricians, such as Alexandre Minkowski, launched clinical research in newborns. Paediatric circles were very favourable to our epidemiological research and gave us active support.

It was different in obstetrics, which, overwhelmed by the baby boom, remained highly traditional. Nearly all women were delivered in obsolescent hospitals or private clinics, many poorly equipped. Nonetheless, several young obstetricians were building the foundations of modern obstetrics, leading a radical evolution that was going to surprise us. Claude Sureau in Paris (Sureau 1956) and Robert Renaud in Strasbourg had begun the electronic study of fetal heart rates and of ultrasound examination. Emile Papiernik began to develop the concept of risk (Papiernik 1969).

How epidemiology interacts with public health services and clinical medicine

These interactions differ according to the type of epidemiology. They also depend on the organization of health care and the status of clinical medicine. Before analysing several examples from the history of perinatal epidemiology, we shall look at the factors that affect these interactions, some of them specific to France.

Factors affecting the interactions

The profession of the epidemiologist is far from uniform. Some epidemiologists are especially attracted by explanatory research on the causes of disease. They tend to work closely with biologists and clinicians. Other epidemiologists turn towards more applied research, defining high-risk populations or evaluating the outcomes of prevention. This group must work with public health services. Several epidemiologists have gone further, defining what they call 'interventional epidemiology', where 'epidemiology is more of a tool for decision than for research'. In this version, ties with the public authorities become still more evident.

The interactions also vary according to the organization of health care in a given country. Before 1983, France was highly centralized: the Ministry of Health was the responsible body. Its officials often called on us to participate in their policy planning. They directly proposed some studies, financed and facilitated them, and then applied their results. Regionalization assigned responsibilities for health to the 22 regions and 96 departments of metropolitan France. They are now responsible for the repartition of hospitals and private clinics, and for maternal and child protection (PMI). Although this regionalization had important advantages, it sometimes complicated the organization of nationwide studies: we had to deal with a multiplicity of people as well as encountering local rivalries.

We must, moreover, underline the particular character of the organization of medicine in France. A few medical doctors have civil service status: public health officials, medical school professors, hospital staff physicians, and researchers in public research institutes. All other physicians, that is, the large majority, are in private practice. Patients are free to choose their practitioners. The cost of the medical procedures, of drugs, and of hospitalization is reimbursed by the national health insurance fund (sécurité sociale). The amount of these reimbursements is fixed by agreements between medical syndicates and the health insurance fund, which in turn is funded by mandatory payments by the insured and their employers. The deficit of the health insurance fund grows larger every year. The government makes up the deficit through taxes, and it intervenes more and more in the system. For example, it has just begun to limit direct access to specialists, setting up a system whereby patients are encouraged (strongly, by the reimbursement schedules) to choose a general practitioner, who is required to follow them and refer them towards any necessary speciality care. These interventions sometimes set off maelstroms in the medical profession, and they can affect the relationship of epidemiologists with physicians.

Interactions during the prospective survey on congenital malformations and perinatal risk factors (1963–70)

This study had two objectives: (1) to study the possible teratogenic effect of drugs and (2) to define the risk factors for perinatal mortality, pre-term delivery, fetal growth retardation, and fetal distress. This prospective study covered 18,000 pregnant women consulting in the public hospitals of Paris before the first trimester of pregnancy. Physician investigators interviewed the women with a predefined set of questions, and paediatricians examined the infants at birth.

Teratogenic effect of drugs

Our results concerning the teratogenic effect of drugs did not influence health policies. We found that there was no significant difference in drug intake between the mothers of malformed infants and the others, except for intake of one neuroleptic in the phenothiazine group (Rumeau-Rouquette *et al.* 1977). Studies in other countries reached similar results and raised the same suspicion about drugs affecting the central nervous system.

The Ministry of Health nonetheless reinforced the protocols for new drug experiments before their approval for marketing and strengthened their subsequent monitoring as well. Women were also advised to limit their drug use at the beginning of pregnancy. The position of the authorities was entirely justified by the time lags between the availability of research results and the need for action. Research and policy decisions take place in different time frames, which do not coincide. Moreover, policy-makers have different responsibilities from researchers. The former are sanctioned more severely for their errors and prefer to adopt what has come to be called the 'precautionary principle', reacting swiftly, without awaiting research results.

Risk factors of pre-term delivery, fetal growth retardation, and perinatal mortality

This research topic nonetheless turned out to be quite fruitful, especially for predicting pre-term delivery (Kaminski *et al.* 1973). Several risk factors were barely known at the time, such as smoking and alcohol (Goujard *et al.* 1978; Kaminski *et al.* 1978). The concept of a high-risk population became popular, and health policy-makers quickly adopted it. In the 1970s, high-risk pregnancies became the object of special measures to reinforce antenatal medical surveillance.

Obstetricians had diverse opinions about the last set of measures. They had long agreed to this monitoring for clinical risk indicators, such as hypertension or vaginal bleeding. On the other hand, consideration of social factors, such as educational level or occupational category, did not seem to them to be within their jurisdiction, so to speak. They further noted that the largest contingent of premature infants and newborns with fetal distress came from what were called 'low-risk pregnancies' because there are so many more of them. They thus feared that focusing care on high-risk pregnancies might lead to inadequate care for the others. This fear was partly justified, and the definition of low risk remains a problem today.

The concept of a high-risk population initially had beneficial effects for epidemiologists, who thus received recognition from policy-makers. It was also easier to approach than causal research. But this research pathway has shown its limitations and may have led some of us to abandon our ambition to contribute to the study of pathophysiological mechanisms.

Interactions increased during the perinatal health programme (1970–81)

The perinatal health programme and the national surveys

In 1969, the minister of health assigned a group chaired by an economist to propose actions to improve the conditions of birth.

In 1970, an inventory of needs and means was established. It was based on health statistics, the results of the prospective study described above, and their comparison with those of the British perinatal surveys conducted in 1958 and 1970. The proposals concerned the training and continuing education of medical professionals, improvement in monitoring pregnancies and deliveries, resuscitation in the delivery room, and intensive care centres.

In 1971 the government adopted a perinatal action programme and budgeted substantial funds for it. These were distributed over the next 10 years, at the same time as the government applied new standards to maternity units. The perinatal action programme also planned for the concomitant development of statistical information and research. The ministry of health asked INSERM to conduct national surveys of births. In 1972, the first survey on a representative sample of 10,000 births was conducted by us. Midwives interviewed the women and collected the clinical information after delivery. Subsequent surveys were conducted in 1976 and in 1981, according to the same procedures. These surveys made it possible to monitor trends in health indicators and to assess the impact of the perinatal action programme (Rumeau-Rouquette *et al.* 1984).

These surveys showed that the rate of pre-term deliveries dropped between 1972 and 1981, and perinatal mortality fell substantially more than expected. Monitoring of pregnancy and delivery clearly improved, at the cost, nonetheless, of an increase in the frequency of Caesarean births (Bréart and Darchy 1983). The closing of 700 maternity units that did not meet the new standards lead to a profound modification of practices.

The analysis of changes in methods of prevention and care was especially interesting, showing that the distribution of the new medical techniques differed according to social status and geographical area (Blondel *et al.* 1980). The new technologies of intrauterine diagnosis spread widely, following a geographical east–west gradient and another gradient from urban towards rural areas. Prevention methods affecting lifestyle and habits entered the population more slowly. These complex mechanisms demonstrated an increase in social inequalities, despite the general improvement in prevention.

Was this improvement in the health status of newborns linked to the prevention and information activities undertaken in 1970? There does appear to be a positive association. In support of this, we note that the government chose not to continue this programme between 1981 and 1994, during which period the pre-term delivery rate increased. Nonetheless, we must not exaggerate the effect of government programmes. The actions begun in 1971 were applied at a moment when obstetrics and neonatal medicine were taking big steps forwards in all the industrialized countries, leading to a general reduction in perinatal mortality. It is nonetheless true that the perinatal action programme had a mobilizing effect that allowed the closing of the smallest maternity units and the rapid modernization of others; it also focused the attention of physicians and prospective parents on these issues.

Relations between epidemiologists and public health services

Epidemiologists were associated with the decision-making, and then with its evaluation, which in turn led in 1976 to new reforms intended to simplify some administrative formalities and introduce a social programme. The concept of risk was widely used by the government, sometimes to extremes that complicated administrative management. Some geographical inequalities in access to care were understood better and sometimes corrected. An effort was made to remedy the class-based inequalities in pregnancy surveillance and delivery.

Nonetheless, the following example shows that some of our conclusions were not taken into account. Since the end of the nineteenth century there has been a prejudice against work during pregnancy. But women's jobs and prevention policies have both developed. During the 1970s, we observed that the risk of pre-term birth was lower for pregnant women with professional activities than for those not employed, except for women with physically demanding jobs (Saurel-Cubizolles *et al.* 1982). We therefore hoped for measures targeted at these kinds of jobs and better follow-up of women without jobs. Instead, pregnancy leave was prolonged for all working women.

Relations between epidemiology and clinical medicine

One of our fears was that national surveys might be considered the equivalent of inspections, at a time when the new standards were going to lead to the closure of several hundred small maternity units. Our analyses did not name specific establishments, and we insisted on our independence from the government agencies normally responsible for inspections.

We quickly developed positive contacts with personnel in maternity units, which was essential since the success of these surveys depended on the cooperation of physicians and midwives. For our part we helped to disseminate information about the trends we observed in France and abroad and about new methods of diagnosis and care. We were thus welcomed by all those obstetricians and paediatricians interested in modernizing their practices.

Effects of these relations on epidemiological research

The first effect was to strengthen our team, and we were able in 1975 to create a new laboratory: Unit 149 (Unite de recherches épidémiologique sur lamère et l'enfant). Moreover, other epidemiologists became interested in the perinatal period, thereby strengthening the potential for research.

But the effort that these surveys demanded took us still further away from basic research on the causes of disease. We analysed the distribution of health care and its changes over time and in different social groups, and we sometimes wondered about the validity of our approach, which led us to the borders of sociology. During the 1970s, though, neither clinical nor laboratory research made many discoveries about the causes of fetal anomalies. We still knew little about the pathogenesis of pre-term birth or, despite the progress in genetics, of many congenital malformations. Epidemiological research must be supported by earlier discoveries in biological research.

Recent development of the interactions between epidemiology and medicine (1981–2000)

This period was characterized by intense research activity in several western countries on the topic of reproduction. In France, research first focused on assisted reproductive technologies, pre-term birth, intrauterine growth retardation, and congenital malformations. Then, at the end of the 1980s, an epidemiology of cerebral palsy and mental retardation was developed.

In vitro fertilization

Assisted reproductive technology led to *in vitro* fertilization and through it to very early diagnosis of genetic anomalies and to the culture of embryonic cells. Epidemiologists have focused especially on the study of the outcomes of children born after *in vitro* fertilization. They contributed, for example, to the discovery of the dangers involved in multiple embryo implantation, a technique that increases the risk of multiple births, pre-term delivery, and handicaps.

Recent progress in cloning and culturing embryonic tissues and questions about their use has raised a number of ethical and technical problems that require substantial reflection, a process in which epidemiologists are involved.

Research on pre-term delivery

Medical research has provided positive results for treatment of threatened pre-term delivery (TPD) and care for newborns. Little progress has occurred, however, in the study of the pathophysiology of pre-term delivery.

The diagnosis of TPD, previously based on clinical signs, has been improved by transvaginal ultrasound. In cases of TPD, randomized trials have shown that administration of cortisone to the mother accelerates fetal maturation and reduces the risk of intraventricular haemorrhage. The *in utero* transfer to well-equipped centres has also improved the management of pre-term babies. Progress in resuscitation had considerably augmented the survival of 'very pre-term infants'.

Epidemiologists working with clinicians have conducted numerous randomized trials to compare different techniques of diagnosis and care and they have brought their results together in meta-analyses. More recently Unit 149 undertook the follow-up of these 'very pre-term children' from birth until the age of 5 or 6 years. The survey also attempted to measure the impact of these problems on the family environment and the special difficulties of these fragile children in very poor populations.

Research on intrauterine growth retardation (IUGR)

In previous decades, intrauterine growth retardation was treated by a variety of methods (no-salt diets, diuretics, etc), all of which have been proven ineffective in randomized trials.

In the 1980s, ultrasound made it possible to monitor fetal growth with ever increasing precision. Another source of considerable progress was Doppler velocimetry, which enabled study of the fetal circulation. It allowed a better understanding of the origin of a disease of which prognosis may be improved by aspirin. In many cases, however, Caesarean delivery remains the only possible solution for avoiding the sequelae of IUGR or even the death of the infant *in utero*. Its implementation ever earlier in pregnancy has increased the number of 'very pre-term babies'.

Epidemiologists have participated very actively in the establishment of fetal growth curves, trials of prevention, and meta-analyses on the usefulness of Doppler testing (Goffinet *et al.* 1997) and of aspirin.

Congenital malformations

Antenatal screening of congenital malformations and of genetically transmitted diseases made considerable progress with the development of amniocentesis, which allows the diagnosis of some genetic anomalies, including trisomy 21, the most frequent anomaly. Very early screening for diseases of genetic origin during *in vitro* fertilization opened up new perspectives. Ultrasound is helpful for malformations affecting fetal morphology; its success varies according to the severity and type of malformation. Early neonatal surgery is another source of considerable progress, especially for cardiac malformations. The contribution of epidemiology is seen in the study of the prevalence of congenital malformations, through district registries, in research into aetiological environmental factors, and by the assessment of the outcome of prevention methods.

Cerebral palsy and mental retardation

In 1980 there was a great contrast, in France, between the plentiful research on congenital malformations and the scarcity of research on cerebral palsies and mental retardation, both of unknown prevalence.

Epidemiology has started to make up for lost time. Cross-sectional regional surveys began in 1984. They concerned children older than 6 years and born between 1972 and 1985. Two district registries were also established. These studies showed that the prevalence of cerebral palsy and mental retardation was not diminishing, despite progress in perinatal prevention (Rumeau-Rouquette *et al.* 1997). This finding is probably associated with the increase in 'very pre-term births' and to the progress in resuscitation, which enables the survival of an increasing number of children at high risk.

Intrauterine screening has progressed for ischaemic and haemorrhagic accidents, ventricular dilatation, and several other anomalies. The most important progress, however, has occurred after birth. Neonatal diagnosis has improved. Magnetic resonance imaging (MRI) and new laboratory tests now complement clinical examinations and electroencephalograms. Follow-up of high-risk groups such as 'very pre-term infants' by transfontanelle ultrasound or MRI allows earlier screening of some cerebral lesions. But the pathophysiology of cerebral lesions is still poorly understood.

Recent relations between epidemiologists and public health services (1981–2000)

The perinatal period was no longer a priority (1981–94)

In 1981, the government, probably reassured by the progress during the preceding period, stopped treating the perinatal period as a high priority. Moreover, the political instability that began at that time was not propitious for the development of long-term health actions.

Without funding from the ministry, the national birth surveys were abandoned between 1981 and 1994. In 1988, a regional survey conducted by our laboratory indicated an increase in pre-term birth rates and raised worrisome questions (Bréart *et al.* 1995). The health statistics were no more reassuring: France had fallen in the rankings for perinatal mortality, and maternal mortality was climbing (Bouvier-Colle *et al.* 1994).

A new perinatal action plan in 1994

These results served as a warning signal to the ministry of health, which in 1994, adopted a new health plan aimed at diminishing maternal and perinatal mortality and reducing the number of both low-birth-weight children and of pregnant women receiving no or inadequate antenatal care. New guidelines for obstetric facilities were promulgated in 1998, and regional networks were established to facilitate *in utero* transfer.

The 1994 government plan also restarted the national surveys. They resumed under the supervision of the ministry of health and take place every 3 years in collaboration with our laboratory. They have not shown particularly reassuring trends in health indicators (Blondel *et al.* 1997). Pre-term birth and its sequelae remain matters of concern.

Some have interpreted the poor results observed since 1980 as an effect of the government's lack of interest between 1981 and 1994. It probably played a role, especially since the regionalization of PMI services had unfavourable results in some geographical areas. Nonetheless those conclusions have to be qualified (Rumeau-Rouquette 2001). The increase in the pre-term birth rate is essentially linked to the increase in age at first pregnancy, to the rise in multiple pregnancies associated with *in vitro* fertilization, and to the performance of Caesareans increasingly earlier to minimize the consequences of intrauterine growth retardation. In addition, the social climate has deteriorated as unemployment and precarious employment have grown sharply.

Possible future of perinatal epidemiology

We will consider here the future development of objectives and several dangers that threaten epidemiologists.

Development of objectives as a function of the population's health status

The long-term trends that predictably affect the population's health status affect the development of objectives. These trends include: fewer and later births, the persistence of unemployment and precarious employment, migration, increased drug use, and smoking. These factors affect the health of the newborn and will continue to be part of the framework of epidemiological research.

But unforeseen events and elements can modify these objectives. Forty years ago, the thalidomide tragedy permanently affected the direction of aetiological research and reporting of adverse drug reactions. The recent eruption of AIDS has incited new studies on maternal–fetal transmission and its prevention. No crystal ball will tell us whether a major risk will appear in the 10 years to come and what its effects on reproduction might be.

Development of objectives as a function of scientific progress

Progress in some fields directly touches epidemiology. As computer science and telecommunications have progressed, they have made possible great strides in epidemiology. Epidemiological methods will continue to evolve, integrating these new possibilities for the collection and analysis of information.

Progress in medicine in the perinatal period has also been essential, in particular in genetics, imagery, *in vitro* fertilization, and neonatal resuscitation. This will probably offer new pathways for epidemiological research. We can also hope that new advances in genetics and biology will improve our knowledge of the origin of congenital malformations, of intrauterine growth retardation, and of pre-term birth. But many aspects of this field remain unpredictable. Biologists sometimes estimate that they cannot forecast what their work will be more than 2 or 3 years in advance, but we expect a lot from them.

Dangers of excessive specialization

Beyond their specialization in a medical area (for example oncology, cardiology, reproduction), epidemiologists have shown a growing trend to work either in clinical research or in large population surveys. Others move closer still towards providing health-care provision, with so-called 'interventional epidemiology', which is more concerned with action than with research.

These orientations must not determine the epidemiologist's job or future. It is useful to recall that epidemiology is a science that involves a common set of methods and that it may be dangerous to limit oneself exclusively to one or other of these directions. Choices may vary according to the epidemiologist's age, the state of the science, and available funding in the field. It may be useful to move from research on the perinatal period to studies of the menopause or cancer, for example. It is often good for a laboratory to conduct hospital-based research and large population surveys simultaneously.

The danger of excessive direction by the authorities

This problem is acute in France, with the creation of a national research agency which will have substantial funding. Some see it as a danger for the research institutes. These fears are probably unfounded, but they accurately express the real difficulties that exist at the interface of political power and research.

This malaise exists at the level of the European Union, where research programmes sometimes show clear evidence of technocratic concerns. Moreover, the desire to attain large international participation often reduces projects to the lowest common denominator.

Perinatal epidemiology is doubly exposed to this danger of political and technocratic development because of its associations with public health and the particular weight accorded to reproduction in Europe, where reproductive rates are decreasing. We have managed to control it in the past. Let us hope the same will be true in the future.

References

Blondel B, Bréart G, du Mazaubrun C *et al*. (1997). La situation périnatale en France entre 1981 et 1995. *Journal de Gynécologie Obstétrique et Biologie de la Reproduction*, **26**, 770–80.

Blondel M, Kaminski M, and Bréart G (1980). Antenatal care and demographic and social characteristics. Evolution in France between 1972 and 1976. *Journal of Epidemiology and Community Health*, **34**, 157–63.

Bouvier-Colle MH, Varnoux N, and Bréart G (1994). *Les morts maternelles en France*. Editions INSERM, Paris.

Bréart G and Darchy P (1983). Evolution de la fréquence des césariennes en France (1972–1981). *Revue d'Epidemiologie et de Santé Publique*, **31**, 483–5.

Bréart G, Blondel B, Turpin P, Grandjean H, and Kaminski M (1995). Did preterm deliveries continue to decrease in France in the 1980's? *Pediatric Perinatal Epidemiology*, **9**, 296–306.

Goffinet F, Paris-Lado J, Nisan I, and Bréart G (1997). Utilité clinique du Doppler ombilical.Résultats des essais controlés sur des populations à haut risque et à bas risque. *Journal de Gynécologie Obstétrique et Biologie de la Reproduction*, **26**, 16–26.

Goujard J, Kaminski M, Rumeau-Rouquette C, and Schwartz D (1978). Maternal smoking, alcohol consumption and abruptio placenta. *American Journal of Obstetric and Gynecology*, **130**, 738–9.

Kaminski M, Goujard J, and Rumeau-Rouquette C (1973). Prediction of low birthweight and prematurity by a multiple regression analysis with maternal characteristics known since the beginning of the pregnancy. *International Journal of Epidemiology*, **2**, 195–204.

Kaminski M, Rumeau-Rouquette C, and Schwartz D (1978). Effects on offspring of maternal alcohol use during pregnancy. *New England Journal of Medicine*, **298**, 55–6.

Papiernik E (1969). Coefficient de risque d'accouchement prématuré. *La Presse Médicale*, **77**, 793–4.

Rouquette C and Schwartz D (1970). *Méthodes en épidémiologie*. Editions Médicales Flammarion. Paris.

Rumeau-Rouquette C (2001). Bien naître. *La périnatalité entre espoir et désenchantement*. Editions EDK, Paris.

Rumeau-Rouquette C, Goujard J, Huel G, and Kaminski M (1977). Possible teratogenic effect of phenothiazines in man. *Teratology*, **15**, 57–64.

Rumeau-Rouquette C, du Mazaubrun C and Rabarison Y (1984). *Naître en France, 10 ans d'évolution*. Editions INSERM, Doin, Paris.

Rumeau-Rouquette C, Grandjean H, Cans C, du Mazaubrun C, and Verrier A (1997). Prevalence and time trends of disabilities in school-age children. *International Journal of Epidemiology*, **26**, 137–45.

Saurel-Cubizolles MJ, Kaminski M, and Rumeau-Rouquette C (1982). Activité professionnelle des femmes enceintes, surveillance prénatale et issue de la grossesse. *Journal de Gynécologie Obstérique et Biologie de la Reproduction*, **11**, 956–67.

Schwartz D (1963). *Méthode statistiques à l'usage des médecins et des biologistes*. Editions médicales Flammarion, Paris.

Schwartz D, Flamant R, Lellouch J, and Rouquette C (1960). *Les essais thérapeutiques cliniques méthode scientifique d'appréciation d'un traitement*. Masson, Paris.

Sureau C (1956). Recherches d'électrocardiographie fœtale au cours de la gestation et du travail. *Gynécologie-Obstétrique*, **55**, 21–33.

11

Epidemiology in war and disasters

Haroutune K. Armenian

Personal experiences

Over the years, whether with my mentors, colleagues, or my own students, I have noted the different pathways that led them to choose epidemiology as a career. My choice for a career in public health and epidemiology was made as a medical student in the mid-1960s at the American University of Beirut. Two experiences were critical for my choice.

First, in the summer of 1965, I joined a small group of my fellow second-year medical students on a research assistanceship with Dr Nadim Haddad in field studies of the epidemiology of trachoma and its vaccine trials in the villages of South Lebanon. As one of the first ophthalmologists ever to become an epidemiologist, Nadim was able to get us excited about the whole field and its potential over sandwiches under an olive tree close to the villages where our field surveys and vaccine trials were taking us. I was soon to realize that epidemiology was as 'scientific' as what we were exposed to in biochemistry and physiology.

Secondly, during the winter of 1966 a major poliomyelitis epidemic was sweeping through Lebanon but more so in some of the poorer areas. As a group of medical students we took the initiative of starting a mass vaccination programme in some of the same villages that we were involved in in our trachoma field research. The faculty volunteered to help us in this effort, and most of our weekends during that winter were spent in this vaccination campaign. In the process we learned a lot about the epidemiology of poliomyelitis, in particular how our preventive strategy could become more effective by using our knowledge of the epidemiology of the disease within that particular socio-cultural environment.

Following graduation from medical school, and after 3 years of residency training in internal medicine, a fellowship from the Commonwealth Fund in 1971 allowed me to spend about 3 years at the Department of Epidemiology at Johns Hopkins University with Abraham Lilienfeld as my advisor and a host of leaders in the field as my professors. My doctoral thesis topic had a specific focus on prostate cancer epidemiology (Armenian *et al.* 1974, 1975) and I was trained probably as one of the first chronic disease epidemiologists from Lebanon and the Arab world.

Within a year of getting back to the American University of Beirut, the civil war erupted in Lebanon. The public health and other issues related to the war were very acute and serious. At this point, a shift of interest towards the use of epidemiological methods for studying war-related issues as well as disasters started to assert itself in my professional reality.

A 2-year stint at the Ministry of Health in Bahrain during the oil boom period allowed me to be engaged in health services research on a number of levels. This was a period where my perspectives in epidemiology and public health were broadened and a number of unique health service developmental experiences streamlined my maturation as an epidemiologist (Armenian 1978, 1980a,b, 1982; Armenian *et al.* 1975, 1981a).

In 1978, back in Beirut as a faculty member, I became the acting and later the Dean of the Faculty of Health Sciences at the American University of Beirut between 1981 and 1986. In partnership with faculty colleagues and students we were able to develop a number of epidemiological studies on the effect of war-related factors on specific diseases as well as general health conditions. This was also an opportunity to develop emergency systems in health monitoring and provide a database for public health decision-making for various agencies in the field like UNICEF.

It was during this period that I developed a personal philosophy that has been an important guideline for my personal and professional life: how to turn a moment of adversity into positive achievement. An adverse and horrible situation, like the civil war around us, had led many of our colleagues into a long period of professional retrenchment. Our alternative to retrenchment at the Faculty of Health Sciences was to initiate a number of investigations as to the short- and long-term effects of the major human disaster that was the civil war. It was important to learn from these disasters and wars to prevent excessive morbidity and mortality in such situations in the future. These were opportunities for learning and information that one may try to take advantage from. A meeting with Dr Jens Amlie from the International Committee of the Red Cross (ICRC) led to our getting engaged as a Faculty of Health Sciences in a historically unique programme of surveillance and monitoring of the health conditions and diseases of the population of a city under siege. West Beirut was under siege from the Israeli army and the university was within the part of the city under siege. All the government services were disrupted or paralysed and the donor agencies and local community groups were in need of a continuous assessment of the health situation in the city under siege. Over a period of 4 months, the school of public health served as the hub where many of the public health activities were being initiated in the city, assisted by our epidemiological surveillance and investigation system (American University of Beirut, Faculty of Health Sciences 1983). As will be described later on in this chapter, our engagement in this epidemiological surveillance and investigation project in a city under siege set the model for a number of population-based projects that the Faculty of Health Sciences carried out in the ensuing two decades.

There are very few individuals, if any, who are full time professionals in disaster epidemiology. Circumstances and situations may require any epidemiologist to work in a disaster situation. Thus, one needs to be well prepared to deal with such situations. Anyone of us may be the next person to be called upon in our communities to render services in a disaster situation and one may be the only epidemiologist available there.

In December 1988 following the massive earthquake in northern Armenia, the Gorbachev's Soviet Union opened up to western assistance. As part of a diasporan Armenian assistance group we were in Yerevan within 3 weeks of the earthquake. While much of the assistance was focused on the delivery of humanitarian aid, and in the absence of any effective health monitoring system in the earthquake zone, we focused with our colleagues from the Computer and Information Services of the Ministry of Health of Armenia on a surveillance and monitoring system of the health of the survivors of the disaster. This was also an opportunity to introduce a number of modern epidemiological methods to a country in the Soviet Union where epidemiology had a very traditional infectious disease–microbiology base.

Some of the issues concerning the development and implementation of appropriate epidemiological investigations in situations of war and disasters will be presented in the follwoing.

The interface of epidemiology and services in disasters

In this section we will start with a review of important landmarks and innovations that have marked the use of epidemiology in disasters over the past 50 years.

Acute problem-solving, like in outbreaks, has been at the core of early epidemiological activity in disasters. Introduced in the late 1950s and early 1960s, this approach improved disaster epidemiology at the operational level. In one of the earliest reviews of the role of epidemiology in disasters, Saylor and Gordon (1957) use the concepts of epidemic investigation in disasters. They propose epidemiological terminology and methods for solving problems in disaster situations. For them, a single-impact disaster can be studied like a point epidemic, and in general the medical problems during the disaster can be studied along distributions of time, place, and persons.

Michel Lechat (1976) introduced multidimensional models in disaster epidemiology. He proposed a model for the purposes of organizational planning, and for the long-term evaluation of disaster prevention programmes in public health. Lechat classified the time frame for studying problems of disasters as during impact, post-impact, and in the long term.

War and its long-term impact on human health have catalysed interest towards longitudinal methods in the epidemiology of disasters. The best-studied cohort of a population exposed to a disaster is the longitudinal cohort studies of the Atomic Bomb Casualty Commission in Hiroshima and Nagasaki. Other longitudinal studies of the long-term health effects of war include studies of concentration camp survivors and psychological studies of other subgroups exposed to the major trauma of war and other violence (Eitinger and Strom 1973; Finch 1984).

Over the past four decades, a special unit at the Pan American Health Organization, under the leadership of Claude de Ville de Goyet (1979), has produced some important literature dealing with various aspects of disasters including the use of epidemiological methods. As proposed by de Ville de Goyet, epidemiology needs to be involved at all levels of disaster relief operations.

Thus, the role of epidemiology in disaster situations should include:

◆ surveillance and development of an action-oriented information system;

◆ disease control strategies for well-defined problems;

◆ assessment of the use and distribution of health services facilities;

◆ aetiological research on conditions related to disasters and related issues;

◆ initiation of efforts for the long-term development of surveillance and investigation systems in the community.

The following are some examples of projects that were conducted in wartime and during disasters that highlight the role of epidemiology in such situations.

Emergency health surveillance and monitoring programme in Beirut

Within days of the siege of West Beirut by the Israeli army in the summer of 1982, the international agencies became cognizant of the lack of data and reliable information about the health conditions in the city under siege. A programme was funded by the United States Agency for International Development (USAID) and carried out by the faculty and students of the Faculty of Health Sciences at the American University of Beirut, to assess the health situation and identify major health problems for intervention and assistance. The four components of the programme included: (1) continuous surveillance and monitoring of hospitals and dispensaries; (2) a population-based residential morbidity survey; (3) the setting up of an epidemiological investigation unit; (4) a system for continuous data analysis and reporting. Organizationally, a project management team had daily meetings to oversee problems and a total of 35 people worked on the project at any one time (American University of Beirut, Faculty of Health Sciences 1983).

One of the interesting observations from this programme was that the major problems of acute morbidity in this population were diarrhoea and respiratory and childhood infections. There were no epidemics of major reportable communicable diseases. As per our household surveys, mental health problems were rampant in the population at large (Lockwood Hourani *et al.* 1986). Three-monthly reports were produced in addition to other reports produced for special purposes. The findings were directed to a citywide public health action committee that met regularly with participation from local groups as well as international agencies working in the city. As part of the programme a mobile laboratory was established to monitor water quality in all the neighbourhoods and this helped direct UNICEF's safe water distribution project.

As part of this programme, a study was conducted of all the agencies providing emergency aid in the summer of 1982 in Lebanon. The analysis included an assessment of the approaches for material, personnel, and cash flow in these organizations. Bottlenecks were identified, and unnecessary duplication of effort and other problems were listed. As a conclusion it was proposed to develop an interagency database geared towards disaster management (Matta *et al.* 1982).

Etiological research

While the civil war was in progress in Lebanon, the faculty and students of the Faculty of Health Sciences conducted a number of analytical epidemiological studies to investigate the effect of war-related factors on various conditions of morbidity.

In 1975–76 while studying patients delivering at the university hospital, we observed with the medical students that during the war period patients required significantly less post-partum analgesia. The literature review revealed one previous report by Beecher (1956) of a similar observation in American soldiers post-operatively during the Second World War. Using appendectomy as a model, and after adjustment for a number of variables, we were able to confirm that patients undergoing uncomplicated appendectomies during the war required significantly fewer analgesics and narcotics than patients undergoing the same operation in peacetime (Armenian *et al.* 1981b).

A case–control study was conducted of determinants of arteriographically assessed coronary artery disease (CAD) in wartime Beirut. Compared to normal controls, patients who had experienced two and more major war events had an odds ratio of 2.4 for severe CAD. Daily exposures, like crossing the green line separating the fighting groups, had a similar adverse effect in the development of CAD (Sibai *et al.* 1989).

Other analytical studies assessed the effect of wartime stressors on rheumatoid arthritis, enuresis in children, and breast cancer. None of these studies identified any significant associations with wartime stressors.

Epidemiology following the earthquake in Armenia

As part of our assessment of the health conditions in the population surviving the 1988 earthquake in Armenia, we initiated first a rapid case–control study of determinants of hospitalized injuries from Leninakan (Giumri). As a result of this study we were able to identify protective behaviours during the earthquake as well as factors like building type and location during the earthquake as determinants of serious injury (Armenian *et al.* 1992).

The monitoring of the health of the population was conducted through a special cohort of 33,000 employees of the Ministry of Health from the earthquake region and their families. Following the collection of baseline epidemiological and disaster experience data, this cohort was followed up for 4 years as to the long-term effects of the earthquake. The longitudinal follow-up of the population revealed that much of the excess long-term mortality and morbidity was limited to the first 6 months following the disaster; an observation that was partially made previously following the earthquakes of Thessalonica in Greece and Naples in Italy (Armenian *et al.* 1997, 1998).

A geographically stratified subsample of 1785 adults were the respondents to a psychiatric questionnaire that assessed mental health problems about 2 years following the earthquake. This longitudinal cohort approach was unique for Armenia and the Soviet Union but had also never been done on this scale in previous earthquakes. During the 2 years following the earthquake, about 60% of this adult population had symptoms that could fulfil the diagnosis of either post-traumatic stress disorder (PTSD) or depression; the risk of PTSD and depression was related to the amount of loss in an individual's family. Sharing the experience at the moment of disaster with someone else and receiving support early on were protective factors for mental illness (Armenian *et al.* 2000, 2002).

Information for decision-making

Epidemiology is an information science, since, as a discipline, it aims at influencing *decision-making* in a number of situations. Individuals, health professionals, and policy-makers use data

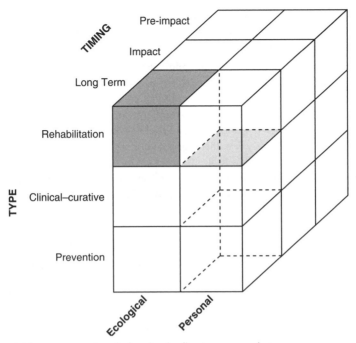

Fig. 11.1 A model for assessment and planning in disaster preparedness.

generated in epidemiology as information, albeit in a transformed format, for making decisions in dealing with various problems. The value of information is a function of its validity, its utility to multiple users, the ability to use it in multiple situations (generalizability), the timeliness with which it is provided, its distribution, its amount, and the cost of producing it. These same principles apply when dealing with data generated during war and disasters.

The test of the work conducted by epidemiologists is in the appropriate use of the information generated. The examples provided in the previous section have highlighted the potential utility of such information. An organized approach to data collection in disaster situations assists us to improve decision-making and predict a variety of options we need to face. As presented in Fig. 11.1, a three-dimensional conceptual matrix assesses disasters along *levels of action* (ecological and personal), *type of action* (preventive, curative, and rehabilitative), and *timing of action* (pre-, during and post-impact). Such a three-dimensional matrix will be useful for analysis, planning, and research in epidemiology during disaster situations.

Based on this model, we developed two-dimensional matrices that can be used to list the various decisions that one may need to make in the different phases of the disaster. Thus, at the pre-impact phase, the decisions are concerned with delineating the at-risk subgroups of the population and assessing the emergency preparedness and the flexibility of the existing surveillance system. During impact, characteristics of the affected population and the need for services have to be assessed quickly, while the post-impact phase needs information on long-term rehabilitation and reconstruction of health services. The epidemiological investigation has to cater to the information needs of the decision–action process of the specific disaster, and thus it cannot be detached from it (Armenian 1989a, 1996).

The problems related to implementing epidemiological investigations under conditions of war and disaster have been described in previous publications and will be briefly summarized.

Having presented in the previous section investigations during war and a natural disaster, we will next highlight some of the differences between these situations in particular relating to the difficulties facing the epidemiologist:

- Disaster epidemiology, in particular epidemiology in wartime, provides the opportunity for the professional to be involved in acute problem-solving situations and to be instrumental in having a direct impact in relieving human suffering. We have heard in the past some criticism of epidemiological investigations in disasters, and in particular in wartime, on moral grounds. If war is considered a disease at the societal level that causes death and suffering to millions of human beings every year, then war is an important problem that needs to be studied by epidemiologists at various levels of operation (Armenian 1986). Following the principle that the epidemiological investigation will have to serve the needs of decision-makers in such situations, and that the information generated could be used for preventive action for future disaster situations, should dampen such criticism.

- Compared with natural disasters where events are more acute, war has both epidemic and endemic presentations as exemplified by the endemic civil wars of the Third World, in particular in sub-Saharan Africa. In many of these endemic war situations the acute single impact or point epidemic model of disaster epidemiology does not apply. In most wars, we are dealing with a situation that is constantly and dynamically changing with periodic exacerbations and remissions.

- In wartime, the personal risk for injury and harm during collection of data and fieldwork is very real and serious. There is more than a moral responsibility that one carries in initiating epidemiological investigations under conditions of war. Thus, the first decision one has to make is whether the data collected will influence significantly decision-making to the extent of saving lives. Such a risk–benefit analysis is important, particularly as it relates to the immediate needs of the situation rather than potential benefits at some future time and place. Thus, in both Beirut during the civil war and in post-earthquake Armenia, our investigations were part of a surveillance and monitoring system of the health of the population and would serve the needs for decision-making of public health programmes in the short and long term (Armenian 1989b, 1999).

- If we are interested in the determinants of injuries and death during war, we may be hampered by inappropriate or inadequate data because of the sensitive military nature of such information. It may be difficult to conduct liberal interviewing of the affected population.

The will and the challenge for action

Considering that as health professionals we are under a moral obligation to provide humanitarian assistance and relief in a disaster situation, most epidemiological initiatives have been primarily used to assist in disaster relief efforts rather than to address some basic research concerns related to the disaster and the prevention of morbidity and mortality in future disasters. Thus, because of our primarily utilitarian concern, methodological innovations have been relatively few in disaster epidemiology over the past 50 years.

Although, over the past couple of decades efforts have been made to develop rapid and valid epidemiological assessment techniques to be used under such circumstances, the majority of epidemiologists are ignorant of these techniques and standard epidemiological textbooks have shunned away from presenting such approaches.

Epidemiologists have traditionally focused on issues of validity and reliability of data in ascertaining various sources. No systematic effort has been made to assess such issues of validity and reliability of data sources in a disaster situation in addition to the completeness, accessibility, and timing of these sources.

In this chapter we have highlighted some of the responsibilities that epidemiologists may carry during disasters and wartime. However, much of what is being done in this area is palliative rather than preventive. Philosophically we may have no difficulty in accepting a role as public health professionals in the prevention of disasters, in particular man-made ones, but when we get to wars as a disaster situation, we may not be as clear about our commitment in its prevention. This is where we need to have concerted action by all health professionals in order to influence the political process and milieu that leads to such wars. Developing a consensus within and between our international professional organizations is a good place to start. Assisting other organizations working for peace and justice is another option.

The will to be involved in action during disasters and wars is what probably most epidemiologists have. Getting involved is a challenge very few of us will actually get the opportunity to undertake.

References

American University of Beirut, Faculty of Health Sciences (1983). Emergency health surveillance project. July–November 1982. *Weekly Epidemiologic Record*, **58**, 7–9.

Armenian HK (1978). Developing a quality assurance program in the state of Bahrain. *Quality Review Bulletin*, **4**, 9–11.

Armenian HK (1980a). Model systems for primary health care in developing countries. In *Human resources for primary health care in the Middle East*. American University of Beirut, Beirut, pp. 194–204.

Armenian HK (1980b). Evaluation and projections for the primary health care system in Bahrain. *Bahrain Medical Bulletin*, **2**, 71–5.

Armenian HK (1982). The office of professional standards and systems analysis, a model for a university extension program. In *The role of the university in extension education*. American University of Beirut, Beirut, pp. 142–9.

Armenian HK (1986). In wartime: options for epidemiology. *American Journal of Epidemiology*, **124**, 28–32.

Armenian HK (1989a). Methodologic issues in the epidemiologic studies of disasters. In *Proceedings of the International Workshop on Earthquake Injury Epidemiology for Mitigation and Response* (ed. N Jones, E Noji, G Smith, and F Krimgold), pp. 95–106. Johns Hopkins University, Baltimore.

Armenian HK (1989b). Perceptions from epidemiologic research in an endemic war. *Social Science and Medicine*, **28**, 643–7.

Armenian HK (1996). Epidemiological issues in disaster situations. In *Proceedings of WHO/HICARE Symposium on Radiological Accidents and Environmental Epidemiology: a Decade after the Chernobyl Accident, Hiroshima, Japan 24–25 August*, pp. 149–57.

Armenian HK (1999). From war to disasters: threads of epidemiologic research and public health action in the Middle East. In *Studies in Middle Eastern health* (ed. JW Brown and R Barlow). The University of Michigan. Ann Arbor, Michigan, pp. 29–38.

Armenian HK, Lilienfeld AM, Diamond EL, and Bross IDJ (1974). Relation between benign prostatic hyperplasia to cancer of the prostate. A prospective and retrospective study. *Lancet*, **2**, 115–17.

Armenian HK, Lilienfeld AM, Diamond EL, and Bross IDJ (1975). Epidemiologic characteristics of patients with prostatic neoplasms. *American Journal of Epidemiology*, **102**, 47–54.

Armenian HK, Dajani AW, and Fakhro AM (1981a). Impact of peer review and itemized medical record forms on medical care in a health center in Bahrain. *Quality Review Bulletin*, **7**, 6–11.

Armenian HK, Chamieh MA, and Baraka A (1981b). Influence of wartime stress and psychosocial factors in Lebanon on analgesic requirements for post-operative pain. *Social Science and Medicine*, **15E**, 63–6.

Armenian HK, Noji EK, and Oganesian AP (1992). A case-control study of injuries due to the earthquake in Armenia. *Bulletin of the World Health Organization*, **70**, 251–7.

Armenian HK, Melkonian A, Noji EK, and Hovanesian AP (1997). Deaths and injuries due to the earthquake in Armenia: a cohort approach. *International Journal of Epidemiology*, **26**, 806–13.

Armenian HK, Melkonian AK, and Hovanesian AP (1998). Long term mortality and morbidity related to degree of damage following the 1988 earthquake in Armenia, *American Journal of Epidemiology*, **148**, 1077–84.

Armenian HK, Masahiro M, Melkonian AK, *et al.* (2000). Loss as a determinant of PTSD in a cohort of adult survivors of the 1988 earthquake in Armenia; implications for policy. *Acta Psychiatrica Scandinavica*, **102**, 58–64.

Armenian HK, Morikawa M, Melkonian AK, Hovanesian A, Akiskal K, and Akiskal HS (2002). Risk factors for depression in the survivors of the 1988 earthquake in Armenia. *Journal of Urban Health: Bulletin of the New York Academy of Medicine*, **79**, 373–82.

Beecher HK (1956). Relationship of significance of wound to pain experienced. *Journal of the American Medical Association*, **161**, 1609–72.

De Ville de Goyet C (1979). Maladies transmissibles et surveillance epidemiologique lors des desastres naturels. *Bulletin of the World Health Organization*, **57**, 153–65.

Eitinger L and Strom A (1973). *Mortality and morbidity after excessive stress*. Humanities Press, New York.

Finch S (1984). Leukemia and lymphoma in atomic bomb survivors. In *Radiation carcinogenesis: epidemiology and biological significance* (ed. JD Boice and JF Fraumeni), pp. 37–44. Raven Press, New York.

Lechat MF (1976). The epidemiology of disasters. *Proceedings of the Royal Society of Medicine*, **69**, 421–6.

Lockwood Hourani L, Armenian H, Zurayk H, and Afifi L (1986). A population-based survey of loss and psychological distress during war. *Social Science and Medicine*, **23**, 269–75.

Matta NF, Armenian HK, and Jarawan E (1982). *A framework of a database for disaster management: the case of Lebanon, 1982*. Faculty of Health Sciences, American University of Beirut, Beirut.

Saylor LF and Gordon JE (1957). The medical component of natural disasters. *American Journal of Medical Science*, **234**, 342–62.

Sibai AM, Armenian HK and Alam S (1989). Wartime determinants of arteriographically confirmed coronary artery disease in Beirut. *American Journal of Epidemiology*, **130**, 623–31.

12

Emerging infectious diseases

Roger Detels

Microbes and vectors swim in the evolutionary stream and they
swim faster than we do. Bacteria reproduce every 30 minutes.
For them, a millennium is compressed into a fortnight; they are
fleet afoot, and the pace of our research must keep up with them,
or they overtake us. Microbes were here on earth 2 billion years
before humans arrived, learning every trick for survival, and
it is likely that they will be here 2 billion years after we depart.
Krause (1998)

Personal experiences

As a young medical student at New York University in the early 1950s, I wanted to 'save the world' by
becoming a medical missionary. In my third year, through the courtesy of Professor Harry Most, a
leading parasitologist, I was able to work for 6 months in 1960 at the Naval Medical Research Unit #2
in Taipei, Taiwan, then a developing country. Once there, I attached myself to the busiest investigator,
J. Thomas Grayston, an epidemiologist who subsequently founded the School of Public Health at the
University of Washington, and Dr San-Pin Wang. During my 6 months there, I participated in studies
of trachoma and cholera. That experience made me realize that one-on-one treatment of patients had
a minimal impact on improving the health of people in developing countries. I came to the conclusion
that public health was a far more effective way to contribute to the health of society, and that research
in public health issues could have a lasting impact. Through the example of Professors Grayston and
Wang, I realized that epidemiology was an exciting strategy for identifying health problems and investigating their causes, distribution, transmission, and control. After completion of medical school and
an internship, I took a post-doctoral fellowship in epidemiology in the Department of Preventive
Medicine at the University of Washington under Professors Grayston and E. Russell Alexander. I have
been in epidemiology and public health ever since, and continue to find the field challenging, exciting,
and very rewarding.

The twentieth century witnessed both the recognition of many new infectious diseases and
agents and a host of new vaccines and antimicrobial agents. By the late 1960s, the Surgeon
General of the United States and one of the leading infectious disease researchers in the USA
(who would prefer not to be identified) both declared infectious diseases conquered!

Then came HIV/AIDS, reminding us that infectious diseases would be a constant threat as new
agents emerged and old agents mutated to become resistant to the cures and treatments we had
developed.

Types of emerging diseases

Emerging diseases can be divided into four major groups. (1) Newly emerging diseases not previously known (e.g. hantavirus, Ebola virus, and human immunodeficiency virus/acquired immune deficiency disease (HIV/AIDS)); (2) re-emerging diseases (e.g. tuberculosis and malaria); (3) new manifestations of known disease agents (e.g. genital, respiratory, and cardiac manifestations of chlamydiae); and (4) introduction of known agents into new territories (e.g. the rapid spread of West Nile virus in the United States in the last decade of the twentieth century).

Another strategy for classifying emerging diseases was proposed in the US Institute of Medicine report on emerging infections (Lederberg *et al.* 1992). This classification grouped emergent diseases by the most likely cause of their emergence or re-emergence. These are: (1) changes in human demographics and behaviour (HIV/AIDS, dengue virus); (2) technical and industrial advances (vulnerable populations and nosocomial infections, food processing and *Salmonella agoni*); (3) economic development and changes in land use (reforestation and Lyme disease); (4) international travel and commerce (sudden acute respiratory syndrome (SARS)); (5) microbial adaptation and change (influenza, drug-resistant organisms); and (6) breakdown of public health measures (resurgence of *Vibrio cholerae* in the Americas in the early 1990s).

Causes of emerging diseases

The reasons for the emergence of new agents and the resurgence of known agents are complex, and involve the many changes occurring as society modernizes and becomes more affluent. These changes are discussed below, using a modified version of the classification strategy proposed by the Institute of Medicine. There is, however, considerable overlap between the two classification schemes. Examples are provided for each factor.

Changes in human behaviour

Although people have engaged with multiple sexual partners for centuries, there were dramatic changes in sexual behaviours in the twentieth century. Whereas having multiple sexual partners was socially unacceptable in the early twentieth century and only covertly practiced, having multiple sexual partners had not only became acceptable by the latter half of the twentieth century, but became the norm in many societies. As cures for the known sexually transmitted diseases (STDs) became available, the constraints against multiple partners were reduced. Getting an STD became a treatable inconvenience, not a life-compromising event. Multiple partners became the rule in some subpopulations, such as men-who-have-sex-with-men (MSM). A MSM going to a bathhouse could engage in oral and anal sexual intercourse with as many as 10–20 partners in a single evening. Among heterosexuals, the barrier of unwanted pregnancy was reduced by effective contraceptive methods. In many societies, recreational drug use became common. Because of rising drug costs, many users switched to injecting, which requires lower doses of expensive drugs to achieve a 'high'. Because of constraints against obtaining clean needles and syringes, injecting drug users (IDU) often share injection paraphernalia with other injectors. The increase in sexual mixing and syringe/needle-sharing promoted the rapid spread of many infectious disease agents, including human immunodeficiency virus (HIV), hepatitis C (HCV), herpes simplex type II, and genital chlamydiae, which were unknown in the early part of the century but were identified during the twentieth century.

Changes in the environment

Increasingly, the growth of the population and the concomitant release of pollutants into the air have modified the environment. As people seek respite from the crowding of the cities by moving into rural environments, they are increasingly exposed to zoonotic agents such as hantaviruses, not previously recognized as human pathogens. The reforestation of areas previously devoted to farming, a result of the increased efficiency of agriculture, also results in the reintroduction of animals such as deer and arthropod vectors, which introduce zoonotic diseases such as Lyme disease into new areas. During the twentieth century, there have been an extraordinary number of new chemical agents developed to 'improve' the quality of life. Eventually these agents find their way into the air and water supply, adversely affecting the increasing number of vulnerable persons in society and making them more susceptible to agents previously thought to be benign. The rapid urbanization of populations all over the world has put tremendous pressure on cities to maintain effective waste disposal systems. Often these systems cannot keep up with the demand, and breakdowns occur, exposing residents to infectious disease agents. 'Global warming' due to the promiscuous release of chlorofluorocarbons and other gases may also promote the breeding of disease-bearing mosquitoes in areas previously not experiencing mosquito-borne diseases.

Promiscuous use of antibacterial and antiviral drugs

One of the great advances of the twentieth century has been the development of drugs against a wide range of bacterial, viral, and other agents. Unfortunately, improper and over-use of these drugs has resulted in the evolution of drug-resistant agents of diseases that we thought we had under control, such as tuberculosis. This problem has been compounded by the widespread addition of antibiotics into the feed of livestock, including chickens and cattle, to control disease amongst them, further promoting the evolution of resistant strains of organisms.

Changes in health care

Advances in health care have increased the number of vulnerable people surviving life-threatening diseases. Procedures such as bone marrow replacement for leukaemia patients have produced temporarily vulnerable patients in hospitals, which tend to be repositories of drug-resistant infectious disease agents. The stringent procedures to isolate these vulnerable individuals are not always successful. Other changes, such as the assignment of multiple patients to a single nurse, possible because of technical advances increasing nursing efficiency, provide an opportunity for inadvertent transmission of agents between patients. Other individuals with immunodeficiency diseases such as AIDS or who are undergoing chemotherapy for malignancies are kept alive through the 'miracle' advances developed in the twentieth century, but are susceptible to opportunistic organisms such as *Pneumocystis carinii*, which do not cause disease in healthy individuals.

Antigenic drift and shift

Some organisms, most notably the influenza virus, respond to selective pressures such as high proportions of immunes in society due to previous epidemics or vaccination programmes, by undergoing genetic changes that overcome specific human immune responses to previous influenza strains. Sometimes these agents can also undergo genetic exchange if two different strains of the agent simultaneously infect natural reservoirs such as pigs. Thus the mixing of avian and human strains of influenza in pigs is thought to have been responsible for the lethal 1917–18 swine flu pandemic that killed millions worldwide, and is a concern regarding the recent H5N1 influenza outbreak in birds and humans.

Lapses in public health vigilance

Complacency with accepted public health measures can result in the resurgence of diseases previously brought under control. An example is the resurgence of measles in Los Angeles, San Diego, and Dallas 20 years after the implementation of an effective vaccine. Immunization rates had been allowed to decline, particularly in minority populations, resulting in over 1000 cases of measles in each of these cities in 1990. The succumbing of public health professionals to public pressure by specific interest groups can also result in breakdowns of public health vigilance. Thus, MSM groups in the early 1980s successfully pressured public health officials to not screen blood donors to exclude individuals practicing male-to-male sex. Because public health officials forgot that their first obligation was to protect the uninfected, thousands of blood recipients and haemophiliacs were infected with HIV (Leveton *et al.* 1995). In 1993, there was a breakdown in the water supply to Milwaukee, Wisconsin, resulting in a huge outbreak of cryptosporidiosis that infected half a million people and resulted in 100 deaths, underscoring the need to avoid complacency regarding long-established public health interventions.

Advances in food processing

Food preparation, a time-consuming task in the early part of the twentieth century, has been revolutionized with the introduction of processed foods and 'fast food' restaurants. However, introduction of a disease agent into the food processing chain can occur, as happened with the distribution of frozen strawberries from Mexico through a US Department of Agriculture (USDA)-sponsored school lunch programme in 1997, which resulted in the infection of many children with hepatitis A from a single event. Introduction of contaminated food into a fast food restaurant can cause illness in large numbers of people served by the restaurant. An example of this was the outbreak of *Escherichia coli* O157:H7 in Seattle in 1993.

Internationalization of the food supply and laboratory animals

With the development of rapid means of transportation and better preservation of food (e.g. refrigeration), food can be imported great distances both within countries and from country to country. Thus, fresh fruits from Mexico and Chile are commonly consumed in the winter in the USA, and those from Israel and other countries in Europe. Similarly, meat from Argentina, Canada, and Australia is consumed in many countries of Europe and in the USA. Thus, organisms occurring in the producing countries can cause diseases not usual in the consuming countries, as happened in October 1994 with a snack food produced in Israel, which caused an outbreak of *Salmonella agona* in both Israel and the UK. In modern research, there is an increasing need for monkeys and other laboratory animals for the development of laboratory models of disease and evaluation of potential vaccines. This has necessitated the importation of these animals into those countries most actively involved in research. Thus, monkeys imported from Uganda were responsible for the introduction of Marburg virus into Marburg, Germany in the late 1960s, causing many deaths.

International travel

Since the third quarter of the twentieth century, individuals have been able to travel huge distances in a matter of hours, well within the incubation period of many infectious diseases. Thus, an individual acquiring influenza, dengue, or malaria in an endemic area can transport the causative agent to new areas with many susceptibles and, in the case of malaria, dengue, and other arboviruses, to many vectors capable of transporting the agent to new susceptibles.

War

Although not a new phenomenon, in the twentieth century, war continued to promote the exposure of troops to new agents that they can introduce into their home country upon return.

Further, war promotes the breakdown of public health measures and usually creates thousands of refugees who are herded into refugee camps that are crowded and lack sanitary facilities, ideal conditions for the spread of many infectious diseases. War also promotes lapses in behavioural constraints regulating disease-spreading behaviours, most notably sexual constraints. Thus, thousands of women were raped, and they and their resulting children were tragically infected with HIV during the Rwandan civil war.

As pointed out in the quote from Richard Krause at the beginning of this chapter, disease agents respond rapidly to the opportunities presented by these events and social changes that occurred in the twentieth century, adapting their modes of spread, host requirements, etc., to thrive in the new environments presented by these changes. Thus, it is reasonable to expect the emergence of even more new diseases, re-emerging diseases, and resistant agents as we progress into the twenty-first century. For example, we have already seen the emergence of two new threatening agents, SARS and H5N1 avian influenza, and the new century is only 6 years old!

Examples of disease emerging in the twentieth century

It is impossible in a single chapter to discuss all the agents and diseases that emerged or re-emerged as problems in the twentieth century. A list of emerging diseases from 1980–2004 provides a sense of the magnitude of the problem (Table 12.1). Two major re-emergent diseases, tuberculosis and malaria, are discussed elsewhere in this volume, and therefore will not be discussed further in this chapter. Below is a more detailed discussion of five emergent diseases as examples of the range of diseases and control strategies implemented in the twentieth century. These are HIV/AIDS, Ebola, kuru, and dengue haemorrhagic fever, all new diseases, and the new manifestations of chlamydiae infection, as examples of major emergent diseases of the twentieth century.

Table 12.1 Newly identified infectious diseases and pathogens

Year	Disease or pathogen
1980	Human T-lymphotropic virus
1982	*Escherichia coli* O157:H7, Lyme borreliosis, human T-lymphotropic virus type 2
1983	HIV
1988	Hepatitis E, human herpesvirus 6
1989	Hepatitis C
1991	Guanarito virus
1992	*Vibrio cholerae* O139
1993	Hantavirus pulmonary syndrome (Sin Nombre virus)
1994	Savia virus, Hendra virus
1996	New variant Creutzfeldt–Jakob disease, Australian bat lyssavirus
1997	H5N1 (avian influenza A virus)
1999	Nipah virus
2003	SARS
2004	Avian influenza

Source: Workshop presentation by David Heymann, World Health Organization (1999).

HIV/AIDS

Perhaps the most significant new disease of the twentieth century was HIV/AIDS, which accounted for approximately 80 million cases and over 36 million deaths between its first recognition by Michael Gottlieb at the University of California, Los Angeles (UCLA) in 1980 and the end of 2006. Because it attacks primarily individuals in groups shunned by mainstream society, it is probably the most politicized disease of the twentieth century.

In 1980, Dr Michael Gottlieb, then a young assistant professor of medicine at UCLA, identified three young men with severe immune deficiency without any apparent underlying cause. Dr Gottlieb noted that all three men engaged in male-to-male sexual intercourse. He suggested that the disease in these young men was a new disease not previously recognized. Once he published these cases reports, other homosexual men with a similar unexplained immune deficiency were reported in New York City and San Francisco. Within a year, cases were also reported among haemophilia patients, and not long after, among IDU. Because two of the major groups suffering from the disease were marginalized, there was considerable political manoeuvring before the American government responded to the epidemic. The American president at the time, Ronald Reagan, did not mention the disease in public statements until 1986. It was not until late 1983 that blood banks initiated screening to eliminate blood donated by members of risk groups. Not long after recognition of the disease in the USA, reports of a similar disease were reported from Haiti and countries of sub-Saharan Africa. However, very few of the cases reported from these countries were among homosexual men or IDU; most were heterosexual. With the recognition that the epidemic affected not only marginalized groups, more action was taken by the US government, and funds were allocated by the National Institutes of Health to study this new disease.

Although the disease was first recognized and reported in the USA, over 90% of new infections occur in developing countries and in persons 15–45 years, the most productive segment of the population (Phoolcahroen and Detels 2002). Although the prevalence in the USA has remained under 1%, in some areas of sub-Saharan Africa, the hardest hit area, the prevalence has reached 30% or more among the adult population. As a result, the HIV/AIDS epidemic has had a strong negative impact on the economic and political stability of these countries. The epidemic did not take hold in Asia until the late 1980s, fuelled initially by the epidemic of injected drug use, occurring primarily in the countries of the 'Golden Triangle', Thailand, Burma, northeast India, and southern Yunnan, China. However, it was not long before heterosexual intercourse became the major mode of transmission in all of these countries. There is major concern about the spread of the epidemic in China and India, the most populous countries in the world. By 2005, there were more cases of HIV/AIDS in India than in any other country in the world. Although the potential for spread is great in China, the government has recently implemented strong intervention programmes to stop the epidemic while the prevalence is still low (Wu *et al.* 2007). Russia, another large country recently experiencing the epidemic, has been slower to implement strong intervention measures. In Latin America, the epidemic has spread less rapidly, although in the mid-1980s Brazil had the third highest number of cases. The Brazilian government, however, has taken strong action to slow the epidemic by making treatment available to those HIV-infected individuals in need of treatment.

It was not until 1984 that the cause of the new disease was recognized by Robert Gallo at the US National Institutes of Health, although the causative agent, the human immune deficiency virus, was isolated from an individual with early signs of AIDS by Luc Montagnier and his group at the Pasteur Institute in 1983. Once HIV was isolated, it became possible to identify subclinical infections and to describe the natural history of HIV infection leading to clinical AIDS and death. Work began immediately on the development of a vaccine.

There has been considerable controversy over the origins of the virus. It is now accepted by most scientists in the field that HIV probably evolved from similar retroviruses infecting monkeys, probably in Africa, and spread to humans through butchering of infected monkeys for food and monkeys kept as pets. Thus, it represents a new agent evolving in the twentieth century.

HIV is actually a relatively non-infectious disease agent. It is estimated that infection in individuals without concurrent STDs may occur only once in 500–1000 exposures. Once successful infection occurs, the incubation period to onset of clinical AIDS is approximately 9 years, although some infected individuals develop clinical AIDS within 1 year, and others may be infected for 20 years or more without signs of clinical AIDS. Once AIDS occurs, patients survive on average 6–12 months in the absence of treatment. HIV manages to evade the human immune response by changing its antigenic structure during each replication cycle. The human immune response is absolutely subtype-specific, and the newly replicated virus with the minor mutations can successfully evade the immune response to the parent virus. Thus, the immune response is always several weeks behind the HIV strain currently circulating in the infected individual.

Currently there is no cure for HIV/AIDS and no vaccine. However, by 1995, three different classes of drugs had been developed which, in combination, reduced the amount of HIV circulating in the infected individual and partially restored the level of circulating CD4+ cells, the target cell of the virus. From the perspective of the infected individual, this was a great advance, which converted a 100% lethal disease to a chronic, treatable disease, albeit with problems of side-effects and development of resistance to specific drugs. On the other hand, for society, it meant that infected persons who would have died would live indefinitely, but would require continuing expensive treatment. This presents a particularly difficult burden on the health-care systems of developing countries, where the majority of cases occur.

HIV/AIDS was able to take hold and to be sustained because of the major social changes that occurred globally in the twentieth century. Since the first cases were recognized, stigmatization has been a major barrier to control, and has caused some countries to attempt to ignore the epidemic. The major barrier to control was a lack of political commitment by governments at the highest levels to recognize the epidemic and to take action. In those countries where the government has made a major commitment, considerable progress towards control of the epidemic has been achieved.

Control of the HIV/AIDS epidemic presents a unique challenge to public health professionals. Unlike cholera and plague, major epidemics of the past, HIV is not manifested as clinical disease for an average of 9–10 years, and can only be recognized by laboratory testing prior to onset of symptoms. Typically, by the time the first cases of AIDS are recognized, there are usually several thousand HIV-infected individuals for every clinical case of AIDS. Thus, the epidemic is already far advanced before the need for intervention is recognized. Although HIV/AIDS is a sexually transmitted disease, unlike syphilis and the majority of the other sexually transmitted diseases, it does not present symptoms during the acute stage, and cannot be cured through treatment.

An effective vaccine has not been developed, and is unlikely to be developed within the next decade. Thus, the major intervention strategies have relied on behaviour change and harm reduction. Although the US government has emphasized sexual abstinence and monogamy, it is clear that there is a major segment of the population that either cannot adopt these strategies (e.g. impoverished, powerless women driven to sex work) or will not. Thus, behavioural interventions to increase the use of condoms have been emphasized. This strategy (the 100% condom programme) has been successful in Thailand and Cambodia with men patronizing brothels, but has been less successful with casual partners and spouses, and has not been very effective in Africa.

Before treatment became available, the fear of stigmatization caused people to avoid testing and promoted continued risky behaviour and transmission of the virus. With the development of effective treatment, there is a strong rationale for persons suspecting that they are infected to get tested. Numerous studies have demonstrated that both infected and uninfected individuals reduce their risky sexual behaviour once they know their status.

Health education alone has been shown not to be effective. However, early education of children, not just about the risks of HIV/AIDS but also about coping strategies to resist peer pressure, may be effective and have been implemented in many countries. Because in many developing countries those most vulnerable to HIV/AIDS are most likely to leave school after 6 years, it is important to implement these programmes in elementary school. Cuba used widespread compulsory testing and 'quarantine' as a strategy to contain the spread of HIV. To some extent this worked, because Cuba is an island with strictly controlled and limited entry and departure of travellers. These conditions clearly do not exist for the majority of countries worldwide and, thus, are not appropriate as a major strategy for containment of the virus.

For transmission by sharing of injecting equipment, 'harm reduction' strategies have been promoted. These include needle/syringe exchange programmes and drug replacement therapy. Needle exchange programmes have little effect on drug use, but reduce the likelihood of exposure to HIV-contaminated needles and reduce the amount of HIV circulating among IDU in the community. Drug replacement programmes provide oral drugs, usually methadone or bupremorphine, which reduce the craving for injecting. Thus, exposure to contaminated needles is eliminated or reduced. Neither of these programmes treats the drug addiction, but they do reduce exposure to HIV and other pathogens such as hepatitis C virus.

Ultimately, a combination of political pressure and community involvement is likely to be the most effective strategy for containing the epidemic. For example, a community intervention study that mobilized the community to recognize that injecting drug use was a problem in their community and to take the initiative to address the problem resulted in a drop of new drug-using youth by two-thirds within 2 years.

The HIV/AIDS epidemic has, however, also advanced the fields of epidemiology, immunology, and virology through the massive amount of research funding that has been allocated. This research has refined the strategy of sentinel surveillance, and provided opportunities to improve the 'nested case–control' design used in epidemiology, the understanding of the advantages and limitations of epidemiological modelling, and the understanding of the response of the immune system, particularly the cellular immune response, to foreign agents and the strategies used by viruses to avoid the immune system response. Thus, research on HIV/AIDS has benefited the entire field of science and the public's health.

Ebola

Ebola virus disease was first identified concurrently during epidemics in Zaire (now the Democratic Republic of the Congo) and Sudan in 1976, but there is serological evidence of an earlier epidemic in 1972 in Zaire. Both of the 1976 epidemics were first recognized among patients entering local hospitals in the two countries. The causative agents in the two epidemics, Ebola-Zaire and Ebola-Sudan, differed slightly, perhaps explaining the lower case fatality in Sudan (54%) than in Zaire (88%) (eMedicine.com 2005). The transmission in Zaire occurred primarily through reuse of unsterilized needles and syringes, whereas in Sudan transmission was primarily through close personal contact with a patient. Both epidemics died out when strict containment procedures were implemented. Containment requires universal precautions and barrier nursing care, including the use of latex gloves, masks, and gowns, and isolation of patients. The common practice in Africa of open-casket funerals, with extensive cleansing and preparation of the body by relatives and close friends, had to be stopped, and closed-casket ceremonies substituted.

Fifteen subsequent outbreaks of Ebola have occurred in Gabon, Côte d' Ivoire, Liberia, South Africa, Uganda, and the latest in 2004 in Sudan. There have been a total of 1848 known cases, with 1287 (69.6%) deaths. Secondary transmission occurs primarily to caregivers, hospital personnel, and immediate family members through direct exposure to blood, other bodily secretions, and infected organs. Implementation of strict infection precautions and changes in burial customs usually resulted in the containment of each of the epidemics. Fortunately, Ebola does not appear to spread via the respiratory route.

The source of the initial cases in each of the epidemics is unknown, but most cases have been in proximity to African tropical forests. Ebola has been isolated from carcasses of chimpanzees, gorillas, monkeys, forest duikers, and porcupines found dead in the forests, but it is not known whether they are the primary reservoir. Presumably the primary reservoir is a dweller of the tropical forests of sub-Saharan Africa. The origins of the virus are also unknown.

The usual incubation period ranges from 2–21 days. The initial symptoms include sudden malaise, headache, and muscle pain, progressing to high fever, vomiting, and bloody diarrhoea. Patients are most infectious during the phase of vomiting and diarrhoea. Patients die from haemorrhaging of internal organs. The case fatality ranges from about 50% to over 89%, and appears to be somewhat lower for Ebola-Sudan than Ebola-Zaire.

Ebola belongs to the newly described genus, filovirus (Feldmann *et al.* 1996). Two other filoviruses were recognized in the twentieth century, Reston virus and Marburg virus, both initially causing outbreaks in laboratories (World Health Organization 1992). The Reston virus appears to be less virulent than the other two members of the family. Recently, in 2005, Marburg caused an epidemic of 351 known cases in Angola, with a case fatality rate of 88.8%. This epidemic was larger than most of the known Ebola outbreaks, and suggests that Ebola and Marburg viruses may cause more substantial epidemics in the future unless more effective prevention and containment strategies can be developed and implemented.

Kuru

In the early 1900s, a fatal neurodegenerative disease appeared in the South Fore people of the New Guinea Highlands. The disease was eight times more common among women than men. Children were also victims of the disease. At first the disease was thought to be a genetic disease.

Ritual mortuary cannibalism was practiced by the South Fore people. When one of them died, they would be butchered, and the brain and innards consumed by women who were in charge of preparing the body for consumption. The men, who preferred muscle to brain tissue were less affected. Gadjusek, Gibbs and Alpers (1996) were able to transmit the disease from chimpanzees injected with tissue from kuru victims to chimpanzees never exposed to tissue from kuru victims, demonstrating that the causative agent could be transmitted.

Subsequently, Prusiner (1995) was able to identify the causative agent, and to demonstrate that it did not contain nucleic acids, indicating that the agent was not a virus but a newly recognized agent, a 'prion'. Further work by Prusiner and others confirmed that the prion was a cellular protein variant of a gene found in humans called PrPc, caused by a single point mutation. The variant, labelled PrPSc, recruits normal proteins by 'flipping' them into a prion-like shape that can then infect other cells and animals. Thus, the prion is able to replicate in the absence of nucleic acid genetic material through a chain reaction-like mechanism. The normal PrPc gene does not appear to be essential for humans; thus, treatment may be possible through agents targeting the PrPc and its variant prion. The biological mechanisms of prion disease, however, are still not fully understood, and present a challenge to future scientists.

Gadjusek hypothesized that the disease was caused by a slow virus with an incubation period of 2–25 years. On the basis of these studies, he was the first epidemiologist to be awarded a Nobel prize. The discovery that the cause of kuru is a prion was important because it defined an entirely new class of infectious agents that are the cause of many neurodegenerative diseases, including 'mad cow disease' (bovine spongiform encephalitis), the probable cause of variant Creutzfeldt–Jakob disease in humans, which has caused so much concern and economic loss in the last decades of the twentieth century.

Thus, kuru and the work by Gadjusek, Prusiner, and colleagues is significant because it identified an entirely new class of infectious agents that do not depend on nucleic acids for replication and transmission. Prions have now been recognized as the causative agent of many neurodegenerative disorders, but it is possible that as the twenty-first century progresses, we may find other diseases caused by this new class of infectious agent.

Dengue haemorrhagic fever

The first reported epidemics of dengue fever occurred in 1779–80 in Asia, Africa, and North America. The disease was described by Benjamin Rush, a Philadelphia physician, as 'break bone fever' in 1780. The causative agent, dengue virus, was not isolated until 1943. Dengue virus causes an acute febrile illness with severe symptomatology, but is self-limiting and seldom results in death. The haemorrhagic complications of infection with the dengue virus, dengue haemorrhagic fever (DHF), were not described until the 1950s in the Americas and Southeast Asia. Unlike dengue fever, DHF is associated with serious morbidity and a high case fatality. Volumetric fluid replacement and supportive care can reduce the case fatality from 40–50% to 1–2%. Although an attenuated vaccine to dengue has been developed, it has not been subjected to efficacy trials in humans as yet. It is unlikely that an effective vaccine will be available for public health use in less than a decade. From a public health perspective, it is essential that vaccination results in protection against all four subtypes, as protection against only one or two subtypes may result in more serious disease due to subsequent infection with the other subtypes. By the end of the twentieth century, DHF had become a major cause of morbidity and mortality in children in many of the countries of these two regions (World Health Organization 2002).

There are four subtypes of dengue virus, types 1, 2, 3, and 4. Infection with a particular subtype of the virus provides lifelong protection against that subtype, but not against the other subtypes (Centers for Disease Control 2005). It has been suggested by Scott Halstead that sequential infection with different subtypes may result in haemorrhagic fever. However, some epidemics of DHF have been reported to be associated with subtypes 2 and 3.

The resurgence of dengue fever and the emergence of DHF can be ascribed to the rapid urbanization that has occurred in the second half of the twentieth century. The usual mosquito vector, *Aedes aegypti*, breeds in urban water sources, such as water collected in discarded tyres, water containers, and other urban locales where standing water collects long enough for the breeding of mosquitoes. The rapid growth of cities of Latin America and Southeast Asia has led to the building of impromptu slums, which have inadequate housing and no water, sewerage, or waste management systems. These slums usually contain many sources of standing water ideal for breeding of the dengue vector. In the absence of an effective vaccine control, efforts must concentrate on eliminating the vector. However, vector control is essentially absent in the rapidly growing urban areas of developing countries, which are often concerned with other pressing problems. The rapid increase in international travel, possible with the introduction of jet aircraft, has allowed the transmission of dengue to new locations that may have vectors capable of transmitting the virus. Control of dengue and DHF in the twenty-first century, in the absence of a vaccine, will require surveillance to identify areas in which dengue is occurring and vigorous efforts to control the breeding of the vector. Health education efforts to induce the public to reduce the sources of standing water around their homes will also be a key factor.

Chlamydiae

Trachoma, an ocular disease caused by *Chlamydia trachomatis*, was known in ancient China and Egypt thousands of years ago, but the causative agent was not isolated until 1957 by Tang and associates in China and confirmed in 1958. Trachoma was the most frequent cause of preventable blindness worldwide. It has been estimated that there are still 70 million active cases of ocular trachoma infection worldwide, including approximately 2 million people with associated conjunctival scarring and eyelid deformities (Dugger 2005). Ocular trachoma is associated with crowding and poor hygiene. Although the disease is curable with vigorous treatment, improved living and sanitary conditions have been the primary cause of the decline in the disease.

The other chlamydial agent known for many years is *Chlamydia psittaci*, a major cause of respiratory disease that occurs primarily among those handling infected birds, including chicken and turkey processing plants. Person-to-person spread is rare, but has been observed in some outbreaks of the disease. In the USA and other countries, psittacosis is a problem because it is repeatedly reintroduced by importation of exotic or psittacine birds.

With the rapid development of new laboratory technologies in the second half of the twentieth century, other manifestations of chlamydiae infection have been recognized (Peeling and Brunham 1996). In the late 1960s, it became clear that *C. trachomatis* could also cause genital disease in sexually active individuals. Clinical manifestations include cervicitis, urethritis, endometritis, pelvic inflammatory disease, and proctitis. Subsequently, *C. trachomatis* has been recognized as one of the major STDs worldwide. The World Health Organization has estimated that there were 95 million new chlamydial infections worldwide in 1995. Unfortunately, the majority of genital chlamydiae infections (50–70%) are asymptomatic, particularly among women. Thus, they are seldom diagnosed and treated before serious complications occur. Current infection can be eliminated by a single dose of azithromycin or a 7-day course of doxycycline, but infection does not confer immunity. Thus, reinfection is common in those who are sexually active and repeatedly exposed. Another manifestation of *C. trachomatis* is lymphogranuloma venereum, which is five times more frequent in men than women, and is also easily treatable.

In the early 1980s, Grayston *et al.* (1986) and Saikku *et al.* (1993) identified another subtype of chlamydiae now known as *Chlamydia pneumoniae*. It is the third most common cause of community-acquired pneumonia, and frequently causes mild respiratory disease. Antibodies to *C. pneumoniae* are found in over 50% of most adult populations worldwide. It is one of the most common causes of pneumonia in early infancy. The onset of asthma and exacerbations of asthma have also been reported to occur in association with *C. pneumoniae* infection.

In 1988, Saikku and colleagues noted that patients with acute myocardial infarction and coronary heart disease often had elevated levels of IgG and IgA antibodies to *C. pneumoniae* (Saikku 1993). Subsequently, *C. pneumoniae* has been linked to atherosclerosis (Kuo and Campbell 2000). However, a recent trial of preventive treatment with antibiotics did not result in a lower rate of myocardial infarction in those treated. However, animal model studies have shown that *C. pneumoniae* respiratory infection can accelerate atherosclerotic formation in hyperlipidaemic mice and rabbits. Thus, the nature of the relationship with *C. pneumoniae* is still not fully understood.

In summary, chlamydiae are a major cause of morbidity worldwide, but only through the development of new laboratory technologies in the twentieth century has the range of diseases they causes become apparent. It is possible that even more manifestations of these ubiquitous agents may be discovered in the twenty-first century.

Prevention of emerging diseases

The US Centers for Disease Control and Prevention (1998) has outlined the objectives for preventing emerging diseases in the future. These are (including examples):

- Enhance global watchfulness for new diseases and agents. The World Health Organization has established the Global Outbreak Alert and Response Network, which is a collaboration of existing institutions and networks worldwide that pool human and technical resources for the rapid identification, confirmation, and response to outbreaks of international importance.

◆ Develop strategies to fight new, previously unknown diseases (e.g. SARS). SARS was contained through a strategy of alerting the public and travellers to the early symptoms, and voluntary quarantine of exposed contacts and isolation of cases.

◆ Protect the blood, food, and water supplies from contamination. Governments in developed countries, and increasingly in developing countries, have established agencies that are responsible for maintaining the quality and safety of blood, food, and water.

◆ Continually develop new antibiotics to organisms that have become resistant to current drugs. A major effort continues to identify new classes of drugs that act at different points in the replication of HIV, e.g. attachment of the virus to the target cell and integration of the virus into the cell genetic material. Similar research is being conducted to overcome resistance to staphylococci and other agents.

◆ Develop new vaccines. There are major efforts being made by scientists to develop effective vaccines to protect against malaria and HIV/AIDS.

◆ Prevent zoonotic diseases from spreading to humans. A major source of SARS, influenza, and other zoonotic diseases from southern China are live animal markets, where animals are crowded together for sale, promoting rapid spread of infectious agents among them. Traditionally, Chinese doubt the freshness of animal produce unless they kill it themselves. Hong Kong has now outlawed live markets.

◆ Protect vulnerable populations, e.g. the sick, the elderly, pregnant women, etc. Many countries have implemented special centres for the elderly that provide activities, exercise, and advice on maintaining health. Facilities for handicapped people are being mandated by law. Antenatal clinics are now found in almost all countries, although the coverage may be inadequate in some developing countries.

◆ Prevent terrorist attacks with microbial agents, and respond quickly and effectively when incidents do occur. Many countries have implemented special procedures for identifying terrorist attacks with microbial agents and implementing containment procedures. The USA and other countries are stockpiling vaccines to likely terrorist agents such as smallpox. Unfortunately there has been relatively little attention paid to resolving the underlying causes of the terrorist attacks (Sorvillo *et al.* 2002).

The CDC proposes four interdependent strategies:

◆ Surveillance for new diseases and agents, and monitoring of their occurrence once recognized.

◆ Applied research to develop new techniques to fight emerging diseases, including identifying new agents and developing new strategies and drugs to control their morbidity and spread.

◆ Infrastructure development to heighten preparedness and to sustain surveillance, applied research, and prevention programmes, as well as training of personnel to implement these activities.

◆ Prevention and control through surveillance, applied research, and infrastructure development.

We were only partially successful at meeting the challenge of emerging diseases in the twentieth century. The twenty-first century will bring new social, economic, and scientific advances and changes that will foster the emergence of new diseases and the re-emergence of diseases we thought we had controlled. The challenge is to do better in this century before us.

References

Centers for Disease Control (1998). *Preventing emerging infectious diseases: a strategy for the twenty-first century*. Centers for Disease Control, Atlanta, GA.

Centers for Disease Control. (2005). *Dengue fever*. Centers for Disease Control and Prevention, Atlanta GA (see www.cdc.gov/ncidod/dvbid/dengue).

Dugger CW (2005). On the brink—trachoma: preventable disease blinds poor in third world. *New York Times*, March 31.

eMedicine.com (2005). *Ebola virus*,www.emedicine.com 2005.

Feldmann H, Slenczka W, and Klenk HD (1996). Emerging and reemerging of filoviruses. *Archives of Virology*, **11**, S77–S100.

Gadjusek DC, Gibbs CJ, and Alpers M (1966). Experimental transmission of a kuru-like syndrome to chimpanzees. *Nature*, **209**, 794.

Grayston JT, Kuo CC, Wang SP, and Altman J (1986). A new Chlamydia psittaci strain, TWAR, isolated in acute respiratory tract infections. *New England Journal of Medicine*, **315**, 161–8.

Krause RM (1998). *Emerging infections*, pp. 20–21. Academic Press, New York.

Kuo CC and Campbell LA (2000). Detection of *Chlamydia pneumoniae* in arterial tissues. *Journal of Infectious Diseases*, **181**, S432–S436.

Lederberg J, Shope RE, and Oaks SC (1992). *Emerging infections*. National Academy Press, Washington, DC.

Leveton LB, Sox HC, and Seto MA (1995). *HIV and the blood supply: an analysis of crisis decision making*. National Academy Press, Washington, DC.

Peeling RW and Brunham RC (1996). Chlamydiae as pathogens: new species and new issues. *Emerging Infectious Diseases*, **2**, 307–19.

Phoolcahroen W and Detels R (2002). Acquired immunodeficiency syndrome. In *Oxford textbook of public health*, 4th edn, pp. 1453–80. Oxford University Press, Oxford.

Prusiner SB (1995). Prion diseases. *Scientific American*, **272**, 48–56.

Saikku P (1993). Chlamydia pneumoniae infection as a risk factor in acute myocardial infarction. *European Heart Journal*, **14**, S62–S65.

Saikku P, Ruutu P, Leinonen M, Kleemola M, Paladin F, and Tupasi TE (1993). *Mycoplasma pneumoniae* and *Chlamydia trachomatis* in acute lower respiratory infections in Filipino children. *American Journal of Tropical Medicine and Hygiene*, **49**, 88–92.

Sorvillo F, Greenwood JR, and Detels R (2002). Bioterrorism. In *Oxford textbook of public health*, 4th edn, pp. 1947–55. Oxford University Press, Oxford.

World Health Organization (1992). Viral haemorrhagic fever in imported monkeys. *Weekly Epidemiological Record*, **67**, 142–3 (based on Department of Health, Communicable Diseases New Zealand, 1991).

World Health Organization (2002). *Dengue and dengue hemorrhagic fever*, Fact Sheet No 117. WHO, Geneva (available at www.who.int/mediacentre/factsheets/fs117/en/).

Wu Z, Sullivan SG, Wang Y, Rotheram-Borus MJ, and Detels R (2007). Evoluation of China's response to HIV/AIDS. *Lancet*, in press

13

Tuberculosis

George W. Comstock

Personal experiences

My introduction to epidemiology came long before I had heard or seen the word.

During my years at Antioch College, I had a cooperative job in the research laboratories of Eli Lilly and Company. One of their major activities was the search for the pellagra preventive factor. I recall being impressed by the different conclusions reached by the US Public Health Service investigators, Joseph Goldberger and Edgar Sydenstricker, and a competing group who were studying the same group of southern mill villages. The latter, using a largely qualitative dietary history, came to the conclusion that pellagra was not a dietary disease because pellagrins and normal persons ate similar foods. Goldberger and the economist Sydenstricker showed that pellagrins ate much less of the protective foods, particularly in the months preceding the pellagra season (Kraut 2003). This was my introduction to the US Public Health Service and the importance of quantitative data.

Following my graduation from Harvard Medical School in 1941, I became a Commissioned Officer in the Service. On completion of a tour of sea duty, I had the good fortune to be assigned to the newly created Tuberculosis Control Division whose director, Herman Hilleboe, had an uncanny ability to impress his superiors and Congress with the importance of tuberculosis and the necessity for adequate funding. In 1946, I was assigned to the Muscogee County Health Department in Columbus, Georgia to conduct long-term follow-up studies of the kinds of tuberculosis suspects that were being detected in great numbers in the mass chest X-ray surveys being conducted at that time.

The Muscogee County Tuberculosis Study was one of three 'facilities' with which I have been associated. (Facility is a word used by Carroll E. Palmer to mean a study situation where a variety of epidemiological studies can be carried out with minimal difficulty.) The other two are the Bethel area of Alaska, and Washington County, Maryland. In each of the three areas, a community health-oriented private census provided baseline data.

Along the way, I inherited the follow-up of the BCG vaccination trial in Puerto Rico and a study of tuberculosis among US Navy personnel (Comstock *et al.* 1974a,b). However, the most important aspect of my Public Health Service career was my close association with Carroll E. Palmer and Shirley Ferebee Woolpert, two of the best epidemiologists I have ever known. I owe much to their examples and tutelage.

Prior to the last two decades of the nineteenth century, the study of tuberculosis was based on the shaky foundations of historical, physical, and autopsy findings. In 1882, Robert Koch's discovery of methods to demonstrate mycobacteria on microscopic examination set the stage for modern diagnosis (Koch 1932). A few years later, his 'heilmittel', a crude extract of the broth in which tubercle bacilli had been grown, was found to cause delayed inflammatory reactions when injected intracutaneously into persons who had been infected with *Mycobacterium tuberculosis* or related mycobacterial species (Koch 1890). When Roentgen's discovery of X-rays in 1895 made chest radiography possible, basic tools for the diagnosis of pulmonary tuberculosis were at hand. It was now possible to assess the importance of various risk factors in the chain of events that could lead from exposure to a person with infectious tuberculosis to death from tuberculosis. Only then could the epidemiology of tuberculosis be established on a reasonably solid basis.

More recent improvements in the diagnostic armamentarium, such as the ability to culture mycobacteria and assess their sensitivity to various drugs, and the identification of specific strains of tubercle bacilli by genotyping, have made diagnoses more precise and epidemiological knowledge more certain.

The first major study to make use of the early improvements in diagnosis was the Framingham Community Health and Tuberculosis Demonstration (Dublin 1952; Comstock 2005). A remarkably complete tuberculosis control programme was established in Framingham, Massachusetts in 1917 by the Metropolitan Life Insurance Company and continued for several years thereafter. Tuberculosis case rates dropped markedly soon after the start of the programme, considerably more than in several control villages. Its major legacy was the finding that there were nine unrecognized cases in the community for every reported case. This ratio was used for planning tuberculosis control programmes in the USA for several decades.

Nearly 50 years later, a study that had many similarities to the first Framingham Study was conducted in Kolin, Czechoslovakia during the period 1960 to 1972 (Styblo et al. 1967). Because the epidemiological situation in Europe had changed greatly during the 1950s, 'Czechoslovakia agreed to collaborate with WHO in a complex long-term experimental, epidemiological and clinical study of tuberculosis in a representative sample of the population'. The principal difference from the Framingham Study was that in Kolin the purpose was only to describe the tuberculosis problem and the practices used to control it in an area similar to most of central Europe. There were no control populations as in the Framingham Study. Preventive procedures at that time were BCG vaccination, case-finding, including repeated mass chest X-ray surveys, and chemotherapy (streptomycin, para-aminosalicylic acid (PAS), and isoniazid for the most part) initiated in the sanatorium and continued as self-medication at home for 18–24 months. Continued follow-up in the Kolin District for a total of 12 years showed that there had been a considerable decrease in the prevalence of tuberculosis but a steady development of new cases, particularly among the middle-aged and elderly population (Krivinka et al. 1974). It is disappointing that there was no comparison with other programmes and places.

In England, another pioneering study was the Prophit Tuberculosis Survey, conducted over a 10-year period from 1933 to 1944 (Daniels et al. 1948). Its major finding was that subsequent case rates for young adults were three times higher for those who were tuberculin negative at entry to the study than the rates for the tuberculin-positive reactors. This excess was greater for females than for males, and was related to intensity of exposure. Tuberculosis was most likely to develop among persons with the strongest reactions to tuberculin and the high risk of developing tuberculosis shortly after becoming infected was clearly established.

In the nineteenth century, European ideas about the nature of tuberculosis were split. In the north, it was considered to be hereditary while residents of southern Europe feared it as contagious. When George Sand took Chopin to Mallorca for his health, the villagers forced the couple to leave, considering Chopin's tuberculosis to be dangerous to society (Daniel 1997). As things have turned out, there is a degree of truth on both sides. There is now no doubt that tuberculosis is contagious. Thanks largely to the Prophit Committee of the Royal College of Physicians of London, there is good evidence that there is a degree of hereditary susceptibility as well. Barbara Simonds was recruited to gather and analyse data on twin pairs in which at least one had tuberculosis (Comstock 1978). By searching all the tuberculosis case registers in England she was able to identify 205 such pairs. All but three pairs had sufficient information about zygosity and risk factors to be included in the study. Sadly, the report had to be completed while Dr Simonds was on her deathbed. The finished report concluded that zygosity was not important.

Fortunately, the report included an appendix with considerable clinical and socio-economic information on each twin. Some years later when methods of accounting for the effects of confounding variables became available, the data were reanalysed using binary variable regression. It then became apparent that if one twin of a pair had tuberculosis, the risk of the other twin developing the disease was considerably greater among monozygotic than dizygotic pairs. This was strong evidence that 'inherited susceptibility is an important risk factor for tuberculosis among twins' (Comstock 1978).

Methods for analysing tuberculosis trends were developed in the 1930s. Cohort analysis, namely the study of disease or death among a hypothetical group of persons born in the same place and time period was introduced by a Norwegian, Kristian Andvord (Andvord 1930). It did not come to general attention, however, until Wade Hampton Frost independently developed the same method of analysis (Frost 1939). Even then, the idea narrowly escaped oblivion, for Frost was apparently concerned by his belated discovery of Andvord's work, and had set his own paper aside. It was not discovered and published until after Frost's death.

Frost made other important contributions to the epidemiology of tuberculosis. When E. L. Bishop, the Commissioner of Health for the State of Tennessee, wished to set up a major community-based study of tuberculosis, he asked his former professor for advice. Frost suggested a pilot study in a smaller county, a retrospective study of tuberculosis cases for the past several decades, an approach now known as a historical cohort study (Frost 1933). In addition to this unique approach, he made an adaptation of the secondary attack rate for acute infectious diseases developed by C. V. Chapin, Health Commissioner for Providence, Rhode Island (Cassedy 1962). In a chronic disease like tuberculosis, it was often impossible to identify the primary case in a household. Frost suggested that the first case to be reported be called the 'index case'. If index cases were excluded from the calculations, a measure of the risk of developing tuberculosis for other household members could be developed that was analogous to the secondary attack rate (Frost 1933).

Cohort analyses of tuberculosis deaths clearly showed that there was a peak of mortality among young adults, earlier in life and more marked among females than males. Such a peak was so prominent in the early decades of the twentieth century in the USA that it was easily seen even in cross-sectional graphs. These graphs for the 3-year periods around 1920, 1930, and 1940 were published in considerable detail in monographs by the US Public Health Service (Federal Security Agency, US Public Health Service and Medical Research Committee, National Tuberculosis Association 1943). Unfortunately, like most monographs, this series attracted little attention and was soon forgotten. A peak of mortality in the age group 25–29 years was most prominent among non-whites, females, and residents of states that most people would judge as the least prosperous. By 1940 the peak had disappeared for males, and had become much less prominent for the other sex–age groups. Similar findings were noted among European nations (Holland 1997).

During the 1930s it was generally believed that two findings were pathognomonic of a previous infection with tubercle bacilli—pulmonary calcifications and positive reactions to any of the commonly used doses of tuberculin. It came as a shock when L. L. Lumsden, an American shoe-leather epidemiologist and a bit of an iconoclast, announced the results of his studies in the states of Tennessee, Alabama, and Mississippi in the southeastern USA. Particularly in Tennessee, people with pulmonary calcifications often did not react to tuberculin, and in the more southern states of Alabama and Mississippi, reactions to strong doses of purified tuberculin did not correlate with other indices of tuberculosis prevalence (Lumsden and Dearing 1940).

To confirm and understand these apparently contradictory findings, a meeting of experts in the fields of radiographic diagnoses or tuberculin testing was arranged in Hagerstown, Maryland, USA in 1939 (Comstock 1969). Under the watchful eyes of the experts, school children and food handlers were tuberculin tested and had chest radiographs interpreted. When the findings were presented to the meeting, it was found that Lumsden was correct. The two 'pathognomonic' findings disagreed more often than not. Most of the experts left the meeting, puzzled perhaps, but without plans for further investigations. Only Esmond Long, Head of the Phipps Institute in Philadelphia, and Carroll Palmer, a junior investigator from the US Public Health Service, decided that the only solution to the dilemma was that there had to be more than one cause for pulmonary calcifications and also for tuberculin sensitivity. Long did not investigate the matter further; Palmer set up large studies to look into this apparent contradiction. That pulmonary calcifications could also be caused by histoplasmosis was first reported by Christie and Peterson, physicians in Tennessee (Christie and Peterson 1945), a finding confirmed later by Palmer's much larger study among student nurses (Palmer 1945; Goddard *et al.* 1949). Histoplasmosis is primarily an infection of middle North America, where pulmonary calcifications are most likely to result from infections with *Histoplasma capsulatum*. In the rest of the world, histoplasmosis is rare or absent, and calcifications may safely be considered as indicating healed primary tuberculosis. Answers to the significance of reactions only to the strong dose of tuberculin would come largely from another of Palmer's facilities: US naval recruits tuberculin tested by specially trained nurses (Palmer *et al.* 1959) and from results of the International Tuberculosis Campaign.

The International Tuberculosis Campaign was the first major disease control programme of the World Health Organization (WHO) (Comstock 1994a). It was planned and directed by Johannes Holm as the only feasible mass programme for combating the threat of an epidemic of tuberculosis in the areas devastated by the Second World War. Millions of children and young adults in many countries around the world (but primarily in Europe) were tuberculin tested and if they were negative reactors, were vaccinated with BCG. Palmer recognized the research potential of this vast database, and with Knud Magnus, Johannes Guld, and Lydia and Phyllis Edwards (not related), established the WHO's Tuberculosis Research Office. During the early days of the campaign, people to be vaccinated were tested first with a weak dose of tuberculin. Two days later, non-reactors to that dose were tested with the strong dose, and 2 days after that, those who were still tuberculin negative were vaccinated. This was obviously cumbersome and time-consuming. Eventually, it was shown that preliminary tuberculin testing was unnecessary since needless vaccination of positive reactors or tuberculosis patients caused no harm other than lost time and inconvenience for patients and personnel (Raj Narain and Vallishayee 1976).

When the characteristics of persons who reacted only to the strong dose were compared with those who reacted to the weaker dose, it was found that only the latter reactions indicated exposure to tuberculosis. Reactions only to the stronger doses of tuberculin were more frequent among persons who lived at lower latitudes and altitudes; in those areas they were unrelated to tuberculosis.

Another of Palmer's facilities that contributed to the understanding of the significance of strong dose reactions came from the work of the tuberculin testing teams of trained Public Health Service nurses at the US Naval Training Centers at Chicago and San Diego (Edwards and Palmer 1969). From 1958 to 1964, more than 600,000 recruits were given a standard tuberculin test and tests with sensitins from three other mycobacteria—PPD-B from *Mycobacterium avium/intracellulare*, PPD-G from *Mycobacterium scrofulaceum*, and PPD-Y from *Mycobacterium kansasii*. Results were classified by which sensitin gave the largest reaction. Reactions to PPD-B were most common south of a diagonal line drawn from New England to southern California. Reactions to PPD-G were even more common in the southeastern-most states, and reactions to PPD-Y were common in the northern Midwest. Reactors only to the second dose of tuberculin were very likely to react to one of these non-tuberculous mycobacterial antigens. Studies of non-tuberculous mycobacterial infections outside of the USA have relied almost entirely on comparisons of reactions with purified tuberculin (RT-23 or PPD-S) and PPD-B. Because PPD-B has a broad antigenic spectrum, reactions to it are a good indicator of the frequency of non-tuberculous mycobacterial infections. Like reactions only to the strong dose of PPD-S, they tend to be most common at low latitudes and altitudes, and absent at very high altitudes and in the high Arctic.

Follow-up of controlled trials of BCG vaccination has yielded much useful epidemiological knowledge, notably studies conducted by the British Medical Research Council, the US Public Health Service, and the Indian Council of Medical Research. All showed that reactors to the weaker dose of tuberculin were at considerable risk of developing tuberculosis and that reactors only to the strong dose of tuberculin had some degree of protection against subsequent tuberculosis (Hart and Sutherland 1977; Comstock and Webster 1969; Datta *et al.* 1999).

While it has been clear for a long time that some BCG vaccines can prevent tuberculosis disease, little attention has been paid to their ability to prevent vaccinees from becoming infected after exposure. While this additional mode of protection has seemed entirely reasonable, it has only recently been confirmed. Using ELISpot to differentiate vaccinated from naturally infected children in Turkey, Soysal and colleagues produced evidence that their strain of BCG also protected children against tuberculosis infection (Soysal *et al.* 2005).

Proof that tubercle bacilli could be spread as droplet nuclei by the airborne route was clearly demonstrated by Riley and his associates in 1959 (Riley *et al.* 1959). Individual tuberculosis patients were housed in one of the six rooms that had been built as a sort of penthouse on the roof of a Veterans Administration hospital in Baltimore, Maryland. Air from these rooms was exhausted through a space containing cages of guinea pigs. The animals were tuberculin tested monthly and sacrificed when they developed a positive reaction. The lungs were carefully examined for evidence of tubercles. During the 2 years of the experiment, almost half of the guinea pigs became infected. The patients responsible for the infection could be determined by the timing of the infection and the drug sensitivities of the organisms. Two patients were highly infectious; some others infected no guinea pigs. Riley's work proved beyond any doubt that tuberculosis could be spread by the airborne route. He also showed that infections ceased when the exhausted air was exposed to strong ultraviolet irradiation before it reached the guinea pigs.

The Danish Tuberculosis Index was created to keep track of tuberculosis that developed among the 783,000 persons between the ages of 15 and 35 years who were the principal targets of a tuberculosis mass screening programme conducted in 1950–52. Follow-up results were limited by the untimely deaths of its directors, E. Groth-Petersen and his successor Ole Horwitz. One of the last studies from the Index was a report of tuberculosis incidence and mortality among males in the Index population during the 6 years after the initial screening examination (Horwitz and Knudsen 1961). Tuberculosis rates were presented only by broad occupational groups. Males employed in agriculture had tuberculosis rates approximately 20% lower than males in other occupational–social groups, among whom only trivial differences were found. There was no analysis by smaller occupational groups.

A later study of occupational tuberculosis in the USA used a much more detailed grouping (McKenna *et al.* 1996). Tuberculosis case rates were inversely associated with presumed socio-economic status, with two striking exceptions. High case rates were found, not unexpectedly, among personnel engaged in inducing sputum from tuberculosis suspects with non-productive coughs. A surprise was the high rate among funeral directors. A follow-up investigation of this finding showed that the frequency of positive tuberculin reactors was directly associated with the number of embalmings they had done, almost universally without any respiratory protection (Gershon *et al.* 1998). Aerosols are apparently produced during the embalming process, and tubercle bacilli, if present, are at least temporarily protected against the bactericidal properties of embalming fluids by mucoid secretions.

There has been a relative flurry of interest recently in the association of smoking and tuberculosis. In addition to the study by Soysal *et al* (2005) mentioned earlier, three others have appeared since 2004. In a retrospective cohort study of 42,655 clients registered with the Hong Kong Elderly Health Services, smoking was significantly associated with the development of tuberculosis disease (Leung *et al.* 2004). Similarly, in three countries of West Africa, a case–control analysis found the same association (Lienhardt *et al.* 2005). The last of this trio looked at the association of smoking with tuberculosis infection, finding a significant association. The authors speculated that production of cigarette smoke 'may favor persistence and replication of ingested mycobacteria by improving the macrophage or dendritic cell factors' (den Boon *et al.* 2005). An editorial reviewing the evidence concluded that there was little evidence to support a direct effect of smoking on tuberculin sensitivity but that available data 'are consistent with the hypothesis both a long duration of smoking and current smoking might be related to the development of active pulmonary tuberculosis' (Bothamley 2005).

In the tuberculosis literature there are scattered accounts of the association of mental distress and depression with a predisposition to tuberculosis (Holmes 1956). More direct evidence comes from a study conducted by Lydia Edwards (Comstock *et al.* 1974a). She was able to follow an almost complete cohort of enlisted men in the US Navy during the 4 years of their initial enlistment. Among those who were tuberculin negative on enlistment, there was very little tuberculosis during the next four years. Rates were very much higher among the positive reactors, somewhat higher among Blacks than Whites, with both showing a slight decrease over the next 4 years. Among Asians reactors, almost all of whom were Filipinos, case rates became very high by the second year and remained high during the remaining 2 years of their first enlistment. Filipinos were subject to much more mental and social stress than Blacks or Whites. The latter two groups were US citizens. To rejoin their families at least periodically when not at sea was relatively easy for them. Furthermore, if they did not like the navy, they did not have to re-enlist when their 4 years of service was completed.

The Filipinos almost always stayed in the navy for 20 years, looking forward to the time when they could come home with a retirement income that made them relatively rich men. However, for 20 years they were isolated from family and friends. Because most of their pay was sent home for family support, they could not afford the expensive fare home for a visit. In all other ways— ecological, occupational, financial, and medical—Whites, Blacks, and Filipinos were equal. The most plausible explanation for the increased risk among tuberculin-positive Filipinos is that stress increased the probability of reactivation of latent tuberculosis infections.

A finding of importance for tuberculosis control in poor nations was reported by two sociologists, D. Banerji and S. Andersen, based on their work in south India (Banerji and Andersen 1963). Almost all highly infectious cases of tuberculosis, those with tubercle bacilli in the sputum so numerous that they are demonstrable by simple microscopic examination of stained smears, had chest symptoms, notably cough, that had persisted for 3–52 weeks. Coughs of shorter duration were almost always due to acute infections; few undiagnosed and hence untreated tuberculosis cases lived longer than a year. A cough history is still a practical method of case-finding in poor countries even though the advent of AIDS as a major complication of tuberculosis has made cough histories less useful since the symptoms of combined tuberculosis and AIDS are so different from uncomplicated tuberculosis.

Genotyping is the latest group of procedures to help our understanding of tuberculosis. The development and use of various methods of genotyping are still evolving (Daley 2005). There are several complementary procedures. Restriction fragment-length polymorphism (RFLP), using the insertion sequence 6110 is the most common. Spoligotyping is less discriminating, but can be used when only small amounts of DNA are available. The most recently introduced method is MIRU-VNTR (mycobacterial interspersed repetitive units–variable number tandem repeats). The Centers for Disease Control and Prevention are said to be planning to use the last two methods to characterize the strains of tubercle bacilli submitted to them as a national sample. A major contribution of genotyping has been to demonstrate that various strains of BCG vaccines have unique 'fingerprints' (Behr *et al.* 1999). This finding adds convincing evidence to earlier reports that BCG strains varied in every characteristic on which they had been compared, including the ability to protect against tuberculosis (Comstock 1994b).

It is now possible to study the ability of BCG vaccination to protect not only against tuberculosis disease but also against acquiring tuberculous infection. A recent study from Turkey has shown that a T-cell-based enzyme-linked immunospot assay (ELISpot) can indicate which children exposed to infectious tuberculosis in the household had become infected. Those who had been vaccinated with BCG were considerably less likely to have been infected with tubercle bacilli (odds ratio = 0.60, 95% confidence limits 0.43–0.83). While this has always seemed reasonable, the Turkish study provides the first evidence of an additional protective effect of BCG vaccination. (Soysal *et al.* 2005).

Genotyping has also confirmed the long-held suspicion that exogenous reinfection is a reality. In fact, more than one strain of tubercle bacilli has been found in the secretions of a number of individual patients. However, the most exciting use of genotyping has been to trace the transmission of tuberculosis within communities (Kunimoto *et al.* 2004). For years it has been the belief that close contacts of a case of tuberculosis contracted the disease because of transmission from case to contact, leading to the traditional case-finding procedure of concentrating first on the closest contacts, the so-called stone-in-the-pond or concentric circle approach. While this is still general policy in the USA, genotyping is now recognized as 'integral to the detection and control of TB outbreaks... and to identify the site or sites of transmission' (American Thoracic Society, Centers for Disease Control and Prevention and Infectious Diseases Society of America 2005).

Genotyping is barely out of its infancy and appears to be starting an adolescent growth spurt. It has already forced changes in and broadening of some ideas about the epidemiology of tuberculosis, and there are undoubtedly more to come. Its contributions to our understanding of the epidemiology of tuberculosis are rivalled only by Koch's discovery of the tubercle bacillus and tuberculin. These older basic tools yielded a 'broad brush' picture of tuberculosis epidemiology. Genotyping is filling in the details, creating a more distinct picture, thereby making an invaluable contribution to the epidemiology of tuberculosis.

References

American Thoracic Society, Centers for Disease Control and Prevention and Infectious Diseases Society of America (2005). Controlling tuberculosis in the United States. *American Journal of Respiratory and Critical Care Medicine*, **172**, 1169–227.

Andvord KF (1930). What can we learn by following the development of tuberculosis from one generation to another? [English translation by G. Wijsmuller]. *International Journal of Tuberculosis and Lung Disease*, **6**, 562–8.

Banerji D and Andersen S (1963). A sociological study of awareness of symptoms among persons with pulmonary tuberculosis. *Bulletin of the World Health Organization*, **29**, 665–83.

Behr MW, Wilson MA, Gill WF, *et al.* (1999). Comparative genomics of BCG vaccines by whole genome DNA microarray. *Science*, **234**, 1520–3.

Bothamley GH (2005). Editorial. Smoking and tuberculosis: a chance or causal association? *Thorax*, **60**, 527–8.

Cassedy JH (1962). *Charles v. Chapin and the Public Health Movement*. Harvard University Press, Cambridge, MA.

Christie A and Peterson JC (1945). Pulmonary calcifications in negative tuberculin reactors. *American Journal of Public Health*, **35**, 1131–47.

Comstock GW (1969). The Hagerstown Tuberculosis Conference of 1938: a retrospective opinion. *American Review of Respiratory Diseases*, **99**, 119–20.

Comstock GW (1978). Tuberculosis in twins: a re-analysis of the Prophit Study. *American Review of Respiratory Disease*, **117**, 621–4.

Comstock GW (1994a). The International Tuberculosis Campaign: a pioneering venture in mass vaccination and research. *Clinical Infectious Diseases*, **19**, 528–40.

Comstock GW (1994b). Field trials of tuberculosis vaccines: How could we have done them better? *Controlled Clinical Trials*, **15**, 247–76.

Comstock GW (2005). Commentary: The First Framingham Study—a pioneer in community-based participatory research. *International Journal of Epidemiology*, **34**, 1188–96.

Comstock GW and Webster RG (1969). Tuberculosis studies in Muscogee County, Georgia. VII. A twenty-year evaluation of BCGF vaccination in a school population. *American Review of Respiratory Diseases*, **100**, 839–45.

Comstock GW, Edwards LB, and Livesay VT (1974a). Tuberculosis morbidity in the U. S. Navy: its distribution and decline. *American Review of Respiratory Diseases*, **110**, 572–80.

Comstock GW, Livesay VT, and Woolpert SF (1974b). Evaluation of BCG vaccination among Puerto Rican children. *American Journal of Public Health*, **64**, 283–91.

Daley CL (2005). Molecular epidemiology: a tool for understanding control of tuberculosis transmission. *Clinical Chest Medicine*, **26**, 217–23.

Daniel TM (1997). *Captain of death: the story of tuberculosis.* University of Rochester Press, Rochester, NY.

Daniels M, Ridehalg F, Springett VH, and Hall IM (1948). *Tuberculosis in young adults: report on the Prophit Tuberculosis Survey.* H. K. Lewis & Co., Ltd, London.

Datta M, Vallishayee RG, and Diwakara AM (1999). Fifteen year follow-up of trial of BCG vaccines in South India for tuberculosis prevention. *Indian Journal of Medical Research*, **110**, 56–69.

den Boon S, van Lill SW, Borgdorff MW, *et al.* (2005). Association between smoking and tuberculosis infection: a population survey in a high incidence area. *Thorax*, **60**, 555–7.

Dublin LI (1952). *A 40 year campaign against tuberculosis*, pp. 80–95. Metropolitan Life Insurance Company, New York.

Edwards LB and Palmer CE (1969). Part II. Tuberculosis infection. In *American Public Health Association vital and health statistics monograph, tuberculosis*, pp. 123–222. Harvard University Press, Cambridge, MA.

Federal Security Agency, US Public Health Service, Medical Research Committee, National Tuberculosis Association (1943). *Tuberculosis in the United States, Volume l, mortality statistics for states and geographic divisions,* USPHS, Washington DC.

Frost WH (1933). Risk of persons in familial contact with tuberculosis. *American Journal of Public Health*, **23**, 426–32.

Frost WH (1939). The age selection of mortality from tuberculosis in successive decades. *American Journal of Hygiene*, **30**, 91–6. (Reproduced in *American Journal of Epidemiology*, 1995, **141**, 4–9.)

Gershon RRM, Vlahov D, Escamilla-Cejudo JA, *et al.* (1998). Tuberculosis risk in funeral home employees. *Journal of Occupational and Environmental Medicine*, **40**, 492–503.

Goddard JG, Edwards LB, and Palmer CE (1949). Studies of pulmonary findings and antigen sensitivity among student nurses. IV. Relationship of pulmonary calcification with sensitivity to tuberculin and to histoplasmin. *Public Health Reports*, **64**, 820–46.

Hart PD and Sutherland I (1977). BCG and vole vaccines in the prevention of tuberculosis in adolescence and early adult life. *British Medical Journal*, **2**, 275–93.

Holland WW (1997). *European atlas of 'avoidable death', 1985–1989*, CEC Health Services Research Series No 9, Oxford University Press, Oxford.

Holmes TH (1956). Multidiscipline studies of tuberculosis. In *Personality, stress and tuberculosis* (ed. PJ Sparer), pp. 65–152. International Universities Press, Inc., New York.

Horwitz O and Knudsen J (1961). A follow-up study of tuberculosis incidence and general mortality in various occupational-social groups of the Danish population. *Bulletin of the World Health Organization*, **24**, 793–805.

Koch R (1890). A further communication on a remedy for tuberculosis. *British Medical Journal*, **2**, 1193–5.

Koch RA (1932). *Die aetiologie der tuberkulose* [translation by Berna and Max Pinner with an introduction by Allen K Krause]. *American Review of Tuberculosis*, **25**, 285–323.

Kraut AM (2003). *Goldberger's war. The life and work of a public health crusader*, pp. 101–2. Hill and Wang, New York.

Krivinka R, Drapela J, Kubik A, *et al.* (1974). Epidemiological and clinical study of tuberculosis in the district of Kolin, Czechslovakia. Second report (1965–1972). *Bulletin of the World Health Organization*, **51**, 59–69.

Kunimoto D, Sutherland K, Wooldrage K, *et al.* (2004). Transmission characteristics of tuberculosis in the foreign-born and the Canadian-born populations of Alberta, Canada. *International Journal of Tuberculosis and Lung Disease*, **8**, 1213–20.

Leung CC, Li T, Lam TH, Yew WW, *et al.* (2004). Smoking and tuberculosis among the elderly in Hong Kong. *American Journal of Respiratory and Critical Care Medicine*, **170**, 1027–33.

Lienhardt C, Fielding K, Sillah JS, *et al.* (2005). Investigation of the risk factors for tuberculosis: a case-control study in three countries in West Africa. *International Journal of Epidemiology*, **34**, 914–23.

Lumsden LL and Dearing WP (1940). Epidemiologic studies of tuberculosis. *American Journal of Public Health*, **30**, 219–28.

McKenna MT, Hutton M, Cauthen G, and Onorato IM (1996). The association between occupation and tuberculosis. A population-based survey. *American Journal of Respiratory and Critical Care Medicine*, **154**, 587–93.

Palmer CE (1945). Nontuberculous pulmonary calcifications and sensitivity to histoplasmin. *Public Health Reports*, **60**, 513–20.

Palmer CE, Edwards L, Hopwood L, and Edwards PQ (1959). Experimental and epidemiological basis for the interpretation of tuberculin sensitivity. *Journal of Pediatrics*, **55**, 313–429.

Raj Narain and Vallishayee RS (1976). BCG vaccination of tuberculosis in-patients and of strong reactors to tuberculin. *Bulletin of the International Union against Tuberculosis*, **51**, 242–4.

Riley RL, Mills CC, Nyka WD, *et al.* (1959). Aerial dissemination of pulmonary tuberculosis. A two-year study of contagiousness in a tuberculosis ward. *American Journal of Hygiene*, **70**, 185–96.

Soysal A, Millington KA, Bakir M, *et al.* (2005). Effect of BCG vaccination on risk of *Mycobacterium tuberculosis* infection in children with household tuberculosis contact: a prospective community-based study. *Lancet*, **366**, 1443–51.

Styblo K, Dankova D, Drapela J, *et al.* (1967). Epidemiological and clinical study of tuberculosis in the district of Kolin, Czechoslovakia. Report of the first four years of the study (1961–1964). *Bulletin of the World Health Organization*, **37**, 819–74.

14

Malaria

Richard H. Morrow and William J. Moss

Personal experiences

Richard Morrow: My wife and I went to Ghana in 1962 after I had completed 3 years of internal medicine residency at Strong Memorial Hospital, University of Rochester School of Medicine and a year
working with Walsh McDermott at New York Hospital, Cornell University Medical School. McDermott
arranged for me to join a new National Institutes of Health (NIH) programme, developed jointly with
the recently established Ghana National Institute of Health and Medical Research (NIHMR), under an
agreement reached by Nkrumah and Kennedy to conduct research on important endemic diseases in
West Africa. I was responsible for clinical care on the adult wards of the newly built infectious disease
unit at Korle Bu, the main hospital and national referral centre for Ghana. We rarely saw clinical
malaria on the adult side, although it was a common cause for paediatric admission. As a direct result
of our experience in Ghana (and strongly influenced by two close colleagues—Fred Sai, who later
became the first Professor of Community Health of the Ghana University School of Medicine and
then Minister of Health, and Silas Dodu, later to become the first Professor of Medicine and first Dean
of Faculty for the Ghana University School of Medicine), I became convinced that skills and knowledge in public health, and particularly epidemiology, were critical for solving public health problems
in Africa.

Ghana, like most other African nations, was not involved in the global malaria eradication
campaign. Malaria, although recognized as an important problem in young children, was not considered
a serious disease by most clinicians and was not a research priority. Rather, malaria was accepted as a
fact of childhood that was readily treated with Nivaquine (chloroquine). Although it was appreciated
that malaria contributed to anaemia in women and children, anaemia itself was not considered an
important public health problem. Haemoglobin levels of seven or eight grams per cent were considered 'normal'. Larvaciding was carried out in urban areas at the time of independence, but was largely
abandoned within a few years as too costly. Other approaches to mosquito control were not even
considered. There was no malarial control programme, and the clinical treatment of symptomatic
malaria was the only antimalarial intervention in use.

In 1964, I returned to NIH and was posted to the Harvard School of Public Health to obtain
a Masters Degree in public health. Two events occurred while at Harvard that shaped my future career
path: I came to know Tom Weller, Professor of Tropical Public Health, and I received an invitation to
join the Department of Community Health at Makerere University Medical School in Kampala as
WHO Senior Lecturer in Epidemiology as they began the first post-graduate programme in public
health in East Africa. With the blessings of NIH, which provided research support for clinical and
epidemiological studies of Burkitt's lymphoma in Uganda, I accepted the position. We spent the next
5 years (1966–70) at Makerere, where I first assumed the mantle of epidemiologist. Following in
the footsteps of Denis Burkitt, we found epidemiological associations between Burkitt's lymphoma,
exposure to falciparum malaria and Epstein–Barr virus infection. But malaria in Uganda, as in Ghana,
received scant attention either as a research priority or as a serious public health problem.

In the three decades since leaving Uganda in 1970, I have been involved in research and teaching
concerning the epidemiology of endemic tropical diseases, methods for field trials, epidemiological

approaches to establishing health-care priorities, and health systems issues of quality management, particularly in Africa. It was late in my career before I became directly involved in malaria research. With a doctoral student working in Tigray, Ethiopia, we studied the impact of teaching mothers how to recognize malaria and immediately treat their children with antimalarials kept in the household. Although controversial at the time, our randomized trial demonstrated a 40% reduction in overall under-5 mortality and the approach has won widespread recognition. The study and its results have radically altered my views about malaria pathogenesis and control in areas with intense transmission.

William Moss: William Moss first encountered malaria while working as a paediatrician in Ethiopia in the late 1980s and early 1990s. After several years working at Harlem Hospital in New York City, he returned to Africa to direct a study a sexually transmitted diseases in western Kenya. He then went on to complete a Fellowship in Paediatric Infectious Diseases at Johns Hopkins Hospital and began work with Dr Diane Griffin on the impact of the HIV epidemic on measles control in Zambia. With the increasingly successful control of measles in parts of sub-Saharan Africa, he has turned his attention to the study of malaria control and transmission dynamics in southern Zambia in collaboration with colleagues from the Johns Hopkins Malaria Research Institute.

Malaria and its life cycle

Vertebrates, mosquitoes, and malaria have been evolving together for many thousands of years, and humans have been afflicted with malaria for as long as there have been humans. Four species of protozoan parasites of the genus *Plasmodium* infect humans: *Plasmodium falciparum*, *Plasmodium vivax*, *Plasmodium ovale*, and *Plasmodium malaria*. Although *P. vivax* is the most widespread, *P. falciparum* causes the most severe disease and is responsible for most deaths and morbidity due to malaria. In the 2004 World Health Report, a total of 1,272,000 deaths due to malaria were estimated globally, of which 90% were in Africa. The frequency of sickle-cell trait (haemoglobin AS) in tropical Africa provides an indirect indicator of the burden of malaria: to account for a 25% prevalence of AS haemoglobin in adults, the historical case fatality rate attributed to malaria must be 15–20% for children with AA haemoglobin (Morrow and Moss 2006).

The malaria parasite undergoes multiple transformations within the mosquito and human hosts and at least a dozen separate steps have been defined. The sporozoite form is transmitted to humans in the saliva of an infected female anopheline mosquito taking a blood meal, enters the venous blood system, and invades a liver cell where it replicates thousands of times. Merozoites, released from infected liver cells, penetrate red blood cells, ingest haemoglobin and replicate. The infected red cells burst, releasing the next batch of parasites that penetrate new red blood cells and begin the cycle again. A single *P. falciparum* parasite can potentially lead to 10 billion new parasites through these recurrent cycles (Bruce-Chwatt 1988). After a number of cycles within red blood cells, some parasites differentiate into sexual forms, gametocytes, to be ingested by an anopheline mosquito during its next blood meal.

In the mosquito, the male and female gametocytes fuse and undergo several transformations leading to the sporozoite forms to be injected back into the human host. Once infected with malaria, a female anopheline mosquito remains infected for life and transmits sporozoites with each blood meal (Russell *et al.* 1963; Garnham 1966). Parasite development within the mosquito comprises the extrinsic cycle and takes 7–12 days. Each pair of gametocytes can produce over 10,000 sporozoites, but generally only a few dozen are injected with a single bite (Pringle 1966; Beier *et al.* 1991).

The epidemiological understanding of malaria in the twentieth century was based upon the ever increasing scientific knowledge of the malaria parasite, the anopheline vector, and the pathogenesis of malaria in the human host. This epidemiological understanding formed, in turn, the foundation for the development and implementation of a variety of malaria control strategies. Successes and failures in malaria control led to further insights into the epidemiology of malaria as hypotheses and conceptual frameworks were tested against the complex realities of local ecological conditions and programmatic constraints.

The epidemiology of malaria at the turn of the twentieth century

Knowledge of the biology and epidemiology of malaria in the twentieth century was made possible by the discoveries of the last two decades of the nineteenth century. These fundamental discoveries were the identification of the malaria parasite and its transmission by mosquitoes. For centuries prior to these discoveries, malaria was associated with bodies of water and control efforts consisted of draining swamps and marshes. The name 'malaria' comes from the Italian and means 'bad air', reflecting the association with foul-smelling stagnant water. Chemotherapy also preceded a basic understanding of malaria epidemiology by hundreds of years. Extracts from the wormwood plant, *Artemisia annua*, had been used for centuries in China. Cinchona bark was used to treat fevers in Peru and Ecuador prior to the arrival of Europeans, and its therapeutic properties were carefully investigated by European explorers in the seventeenth century (Desowitz 1991). Quinine was first extracted from cinchona bark in the early nineteenth century, and by the turn of the twentieth century was the only available antimalarial drug.

From the perspective of the early twenty-first century, an important epidemiological feature of malaria in the nineteenth and early twentieth centuries was the extent of its geographical spread. Malaria was not restricted to the tropics but extended far into North America and into northern and western Europe, prompting large-scale public health interventions in, among other places, southern Italy and the USA. This, in conjunction with the expansion of colonial powers into the tropics, created urgency in understanding the epidemiology of malaria and in developing effective control strategies.

In 1880, the understanding of malaria changed when Laveran, a French army physician working in Algeria, first identified the causative agent of human malaria. Using a crude microscope, Laveran identified gametocytes in the blood of a soldier infected with *Plasmodium falciparum*. However, it took many years, the development of the oil immersion microscope lens by Zeiss, and specific staining techniques by Romanowsky, for malariologists to accept Laveran's discovery. For his work, Laveran received the Nobel prize in 1907. Laveran's initial description of the malaria parasite in 1880 followed by 1 year a description of the 'bacterial cause' of malaria by Klebs and Tomasi-Crudeli (Desowitz 1991). Within the scientific community dominated by the discoveries of Louis Pasteur and Robert Koch, there was widespread belief that bacteria were the causative agents of infectious diseases. Klebs and Tomasi-Crudeli injected marsh water into rabbits, which became ill with fever. A bacterium, named *Bacillus malariae*, was isolated from the sick rabbits and assumed to be the cause of malaria. Among some malariologists, this evidence was sufficient to establish the bacterial aetiology of malaria and disprove Laveran's crude observations.

More controversial were debates about how malaria was transmitted and who was to be credited for this discovery. Patrick Manson, who had reported that filariasis was transmitted by mosquitoes while working in China (although incorrectly hypothesizing that it was transmitted by ingestion of infected mosquitoes), first proposed that malaria was transmitted by mosquitoes in 1894 (Desowitz 1991). In 1897, Ronald Ross, an army physician working in India and who trained under Manson, identified oocysts of the malaria parasite in the stomach of a mosquito that had previously fed on a patient with malaria. However, both Ross and Manson were initially convinced that ingestion of the oocyst in water contaminated with infected mosquitoes was responsible for human disease. Transmission of an infectious agent by the bite of an arthropod was a novel epidemiological concept at the turn of the twentieth century. The first demonstration of vector-borne transmission by a blood-sucking arthropod was by Theobald Smith and F. L. Kilbourne in 1893, who reported that babesiosis (involving a protozoan similar to *Plasmodium*) was transmitted by the bite of a tick (Desowitz 1991).

Writing shortly after Ross' observations, William Thayer at the Johns Hopkins Hospital was not yet convinced of the evidence that mosquitoes transmit malaria (Thayer 1897). In his 300-page *Lectures on the malarial fevers* published in 1897, Thayer describes Ross's experiments: 'Ross placed mosquitoes upon individuals whose blood contained crescentric, ovoid, and round bodies, and observed flagellation of these forms in blood taken later from the stomach of the mosquito. This interesting though insufficient evidence has led Manson to assume that the mosquito is a normal intermediate host in the life of the malaria parasite'. More convincing evidence that malaria was transmitted by the bite of mosquitoes came a year later, in 1898, when Ross, then stationed in Calcutta, began studies of avian malaria. Through microscopic examination of infected mosquitoes, Ross was able to follow the life cycle of malaria parasites from the gut wall to the salivary glands. He then demonstrated that mosquitoes with parasites in their salivary glands could transmit malaria to uninfected sparrows.

In 1902 Ross received the Nobel prize for his work. However, as Ross was conducting experiments with avian malaria, the Italian malariologist Giovanni Batista Grassi was elucidating the life cycle of the human malaria parasite *P. falciparum* within anopheline mosquitoes (Desowitz 1991). Grassi's knowledge of entomology was much greater than that of Ross, and he was the first to understand that anophelines are the only species of mosquito capable of transmitting malaria to humans. However, Grassi published his work in 1898 after Ross had made his observations public. Thus began the acrimonious debates as to who deserved credit for the discovery of the transmission of malaria by mosquitoes. Ross received the Nobel prize alone, in part due to the intervention of Robert Koch, whom Grassi had angered and who opposed Grassi's nomination. Later, in 1901, Grassi predicted a third phase in the life cycle of the malaria parasite, distinct from the blood stage described by Laveran and the sexual stage described by Ross. However, the exo-erythrocytic stage in the liver would not be fully characterized until four decades later, in part because of an erroneous report by Schaudinn in 1902 that sporozoites could directly invade red blood cells.

Ross's contributions to the understanding of malaria were not limited to his work with mosquitoes and the mechanisms of transmission. The epidemiological understanding of malaria was first systematized in his mathematical model of malaria transmission developed in 1908. Ross had an interest in mathematics (and poetry) and used equations to describe malaria transmission dynamics. Importantly, Ross formulated the concept of threshold densities of mosquitoes and their relationship to vector control: '. . . to counteract malaria anywhere we need not banish Anopheles there entirely. . . we need only to reduce their numbers below a certain figure' (quoted in McKenzie and Samba 2004) Another implication of his model was that successful malaria control was more likely to result from integrated programmes, combining vector control, treatment of infected persons with quinine, and personal protection through bednets, than from a single intervention. However, this epidemiological insight was not always adhered to in the subsequent development of malaria control programmes.

The discovery of the malaria parasite and its vector-borne transmission are the foundation for any epidemiological understanding of malaria. However, debates flourished after these discoveries on how best to control malaria. On one side were those who believed the burden of malaria could be reduced only through improvements in economic and social conditions. On the other were those who believed that scientific advances led to the rational development of focused public health interventions. This view was in turn divided into those who believed vector control should be the primary strategy and those who favoured treatment of infected individuals with the antimalarial quinine.

The concept that malaria control was linked to improvements in living conditions derived from earlier associations between malaria and swamps. At the turn of the twentieth century, the Italian malariologist Angelo Celli, aware of the recent discoveries regarding the malaria parasite and its transmission by mosquitoes, developed a malaria control strategy for Italy that included economic, agricultural, and social reforms to improve the housing, nutritional status, and health care of the rural poor (Packard and Gadelha 1994; Hamoudi and Sachs 1999). The widespread use of quinine was also part of the Italian control strategy. This epidemiological perspective, which links malaria with broader economic and social conditions, persists in recent arguments that economic development can be enhanced by reducing the disease burden due to malaria (Sachs 2001), but was not the dominant viewpoint after the Second World War.

At the turn of the twentieth century, there were some successful efforts in vector control based upon the recent discoveries in the epidemiology of malaria (Hamoudi and Sachs 1999). In 1901, Malcolm Watson eliminated the vector of malaria in Malaya by altering breeding sites, and thus reduced the burden of malaria on the colonial rubber and tea plantations. But success was temporary, as a large outbreak of malaria occurred 10 years later. Intensive vector control strategies also were used effectively by William Gorgas in 1904 to control malaria in the Panama Canal Zone. However, not all efforts at vector control were successful, including Ross's own effort at eliminating parasite breeding sites in Freetown, Sierra Leone. Between 1902 and 1909, an expensive vector control project established by the British in the city of Mian Mir in India failed to reduce malaria (Bradley 1998). There was more to learn about the epidemiology of malaria.

Advances in malaria epidemiology after the First World War

The social changes that occurred in the wake of the First World War focused malaria control priorities on the USA and Europe. In these regions, rapid economic growth contributed to the decline in malaria, particularly through improved agricultural land use, better access to health care, and urbanization. This decline in the prevalence of malaria, often in the absence of specific vector-control measures, was consistent with the broader epidemiological perspective of malaria as a disease of poverty and underdevelopment. The debate between those who advocated vector control and those who promoted social and economic reforms was taken up by the Malaria Commission established by the League of Nations. In reports published in 1924 and 1927, the Commission favoured the broad malaria control strategies developed in Italy (largely the reclamation of marshlands, leading to economic development of the rural poor, and the widespread use of quinine) as opposed to more focused vector control strategies (Packard and Gadelha 1994).

After the First World War, advances in vector control continued to be made, particularly the development and widespread use of larvicides such as Paris Green. However, the most important advance in the epidemiology of malaria between the two World Wars was in understanding the ecological complexities of *Anopheles* mosquitoes. In the 1920s, several investigators, including Roubaud in France, Swellengrebel and Van Thiel in The Netherlands, and Falleroni in Italy differentiated the subspecies of the *Anopheles maculipennis* complex and described the role of mosquito behaviour in the transmission of malaria. Specifically, strains of *A. maculipennis* (the predominant species complex in Europe) were observed to differ in their feeding, resting, mating, and breeding habits, and these differences accounted for the local epidemiology of malaria and the success or failure of vector control efforts. For example, different species and subspecies of *Anopheles* mosquitoes have varying capacities to transmit malaria to humans depending upon their propensity to bite humans (anthropophilic versus zoophilic) and reside close to human habitations. Until these differences were recognized, the phenomenon of 'anophelism without malaria' (i.e. regions where *A. maculipennis* existed but malaria did not) remained an epidemiological puzzle.

How the local epidemiology of malaria, and specifically the breeding habits of the local *Anopheles* species, determined the effectiveness of vector control efforts was described by Lewis Hackett in 1937. Hackett wanted to explain why larvicides were effective in North America but failed in Europe (Hackett 1937). He argued that larvicides were more effective in eliminating the vector of malaria in North America because it bred in the vegetation of ponds and lakes, whereas the primary vector of malaria in Europe bred at the edges of streams and rivers where larvicides were less effective.

An interesting aspect of the history of malaria between the two World Wars was the increasingly widespread use of malaria as a therapeutic agent; that is, the deliberate infection of persons with malaria parasites to treat other diseases (particularly neurosyphilis). Initially, therapeutic malaria was induced by the injection of infected blood from an infected person; later, beginning in the 1920s, mosquitoes were used frequently to infect the patient. Because of its relatively benign course, the malaria parasite most commonly used for therapeutic purposes was *P. vivax*. The deliberate infection of persons with malaria parasites allowed careful measurement of the incubation period and its relationship to the number of infecting parasites, as well as the discovery of the hypnonzoite liver stage of *P. vivax*.

The Second World War and progress in the fight against malaria

In the years preceding the Second World War progress was made in the development of important tools in the fight against malaria, including the insecticide DDT and new synthetic antimalarial drugs to reduce dependence upon Cinchona plantations. DDT, originally synthesized in Germany in 1874, was recognized as a useful insecticide during the late 1930s. Synthetic antimalarials, largely developed in Germany during the 1920s and 1930s, included pamaquine, mepacrine, and, most importantly, chloroquine. Chloroquine provided a safe and inexpensive drug for both treatment and chemoprophylaxis that would be widely used for decades until resistance reduced its effectiveness.

The impact of these technological advances on the epidemiology of malaria was to again focus attention on large-scale vector control programmes. The best example of this approach, and one that had a profound influence on subsequent efforts to eradicate malaria, was the successful vector control programme led by Fredrick Soper of the Rockefeller Foundation's International Health Division to eradicate *Anopheles gambiae* from northeast Brazil between 1939 and 1941 (Packard and Gadelha 1994). *Anopheles gambiae*, an extremely efficient transmitter of malaria to humans, was introduced into Brazil from West Africa in 1930 and was responsible for several large outbreaks of malaria. Using vector control methods to eliminate breeding sites and fumigate homes, Soper and his team were able to eradicate *A. gambiae* from Brazil within 2 years. A similar programme, also led by Soper, eliminated *A. gambiae* from Upper Egypt. Although social and economic factors may have contributed to malaria control in Brazil (Packard 1998), the success of these programmes was critical in directing malaria control after the Second World War.

The era of hope after the Second World War and the great malaria eradication campaign

With the conclusion of the Second World War in 1945, the world settled into an era characterized by international hope, optimism, and idealism. Almost immediately following the surrender of

Japan, the United Nations Charter was ratified by 51 nations on 24 October 1945. The World Health Organization (WHO), the United Nations specialized agency for health, was established in April 1948 with the objective that all people should attain 'the highest possible level of health'. From its very beginning, the WHO recognized that malaria was of great importance to human health and well-being. The commission responsible for drafting the WHO constitution and launching its antecedent activities in 1947 declared that: '... Apart from its ... fundamental work ... meeting its statutory obligations, the Commission was confronted with the task of initiating a direct attack on the diseases which were the principal cause of wastage of human life and effort. Of these, malaria, tuberculosis, and venereal disease were ... paramount importance .... The Expert Committee on Malaria was ... to advise on a general plan for the world control of malaria ...'.

As experience increased in the post-war period with the magic of DDT, the broad array of malaria control efforts shifted to the narrow focus of eliminating anopheline vectors. The culmination of this shift was the adoption of a most ambitious and dramatic plan for global malaria eradication by the 8th World Health Assembly in 1955. The Director General of WHO in making the case for the plan put forth the following information:

- ◆ Tremendous success had been achieved in controlling malaria through the use of DDT in a variety of countries.

- ◆ Evidence from several countries indicated that malaria eradication by residual spraying was technically and economically feasible.

- ◆ There was growing evidence that vector resistance was increasing to DDT and other pesticides.

The Director General concluded that 'there is no other logical choice: malaria eradication is clearly indicated, presents a unique opportunity and should be implemented as rapidly as possible. Time is of the essence'. The decision to launch the plan was based upon a conviction that eradication was possible and that it should be carried out before vector resistance precluded the possibility (Packard 1998).

By 1958 the most inspirational, ambitious, complex, and costly health campaign ever undertaken was well under way (Russell *et al.* 1963). Eradication using DDT residual spraying was estimated to cost less than 25 cents per person per year. The total cost for the first 5 years would be half a billion US dollars (International Development Advisory Board 1956). The four-phase strategy of the global eradication programme (preparation, attack, consolidation, and maintenance) was designed to make maximum use of the continually shrinking time frame of DDT effectiveness. Agricultural use of the insecticide had already begun to select for resistance before the eradication programme began. The goal of the attack phase of the programme was to use residual application of DDT on the walls of houses to reduce Macdonald's variable, p, related to the lifespan of the vector (Hamoudi and Sachs 1999). Emilio Pampana emphasized that the extrinsic incubation period of the parasite requires several days and that during this period, as most anophelines feed every 48 hours, the infected mosquito would come back repeatedly and each time risk being killed. If all houses have their inner walls appropriately sprayed with insecticide, transmission of malaria will be stopped (Pampana 1969). Although the designers of the programme understood the ways in which topography, geography, climate, evolutionary history, and many other local factors influenced the dynamics of malaria transmission, these factors were considered irrelevant in comparison to the enormous power of DDT to reduce mosquito longevity. Most European countries and many across Asia and Latin America joined the programme and many achieved outstanding success. In Malta, the anopheline vector was completely eliminated (Russell *et al.* 1963) and during the first few years of the programme malaria was fully eliminated from Europe (Hamoudi and Sachs 1999).

A new approach to malaria surveillance

National malaria eradication programmes began in the period 1957 to 1960. The four-phase strategy achieved rapid reduction in malaria, often with parasite rates dropping to less than 2%. Standard malariometric surveys that provided population-based parasitaemia prevalence rates were not sufficiently sensitive to measure continuing progress. It became critical to develop a new surveillance system based on the detection of incident cases of malaria disease rather than the prevalence of parasitaemia. Reliable evidence was required to ensure that spraying could be safely discontinued following the consolidation phase. During consolidation every case detected was given radical treatment (chloroquine plus primaquine to ensure elimination of possible relapse), a careful epidemiological investigation of the case and surroundings with focal spraying as needed, and antimalarials to anyone with fever in the neighbourhood. Thus, surveillance in the consolidation phase consisted of two kinds of activities: epidemiological and clinical evaluation plus action to remedy the spread of infection. For malaria eradication, a case of malaria was defined as the presence of a microscopically confirmed malaria parasite regardless of symptoms. In those countries successfully achieving the consolidation phase, this finding was considered highly specific (with few false positives), although not very sensitive since false negative tests occurred at low levels of parasitaemia. Surveillance was carried out both by periodic blood smear population-based surveys (active case-finding) and through blood smear examination of patients presenting with fever at health facilities (passive case-finding). It was recognized that in highly endemic areas, not yet in the consolidation phase, a large proportion of the population might have asymptomatic malaria and that this case definition would not be useful (see also below about the situation in holoendemic Africa). However, in those countries progressing toward eradication, the case definition was useful and an essential component of eradication programmes (Yekutiel 1965).

The role of mathematical modelling

In the 1950s, George Macdonald returned to England from years of work in the tropics and began to build on Ross's mathematical models of malaria transmission (McKenzie and Samba 2004). Macdonald's models indicated that, at equilibrium, the weakest link in the chain of malaria transmission was the survival of adult female *Anopheles* (Macdonald 1957). Macdonald defined the basic reproduction number (R_0) as the number of secondary infections which result from a single infection over the period of infectivity. R_0 depends on many factors, including the abundance of vectors, the propensity of a vector to bite humans, the proportion of bites that are infectious, the lifespan of the vector, and the time to reproduce in the vector. The most important of these is the lifespan of the vector. As the R_0 increases, it becomes more difficult to protect a community from infection, since each case poses a danger to a larger proportion of the community. On the other hand, the incidence of malaria decreases when R_0 is less than 1. Therefore, it is theoretically possible, by manipulating one or more of the determinants of the basic reproduction number, to eradicate malaria. In this context, DDT emerged as a potential panacea, which could sufficiently reduce the vector's lifespan to hold R_0 at less than 1 for several years and eliminate malaria. This was the basis of the Global Malaria Eradication Program launched by the World Health Organization in the late 1950s.

Given that Macdonald's models were published at about the time the global eradication campaign based on DDT began, it is not surprising that this conclusion was recruited to the cause. What Macdonald actually wrote suggests more insight and caution, but it may be that he too was caught up in the appeal of DDT as a 'silver bullet'. Careful study of the consequences of the very high vectorial capacity in Africa as done by the Garki Project provide a powerful argument against eradication attempts and demonstrated how futile such a global effort would be (Molineaux and Gramiccia 1980). It is particularly interesting to examine the conceptual basis for case definition, incidence, and prevalence of malaria in the ecological and epidemiological circumstances in the countries in which eradication programmes were undertaken as discussed above, and contrast these with the situation in holoendemic malaria in tropical Africa where everyone is inoculated with sporozoites several times a week and virtually all are infected with malaria all the time. Here neither incidence nor prevalence have much meaning and a case definition is based on clinical criteria and parasite density.

The era of disillusionment

With the urgent military-style campaign mentality, however, those conducting the global eradication campaign overlooked knowledge of the times. A sense of urgency overruled practicality, and sometimes Cold War politics dictated its direction (Litsios 1996). Much was known not to be known, including the absorption of DDT on mud-wall surfaces, and the biting and resting habits of important vectors. Indeed, the last Expert Committee meeting on malaria before the eradication plan was adopted by the WHO Assembly advocated a broad range of approaches and concluded that 'it is not likely that any single policy will be generally applicable. . .' (Packard 1998).

Despite the dramatic success in a number of countries, little impact was seen in many continental tropical countries of Asia and South America. In Africa, where malaria was of greatest importance by far, virtually nothing was even attempted. Unfortunately, with the emphasis on logistics and organizational activities, there seemed a comparable de-emphasis of scientific research. Fred Soper of the Rockefeller Foundation argued against 'long-term detailed entomological or malaria studies . . . unless residual DDT fails to greatly reduce [mosquito] densities which will be contrary to all previous experience' (Stapleton 2004). The general opinion frequently and loudly expressed was that 'We know what has to be done; let us get on with it!'

The eradication approach—a single-minded, insecticide-based attack on malaria—may have been the most successful antimalaria strategy of all time. Yet it contributed to a legacy of insecticide-resistant anophelines and single-purpose health cadres. Of even greater importance, over a period extending for 20 years, virtually no innovative research on malaria was undertaken. An entire generation of malaria researchers was lost.

Even by the early 1960s, it was clear that eradication would fail. The complex logistical and operational needs for the eradication effort were too much for the weak infrastructures in most tropical countries; moreover, the parasite and vector were evolving, including anopheline resistance to insecticides and parasite resistance to antimalarials (World Health Organization 1969; Krishna 1997). A further problem was that the exclusive use of household residual insecticide spraying failed to account for vital differences in anopheline behaviour. Some mosquito species bite outdoors and others do not rest indoors after feeding, avoiding contact with residual insecticides. Additionally, the organizational design of national eradication programmes became extremely centralized, often with malaria eradication offices located outside established health ministries. The infrastructure and trained personnel were then unavailable for the transition to the consolidation phase based upon the diagnosis and treatment of suspected cases. As long as even a small parasite reservoir remained, the programme could not be stopped without malaria transmission recurring. As hope of eradication and international commitment waned, this vicious cycle was repeated in more and more countries. Many communities abandoned their antimalaria efforts. In some regions, notably in southern Asia, where the prevalence of malaria remained low and the community rendered immunologically naïve, devastating resurgences occurred throughout the 1970s. Entire communities fell ill in ever-increasing waves until communal immunity was re-established and malaria achieved its relatively silent endemic equilibrium.

By 1969, the malaria eradication campaign was viewed as a major failure and was abandoned. In the wisdom of hindsight, the failure was seen as a result of scientific arrogance and lack of foresight. In truth, large numbers of lives were saved in many countries and major economic activities were spurred. With the formal declaration ending the global eradication programme, the substantial multilateral funds that had gone to support local malaria control programmes were withdrawn. At the same time, each country was forced to develop its own control programme based upon local ecology and resources. To do so, countries required a much greater level of epidemiological and ecological expertise. Since virtually all resources had been single-mindedly put into the logistics of DDT residual spraying, such expertise was lacking.

A few countries, such as Mauritius and some Caribbean islands, successfully continued malaria eradication. Some countries, such as Nepal, converted their armies of spray-teams into multipurpose health workers. But most countries simply ceased malaria control activities. In Asia, many countries had devastating resurgences and then settled back into their previous state of endemic transmission. Malaria remained endemic in about 100 countries. These countries faced enormous challenges: vector control strategies hindered by the rapid spread of insecticide-resistant mosquitoes; strategies based on reduced vector–human contact hindered by poorly constructed dwellings, outdoor feeding and resting vectors, and limited compliance with bednet strategies; drug treatment strategies overcome not only by the explosion of drug resistance but also hampered by inadequate health-care infrastructure, poor distribution systems, and inadequate self-treatment education of the community (Hamoudi and Sachs 1999).

'Peaceful coexistence' and focus on disease control

As countries struggled with developing their national control programmes under the new WHO Global Malaria Control Program, the notion that peaceful coexistence between humans and malaria parasites would have to be worked out was gradually accepted. A major revolution in ideas about what could be done about malaria control was fostered. Investigators went back to back to basic research to improve understanding of the pathogenesis, immunology, and transmission dynamics of malaria, to develop new vaccines, new approaches to vector control, and innovative approaches for household and community interventions.

The major challenges remain in Africa where malaria control has never been achieved and, except for parts of southern Africa and highland Ethiopia, generally never even attempted. The first 25 years of global malaria control coincided with the horrors of the HIV/AIDS epidemic in Africa, and ministries of health along with major donors focused attention and efforts on mitigating this epidemic. Only with the establishment of the Roll Back Malaria initiatives beginning in 1998 has serious attention been given to malaria. Despite the recent sharp criticism of the very slow pace and paucity of achievement (much of it related to the complicated issues of drug resistance and determining an affordable approach), much can be done to reduce the consequences of malaria through personal and household protection from vectors by the use of insecticide-treated bednets, prompt treatment with artemisinin-based combination therapy (ACT) at early signs of malaria, and by intermittent presumptive therapy with ACT for pregnant women and children less than 5 years of age. The relatively high costs of these approaches, and who should pay, remain major issues to be resolved. The cost is high relative to current expenditures on health in African countries, but not compared to global expenditures on virtually anything else (e.g. video games!). In addition, the logistics and infrastructure needed to provide therapy still lags behind the demand. Nevertheless, there is progress in some African countries and now sufficient experience with successful programmes to know that it can be done.

The era of molecular biology

Molecular tools have allowed for epidemiological investigations of malaria on temporal and spatial scales that were not previously possible. These tools have been used in studies of the evolutionary relationships between malaria parasites, parasite and mosquito population structures, co-infection with the same or different species of *Plasmodia*, and the evolution and spread of drug-resistant strains.

One example of how molecular tools have advanced our understanding of malaria is by elucidating the evolutionary relationships between malaria parasites. Phylogenetic analyses demonstrate a close relationship between *P. faciparum* and a malaria species found in chimpanzees (Carter and Mendis 2002). These closely related human and chimp species, along with avian malaria species, diverged from the other mammalian malaria species, including *P. vivax*, *P. ovale*, and *P. malariae*, about 130 million years ago. *Plasmodium falciparum* then diverged from chimp malaria approximately 5 million years ago, about the time human ancestors diverged from the African great apes. Thus, *P. falciparum* is by far the most recent human malaria species, and *P. vivax*, *P. ovale*, and *P. malariae* co-evolved with hominid ancestors over millions of years.

Simultaneous with the publication of the genome sequence of *P. falciparum*, a first draft of the genome sequence of *Anopholes gambiae* was published in 2002. Identification of polymorphisms within the *A. gambiae* genome permit epidemiological studies of insecticide resistance, transmission efficiency of malaria parasites, and gene flow within mosquito populations (Morrow and Moss 2006). Knowledge of gene flow within mosquito populations is critical to assessing the potential effectiveness of introducing genetically modified *Anopheles* mosquitoes that fail to transmit malaria.

The epidemiology of drug-resistant strains can be investigated using genetic polymorphisms associated with drug resistance, which are best characterized for chloroquine and sulfadoxine–pyrimethamine (Morrow and Moss 2006). Chloroquine resistance is conferred by a complex set of genetic mutations, making multiple independent origins unlikely. Resistance to chloroquine appears to have originated only four times, and to have spread from Asia to Africa. Because of the less complex nature of resistance to sulfadoxine–pyrimethamine, and the ease in which resistance mutations can be induced in the laboratory, resistance to sulfadoxine–pyrimethamine was thought to have multiple, independent origins. However, genotyping of microsatellite markers flanking the *dhfr* gene suggests that high-level resistance to sulfadoxine–pyrimethamine (i.e. triple or quadruple mutant *dhfr* alleles) also originated in southeast Asia and subsequently spread to Africa.

An unresolved question regarding the epidemiology of malaria is whether drug resistance evolves faster in areas of high or low malaria transmission (Morrow and Moss 2006). This question has important public health implications, as interventions to reduce transmission could impact on rates of drug resistance. Lower transmission was hypothesized to increase rates of drug resistance by enhancing parasite inbreeding, thereby increasing the probability that drug resistance mutations would spread in the parasite population. The frequent emergence of resistance along the Thai–Cambodian border supports the hypothesis that lower transmission facilitates the emergence of drug resistance. Further epidemiological studies are needed to resolve this issue. The history of the epidemiology of malaria teaches that the answer may not be the same in all places and at all times.

The future of malaria epidemiology

The failure of malaria eradication in the mid-twentieth century makes it highly unlikely that any single approach to malaria control will be attempted again. Successful control will require deeper understanding of the local epidemiological and ecological interactions between malaria parasites, anopheline vectors, and human hosts. Such an understanding will be enhanced by the use of molecular tools to study the population structure and evolution of malaria parasites and anopheline vectors. As vaccines against malaria are developed and tested under different ecological conditions, new insights will be gained into the epidemiology, transmission characteristics, and population immunity of malaria, insights that will build upon the seminal discoveries of Laveran, Ross, and Grassi at the turn of the twentieth century. But the old insight of Angelo Celli and others, that malaria control is dependent upon social and economic development, should be kept alive. Malaria and its consequences differentially burden the impoverished rural populations of Africa and contribute to a vicious cycle of poverty, misery, and injustice. The history of the epidemiology of malaria shows that the international cooperation needed to break this cycle is achievable.

References

Beier JC, Onyango K, Ramadhan M, *et al.* (1991). Quantitation of malaria sporozoites in the salivary glands of wild Afrotropical *Anopheles. Medical and Veterinary Entomology*, **5**, 63–70.

Bradley DJ (1998). The particular and the general. Issues of specificity and verticality in the history of malaria control. *Parassitologia*, **40**, 5–10.

Bruce-Chwatt LJ (1988). History of malaria from prehistory to eradication. In *Malaria: principles and practice of malariology* (ed. WH Wernsdorfer and I McGregor), pp. 1–69. Churchill Livingstone, Edinburgh.

Carter R and Mendis KN (2002). Evolutionary and historical aspects of the burden of malaria. *Clinical Microbiology Reviews*, **15**, 564–94.

Desowitz RS (1991). *The malaria capers. Tales of parasites and people.* WW Norton & Company, Inc. New York.

Garnham PCC (1966). *Malaria parasites and other hemosporidia.* Blackwell Scientific Publications, Oxford.

Hackett L (1937). *Malaria in Europe: an ecological study.* Oxford University Press, London.

Hamoudi A and Sachs JD (1999). *The changing global distribution of malaria: a review,* Working Paper No 2. Center for International Development, Harvard University.

International Development Advisory Board (1956). *Malaria eradication: report and recommendations of the International Development Advisory Board.* International Development Advisory Board. Washington, DC.

Krishna S (1997). Malaria. *British Medical Journal*, **315**, 730–2.

Litsios S (1996). *The tomorrow of malaria.* Pacific Press, Wellington.

Macdonald G (1957). *The epidemiology and control of malaria.* Oxford University Press, Oxford.

McKenzie FE and Samba EM (2004). The role of mathematical modeling in evidence-based malaria control. *The American Journal of Tropical Medicine and Hygiene*, **71**, S94–S96.

Molineaux L and Gramiccia G (1980). *The Garki Project: research on the epidemiology and control of malaria in the Sudan savanna of West Africa.* WHO, Geneva.

Morrow RH and Moss WJ (2006). The epidemiology and control of malaria. In *Infectious disease epidemiology*, 2nd edn (ed. KE Nelson, CM Williams, and NMH Graham). Jones and Bartlett, pp. 1079–1130. Boston.

Packard RM (1998). 'No other logical choice': global malaria eradication and the politics of international health in the post-war era. *Parassitologia*, **40**, 217–29.

Packard RM and Gadelha P (1994). A land filled with mosquitoes: Fred L. Soper, the Rockefeller Foundation, and the *Anopheles gambiae* invasion of Brazil. *Parassitologia*, **36**, 197–213.

Pampana E (1969). *A textbook of malaria eradication.* Oxford University Press, Oxford.

Pringle G (1966). A quantitative study of naturally acquired malaria infections in *Anopheles gambiae* of East Africa. *Transactions of the Royal Society of Tropical Medicine and Hygiene*, **60**, 626–32.

Russell PF, West LS, Maxwell RD, and Macdonald G (1963). *Practical malariology*, 2nd edn. Oxford University Press, Oxford.

Sachs JD (2001). *Macroeconomics and health: investing in health for economic development*, Report of the Commission on Macroeconomics and Health. WHO, Geneva.

Stapleton DH (2004). Lessons of history? Anti-malaria strategies of the International Health Board and the Rockefeller Foundation from the 1920s to the era of DDT. *Public Health Reports*, **119**, 206–15.

Thayer WS (1897). *Lectures on the malaria fevers*. D. Appleton and Co., New York.

World Health Organization (1969). Re-examination of the global strategy of malaria eradication. *Official Records of the World Health Organization*, **176**, 106–26.

Yekutiel P (1965) Basic principles. Comparability in international epidemiology. *The Milbank Memorial Fund Quarterly*, **XLII.**

Section 3

Applications and role of epidemiology in related domains

15

Public health and epidemiology

Lester Breslow and Roger Detels

Personal experiences

Having entered the University of Minnesota Medical School to become a psychiatrist, I [Lester Breslow] spent the summer after my third year of medical school as a medical extern in a state mental hospital. Observing that almost nothing useful could be done then (1937) for the thousands of severely ill patients, I returned to my final year in medical school completely disenchanted with psychiatry and confused as to my career direction.

A friendly young faculty member, hearing my lamentations, suggested that with my ideology, I consider public health, and encouraged me to enter the field. Following that lead brought me into contact with the newly arrived professor of preventive medicine and public health who inspired me with the opportunity to do what I really wanted to do—help bring people *en masse* to better health. After clinical training at a US Public Health Service Marine Hospital, but rejected as an officer in the Corps (I later learned because of my ideology, not my medical record), I returned to Minnesota for a Master of Public Health degree.

Thereafter, I joined the Minnesota State Department of Public Health as an epidemiologist. After some satisfying experience with communicable disease outbreaks and tracking tuberculosis and syphilis cases, which concretely taught me the value of approaching health on a population basis, I was assigned as the health officer to a six-county rural region. The advances of Nazi and Japanese forces in the Second World War, however, induced me to serve in the US Army as a preventive medicine officer for the seventh infantry division during the Leyte and Okinawa campaign.

Returning from the Pacific in 1945 and recognizing the increasing significance of the epidemics of non-communicable disease then becoming apparent, I was determined to apply epidemiology and public health to them. I founded the Bureau of Chronic Disease in the California Department of Public Health, which provided an opportunity to initiate epidemiological studies, for example, of lung cancer, obesity, occupational disease, and morbidity measurement, work that led to my being invited to the 1957 Netherlands meeting that established the International Epidemiological Association. Acquaintance there with Richard Doll, John Pemberton, Archie Cochrane, Jerry Morris, and other British luminaries in epidemiology during the post-Second World War period greatly encouraged me to continue in that field, as well as in public health administration.

[See the introduction to Chapter 12 for the story of how Roger Detels became involved in epidemiology.]

Epidemiology as the basic science of public health

Epidemiology constitutes the basic science of public health. This is particularly true if one accepts the mission of public health to be that delineated by the US Institute of Medicine, National Academy of Sciences; namely, 'fulfilling society's interest in assuring conditions in which people can be healthy' (Institute of Medicine 1988). In its relationship to public health, the basic mission of epidemiology is to determine the conditions that influence health to be better or worse. Thus, just as medicine takes anatomy, physiology, bacteriology, etc. to be its basic sciences, so public health depends on epidemiology.

Table 15.1 Selected communicable disease case rates per 100,000 population: USA, selected years, 1950–2000

Disease	1950	1970	1990	2000
Diphtheria	3.83	0.21	0.00	0.00
Pertussis	79.82	2.08	1.84	2.88
Poliomyelitis	22.02	0.02	0.00	0.00
Measles	211.01	23.23	11.17	0.03
Tuberculosis	–	18.28	10.33	3.01
Syphilis	146.02	45.26	54.30	11.58

Source: National Center for Health Statistics, United States, 2002. Hyattsville, MD.

Examples abound indicating the crucial contributions of epidemiology to public health: the identification of polluted water, asbestos fibres, cigarette smoke, and myriad other conditions that injure health, as well as the social network, availability of appropriate foods, and many other factors that favour health. Epidemiologists usually initiate studies in which they seek to ascertain the causes of disease, although recently they have also looked for determinants of health. In so doing, they identify the conditions for which public health can intervene to support health. The results of epidemiological work thus comprise the underpinnings of public health.

Hence, public health administrators turn to epidemiologists to reveal the facts concerning the conditions that lead to disease or health upon which to proceed with interventions. Appropriate action, based on epidemiological findings, has been largely responsible for the huge successes against the communicable diseases and, more recently, against the non-communicable diseases (Tables 15.1 and 15.2).

Thus, epidemiologists (especially Bradford Hill and Richard Doll) determined, using case–control and then cohort studies, the major cause of the lung cancer epidemic during the first half of the twentieth century, namely cigarette smoking (Surgeon-General, U.S. Public Health Service 1964). Public health administration has used that knowledge for effective action in controlling the disease: for example, in California the lung cancer mortality rate has declined from more than 40 deaths per 100,000 in 1950 to fewer than 16 in 2004.

After laboratory scientists discovered the viral agent of poliomyelitis and developed vaccines against it, epidemiologists (especially Thomas Francis) conducted large-scale field studies demonstrating the vaccine's effectiveness. Subsequent immunization programmes have eliminated poliomyelitis from Europe, the Americas, and other parts of the world (Thuriaux 2002).

Table 15.2 Age-adjusted death rates, selected causes of death, USA, selected years, 1950–2005

	1950	1970	1990	2000	2002
All causes	1446	1223	939	869	845
Heart diseases	586	493	322	258	241
Malignant neoplasms	194	199	216	200	194
Cerebrovascular disease	181	148	65	61	56

Source: National Center for Health Statistics. Health, United States, 2002. Hyattsville, MD.

The 'epidemiological transition' during the twentieth century, from the era in which the communicable diseases dominated the health scene to that in which non-communicable diseases have been most prominent, increasingly influences what public heath can do and in fact does.

Because epidemiology is a basic science, it maintains close links with universities, where it is continually advanced and taught. Public health administrators, some of whom have migrated from epidemiology, have included personnel trained in epidemiology as prominent staff members because of their expertise in connection with many public health responsibilities. This includes: investigating untoward health events in the population being served (for example outbreaks or other unusual occurrences of disease); working with biostatisticians and others in the health department to maintain surveillance of health, disease, and the factors influencing health; conducting research appropriate to the agency's mission; providing appropriate data to facilitate the work of the agency's leaders; serving as epidemiological consultants to community public health activists outside the agency; and maintaining links with university-based epidemiologists.

Thus, epidemiologists in the industrialized nations alerted public health administrators in the mid-twentieth century to the emerging epidemics of non-communicable chronic disease and the causes thereof, and guided public health programmes for their control (Breslow 1947). Those contributions by epidemiologists, in collaboration with laboratory scientists, have led to the increasing focus of public health on such problems as obesity, hypercholesterolaemia, hyperglycaemia, and their disease consequences.

Studies in Alameda County, California exemplify the behavioural approach, especially to the chronic diseases that, by the mid-twentieth century, were dominating the health scene (Breslow and Breslow 1993). In what was called the Human Population Laboratory, epidemiologists in the State Department of Health found that seven habits of daily life profoundly influenced mortality and disability: not smoking, moderate or no use of alcohol, moderate exercise, sleeping seven or eight hours per night, maintaining a moderate weight, eating breakfast, and eating regular meals. In a general population sample of adults compared with several major appropriate controls, those who had six or seven of these habits suffered only half the subsequent mortality and disability compared with those who had none or only one to three of these habits; those with four or five suffered intermediate consequences. That series of epidemiological studies and others that were similar led to the public health concern (and increasingly, popular concern) and action to adopt lifestyles that are conducive to good health. For example, major campaigns have been mounted by governmental and non-governmental agencies to decrease smoking, obesity, and excessive alcohol consumption, and to increase exercise.

The role of epidemiology in public health

In carrying out its mission, public health performs several functions utilizing epidemiological expertise: surveillance of the population's health and the conditions that are responsible for it, designing studies and providing for formulation of strategy and policies to improve health and seeking their implementation, developing and conducting programmes, and evaluating their effectiveness and modifying them as necessary.

Surveillance constitutes a fundamental aspect of epidemiology, because the information derived from it guides the entire effort. To keep abreast with health problems, public health agencies use several instruments, including birth and death registration, reporting of communicable diseases and certain other conditions affecting people (for example genetic and occupational diseases), population surveys to determine health problems and their related behaviours, registration of certain chronic disease cases (for example cancer and myocardial infarction), and ascertaining environmental conditions that influence health (for example air pollution and food and water). Analysis of data from these sources is used for determining priorities and policy and programme development.

While public health agencies have the responsibility for strategy and policy, their authority is designated by legislative and executive bodies and governing boards. Hence, public health leaders must not only formulate and implement strategy, but must also use their expertise to design policies for health that go beyond their established authority and require the approval of higher governing bodies. Willingness and effectiveness in doing so, based on knowledge derived from epidemiological studies, are the hallmarks of good public health leadership.

Public health programmes reflect that knowledge and incorporate three ways to improve the population's health: medical services, with an emphasis on prevention; environmental control measures; and social efforts to influence health-related behaviour:

1. Medical services have achieved considerable health improvement through immunization, as well as through drugs, surgery, and other treatments. Although industrialized societies spend the most money on medical services and people in those nations look to medical services for health maintenance, they may not carry as much weight as popularly supposed (Bunker 1995).

2. Environmental measures are historically the most effective, because they are generally based on well-understood scientific principles and, once in place and maintained, do not depend for their effectiveness upon further action by individuals. However, they do require constant monitoring. Examples are milk pasteurization, fluoridation of water, minimizing air pollution, and occupational safety.

3. Health-related behaviour is now recognized as a major influence on health; social opportunities for and pressure to improve behaviour hence constitute highly significant actions for promoting health. Tobacco use and lack of physical exercise exemplify the harmful consequences of lifestyle in recent decades. A strong social network also demonstrates the positive effect that a social condition exerts on health. Table 15.3 indicates how public health incorporates all three modalities—medical, environmental, and socio-behavioural—into a strategy for controlling health problems.

Table 15.3 Ways of maintaining and improving health: approaches to specific problems

Problem	Environmental	Medical	Socio-behavioural
Automobile trauma	Safe automobiles, safe highways	Ambulance services, emergency medical services	Avoidance of drugs and alcohol when driving, and not exceeding speed limits
Loss of teeth	Fluoridation, reduced production and promotion of refined sugars	Repair dental caries, remove calculus	Prudent diet, encouragement of tooth brushing and flossing
Infant mortality	Home hygiene, reduced exposure to toxic agents	Pre-natal and paediatric care	Breastfeeding, parent education
Ischaemic heart disease	Minimize availability of tobacco, make physical activity available	Emergency medical services, treatment of hypertension and hypercholesterolaemia, and use of aspirin	Minimize fats, avoid cigarettes, and get physical exercise
Lung cancer	Reduce occupational exposure to pulmonary carcinogens	Detect and treat disease early	Curtail promotion of cigarettes, and encourage non-smoking.

Source: National Center for Health Statistics. Health, United States, 2002. Hyattsville, MD.

Epidemiological investigations have contributed substantially to the items in Table 15.3. For example, Ancel Keys noted differences in cardiovascular disease rates around the world, and helped establish the relationship between excessive fat consumption and ischaemic heart disease, thus leading to a major element in the control of that condition (Keys 1970). Epidemiologists have determined that occupational exposure to asbestos has been responsible for many lung cancer deaths, as well as other pathology. Epidemiological observations of the association between naturally occurring fluoride in the water and dental caries resulted in the addition of fluoride to the water supply in several cities and the subsequent great decline in the disease compared with other cities with low levels of fluoride. Gradual spread of fluoridation and the ensuing improvement in oral health has been one of the greatest public health achievements in the second half of the twentieth century.

The mission of public health professionals is to maintain an overview of the population's health and health conditions, decide on priorities, formulate strategies, develop and implement programmes, and deal with external forces, including industrial, medical, and political pressures.

To be most effective, epidemiology should address local, state, national, and world public health problems, both present and anticipated. In that way, it can maintain close connections with what is happening in health and participate in responding. Thus, the International Epidemiological Association (IEA), organized on a global basis and recognized as a non-governmental organization (NGO) by the WHO, has developed regional bodies paralleling the comparable WHO regional structures. Regional activities have thus flourished in several parts of the world, and each regional body is represented on the IEA Council (Breslow 2005). National, state, and local public health agencies generally include substantial epidemiological resources that are supplemented by academic epidemiological departments, often supporting governmental public health efforts.

These associations are vital to ensure the major contributions to public health that epidemiology can and should make. We now turn to the broad functions of epidemiology in support of health.

Functions of epidemiology

Epidemiology can be used in many ways to help establish and achieve public health goals. Professor J. N. Morris outlined some of these in his book, *Uses of epidemiology* (Morris 1957). We have taken the liberty of paraphrasing these and adding to them in the light of additional contributions to science and public health that have been made since he first put forward these functions. For each, we have given examples taken from advances during the twentieth century. They are:

1. *To establish the natural history of a disease in a population.* An example of this function was the use of epidemiology to document the 10-year cycle of rubella epidemics in Taiwan, which permitted the evaluation of the rubella vaccine in the 1960s, just prior to the anticipated epidemic that typically occurred every 10 years (Grayston *et al.* 1972).

2. *Community diagnosis.* Epidemiological surveys are often used to establish the morbidity and mortality from specific diseases allowing efficient use of limited public health funds for control of those diseases, having the greatest negative impact on the health of the community. For example, an epidemiological survey in one area of China identified the epidemic of HIV due to plasma donations in villages of the area (Wu and Detels 1995; Wu *et al.* 2001; Ji *et al.* 2006).

3. *To identify the natural history of disease in the individual.* Cohort studies have been used to describe the progression of HIV infection through the acute syndrome, the latent period, the early prodromal period, clinical AIDS, and death (Kaslow *et al.* 1987; Detels *et al.* 1992).

4. *To describe the clinical picture of a disease.* Epidemiological strategies can identify who is likely to get a disease such as capillariasis, the characteristic symptoms and signs, the extent of the

epidemic, the risk factors, and the causative agent, and can help to determine the effectiveness of treatment and control efforts (Detels *et al.* 1969).

5. *To identify the factors associated with risk of disease acquisition.* Cohort studies have established the important risk factors for such diseases as heart disease and many of the cancers, for example smoking and diet (Dawber 1980; see also Chapter 7).

6. *To identify factors associated with good health.* Cohort studies have been used by Breslow and Breslow (1993) to establish behavioural/social practices that favour low morbidity and mortality.

7. *To identify precursors of disease and syndromes.* High blood pressure, a treatable condition, has been identified through case–control studies and cohort studies as a precursor to heart disease, stroke, and kidney disease (Joint National Committee on Prevention, Detection, Evaluation, and Treatment of High Blood Pressure 1997).

8. *To evaluate prevention/intervention/treatment programmes.* An excellent example of this is the evaluation of the many vaccine programmes in the 1950s and 1960s which reduced the prevalence, morbidity, and mortality of childhood diseases such as polio, measles, mumps, chicken pox, etc., and studies to evaluate the effectiveness of new treatments such as highly active antiretroviral therapy (HAART) on HIV/AIDS (Detels *et al.* 1998).

9. *To investigate epidemics of unknown aetiology.* Epidemiological strategies were used to establish the cause, modes of transmission, and risk factors for Ebola haemorrhagic fever, which first occurred in the Congo in 1976 (Feldmann *et al.* 1996; eMedicine.com 2005).

10. *To elucidate the molecular determinants of disease progression.* Epidemiological strategies can help to elucidate the changes in the human immune response which accompany infection by disease agents, for example the initial immune response to HIV infection (Detels *et al.* 1983; Fahey *et al.* 1984; Ho *et al.* 1995).

11. *To better measure morbidity as well as mortality.* Until the latter half of the twentieth century, disease occurrence was largely characterized by mortality rates. The development of parameters such as 'years of healthy life lost' and 'disability-adjusted life years' (DALYs) have significantly increased our capacity to consider the ability to function normally as an important element of health, and have resulted in a reordering of diseases of major health significance (Murray 1994).

From the examples given above, it should be clear that epidemiology functions as the backbone or core of evidence-based public health practices, as well as a key strategy for evaluating the effectiveness of both clinical and public health interventions.

Significant contributions of epidemiology to public health

Viewed in retrospect, the pace of new advances in public health attributable to the innovative use of epidemiology in the twentieth century, assisted by advances in the laboratory sciences, was truly astounding. As a result of epidemiological research and interventions based on them, the average life expectancy in the USA, for example, increased from 47.3 years at the beginning of the century to 77.2 years by the end of the century. Most diseases that were common causes of death early in the century were brought under control or, in the case of smallpox, eliminated completely. Children in many parts of the world no longer expect to have measles, mumps, rubella, and chicken pox, childhood diseases that were common in the early part of the century. The so-called 'epidemiological transition' meant that the major causes of death had changed from infectious diseases in the early part of the century to chronic diseases in the latter part. Even in most developing countries, chronic diseases accounted for more than half of the deaths by the end of the century.

Below we would like to discuss a few of the outstanding examples of the contributions of epidemiology that resulted in these dramatic improvements in the health of the public:

◆ *Smallpox*. The elimination of this terrible epidemic disease is perhaps the best example of the contribution of epidemiology to health in the twentieth century. An effective vaccine against smallpox was invented in the late eighteenth century, but epidemic smallpox persisted for another 160 years, killing millions of people until it was eliminated globally in 1977. Why were we able to eradicate smallpox only 160 years after the development of an effective vaccine? The reason was that it took that long to devise and implement a rational intervention strategy based on sound epidemiological principles. In the middle of the twentieth century, epidemiologists proposed a new strategy to replace the old practice of trying to vaccinate a high enough proportion of the population to prevent transmission. The latter strategy failed in part because of the repeated reintroduction of the agent from parts of the world with low vaccination rates. Epidemiologists realized that a global approach was needed to eliminate the disease. Because the incubation period (7–19 days) is sufficiently long to allow action to be taken after discovering a case, there are very few subclinical cases, and because the agent has low transmissibility, a group of epidemiologists proposed using a strategy of 'search and containment'. Thus, a vigorous surveillance programme was initiated globally in every country. Once a case was found, all known contacts were immediately vaccinated, preventing the further spread of the virus (Henderson 1998). This same strategy is now being implemented to eliminate polio worldwide. Although polio has been eliminated from most countries of the world, it persists in a few. Polio is a greater challenge because there are many subclinical cases of the disease, and it is highly transmissible. On the other hand, the availability of a lyophilized oral vaccine greatly facilitates vaccination programmes, particularly in remote areas.

◆ *The health hazards of smoking*. The traditional approach to disease investigations in the early twentieth century was to identify a disease, then to use different strategies to describe the clinical symptoms, disease course, modes of spread (if infectious), and other relevant characteristics of the disease and the causative agent. However, some agents cause a wide spectrum of disease. Sir Richard Doll and Bradford Hill dramatically demonstrated the relationship of smoking to lung cancer (see Chapter 6). However, the large longitudinal studies of cardiovascular disease in the mid-twentieth century, including Framingham, Tecumseh, and others, demonstrated that smoking was also a risk factor for cardiovascular diseases (see Chapter 7). Subsequent cohort studies comparing health outcomes among smokers with those among non-smokers not only identified a wide spectrum of diseases that were associated with smoking, but also identified smoking as the single most important health hazard of the twentieth century, accounting for about one-fifth of all deaths in the USA (McGinnis and Foege 1999).

◆ Kuru. One of the most important discoveries of the twentieth century was diseases caused by 'prions', a newly recognized class of disease agents that caused disease only after an incubation period often lasting decades. The epidemiological investigation by Carleton Gajdusek and Joseph Gibbs (Gajdusek *et al.*1966) of kuru, a rare neurological disease occurring in the eastern New Guinea Highlands, primarily among women and children, resulted in the discovery of prions as disease agents. Gajdusek noted that New Guinea highlanders engaged in ritual eating of their recently deceased relatives. This was viewed as a sign of respect and regeneration by the highlanders. Traditionally the male members of the family ate the muscles, leaving the internal organs and brain to be consumed by the women and children. The disease, a neurological disease with a slow degenerative course, was noted to occur primarily among the women and children. Suspecting that the brains of the deceased might contain a disease agent, Gajdusek sent specimens of the brains of the deceased to his colleague, Joseph Gibbs at the US National Institutes of Health, to inject into the brains of monkeys. Gibbs kept the monkeys under observation for years, and noted that many of the monkeys injected with the brain material eventually developed neurological symptoms and died, whereas control monkeys did not. Injection of brain material from these diseased monkeys into other monkeys, who subsequently developed neurological disease, demonstrated the presence of a transmissible agent in the brain. Microscopic inspection of the diseased monkey brains revealed small particles unlike any known organisms. Gajdusek and Gibbs thought these were virus particles, but subsequently they were shown to be prions, which are also the causative agent of other slow diseases, including Creuzfeldt–Jakob disease and 'mad cow' disease (bovine spongiform encephalopathy), recently plaguing Europe and North America (Prusiner 1995). This discovery led to the first award of a Nobel prize to an epidemiologist, Carleton Gajdusek, in 1976 (see Chapter 12 on emerging diseases for a more detailed description).

◆ *The Alameda Health Study*. In the first half of the twentieth century, as in previous centuries, scientists, as well as the public, felt that diseases had a biological causation minimally influenced by psychosocial factors not associated with exposure to the causative agent (Breslow and Breslow 1993). These landmark studies (described above) provided evidence for the development and implementation of successful behavioural interventions, now one of the mainstays of the public health armamentarium.

◆ *Injuries*. In the early part of the twentieth century, public health professionals, including epidemiologists, were primarily concerned about diseases, but as high-speed modes of transportation, primarily automobiles, became available, injuries became an increasing cause of serious morbidity and death. As epidemiological studies demonstrated the underlying causes of many injuries, it became apparent that better design of cars, ladders, and other tools of modern society, as well as policy decisions, were required to reduce accidents and injuries resulting from them. Epidemiologists have played an important role in demonstrating that interventions such as seat belts and air bags in automobiles, helmets required of motorcyclists, and lower speed limits have reduced the incidence of accidents and of serious injuries associated with them. Automation of assembly lines, long hours of computer usage, and other advances in the twentieth century have introduced injuries such as carpal tunnel syndrome, which have been elucidated by epidemiological studies.

◆ *Environmentally induced diseases*. Although many areas of the world suffered from terrible environmental conditions in the nineteenth century, there was little scientific evidence demonstrating that the deterioration of the environment (for example, the notorious pea soup fogs of London) were associated with significant, non-reversible health impacts. Epidemiological studies in the twentieth century established that significant reduction in respiratory function was associated with childhood exposure to high levels of photochemical pollutants, and that increased mortality is associated with residence in areas with high levels of petrochemical air pollutants (Detels *et al.* 1991). Similar studies have demonstrated the harm caused by pollution of ground water and the oceans. These studies of the impact of polluted air and water have provided the scientific evidence to legislate stringent policies in many cities to reduce the release of pollutants into the air and water by automobiles and industry in developed countries. Unfortunately, many developing countries and some developed countries still suffer from severe environmental pollution because of the economic competition between production of cheap goods and the cost of prevention and control of environmental pollutants.

◆ *Methodological advances*. Although the origins of epidemiology can be traced back to John Snow's elegant investigation of the cholera epidemics in nineteenth-century London, major advances in epidemiological methodologies were also made in the twentieth century. These new methodologies were made possible in part by the development in the twentieth century of new technologies, such as the computer. For example, it became possible to model the possible course of an epidemic by varying transmission probabilities, etc. By the middle of the twentieth century, it became apparent to epidemiologists that different strategies for selection of study subjects and populations influenced the likelihood of finding epidemiological correlations, and could result in observations of associations that were spurious. Further, as it became apparent that multiple factors such as age and gender were associated with the occurrence of disease and morbidity, epidemiologists recognized the need to control for these multiple factors confounding the relationship between exposure and an outcome, and to document the independent contributions of each factor. In the last quarter of the twentieth century, epidemiologists, including Miettinen, Greenland, and Rothman, developed important strategies to address these issues. These are documented in Chapter 20.

The above represent only a few of the major contributions to public health made by epidemiologists in the twentieth century. Many more significant contributions were made, but the required brevity of this chapter precludes mention of all of them. It is, however, clear that epidemiology will remain the backbone of public health, and will continue to contribute significantly to the health of the public.

References

Breslow L (1947). Chronic disease in the modern public health program. In *California's health*. California State Department of Public Health, Berkeley, CA.

Breslow L (2005). Origins and development of the International Epidemiological Association. *International Journal of Epidemiology*, **34**, 725–9.

Breslow L and Breslow N (1993). Health practices and disability: some evidence from Alameda County. *Preventive Medicine*, **22**, 86–95.

Bunker JJ (1995) Medicine matters after all. *Journal of the Royal College of Physicians London*, **29**, 105–12.

Dawber TR (1980). *The Framingham Study*. Harvard University Press, Cambridge, MA.

Detels R, Gutman L, Jaramillo J, *et al.* (1969). An epidemic of intestinal capillariasis in man: a study in a barrio in northern Luzon. *American Journal of Tropical Medicine and Hygiene*, **18**, 676–82.

Detels R, Fahey JL, Schwartz K, Greene RS, Visscher BR, and Gottlieb MS (1983). Relation between sexual practices and T-cell subsets in homosexually active men. *Lancet*, 1(8325), 609–11.

Detels R, Tashkin DP, Sayre JW, *et al.* (1991). The UCLA population studies of CORD: X. A cohort study of changes in respiratory function associated with chronic exposure to SOx, NOx, and hydrocarbons. *American Journal of Public Health*, **81**, 350–9.

Detels R, Phair JP, Saah AJ, *et al.* (1992). Recent scientific contributions to understanding HIV/AIDS from the Multicenter AIDS Cohort Study. *Journal of Epidemiology [Japan]*, **2**, S11–S19.

Detels R, Munoz A, McFarlane G, *et al.* (1998). Effectiveness of potent antiretroviral therapy on time to AIDS and death in men with known HIV infection duration. Multicenter AIDS Cohort Study Investigators, *The Journal of the American Medical Association*, **281**, 1696–7.

eMedicine.com (2005). Ebola virus. November 2003, updated 2005. www.eMedicine.com.

Fahey J, Prince H, Weaver M, *et al.* (1984). Quantitative changes in T helper or T suppressor/cytotoxic lymphocyte subsets that distinguish acquired immune deficiency syndrome from other immune subset disorders. *American Journal of Medicine*, **76**, 95–100.

Feldmann H, Slenczka W, and Klenk HD (1996). Emerging and reemerging of filoviruses. *Archives of Virology*, **11**, S77–S100.

Gajdusek DC, Gibbs CJ, and Alpers M (1966). Experimental transmission of a kuru-like syndrome to chimpanzees. *Nature*, **209**, 794.

Grayston JT, Gale JL, and Watten RH (1972). The epidemiology of rubella on Taiwan. I. Introduction and description of the 1957–1958 epidemic. *International Journal of Epidemiology*, **1**, 245–52.

Henderson DA (1998). Smallpox eradication – a cold war victory. *World Health Forum*, **19**, 113–19.

Ho DD, Neumann AU, Perelson AS, Chen W, Leonard JM, and Markowitz M (1995). Rapid turnover of plasma virions and CD4 lymphocytes in HIV-1 infection. *Nature*, **373**, 123–6.

Institute of Medicine (1998). *The future of public health*. National Academy Press, Washington, DC.

Ji G, Detels R, Wu Z and Yin Y (2006). Correlates of HIV infection among former blood/plasma donors in rural China. *AIDS*, **20**, 585–91.

Joint National Committee on Prevention, Detection, Evaluation, and Treatment of High Blood Pressure (1997). The Sixth Report of the Joint National Committee on Prevention, Detection, Evaluation and Treatement of High Blood Pressure. *Archives of International Medicine*, **157**, 2413–46.

Kaslow RA, Ostrow DG, Detels R, Phair JP, Polk BF, and Rinaldo CR (1987). The Multicenter AIDS Cohort Study: rationale, organization, and selected characteristics of the participants. *American Journal of Epidemiology*, **126**, 310–18.

Keys A (1970). *Coronary heart disease in seven countries*, Monograph 29. American Heart Association. Futura Publishing Co., Armonk, NY.

McGinnis JM and Foege WH (1999). Mortality and morbidity attributable to use of addictive substances in the United States. *Proceedings of the Association of American Physicians*, **111**, 109–18.

Morris JN (1957). *Uses of epidemiology*. Churchill Livingstone, Edinburgh.

Murray CJ (1994). Quantifying the burden of disease: the technical basis for disability-adjusted life years. *Bulletin of the World Health Organization*, **72**, 429–45.

Prusiner SB (1995). Prion diseases. *Scientific American*, **272**, 48–56.

Surgeon-General, US Public Health Service (1964). *Smoking and health*. US Departments of Health Education and Welfare, Washington, DC.

Thuriaux MC (2002). Epidemiologic transition. In *Encyclopedia of public health* (ed. L Breslow). Macmillan Reference, New York, pp. 397–8.

Wu Z and Detels R (1995). HIV-1 infection in commercial plasma donors in China. *Lancet*, **346**, 61–2.

Wu Z, Rou K, and Detels R (2001). Prevalence of HIV infection among former commercial plasma donors in rural Eastern China. *Health Policy and Planning*, **16**, 41–6.

16

Health services research and epidemiology

Kerr L. White

Personal experiences

Immersion in economics, especially the views of John Maynard Keynes, Eliot Dunlap Smith, Ida M. Tarbell, and Thorstein Veblen, at McGill and Yale universities as an undergraduate and graduate student in the 1930s stimulated my curiosity about the impact of social and economic factors on health and disease. A stint in a factory personnel department, organization of a successful employees' strike and Second World War army experiences abroad under-girded my decision to study medicine. In the late 1940s McGill provided superb clinical education but painfully tedious public health lectures that featured detailed specifications for digging pit privies and canning tomatoes. In my final year, however, I encountered John Ryle's (1889–1950) slim volume *Changing disciplines* (Ryle 1948). Here was the former Regius Professor of Physic (Medicine) at Cambridge embracing both clinical and population perspectives in his new Institute of Social Medicine at Oxford. We corresponded about my spending a year with him but sadly he died prematurely.

Ryle's example strengthened my resolve to complete residency and fellowship training in internal medicine; that was where the profession's intellectual and academic power resided. Prior to the advent of the randomized clinical trial (RCT), 'tests' of the benefit of cortisone involved asking patients hourly whether they 'felt better' or advising them to 'take this—you'll feel better'. The Professor of Medicine, J. S. L. Browne, encouraged my unorthodox interests in questioning the therapeutic impact of physicians' authoritarian certitude about many interventions. He introduced me, a Canadian, to Lester Evans of the Commonwealth Fund in New York who, in turn, referred me to the first new post-war medical school at the University of North Carolina (UNC) where the opening gambit was a 1952 seminar on 'Needed research in health and medical care'. Jerry Morris gave the key-note address which he later enlarged in his classic volume *Uses of epidemiology* (Morris 1957).

Joining UNC's Department of Internal Medicine without formal training in epidemiology (i.e. the study of that which is upon the people) it was my good fortune to work with such innovative investigators as epidemiologists Sydney Kark and John Cassel and biostatistician Bernie Greenberg. They indoctrinated me into the concepts and methods of epidemiology and health statistics. Early publications in the 1950s included the first population-based survey of cardiac failure (with Michel Ibrahim); the first analysis of outpatient medical errors disclosed by record audits (with Bob Huntley); and the first state-wide investigation of patient referral patterns to consultants and academic medical centres (with Frank Williams). These were not problems that appealed to our biomedically oriented colleagues who considered them 'weird'.

The evolution of health services research (HSR) has had many twists and turns. It is the purview not of a single discipline but rather of a wide range of scientists with varied skills whose task is to investigate a hugely expensive and mal-distributed essential human service enterprise. Of the three venues for investigating problems of health and disease—the individual, the laboratory, and the population—the great bulk of HSR has in common the population perspective. Epidemiological methods and 'epidemiological thinking', based on fundamental contributions of earlier French,

Belgian, and British statisticians, are central features. In addition to trained, certified, and self-proclaimed physician and non-physician epidemiologists, HSR is conducted by administrators, anthropologists, clinicians, demographers, economists, nurses, political scientists, psychologists, social workers, sociologists, statisticians, and others. Although the majority embraces the population perspective, most also incorporate one or more of the administrative, biomedical, clinical, financial, organizational, psychological, and socio-economic world views (White *et al.* 1992).

The United States National Academy of Sciences' Institute of Medicine defined HSR in 2000—its most recent iteration—as 'the multidisciplinary field of inquiry, both basic and applied, that examines the use, costs, quality, accessibility, delivery, organization, financing, and outcomes of health-care services to increase knowledge and understanding of the structure, processes, and effects of health services for individuals and populations'. At its founding in 1957, the British Society for Social Medicine stated that its turf encompassed 'epidemiology, the study of the medical and health needs of society, the study of the provision and organization of health services and the study of the prevention of disease'. The terms employed in the overlapping sub-fields of HSR include in alphabetical order: clinical economics, clinical epidemiology, clinical evaluative sciences, evaluative health sciences, evidenced health care, evidenced based medicine, health economics, health policy research, health systems research, health-care research, medical care research, outcomes research, patient care research, population health research, technology assessment, translational research, and probably others. They are used alone or in combination; distinctions are often difficult and there is little point in trying since labels come and go—as many have (Daly 2005).

Initially epidemiological concepts and methods were employed by physicians without formal training. The latter only began in 1918 with Wade Hampton Frost (1889–1938) at Johns Hopkins and in 1928 with Major Greenwood (1880–1949) at the London School of Hygiene and Tropical Medicine (LSHTM). From its earliest days epidemiology buttressed by the mounting importance of bacteriology had focused largely on communicable diseases—then and still an enduring 'bug hunt'. Only later, primarily in Britain, did epidemiologists start tackling non-communicable disorders. Academic interest in evaluating medical care manoeuvres and the workings of health services was minimal until mid-century.

Ideas for evaluating the relative benefits, risks, and, only recently, the costs of medical interventions and health services are, however, not entirely new and they are far from free of political reverberations. The first twentieth-century manifestations of curiosity about clinical ministrations in medicine's hallowed halls are attributed to the Boston surgeon, Ernest A. Codman (1869–1940). Shunned by Harvard's Massachusetts General Hospital for attempts to document hospital surgical outcomes he resigned to start his own 'End Result Hospital' from whence he published all errors (e.g. 123 in 337 patients). Later J. Alison Glover (1876–1963), a UK Health Officer, identified wide disparities in children's tonsillectomy rates among otherwise similar geopolitical jurisdictions—the 'Glover phenomenon' (Glover 1938). Paul A. Lembcke (1908–64), a distinguished epidemiologist at Johns Hopkins in the 1950s, is best remembered for reintroducing Florence Nightingale's and Codman's insistence on auditing hospital outcomes (Lembcke 1956). Sadly Glover's and Lembcke's findings attracted little interest from the broader medical profession.

Times have changed, and now most medical and public health schools in the developed world, and many elsewhere, have units or departments whose titles vary but whose major function is HSR. In the latter part of the twentieth century epidemiological, i.e. population-based, thinking in one guise or another played a necessary, if not always sufficient, role in the rapid ascendancy of HSR. Its origins warrant recounting.

In 1946 the United States Congress passed the Hill-Burton Hospital Construction Act to improve services nationally, especially in underserved areas. Research directed at improving hospital facilities began in 1949, but not until 1955 did Congress provide the first $1.5 million for 'research in hospital *operation and administration*'. Two unsung Federal bureaucrats persuaded Congress to add these funds and a new mandate that included something called 'medical care research':

> The widest latitude is allowed by the wording of the law to permit such research and demonstrations in the hospital *and related fields* [emphasis added]. There is almost universal agreement that required information is lacking in many unexplored areas. At the same time, it is recognized that there are few current methods that are not susceptible to improvement
>
> (Cronin and Block 1956).

About 1956 a small body conducting what we called patient care research (later medical care research), supported by the new Hill-Burton research funds, started meeting periodically to discuss findings. The largest group (Bernard Greenberg, Robert Huntley, Frank Williams, and the present author) was at the University of North Carolina; others were at Cornell University Medical School (Barbara Korsch, George Reader, and Doris Schwartz), the New York City Health Department (Paul Densen and Sam Shapiro), and Harvard's Beth Israel Hospital (Sydney Lee, Cecil Sheps, and Jerry Solon). Later the renowned annual Atlantic City Meeting was added to our venues. There, amidst gatherings of the major medical scientific bodies, we presented our work at the 'patient care research section'. By the 1960s, however, our enthusiasm for this grand venue had waned as biomedical research increasingly dominated the interests of most attendees. There was no longer an academic meeting place or professional home for the expanding band of young academics exploring the workings of patient care and health services.

Responsibility for reviewing applications for the new Hill-Burton research funds was assigned in 1955 to the US National Institutes of Health's (NIH) Division of Research Grants. A mixed bag of study sections with such labels as sanitation, public health methods, and nursing (concerned with patient care) existed and now there was to be a newly established Hospital Facilities Research Study Section; I joined it in 1957. These and seven barely related study sections were designated the 'Health Services Group'.

To consider future research needs bearing on provision of health care the Hospital Facilities Research Study Section took the initiative by establishing a subcommittee. In March 1959 responding to its solicitation for ideas I wrote:

> Should we not encourage the redefinition of 'hospitals' and possibly of the [Hospital Facilities Research] Study Section's functions? ... Should we not spell out what is either stated or implied in the Hill-Burton Act that we are concerned with all facilities, including private physicians' offices, health centers, clinics, diagnostic facilities, industrial health offices, rehabilitation centers, health departments, outpatient departments and inpatient services, both general and specialized, to the extent that they contribute to the medical care needs of society? We have certainly reviewed and sponsored grants in many of these areas.
>
> Should we not encourage studies and approaches that have as their base the health problems of the populations concerned rather than the institutions currently serving those needs? What are the medical care needs of various groups? Who are the patients? Which populations need care—preventive, diagnostic, therapeutic, and rehabilitative?
>
> What economic, social, psychological, cultural, and informational factors inhibit or facilitate access to the best medical care at the earliest phases of disease? Who is to render this care? What health personnel must be educated or trained? How can these professional workers best be organized? What facilities are needed for them?
>
> Perhaps the Study section should have its name changed to the Health Facilities Research Study Section or the Medical Care Research Study Section.

Later in the spring of 1959, following deliberations of that subcommittee, a joint meeting of the Nursing and Hospital Facilities Research Study Sections considered their missions. In 2000 no minutes of that historic meeting could be found in the NIH archives but Cecil Sheps (another Canadian), former Chair of the latter study section, and I, the only living members of that gathering, compared recollections. Neither recalled who introduced the term 'health services research' but both enthusiastically favoured it and are certain the new label arose at that meeting. The group unanimously recommended that it supplant the current term Hospital Facilities Research Study Section, much preferring it over other labels such as medical care research, health facilities research and health resources research. On 1 September 1960, James Shannon, Director of NIH, officially decreed the change to Health Services Research Study Section. But a name change does not a research 'field' create and certainly not a distinct 'discipline'.

In the interim, my 1959–60 sabbatical year had included formal courses in epidemiology and health statistics at the LSHTM with Donald Reid and Bradford Hill, an intellectual base with Jerry Morris at the London Hospital, extensive visits throughout the UK and Europe to individuals concerned with health services and related epidemiological research, and induction into the International Epidemiological Association (IEA) which had been founded in 1954. To these collective experiences and the friendships established I owe most of the ideas and methods used in attempts in the USA to 'spread the gospel' of HSR—a phrase employed by Robert Cruikshank, the IEA's first president.

In the UK, Walter Holland, trained at the LSHTM and Johns Hopkins was a leading player in broadening the applications of epidemiology and especially its role in HSR. In 1962 he joined St Thomas' Hospital's Medical School, London and in 1964 founded the first ever Department of Clinical Epidemiology and Social Medicine. A majority of its many publications, especially those dealing with outcomes, are best categorized as HSR. One of Holland's more influential contributions questioned the benefits of multiphasic screening—a notion being aggressively touted in the USA. Over the decades, in addition to fostering the development of HSR, Holland has trained and mentored numerous distinguished UK epidemiologists as well as others from distant lands, including the USA (Holland 2002).

Meanwhile, in 1962, on assuming chairmanship of the Health Services Research Study Section (the only member with training or experience in epidemiological research), I selected as its new Executive Secretary, Thomas McCarthy PhD. During our initial discussions McCarthy, having just completed an NIH grants associates training programme, emphasized that study sections in addition to 'reviewing research grant applications' were responsible equally for 'defining and developing their respective field, stimulating needed research and improving the field's quality and credibility'. McCarthy was impressed by the work of the Biophysics and Biophysical Chemistry Study Section in developing its new and comparatively unknown field. Based on their experiences we proposed strategies for promoting the strange new arena of HSR. Our ideas were endorsed enthusiastically by all study section members save one—a state Commissioner of Public Health. He argued that 'the government' had no business investigating the clinical activities of doctors and hospitals.

Pursuing five major initiatives over several years we:

1. developed criteria for and funded four types of research—exploratory, pilot, project, and program grants;

2. made 'evangelical' site visits to educate applicants who proposed tackling complicated problems with trivial methods and vice versa;

3. developed criteria for and generously funded a core of health services research centres at major research universities;

4. described the field's current status by commissioning and publishing 14 papers by eminent academics delineating many facets of health services amenable to scientific and scholarly inquiry (Mainland 1966);

5. visited major organizations concerned with the provision or over-sight of health services, e.g. the American Medical Association, the American Hospital Association, the US Center for Communicable Diseases, the California Health Department, and Puerto Rico's health department, new medical school, and regionalized health services.

All this was not accomplished easily. Officials of the then US Department of Health, Education, and Welfare (DHEW) denied us permission to visit the American Medical Association claiming we were 'treating with the enemy'. We went anyway and the bill was paid. Similarly we were denied approval to send study section members to visit British and Scandinavian sites of emerging health services research on the grounds that we could contaminate the 'American way' by 'picking up a lot of "socialistic" ideas'. We sent them anyway and the bill was paid (McCarthy and White 2000).

A new field requires several types of enabling 'tools' to thrive. For example, little HSR can be accomplished without primary databases. Florence Nightingale designed the first hospital discharge abstract form in the 1860s and the UK introduced its Hospital In-Patient Enquiry (later the Hospital Activities Analysis) in the 1950s. With these in mind our group at Johns Hopkins organized three international conferences to examine the need for and recommend examples of uniform minimum data sets (UMDS) for ambulatory care visits, hospital discharge abstracts, and long-term care status abstracts. Over the years the DHEW, its National Center for Health Statistics (NCHS), and other bodies adapted and adopted UDMSs; they have made possible much HSR.

Ambulatory care was a black box insofar as medical education and organization of services were concerned. Modelled after early 1950s surveys by the Royal College of General Practitioners and the UK Registrar-General's Office, the NCHS initiated in 1974 the National Ambulatory Medical Care Survey (NAMCS) designed by our group at Johns Hopkins using epidemiological survey methods (Tenney *et al.* 1974). The NAMCS' periodic reports described the largest component of health services—the content of office-based care—and became the most sought after in NCHS history. Ambulatory care research, especially the study of 'episodes of care', stimulated creation of the 'International Classification of Primary Care' (ICPC) to augment the International Classification of Diseases (Lamberts and Wood 1987). It is now incorporated in the US National Library of Medicine's Unified Medical Language System (UMLS).

A new field requires its own journals. The first was *Medical Care* started in 1963 by Bram Marcus, medical correspondent for *The Observer* of London, and published by Pitman's. Unfortunately interest flagged and as an Editorial Board member I learned of its imminent demise and negotiated transfer to the USA for publication by J. B. Lippincott; it flourishes to this day. In 1963 the American Hospital Association sought NIH funds for a new journal to be called *Hospital Research*. A study section team went to Chicago to help them understand that if they wanted the money they should broaden their horizons and call the journal *Health Services Research*. Reluctantly they agreed and the journal flourishes to this day. In 1970 Vicente Navarro, a protégé of John Brotherston's at the University of Edinburgh, my first student at Johns Hopkins, and now a professor there, founded the *International Journal of Health Services*. Although emphasizing policy issues it frequently includes articles that invoke HSR to inform the positions taken.

The 'tools' required by a new field of enquiry are undoubtedly necessary but far from sufficient. Educational opportunities are essential for aspiring young investigators—especially physicians, since clinical activities of all kinds are a central feature of HSR. As an internist with epidemiological training and experience I had concluded that one of the saddest episodes in the annals of medicine's mission to respond to society's health problems was the Rockefeller Foundation's decision in 1916 to establish schools of public health isolated intellectually, physically, and organizationally from medical schools. Although an understandable response by the Foundation to growing concerns about unaddressed public health problems, the unanticipated consequence of the decision was effective segregation of the population from the clinical and emerging biomedical perspectives. The Epidemiological Society of London, founded in 1850, was composed largely of physicians; epidemiology had long roots in clinical medicine. After 1916 in the USA and in many other countries, epidemiology's relegation to the new schools of public health deprived medical students and their faculties of experience with the requisite concepts and methods for examining the risks and benefits of medicine's interventions at both the individual and population levels (White 1991).

To restore this dysfunctional imbalance our Johns Hopkins department created a hybrid educational experience that enabled interested Hopkins' hospital house staff to integrate courses in epidemiology and HSR with their clinical training. This was not done easily. We had to overcome countless conflicting governance rules in Hopkins' separated schools of medicine and public health such as: hours of 'work', clinical rotation and course schedules, conference hours, semester dates, parking regulations, secretarial salaries, and more. We succeeded in attracting many superb candidates who on completing their training received MSc or DSc degrees. Training involved joint exercises with our other departmental graduate students who had prior degrees in, for example, economics, engineering, hospital administration, nursing, and sociology. With initial support from the Carnegie Foundation and the Commonwealth Fund, and then from the Robert Wood Johnson Foundation, the Clinical Scholars Program, as it was labelled, has flourished for over 30 years, spread to other sites and trained almost 1000 physicians in HSR. Most physicians currently leading this field have been Clinical Scholars.

There was also the matter of a Federal institutional research and funding body similar to NIH's components. Following a 1966 study section meeting in Chicago, Tom McCarthy, two other DHEW officials, and I repaired to our hotel's bar. On the back of a paper napkin we drafted a statement of the mission and organizational relationships of such an entity and labelled it the National Center for Health Services Research (NCHSR). We hastened to Washington, DC where the Association of American Medical Colleges (AAMC) was holding its annual conclave. Over the weekend as McCarthy and colleagues prepared a descriptive brochure I persuaded Bill Hubbard, AAMC president, to let me address the gathering; he agreed. Stony silence met my remarks; strange enquiries labelled 'health services research' should not be allowed to impinge on the deans' growing preoccupation with ever more generous NIH funding for biomedical investigations. A few of the more curious did pick up our brochure.

Nevertheless, all members of the study section supported our proposed NCHSR and I successfully lobbied senior DHEW officials about the need for it. Two exploratory commissions endorsed the idea and my testimony before Senator Ted Kennedy's Congressional Committee was well-received. In 1968 the US Congress established the National Center for Health Services Research and Development (NCHSRD). There is reason to believe that Shannon, a strong supporter of HSR, favoured placing the new centre in NIH where its credibility would be clearly vouchsafed. Unfortunately Shannon became seriously ill and the NCHSRD was placed inappropriately in the newly created and untested Health Services and Mental Health Administration (HSMHA) of DHEW. Paul Sanazaro was appointed founding director and Tom McCarthy his deputy (Flook and Sanazaro 1973).

I chaired the Center's Scientific and Professional Advisory Board (SPAB) that included such eminent scholars as Martin Feldstein, Eliot Freidson, Bob Haggerty, Gordon McLachlan, and Rosemary Stevens (two UK representatives for cross-fertilization). When asked about an early meeting Sanazaro had with then DHEW Secretary Wilbur Cohen he reported that the Center's charge was to 'increase access to health services, improve quality, and reduce costs'. When asked how long Cohen gave the NCHSRD to accomplish all this Sanazaro replied 'six months'. The SPAB was flabbergasted but their advice to avoid over-promising and under-producing was ignored and the NCHSRD plunged ahead. During the ensuing years Congressional dissatisfaction mounted as problems of access, use, quality, outcomes, and costs of care remained unresolved. The Center never really overcame the over-promising. Sanazaro left in 1973 and was succeeded by other directors with limited expertise in research bearing on the provision and evaluation of health services.

During its first 20 years the Center funded much of the seminal research in HSR and initiated many useful contributions. One example was the development of government-wide software for use in the embryonic, but sadly ignored until recently, Electronic Health Record (EHR). Another was creation of the large-scale experimental medical care review organizations—an early national look at 'quality'. Unfortunately the NCHSRD focused excessively on health services investigators as its 'customers' to the neglect of politicians, administrators, other academics, and the public. During the early 1980s annual budgets were reduced by half ($80 to $40 million) with some improvement in 1987 to initiate the Medical Expenditure Panel Survey which, using sophisticated epidemiological methods, continues to this day. Nonetheless, the NCHSRD remained an obscure bureaucratic entity whose mission was poorly understood and whose products were of little help to busy members of Congress and the White House. That is except for the dramatic findings of two of our epidemiologically trained former Hopkins students, financed in part by the NCHSRD, Jack Wennberg and Bob Brook.

In 1962 while at the University of Vermont (in the first US medical school department labelled 'epidemiology') John Last (editor of the IEA's *Dictionary of Epidemiology*) and I, with the help of a generous NHSRD grant, undertook to install in that small state a universal hospital discharge abstract system based on the UK Hospital Inpatient Enquiry. The opportunity to undertake this manageable task had made the Vermont job offer unusually attractive. The objective was to audit Vermont's use of hospitals much as Nightingale, Codman, Lembcke, and Glover had urged for 100 years. It was not an easy task and included my being paraded before the state medical society charged with trying to hatch a communist plot.

After my move to Johns Hopkins in 1965 one of our students, Jack Wennberg (also a McGill medical school graduate), at my suggestion, took a job in Vermont to undertake the hospital studies we had proposed. Wide small-area discrepancies were found not only with tonsillectomies (70% versus 20% by age 12) but also with Caesarean sections, spinal fusions, mastectomies, and coronary by-pass surgeries. His classic 1973 paper in *Science* established the depth and extent of the ubiquitous problems with variations in resources, utilization, and outcomes, demonstrated the practicality of using claims (discharge abstract) data for research, and challenged the received wisdom that 'more treatment is better' (Wennberg and Gittelsohn 1973). Wennberg, cerebral, well-versed in theory, and persistent, pursued path-breaking research and educational programmes as he created his internationally acclaimed Dartmouth Center for Evaluative Clinical Sciences. Among its many publications is the famed *Dartmouth Atlas of Health Care*. Based on Medicare data for the elderly, it graphically depicts nationally unexplained and unwarranted small-area variations in the overall costs of care and the rates for common procedures; the Glover phenomenon writ large. Discharge abstract data for the rest of the US population is still unavailable—a major limitation to investigating hospital activities generated for the entire population.

Bob Brook, a Resident in Internal Medicine at Baltimore City Hospitals (a Johns Hopkins programme), while a Clinical Scholar in our department, wanted to pursue ideas generated by the 1962 UNC analysis of outpatient medical errors. He was forbidden to undertake a similar study at the Johns Hopkins Hospital. Accordingly, he conducted the study at the Baltimore City Hospital—a Hopkins affiliate. Brook's landmark *New England Journal of Medicine* paper, also in 1973, created a substantial stir by setting forth the many serious medical errors uncovered (Brook and Appel 1973). Brook, innovative, persistent, and articulate, mentored numerous acolytes and produced an extensive series of articles documenting dramatic variations in the frequencies, outcomes, and effectiveness of diverse treatments. He established an international reputation from his bases at the University of California (Los Angeles) as Professor of Medicine and Public Health and the RAND Corporation where he is vice-president and director of its health programme.

Wennberg's impressive testimony, bolstered by Bob Brook's equally voluminous studies, was accorded great weight by the US Congress. Together they were largely responsible for renewed and wider Congressional and professional support for HSR as NCHSRD approached a near-death experience. Their strategies with Congressional and White House colleagues enabled Wennberg and Brook to play essential roles in broadening the moribund Center's base and mission. In 1989 Congress substituted the term 'care' for 'services', added 'policy' to its title, dramatically expanded the mandate to include outcomes research and transformed the NCHSRD into the Agency for Health Care Policy and Research (AHCPR). Of greater significance, the enabling legislation elevated AHCPR in the bureaucracy to a par with NIH and increased its budget substantially, albeit to only about 1% of NIH's. Nevertheless, for five more years under the leadership of yet another director with modest experience, AHCPR underwent endless turbulence in productivity and perceptions by politicians and health professionals.

In 1994 Cliff Gaus, former Chief of the Office of Research and Demonstrations in the Health Care Financing Administration (HCFA), and another of our Hopkins' students, was appointed AHCPR's second director. In spite of his epidemiological orientation, extensive research and governmental experience, political astuteness, and gregarious nature, the agency's mission was again brought into question. Many factors were at work, including a dramatic change to Republican dominance in Congress. The tipping point was AHCPR's publication of evidence-based 'best-practice' guidelines for assorted disorders, including 'low back pain'. With devastating effect this treatise was attacked aggressively and relentlessly, both academically and politically, by orthopaedic surgeons, especially the North American Spine Society.

Almost every critic seemed to deplore the government-developed guidelines but believed that the gathering and synthesis of epidemiological and outcome data in advance of promulgating the guidelines was extremely valuable and could not be accomplished without government assistance. After extensive consultation with hospitals, health-care 'plans' and professional groups, Gaus terminated the original guideline exercise and created a new programme consisting of 12 evidenced-based practice centres. With the focus changed and better partnerships achieved with most health-care stakeholders, Congress gave AHCPR a new lease on life and continued funding. The development of evidence-based guidelines by health-care organizations has flourished ever since.

Gaus decided that AHCPR needed new leadership, and in 1997 brokered the appointment of John Eisenberg, Chair of the Department of Medicine and Physician-in-Chief at Georgetown University, as his successor. Eisenberg was a brilliant choice. Not only was he a superb clinician and politically skilful but he was a nationally known health services investigator trained in economics, widely experienced in epidemiology, and former chair of the Physician Payment Review Commission. With yet another name change in 1997 to the Agency for Healthcare Research and Quality (AHRQ), the Federal focus of HSR flourished under Eisenberg as never before; staff, budgets, grants, reports, and support grew rapidly. Both political parties, as well as academic and professional organizations, recognized its critical role in improving the country's increasingly tattered and costly health services. Eisenberg's untimely death in 2002 was a severe blow to the entire HSR establishment but he left an institution (as well as its building named after him) that enjoys well-earned national and international reputations.

Carolyn Clancy, originally appointed by Cliff Gaus as Director of the Center for Outcomes and Effectiveness Research, succeeded Eisenberg. She was trained in clinical epidemiology when both were at the University of Pennsylvania.

AHRQ has done as much as any US Federal or non-profit entity to foster recognition of epidemiologists' essential contributions to the improvement of health services. Its tortuous political, labelling, and budgetary travails are testimony to the need for better professional and political understanding of the population perspective in addition to the biomedical (Gray *et al.* 2003). The Commonwealth Fund, Kaiser Family, Kellogg, MacArthur, Pew, Robert Wood Johnson, and Rockefeller foundations and the Milbank Memorial Fund, have all actively supported HSR and its epidemiological component. The latter foundation during the 1970s and 1980s, under Robert Ebert, former Dean of the Harvard Medical School, had a substantial programme training young American clinicians at the LSHTM under the late Geoffrey Rose—chosen because of his clinical experience and orientation. Many are now leaders in HSR.

Theory is also essential. During the last half century no one contributed more to the underlying theoretical framework for most HSR than the late Avedis Donabedian (1919–2000), an unusually modest and unassuming physician with epidemiological training and a towering intellect. Starting in the 1950s at Harvard and later at the University of Michigan, single-handedly, he wrote numerous papers and a classic three-volume treatise that divides and dissects health services into the basic modalities of 'structures, processes, and outcomes'. Written with unusual insight, clarity, and wit these volumes must surely be the contemporary 'bible' for this nascent brand of scholarship and science (Donabedian 1980, 1982, 1985).

Another requirement for any new field is a 'club'—a professional home. In 1981 two of our epidemiologically oriented Hopkins' students, Cliff Gaus and Bob Blendon, Chair and Professor of Health Policy and Management at Harvard, established the Association for Health Services Research (AHSR) (now Academy Health) with a current membership of over 4000. The AHSR, of which John Eisenberg was also a former president, contributed mightily to building broad-based support for the ever more vigorously focused incarnations of the evolving NCHSRD, AHCPR, and AHRQ. In addition to its annual scientific conferences Academy Health sponsors symposia, conducts short courses, and distributes the field's major journals including *Health Services Research*, *Health Affairs*, and the *Milbank Quarterly*.

Clinical epidemiology, a subset of HSR (or sometimes vice versa), has an illustrious history, although the current label was not formally introduced until 1938 when John Paul, Professor of Medicine at Yale, described the concept and its tasks in his presidential address to the elite American Society for Clinical Investigation (Paul 1938). On several occasions Jerry Morris was a visiting professor at Yale and he and Paul must have exchanged many perceptive clinical and epidemiological insights. These surely were not lost on the late Alvan Feinstein (1925–2001), Sterling Professor of Medicine and Epidemiology at Yale, who in addition to directing one of the most successful Clinical Scholars programmes was a prolific and innovative contributor to the theory and methods of clinical epidemiology. As both a clinician and an epidemiologist he developed, among other metrics, diverse indices for assessing clinical states and the changes wrought by physicians' interventions (Feinstein 1985). Widely regarded as the father of modern clinical epidemiology, Feinstein's neologisms and harsh critiques were not always welcomed by more orthodox epidemiologists based in schools of public health.

In 1979 the Rockefeller Foundation (RF) inaugurated the International Clinical Epidemiology Network (INCLEN), its latest investment in epidemiology and its largest health programme ever. The Foundation had provided the initial funds to found the IEA in 1954 and intermittent support thereafter. Ideas generated during the 1960s and 1970s at IEA seminars in the Caribbean, India, Latin America, and the Middle East that introduced clinicians to epidemiological concepts and methods generated the ideas underlying INCLEN. The RF-funded training centres in medical schools at McMaster and Toronto universities in Canada, the universities of Pennsylvania and North Carolina in the USA and the University of Newcastle in Australia. By 2005 INCLEN had provided master's level training in epidemiology to over 1400 young clinicians, statisticians, economists, and social scientists from over 50 medical institutions in more than 30 largely developing countries on five continents. Working in clinical epidemiology units (CEUs) with about nine members each, their mission is to promote 'equitable health care based on the best evidence of effective and efficient use of resources … and to train leaders in health care research' (White 1991).

Suzanne and Robert Fletcher, both professors and clinicians at the Harvard Medical School (formerly at McGill and UNC) and both our Hopkins Clinical Scholars, have been major contributors to the ever-evolving HSR field. In 1982 they published the first textbook on clinical epidemiology, now in its fourth edition (Fletcher and Fletcher 2005). Their extensive research, consulting, teaching, joint editorship of two major journals (*Journal of General Internal Medicine* and *Annals of Internal Medicine*) and especially their central role in INCLEN's evolution have brought them global recognition. Singly and in tandem they have done as much as any one to generate widespread acceptance by fellow clinicians of the central role that HSR can play in bettering the health-care enterprise.

A Canadian now, David Sackett was American born, educated, and trained. Charismatic, out-spoken, and innovative, he has been a dynamic leader in HSR and clinical epidemiology as well as a leading contributor to INCLEN. He was founding chair of the Department of Clinical Epidemiology and Biostatistics at McMaster University's newly launched medical school in 1967, and a major factor in that institution's rise to global eminence. Sackett credits some of his future educational methods to attendance at one of the annual workshops on HSR and RCTs we held at Hopkins in the late 1960s, co-sponsored with the Association of American Medical Colleges. His accomplishments at McMaster and later at Oxford included training a generation of world-class investigators and teachers in clinical epidemiology. Critical of the limited perspectives of 'public health epidemiology' and 'big E' as Sackett calls them, he may be regarded as a major proponent if not the father of evidence-based medicine (EBM)—a hybrid of epidemiological analysis and clinical insight.

In the UK the Nuffield Trust (founded in 1940 as the Nuffield Provincial Hospitals Trust) under the leadership of Gordon McLachlan, then its secretary (i.e. president) established a field also called medical care research but, as in the USA, later termed health services research. In 1964 he began publishing through Oxford University Press an extensive series of research studies entitled 'Problems and progress in medical care: essays on current research in medical care'. Although initially focused on the workings of Britain's National Health Service they matured into largely generic investigations of problems facing health-care systems in developed countries. Most of the Nuffield-sponsored studies were conducted by epidemiologists in UK departments of social medicine (now public health medicine) and the LSHTM. In addition McLachlan inaugurated regular seminars, symposia, and the annual Rock Carling Lectures that stimulated the field by enabling academicians, practitioners, administrators, politicians, and the public to better understand the problems of health-care organization and services; all these have continued most recently under John Wyn Owen. Epidemiologists sponsored by Nuffield included such pioneering luminaries as Archie Cochrane, Sir John Brotherston, Charles Florey, Walter Holland, George Knox, Bob Logan, Tom McKeown, and Jerry Morris; all produced major contributions to HSR.

Archie Cochrane is best known to the greater medical communities in the UK, USA, and elsewhere for his Nuffield sponsored Rock Carling Lecture 'Effectiveness and efficiency: random reflections on health services' (Cochrane 1972). At the 1974 Annual Meeting of the US Institute of Medicine we distributed a hundred or more copies of Cochrane's classic that McLachlan donated. Among the country's medical establishment these generated unprecedented interest in outcomes research and the need for improved understanding and training in epidemiology, especially as it concerned both clinical and public health interventions.

Another major continuing player in the evolution of HSR in the UK has been the King's Fund through its sponsorship of studies, lectures, publications, and seminars. The Cochrane Collaboration (named after Archie) started by Sir Iain Chalmers is a worldwide collection of entities, usually in academic institutions, dedicated to evaluating and disseminating the 'best' evidence from RCTs to support optimum clinical interventions and health services—EBM. Critical thinking on these matters may have originated with the 1971 report of the WHO Expert Committee on Health Statistics for which Georges Rosch (a Frenchman) and Sakari Haro (a Finn) argued persuasively for the distinctively different definitions of 'efficacy', 'effectiveness', and 'efficiency' (World Health Organization 1971).

Starting in the 1960s the UK National Health Service has devoted increasing resources for studies bearing on staffing, training, institutions, organization, and funding. To these in recent years have been added others focusing on services, safety, quality, and information. The most powerful initiative, light years ahead of similar efforts in the fragmented US 'system', and the largest globally, is directed at the installation by 2010 of an information technology system 'Connecting for Health' (CFH)—that includes electronic health records (EHR)—to link all physicians, hospitals, NHS staff, and 50 million citizens. This cornucopia of privacy-protected world-class epidemiological data should, if exploited creatively, place the UK in the forefront of HSR, to say nothing of health informatics. Another recent UK creation is the National Institute for Health and Clinical Excellence (NICE) which publishes guidelines for the cost-effective management of diverse clinical disorders and public health interventions that are largely evidence-based using epidemiological methods.

The National Centre for Epidemiology and Population Health at the Australian National University, created following recommendations in a 1985 national survey of public health education and research, has an HSR component. There is a Canadian Health Services Research Foundation for conducting and supporting the field and the New Zealand Health Technology Assessment Unit in the Christchurch School of Medicine does outcomes and related research for both New Zealand and Australia. For 40 years Finland's Social Insurance Institution has had a strong HSR component to guide that country's health policies.

The US National Library of Medicine's National Information Center for Health Services Research and Technology Assessment (NCHSRTA) created a video depicting the history of HSR from the days of Sir William Petty (1623–87) and has a website listing three single-spaced pages of US and international entities involved in the field (www.nlm.nih.gov/hsrinfo/alphahsr.html). Many employ epidemiological concepts and methods—even when they don't know they are.

The IEA has been a major player in 'legitimizing' HSR. The earliest members were largely concerned with non-communicable diseases in contrast to others in the USA and Eastern Europe who believed that communicable diseases are the only 'true' province of epidemiology. Gradually the IEA embraced both these areas but not HSR. I vividly recall Archie Cochrane telling me in 1959 that he did not think epidemiology had any role to play in the assessment of medical care; times, problems, and people change. After numerous, often heated, debates the IEA accepted as members those working in the emerging sphere of HSR and related areas. In fact it opened membership to anyone interested enough to complete a brief application form and pay an annual fee for the world-class *International Journal of Epidemiology*.

What then is health services research? It is a broad amorphous field to which many disciplines contribute, but epidemiology with its population perspective and statistical methods is central. As in other applications of epidemiology, the record for HSR is variable. There is an increasing abundance of first-rate work but there is also too much activity directed at unimportant problems where ropey data are massaged with ever-fancier mathematical manoeuvres. Not everything that 'counts' can be counted. Qualitative research can also contribute to *HSR*. At its best this burgeoning field strives to foster and enhance the care of individuals—one by one—as well as the populations from which they come with science-based, compassionate, effective, and efficient services.

Myriads of HSR studies exist. In addition to those already mentioned here are four more, with a salient finding from each, to illustrate the scope of HSR and its potential for impact upon health policies. In 1961 using survey data of our own as well as that from UK and US sources, and a model devised by John and Elizabeth Horder of London, my UNC colleagues (Bernie Greenberg and Frank Williams) and I published an article in the *New England Journal of Medicine*— 'The ecology of medical care' that included a diagram of nested squares. In a population of 1000 adults in the course of a month 750 experienced some kind of health problem, 250 consulted a physician, nine were hospitalized, five were referred to a consultant, and one entered a teaching hospital where the great bulk of medical education takes place. We argued the case for increased emphasis on what we called 'primary medical care' (unaware at the time of the 1918 Dawson Report advocating 'primary care') and more balanced exposure of medical students to the full range of the population's health problems in the community. The results were questioned vigorously at the time but they have been duplicated in several different settings and as recently as 2006. The article and diagram have been widely reproduced in textbooks and anthologies, referenced in many other venues, and used for teaching and policy discussions for over four decades.

In 1971 the RAND Corporation (Joe Newhouse) inaugurated the large-scale Federally funded Health Insurance Experiment by creating an independent health insurance company that covered some 8000 people in 2750 families across the USA. Bob Brook, our Hopkins student, was recruited by Newhouse to head the health and quality parts of the experiment. Families were randomly assigned to policies with either no cost-sharing or 25, 50, or 95% co-payments and a maximum annual payment of $1000. In addition, the maximum amount a family could pay was related to their family income. Another group of families was randomly assigned to one of the country's best health maintenance organizations (HMOs). Their use of health services was recorded and their health status was assessed at entrance, annually, and on termination over 3- to 5-year periods. Multiple reports and articles recounted the experiment's ground-breaking findings. These included demonstrating that cost-sharing reduced equally both 'necessary' and 'unnecessary' use and health-care spending as well. The overall conclusion that cost-sharing did not affect either the quality of care or health status for the 'average' person enrolled in the study was hotly debated but resulted in dramatic changes in classical health insurance plans so that most now include higher cost-sharing. The additional finding that families randomized to the HMO received quality of care equal to those in fee-for-service arrangements resulted in efforts, for better or worse, to increase the 'managed care' market in the USA.

From 1964–76 the World Health Organization/International Collaborative Study of Medical Care Utilization (WHO/ICSMCU) was led from Johns Hopkins but involved essential academic and government colleagues from the seven participating countries: Argentina, Canada, Poland, the UK, the USA and Yugoslavia. We developed instruments and training manuals in four languages and conducted household surveys of almost 50,000 individuals from probability samples of 1000 families in each of 12 study areas in the seven countries; individual area response rates ranged from 90 to 99% and overall was 96.6%. The many relationships among standardized measures of 'need', 'use', and 'resources' were examined extensively. Two volumes, over 60 articles, and countless graduate theses resulted. Among the many findings of imbalances and distortions was demonstration of the relationship between a population's experience of unmet need for a physician (i.e. the percentage of all persons with perceived morbidity of the highest degree of severity within the last 2 weeks who, although wanting to contact a physician for their health problem, were unable to obtain one) and consumption of the area's short-term hospital bed nights (corrected for import and export of hospital use). Regardless of the ratio of short-term hospital beds to the area's population the greater the measure of unmet need the greater the use of hospital bed nights. In other words relatively high rates for the volume of hospital nights are inversely related to the availability and accessibility of ambulatory care. A long-held view that if you build hospital beds they will be filled was contradicted. Adequate access to primary medical care appeared to reduce hospital admissions.

Barbara Starfield, creative, determined, and highly knowledgeable was the first faculty colleague I appointed at Hopkins in 1965. She has had a remarkably productive career with an abiding focus on the content, quality, distribution, and essential role of primary medical care as the underpinning of any balanced health-care system. Of her books and many other publications, documented with exacting details over four decades, those comparing primary-care workforces, costs, and health outcomes in 13 developed countries, if carefully studied by politicians and health 'policy-makers', should have the greatest impact. She found the USA to be in last position, with the lowest ratio of primary-care physicians to specialists and the highest for per capita health-care expenditures. Among the 13 countries, the stronger the primary-care component the lower the costs and the better the outcomes.

Health services research and its analogues are now part of the fabric of the bulk of academic medicine—if not yet universally. A few medical school deans, editors of major journals (*Annals of Internal Medicine* and *The Lancet*) and members of many governmental and philanthropic grant-making bodies have backgrounds in HSR. Hospital and outpatient formal and informal curricula more often than not now incorporate elements of the field.

We may conclude, then, from this half century's scientific odyssey that, by playing a central role in the evolution of HSR, epidemiology has contributed substantially to diminishing the power of authoritarian pronouncements by eminent figures on medical decision-making, therapeutic interventions, health-care organization, resource deployment, and professional education. Biomedicine now has HSR colleagues to ensure that the fruits of its labours are translated effectively and efficiently into better care for individuals and populations. The labels attached to these diverse endeavours will undoubtedly change in the future as they have in the past but epidemiology surely will be the dominant discipline.

Acknowledgements

I thank Bob Brook, Robert Fletcher, Suzanne Fletcher, Cliff Gaus, Tom McCarthy, Gerry Rosenthal, Dave Sackett, Barbara Starfield, and Jack Wennberg for helpful information and thoughtful critiques.

References

Brook RH and Appel FA (1973). Quality-of-care assessment: choosing a method for peer review. *New England Journal of Medicine*, **288**, 1323–9.

Cochrane AL (1972). *Effectiveness and efficiency: random reflections on health services. The Rock Carling Lecture.* Nuffield Provincial Hospitals Trust, London.

Cronin JW and Block L (1956). US grants stimulate hospital research. *Modern Hospital,* January.

Daly J (2005). *Evidence-based medicine and the search for a science of clinical care.* University of California Press/Milbank Fund, Berkeley, CA/New York.

Donabedian A (1980). *Explorations in quality assessment and monitoring, Vol. I The definition of quality and approaches to its assessment.* Health Administration Press, Ann Arbor, MI.

Donabedian A (1982). *Explorations in quality assessment and monitoring, Vol. II The criteria and standards of quality.* Health Administration Press, Ann Arbor, MI.

Donabedian A (1985). *Explorations in quality assessment and monitoring, Vol. III The methods and findings of quality assessment and monitoring: an illustrated analysis.* Health Administration Press, Ann Arbor, MI.

Feinstein AR (1985). *Clinical epidemiology: the architecture of clinical research.* WB Saunders Co., Philadelphia, PA.

Fletcher RH and Fletcher SW (2005). *Clinical epidemiology: the essentials,* 4th edn. Lippincott Williams and Wilkins, Baltimore, MD.

Flook EE and Sanazaro PJ (1973). *Health service research and R & D in perspective.* Health Administration Press, Chicago, IL.

Glover JA (1938). The incidence of tonsillectomy in school children. *Proceedings of the Royal Society of Medicine,* **31,** 1219–36.

Gray BH, Gusmano MK, and Collins SR (2003). AHCPR and the changing politics of health services research. *Health Affairs,* Web Exclusive, **22**(3, June), 284–307. (Available at: http://content.healthaffairs.org/)

Holland WW (2002). *Foundations for health improvement: productive epidemiological public health research 1919–1998.* The Nuffield Trust, London.

Lamberts H and Wood M (ed.) (1987). *International classification of primary care (ICPC).* Oxford University Press, Oxford.

Lembcke PA (1956). Medical auditing by scientific methods illustrated by major female pelvic surgery. *Journal of the American Medical Association,* **162,** 646–55.

Mainland D (1966). *Heath services research I & II.* Milbank Memorial Fund, New York.

McCarthy T and White KL (2000). Origins of health services research. *Health Services Research,* **35,** 375–87.

Morris JN (1957). *Uses of epidemiology.* Churchill Livingstone, Edinburgh.

Paul JR (1938). Clinical epidemiology. *Journal of Clinical Investigation,* **17,** 539–41.

Ryle JA (1948). *Changing disciplines.* Oxford University Press, London.

Tenney JB, White KL, and Williamson JW (1974). *National ambulatory medical care statistics: background and methodology, United States 1967–1972,* DHEW Publication No (HRA), 74–1335, pp.1–76. US Department of Health, Education and Welfare, National Center for Health Statistics, Washington, DC.

Wennberg J and Gittlesohn A (1973). Small area variations in health care delivery. *Science,* **182,** 1102–8.

White KL (1991). *Healing the schism: epidemiology, medicine, and the public's health.* Springer-Verlag, New York.

White KL, Frenk J, Ordonez C, Paganini J, and Starfield B (1992). *Health services research: an anthology,* Scientific Publication No. 554. World Health Organization/Pan American Health Organization, Washington, DC.

World Health Organization (1971). *Statistical indicators for the planning and evaluation of public health programmes, fourteenth report of the WHO Expert Committee on Health Statistics (Brotherston J, Chair and White KL, Rapporteur),* WHO Technical Report Series No. 472. World Health Organization, Geneva.

17

Occupational epidemiology

Malcolm Harrington and Tom Sorahan

Personal experiences

We started from different professional backgrounds, but both of us ended up considering ourselves to be epidemiologists.

Malcolm Harrington: I started in hospital medicine but moved to academic occupational health. During my Master's course in Richard Schilling's department I heard lectures from him on his discovery of byssinosis in cotton workers and from Richard Doll and Bradford Hill. Esme Hadfield described her work on adenocarcinomata of the ethmoid sinus in woodworkers and Robert Case talked about his bladder cancer studies. Later the WHO asked me to act as rapporteur for one of Olli Miettinen's famed epidemiology courses. Two years as a visiting scientist in the Epidemic Intelligence Service at the Centers for Disease Control provided privileged exposure to Alexander D. Langmuir, Joe Fraumeni, and his group, Brian MacMahon and Ken Rothman. *Of course* I became an occupational epidemiologist.

Despite the realization that death certificate studies had some methodological shortcomings, my first survey, a mortality study of sea pilots, was simplicity itself. All sea pilots on the River Thames estuary stayed as sea pilots until they retired or died. For the next of kin, a death certificate was necessary to claim a pension. Thus all study group members were traceable. Later studies of professional groups, such as pathologists, proved equally easy to undertake for similar reasons. Life got harder later when working on company-based records or in field studies of occupational or environmental risks where vital data on illness or exposure were less robust, inaccurate or just missing. But by that time the professional die was cast.

Tom Sorahan: I scraped a degree in physics so plans for becoming a nuclear physicist were put permanently on hold. After a few false starts I found a job as a computing assistant in a department of social medicine, working for Pat Prior and John Waterhouse. I became interested in epidemiological methods and wrote a PhD thesis on the new (now standard) approaches to cohort analysis that were being developed by Duncan Thomas, David Cox, and many other eminent biostatisticians. In later years I also worked with Alice Stewart, George Kneale, and Malcolm Harrington at the University of Birmingham. It could be argued that my career has relied heavily on taking over studies of which others have tired!

My original boss, John Waterhouse, had published a letter in *The Lancet* in 1966 on prostate cancer in nickel–cadmium battery workers (as it happens one of the most widely cited letters concerning occupational cancer ever published) (Kipling and Waterhouse 1967). Some 10 years later I went back to the factory to collect data for a cohort mortality study of all workers at the site. The factory has now closed down but I am still publishing analyses of lung cancer risks in relation to cadmium exposure.

Data sources

Vital statistical databases are fundamental starting points for many types of epidemiological studies. Occupational epidemiologists also use such data but, in addition, they have found useful sources of health and exposure information in professional and other registers, clinical case notes, and company or union records.

Death certificates

Most authorities on vital statistics cite John Graunt (1620–74) and William Petty (1623–87) as early pioneers of the use of such records as the Bills of Mortality for England and Wales. Occupation was added to the United Kingdom (UK) census data in 1851 and the Decennial Supplements on occupational mortality that have been published since then have been a rich source for epidemiologists investigating the effects of occupation on health. Analyses of data for occupations as stated on death certificates have their shortcomings but the UK longitudinal studies that started in 1971 were able to make better use of routinely collected data by linking births, cancer registrations, and deaths to a 1% sample of the population employed at the time of the census.

The accuracy of the information on the cause of death itself varies with age and disease category, while occupation stated on death certificates is often the 'last known' (Harrington 1984a).

Some of these difficulties can be overcome by using other supplementary data sources as described in the next sections.

Professional and other registers

Disease mapping has been a fruitful source of hypothesis-generating exercises, and the US National Cancer Institute maps of cancer registrations by district resulted in a number of important aetiological studies by Fraumeni and colleagues (Devesa *et al.* 1999). Similar maps have been produced in the UK and elsewhere in Europe.

Professional groups rarely change job category, so access to registers of such people can provide evidence of long-term 'exposure' to certain workplaces (see above). The medical profession itself was a crucial database for Doll and Hill's study of smoking habits. In a similar way, studies of formaldehyde exposure were aided by access to anatomists, pathologists, and embalmers, and risks from anaesthetic gases documented in studies of anaesthetists. Other registers have concentrated on exposure including people working with lead or ionizing radiation, whilst other registers have focused on specific health outcomes such as mesothelioma, birth defects, and stillbirths (Harrington 1984b).

Clinical observation leading to epidemiological studies

Clinical hunches that something is amiss after noting a cluster of cases in outpatients or the factory clinic have resulted in some extremely important information linking disease to occupational exposure. Some cases, such as Rehn's suspicion that aromatic amines could cause bladder cancer, took 59 years to be established as fact. At the other end of the spectrum, three shorter intervals—2 years for angiosarcoma of the liver and vinyl chloride monomer, 5 years for mesothelioma and asbestos, and 6 years for nasal sinus cancer and wood dust—are instructive in that epidemiological investigations followed immediately after the first observations by Creech and Johnson, Wagner, and then Hadfield respectively (McDonald and Harrington 1981).

A hospital clinic 'epidemic' of peripheral neuropathy in Ohio was traceable to one workplace and a new fabric-coating agent, ethyl butyl ketone. In another example, one blood sample sent for analysis to the US Centers for Disease Control (CDC), revealed high levels of a persistent organochlorine (Kepone) and the link with sterility in male employees at the manufacturing plant was rapidly followed by closure of the process. In yet another, telephone calls to CDC made by US Veterans complained that they had acquired leukaemia from the atomic bomb testing in Utah and Nevada in the 1950s. This was followed by a study of 3217 nuclear test participants that showed the complainants had correctly identified a link between such exposures and leukaemia.

One cannot rely on such *ad hoc* events to uncover all new occupational diseases but they can be used to support the need to establish surveillance procedures. Reporting networks for possible occupational diseases using occupational physicians and the relevant hospital specialists have now been established in a number of countries.

Company/union-based records

Observations of different health patterns in differing workplace populations is not a twentieth-century phenomenon. In 1831 Thackrah noted astutely the general poor health of workers leaving the Lancashire cotton mills at the end of a shift compared with those workers leaving the Yorkshire woollen mills.

In the twentieth century, factory populations have been studied—where access is granted—in a number of important industrial processes. The rubber industry studies of Veys are described later, but others include the work of McDonald in the Quebec chrysotile mines and mills, Newhouse and the asbestos textile and insulation workers in the UK, Wagoner's studies of the beryllium alloy plants in New England, and the benzene-exposed workers at the Ohio Plioform factory.

Some large organizations, such as Dow, DuPont, and ICI, have been exemplary in monitoring their own employees. So efficient can this exercise be that any suspicion of a new risk or a putative cluster of disease could be investigated immediately and comparisons made with company 'norms' for health data that go back for decades.

Union records may not be so accurate, but Selikoff's crucial studies of asbestos-related diseases in insulation workers relied in large measure on the records of the New York insulation workers' union. Support of the unions was also required for the then nationalized Central Electricity Generating Board in the UK to set up its mortality study in the early 1980s. No particularly risky sub groups were identified in the early years of follow-up (except for mesothelioma in some power station staff) but the suspicion that extremely low-frequency electromagnetic fields might cause brain tumours and leukaemia provided an opportunity to study both power station and overhead line workers in their thousands over decades, supplemented with in-house exposure data supplied by a subsection of the industry.

Finally, even the notoriously inaccurate database that constitutes the average company's sickness absence records can, on occasion, lead to very good epidemiology, as Peter Taylor's ground-breaking studies of Shell's sickness absence records showed (Taylor *et al.* 1972).

Epidemiological and statistical methodology: development and application

Person-years at risk: calculation of standardized mortality ratios using an external standard

It is often difficult to decide who first developed any given technique. Researchers in different parts of the world can appear to converge on a new approach at the same time. Moreover, a statistical technique new to an epidemiologist may be viewed as old hat to an actuary. But to us, the paper that opened up occupational epidemiological enquiry to the importance and scope of person-years at risk and the consequent calculation of expected numbers of deaths based on national or regional mortality rates was that published by Robert Case and co-workers in 1954 on bladder cancer risks in relation to the manufacture of chemical dyestuffs (Case *et al.* 1954). Case was an extraordinarily gifted scientific writer, and he and his colleagues were able to communicate how occupational cohort studies could be carried out. That meant taking into account differences in national rates with age, sex, and calendar year and basing the calculation of the expected numbers of deaths in each period of follow-up on the numbers of the study cohort that were still alive and hence at risk of death at that time.

Person-years at risk: calculation of rate ratios (relative risks) using an internal standard

Case's technique was used for many decades by occupational epidemiologists (and continues to be the mainstay of occupational mortality studies). However, concerns about the relevance of national mortality (and cancer incidence) rates surfaced and attempts were made to develop regional and local rates. But it was never possible to positively identify the 'ideal' reference rate for any given study (national, regional, local), and some aspects of occupational cohort findings such as the healthy worker effect could not be accounted for by the selection of any of these options. There was a need for more flexible forms of analysis, to be able to adjust for any number of variables (not just age, sex, and calendar year), not to have to assume that the 'background' rates in a cohort (i.e. the rates that would have applied if chemical exposures had not been present) are known, and to recognize that cumulative exposure is a time-dependent variable. In the 1970s, there was a series of ground-breaking publications in the fields of survival-time analysis, regression models and life tables, and Poisson regression. Selecting a single paper is unfair to others, but the work on lung cancer risks in relation to asbestos exposure and published by Liddell, McDonald, and Thomas in 1977 communicated very effectively how these new approaches involving internal comparisons were to be applied (Liddell *et al.* 1977). Occupational studies featured strongly in the applied biostatistical literature concerning the treatment of time-dependent variables, partly because of the studies of cancer risks in relation to exposure to ionizing radiation (film badges provided a quarterly dose estimate) and partly because work histories could be translated into exposure histories using job–exposure matrices as an intermediate step.

Mantel–Haenszel and logistic regression techniques applied to case–control studies

The seminal paper on the statistical treatment and interpretation of case–control studies was published in 1959 (Mantel and Haenszel 1959). Some readers were probably not helped by the fact that the first table or figure laying out the basic format of a case–control study (i.e. a 2 × 2 table) did not appear until the twelfth page of this long paper. The reader was given many insights into the nature of epidemiological enquiry and the special (albeit limited) role that 'retrospective' or case–control studies could play. It took many years for most epidemiologists to fully understand the elegant solutions that Mantel and Haenszel had devised both for the calculation of relative risks and for the adjustment of potential confounding variables. The technique made extensive use of stratification, and this could lead to computing difficulties when a large number of variables were being considered. Logistic regression was not prone to such difficulties and was eventually adopted as the technique of choice for the analysis of case–control studies.

Statistical and epidemiological software

Many other techniques have been used by occupational epidemiologists, including cluster analysis and mapping techniques. There is also now extensive computer software available so that the younger epidemiologist is probably no longer writing his or her own FORTRAN software on main-frame computers as we did when we started.

Application and prevention

Whilst epidemiology may be described as the study of the distribution and determinants of disease frequency in human populations, the application of the epidemiological method to working populations has a potentially potent preventive feature. If one can identify a risk factor (or factors) for a noted increased risk of a particular disease in a workforce, then it is theoretically possible to eliminate that risk by removing the hazard from the working environment. Even controlling the exposure could lead to decreased risks. It all depends on the quality of the initial epidemiology, the practicalities of engineering out the risk, and the zeal of those who run the industry to do something to prevent ill-health. Here are four examples.

The rubber industry and bladder cancer

Like so many occupational risks, this one was first noted by astute clinical observation. In 1895 Rehn described three cases of bladder cancer in a group of 45 workers involved in the manufacture of fuchsine—an aniline-based dye. Further clinical reports followed which implicated a number of aromatic amines. In 1938 Hueper induced bladder tumours in dogs following exposure to beta-naphthylamine. This aromatic amine was discovered to be a contaminant of two antioxidants (Nonox S and Agerite resin) used in the vulcanizing of rubber. In the UK these antioxidants were withdrawn from the process in October 1949 having been in continuous use from January 1934. The definitive studies of Case and Hosker in the 1950s showed conclusively that occupational exposure to beta-naphthylamine caused an increased risk of bladder cancer in both the manufacturing and user industries.

Of the various epidemiological studies of rubber manufacturers, perhaps the most complete and comprehensive were those undertaken by Veys at the Michelin tyre factory at Stoke-on-Trent, UK. He recently published the possible final report of his exceptional work carried out over decades. It covers the story of the cohorts of workers from 1945 to 1995 and provides detailed and accurate insight into the risks of bladder cancer in men exposed before 1949 with their unexposed contemporaries as well as the men who followed them in the same jobs but post-1949 (Veys 2004). The standardized registration ratio for bladder tumours was 171 for the 58 tumours in the 2090 men employed from 1945 to 1949 but fell to 102 for the 39 tumours reported in the 3038 men employed from January 1950. Veys was able to pinpoint exactly where each man worked in the plant thus making the task of exposed versus unexposed relatively easy. The superb quality of these studies is modestly ascribed by Veys as due to the demographics of the Stoke population. He describes them as 'being born in Stoke, working in Stoke, retiring in Stoke and dying in Stoke'. Thus a lethal occupational exposure was eliminated from an industry and a town.

Pneumoconiosis in British coal miners

Whilst carcinogenic contaminants of a manufacturing process can be removed and the risk of an occupational cancer eliminated, the same is not true for coal workers' pneumoconiosis which is an inherent risk of inhaling coal dust and thus an ever present hazard to the men working underground. In this case, the best that can be achieved is to reduce worker exposure to coal dust by engineering controls to lower the airborne dust concentrations in the ambient air.

The epidemiological studies of the British coal mining industry began over 50 years ago when it was a nationalized industry. It was the combination of a compliant employer working with a talented team of epidemiologists (including Archie Cochrane), occupational physicians, and engineers that resulted in a series of comprehensive cohort studies of the workforce leading to accurate dose–response measurements. This in turn led to calculations of the dust concentrations needed for each incremental rise in pneumoconiosis rates. Targets were set for dust suppression, and over the period 1960 to 1991 the prevalence of all categories of pneumoconiosis, including the potentially lethal progressive massive fibrosis (PMF), fell from 10.7% (1% PMF) to 0.4% with the disappearance of PMF from the workforce (Parkes 1994).

Differences in prevalence for pneumoconiosis did exist between coalfields—depending on the geology—but the argument over whether coal dust *per se* caused chronic bronchitis raged for decades. Gilson (1970) and others elsewhere asserted that the association was causal, but it was not until the 1990s that sufficiently large studies of non-smoking miners proved Gilson to be correct.

Trawler fishing

Following the sinking of a North Sea trawler with the loss of all hands, a Royal Commission on Trawler safety was set up. Richard Schilling, who was a member of that Commission, had been investigating seafarers' mortality. He discovered that since 1894 there had been two separate sources of registration for fishermen's deaths. The Registrar General's statistics—the main source of mortality data in the UK—did not include deaths at sea. When the two sources were combined and any overlap in reporting removed, Schilling found that the fatal accident rate was 50% higher than the land-based figures would suggest, making fishing the most dangerous of all occupations (Schilling 1971). Further studies revealed that side trawling was much more dangerous than stern trawling. Schilling's work, and the sensational film footage of life on a trawler (filmed surreptitiously by his son-in-law posing as a hired hand) led to the phasing out of side trawlers in the North Sea and the virtual universal switch to stern trawling.

The pharmaceutical industry

Whilst the therapeutic side-effects of oral contraceptive usage were well documented by the 1970s, when one of us (JMH) was asked to study the possible side-effects of occupational exposure to synthetic oestrogens at a plant manufacturing oral contraceptives, we could find no previous studies in the literature. The complaints of the employees were gynaecomastia in males and menstrual irregularities in females. We found that all male employees formulating and drying the powdered product had gynaecomastia and that half the females on the tabletting line had menstrual complaints compared with none elsewhere in the plant. Matched to a non-factory control group, the relative risk for menstrual irregularities was 4.3.

On the face of it, the plant looked clean and local exhaust ventilation seemed efficient. However, detailed measurements of the relevant oestrogens in blood, area dust, and personal dust samplers revealed that, given the biological potency of the dust, a 'no effect' airborne concentration of ethinyl oestrodiol would have to be below 0.2 $\mu g/m^3$ (Harrington *et al.* 1978). Further work showed that such airborne limits could not be reasonably achieved by local exhaust ventilation but would require workers to be enclosed in air-fed suits. Given the potency of all pharmaceutical industry products, this preventive measure was probably required on most production lines whatever the end product might be.

Drivers

Researchers are driven by the desire to discover something new and important, and perhaps for some recognition from their peers. Most occupational epidemiological research, however, requires funding and access; the natural enthusiasm of the researcher may well not be enough to bring the study into the light of day. No doubt there are still some hard-nosed captains of industry who say to researchers 'Here is the money, do whatever you like', but they become more and more difficult to find. Fortunately, there are other 'drivers' that may come into play.

The media

Industry does not like 'health scare' stories in newspapers and television programmes about its products or working practices. Customers may be put off purchasing such products and many questions are difficult to answer (e.g. can you give me a categorical assurance that your product, chemical X, does not cause cancer?). A reply to the effect that 'there is no evidence of any problem but we have now called for a full-scale independent epidemiological investigation into the health of our workforce' may well be enough to silence media attention for some considerable time, and probably forever if no problem is found. If media interest is sufficient, politicians may become involved (e.g. the cluster of childhood leukaemia in the environs of the Sellafield nuclear facility) and research contracts often follow.

However, sometimes, industry abreacts to 'bad news'. In the late 1960s, Tiller, a company doctor for a viscose rayon manufacturer, discovered that carbon disulphide exposure was linked to an excess risk of fatal myocardial infarction in the process workers. The company reputedly threatened Tiller with instant dismissal if he published his findings. He published (Tiller *et al.* 1968).

Worker concerns/trades unions

At the time we started careers in occupational epidemiology, company management often responded to the health concerns of employees by setting up appropriate studies (the study by TS of a semiconductor factory in the West Midlands is a case in point). In the UK, trade unions were starting to employ national health and safety officers who were capable of understanding and interpreting medical publications, and such officials could, like journalists, put difficult questions to management. Sadly, it is our impression that worker concerns do not carry as much weight as they once did.

IARC evaluations and possible regulatory action

The International Agency for Research on Cancer (IARC) carries out hazard identification for occupational carcinogens as part of its 'monograph programme'. These detailed evaluations (with their own well-known terminology, e.g. Group 1 carcinogen) play a prominent role in the later risk quantification (standard setting) exercises and labelling requirements organized by national regulatory agencies. It is not unusual to find cohort studies being updated in time for the latest IARC evaluation.

Mistakes, missed opportunities, and major obstacles

Studies lacking full work histories

The single most important reason for being unable to identify occupational causes of chronic disease from cohort studies is probably the failure to collect full work histories from company records at the outset of the investigations. It is often realized many years later that such data are needed, but by that time the original records may have been destroyed, access is denied by new owners, or research funds have dried up. The most important mistakes are almost always those made at the outset of studies because these are the most difficult to rectify; flawed analyses, after all, can always be replaced by improved procedures. The occupational epidemiology literature is littered with studies that only have data on first job, job in year *x*, or last job. Why was such a decision ever made? Probably to save some funds on data abstraction and because it was never envisaged that researchers would ever be able to achieve more than calculate some overall standardized mortality ratios.

Studies that do not deal with entry cohorts

Entry cohorts refer to all workers who are hired by a company in a specified period, 1970–79 for example. Census cohorts (or survivor populations) refer to all workers in employment on a given date, 1 January 1970, for example, irrespective of the date of hire. The census cohort has some attractions, particularly in the ease of abstracting data from company records. Fox and Collier (1976) provided an elegant description of two selection effects that may well operate in all cohort studies, the healthy worker effect and the survivor population effect. The first effect (low mortality, particularly in early periods of follow-up) is a consequence of selection for health and fitness at the time of hire; the second effect (low mortality in long-term employees) is a consequence of the healthiest members of the cohort tending to remain in the industry (such workers may well attract the heaviest occupational exposures). The problem arises in the interpretation of findings from census cohorts, particularly when the size of the selection effects is comparable with the size of any occupational disease risk. The entry cohort offers some prospect of taking such selection factors into account.

Absence of occupational hygiene data

Even if complete work histories have been collected, the absence of occupational hygiene data will mean that work histories cannot be translated into exposure histories. Such absence will cause problems in the quantifying of occupational risks; it will also make it difficult to carry out meaningful comparisons of different study findings. We have no doubt that occupational hygiene data collected by company personnel have not always been made freely available to epidemiologists. It will of course usually be the case that hygiene data are not available for all areas of the factory or for all time periods under study, and company hygienists may well have had concerns about how epidemiologists will deal with these missing data.

Ignoring confounding

Some occupational epidemiologists (ourselves included) have on occasions fallen into the trap of only collecting data on the main exposure of interest to the researcher (or sponsor); information on other exposure is then limited to listing them in the introduction to the survey report. The hope may well have been that other exposures would not matter, that they would 'average out' in some obscure way. Such hopes are absurd. Equal effort should be placed into characterizing all important exposures. The single most important failure in the epidemiology of metals carcinogenesis (lead, cadmium, nickel, etc.) is probably the failure to control adequately for the effects of arsenic.

Time and effort

Epidemiological cohort studies do require considerable resources of time and effort. For the reasons described above, the key decisions that will determine the usefulness of this time and effort are those made at the outset of the investigation, regarding the definition of the study cohort and the data variables to be collected. There were two large-scale cohort studies of rubber workers organized in the UK in the 1970s, one by the Health and Safety Executive, the other by the British Rubber Manufacturers' Association in conjunction with the University of Birmingham. The first of these studies was a census cohort of all rubber workers employed on 1 February 1967, and work histories were limited to the job being followed in 1967. The second study was an entry cohort of all workers first employed in the period 1946–60, and work histories included all job changes with the participating companies. The first study may well have been able to answer the original study question but the latter study design had the advantage of being capable of answering questions not posed at the outset of the investigation.

Financial support and legislative support

One of the myriad effects of economic globalization has been the outsourcing of occupational health services. This appears to have gone hand-in-glove with a reduction in industry-sponsored epidemiological research. This may not matter in those countries with a strong tradition of government-sponsored OH research, but many countries have relied on industry sponsorship to identify and resolve OH problems. Other dark clouds in the form of privacy laws have moved from the horizon to an overhead position (see below).

The future

The twentieth century was witness to the flowering of occupational epidemiology with the determination of the risks of many occupational diseases from workplace exposures. In the twenty-first century, it will all become a lot more difficult.

The world of work has become more complex. Many workers are 'multi-tasked', on shorter contracts, and with longer and/or vaguer hours of work. Job insecurity is the norm and work-related health issues are focused on illness rather than disease. The main occupational medical issues are now musculoskeletal disorders and stress complaints. Even these two groupings are interrelated for the more diffuse pain syndromes (Buckle 2005).

For occupational medicine, the definition of a 'case' of occupational disease will be more difficult as the 'somatizing tendency' increases. The workplace—at least for the First World countries—is safer than ever before and yet complaints of ill-health abound. There is a real challenge for the epidemiologist to design longitudinal studies to assess the prediction of occupational illness by psychological risk factors and to design intervention trials to review the preventive value of such processes (Coggan 2005).

Again, as real risks to health from workplace exposures fall, the task of clarifying what factors remain to be controlled will stretch the current epidemiological and statistical techniques to the limit. The completion of the Human Genome Project in 2005 has not produced the immediate benefits its more enthusiastic proponents predicted. Gene therapy will come for some disorders, diagnostic techniques will be better delineated for some others, and drug design will, eventually, benefit some chronic disease sufferers and some cancer patients (Steel 2005). For occupational medicine, the discovery of genetic susceptibility to some workplace exposures may lead unscrupulous employers to exclude workers rather than adopt the approach of tightening exposure to safeguard the more vulnerable.

There is a recognizable trend in public fora and in the media to put increasing credence on epidemiological study results whilst, at the same time, epidemiologists are couching their 'results' in more and more caveats. Scientists cannot walk away from the political impact of their work but, for example, despite years of work and hundreds of studies, we are still unable to issue clear guidelines to governments and the public on the risks to human health from extremely low-frequency electromagnetic fields or radio frequencies.

Even the nature of epidemiological studies are under threat from the legislators. As more countries pass privacy laws, restrictions on the availability of health and exposure data could seriously undermine the very existence of some occupational epidemiological studies. General medical practitioners are loath to release patient data and ethics committees are becoming over cautious about study protocols. The argument that these studies are bona fide medical research is cutting little ice in some countries. Even mortality studies may become difficult as the researcher will be unable to get subject consent for inclusion in the cohort!

All this appears to be a daunting start to the twenty-first century or it could be viewed as a challenge to the ingenuity and zeal of the occupational epidemiologist. Challenges should be a spur, not a brake, to endeavour.

References

Buckle P (2005). Ergonomics and musculoskeletal disorders: overview. *Occupational Medicine*, **55**, 164–7.

Case RAM, Hosker ME, McDonald DB, and Pearson JT (1954). Tumours of the urinary bladder in women engaged in the manufacture and use of certain dyestuff intermediates in the British chemical industry. *British Journal of Industrial Medicine*, **11**, 75–104.

Coggan DN (2005). Occupational medicine at a turning point. *Occupational and Environmental Medicine*, **62**, 281–3.

Devesa SS, Grauman DJ, Blot WJ, Pennello G, Hoover RN, and Fraumeni JF Jr (1999). *Atlas of cancer mortality in the United States, 1950–94*, Publication No. NIH 99–4564. US Government Printing Office, Washington, DC.

Fox AJ and Collier PF (1976). Low mortality rates in industrial cohort studies due to selection for work and survival in the industry. *British Journal of Preventive and Social Medicine*, **30**, 225–30.

Gilson JC (1970). Occupational bronchitis. *Proceedings of the Royal Society of Medicine*, **63**, 857–64.

Harrington JM, Rivera RO, and Lowry LK (1978). Occupational exposure to synthetic estrogens- the need to establish safety standards. *American Industrial Hygiene Association Journal*, **39**, 139–43.

Harrington JM (1984a). Occupational mortality. *Scandinavian Journal of Work, Environment and Health*, **10**, 347–52.

Harrington JM (1984b). Epidemiologic study of work related diseases. Methodological problems of register-based studies. *Scandinavian Journal of Work, Environment and Health*, **10**, 353–9.

Kipling MD and Waterhouse JAH (1967). Cadmium and prostatic carcinoma. *Lancet*, **i**, 730–1.

Liddell FDK, McDonald JC, and Thomas DC (1977). Methods of cohort analysis: appraisal by application to asbestos mining (with discussion). *Journal of the Royal Statistical Society*, Series A, **140**, 469–91.

Mantel N and Haenszel W (1959). Statistical aspects of the analysis of data from retrospective studies of disease. *Journal of the National Cancer Institute*, **22**, 719–48.

McDonald JC and Harrington JM (1981). Early detection of occupational hazards. *Journal of the Society of Occupational Medicine*, **31**, 93–8.

Parkes WP (1994). Pneumoconioses associated with coal and other carbonaceous materials. In *Occupational lung disorders* (ed. WP Parkes), 3rd edn, pp. 340–410. Butterworth Heinemann, Oxford.

Rehn L (1895). Blasengeschwülste bei Fuchsin-arbeitern. *Archivfur Klinische Chirurgie*, **50**, 588.

Schilling RSF (1971). The hazards of deep sea fishing. *British Journal of Industrial Medicine*, **28**, 27–35.

Steel M (2005). Molecular medicine: promises, promises? *Journal of the Royal Society of Medicine*, **98**, 197–9.

Taylor PJ, Pocock SJ, and Sergean R (1972). Absenteeism of shift and day workers. A study of six types of shift system in 29 organizations. *British Journal of Industrial Medicine*, **29**, 208–13.

Tiller J, Schilling RSF, and Morris JN (1968). Occupational toxic factors in mortality from coronary artery disease. *British Medical Journal*, **ii**, 407–10.

Veys CA (2004). Bladder tumours in rubber workers: a factory study 1946–1995. *Occupational Medicine*, **54**, 322–9.

18

Social epidemiology

Mervyn Susser and Landon Myer

Personal experiences

The antecedents of Mervyn Susser's interest in social epidemiology began after volunteer service in the South African corps during the Second World War. The post-war period aroused a general spirit of hope and commitment to a socially useful occupation. This gave focus to his medical studies at the University of the Witwatersrand in Johannesburg, where together with his wife Zena Stein, he saw the practice of comprehensive, socially oriented medicine as an important form of activism. At the same time, they learned about social medicine from Sidney Kark, who emphasized epidemiology and the social sciences as valuable research tools for promoting health.

After graduating from medical school in 1950, Susser and Stein implemented this community-oriented approach while directing a primary health-care centre in the Johannesburg slum of Alexandra. Here, they systematically recorded patient contacts in order to describe the morbidity and mortality patterns in an urban African population, and ultimately to document the conditions which shaped the population's health. The experience had a profound impact on their joint vision of epidemiology and its role in improving public health.

By the late 1950s, Susser and Stein's involvement in political opposition to the racist policies of the Nationalist government drew the attention of authorities and eventually led to Susser's removal from the Alexandra Health Centre. Unable to find opportunities to continue their work in social medicine, Susser and Stein left for England in 1959. There, Susser took up a lectureship in the Department of Social and Preventive Medicine at Manchester University, and was exposed to diverse perspectives in both medicine and the social sciences. His work during this period reflected this increasing insight and in 1962 he published *Sociology in medicine* along with social anthropologist William Watson, the first text to integrate sociocultural and epidemiological perspectives on health at both the individual and population levels.

After a sabbatical in the United States, in 1966 Susser and Stein took senior professional positions in the Department of Epidemiology at Columbia University. During their 40 subsequent years at Columbia they continued their work on societal determinants of health, including the roles of social forces in the aetiology and course of mental development and illness, the role of poverty and nutrition in perinatal health, community psychiatry, and the history, philosophy, and general theory of epidemiology.

Landon Myer is a Senior Lecturer in the School of Public Health and Family Medicine at the University of Cape Town. He completed undergraduate and post-graduate studies in social anthropology before undertaking a PhD in epidemiology at Columbia University, where he studied under Mervyn Susser, Zena Stein, and Ezra Susser. His current work focuses on the social, behavioural, and biological determinants of the HIV/AIDS epidemic in South Africa, including both prevention and treatment.

Introduction

The observation that wealth and poverty are strongly associated with disease has been made repeatedly for at least 2000 years. Many early epidemiologists focused on poverty and related social conditions as a powerful determinant of health outcomes during the nineteenth century. But despite these antecedents, social and economic conditions received relatively little attention for much of the twentieth century as epidemiology grew into a mature discipline. Most recently, 'social epidemiology' has experienced a sort of renaissance, as epidemiologists rediscover the powerful effect of social conditions in shaping morbidity and mortality.

We define social epidemiology as the study in populations of those causes of disease centred in societal structure and its gradients of opportunity, resources, and power; in social conditions; and in personal interactions and behaviours. In this chapter, we review the study of these types of causes during the twentieth century, with a basic distinction between the early era (1900–40), the decades after 1950, and recent developments since 1980. For each of these periods, we note important distinctions between the trajectory of social epidemiology in Britain and the USA, as well as how the epidemiological study of social factors has fared under different paradigms of disease aetiology. Throughout, we highlight the fundamentally interdisciplinary nature of social epidemiology, including important contributions from sociology and psychiatry.

'Social' epidemiology in the first half of the twentieth century

Though the term 'social epidemiology', was coined only in 1950, the concepts underpinning the contemporary field can trace roots to the earliest examples of epidemiological thinking. In Paris in 1826, Louis Rene Villermé described the patterns of poverty and mortality across the wards of the city. His finding of a continuous relationship between poverty and mortality—with poorer neighbourhoods having worse health than wealthier ones across all levels of wealth—is the first systematic evidence of a graded class relationship since widely documented. At mid-century, Rudolph Virchow, best known as the father of modern pathology, likewise emphasized the inseparable nature of population health and socio-economic conditions in his advocacy for improved living conditions for the poor in Germany.

An independent strand of the history of social epidemiology stems from the origins of sociology as a discipline in the late nineteenth and early twentieth centuries. The earliest sociologists made important contributions to thinking about how specific aspects of social organization could influence individual health outcomes. In his book *Suicide* (1897), Emile Durkheim investigated the social aetiology of suicide in France. Durkheim emphasized the distinction between societies on the one hand, which manifest group effects and require group analysis of 'social facts' (described as 'ecological variables' in modern epidemiology), and individuals within those societies on the other, who manifest separate individual characteristics. This distinction has received renewed interest among epidemiologists in recent years in the form of multilevel and ecological analyses.

Through the first half of the twentieth century in Europe and North America the revolutionary bacteriological paradigm dominated epidemiological thinking about disease aetiology. With the help of microbiologists, epidemiologists focused on the search for specific infectious agents of disease. By unravelling the modes of transmission, the locus of reservoirs of the pathogen, and the nature of immunity, bacteriologists, epidemiologists, and pathologists together opened the way to effective intervention.

In this period of an epidemiology dominated by bacteriological underpinnings, chronic diseases—with no apparent infection to account for them—were scarcely given analytical attention by epidemiologists. A notable exception was the work on pellagra of Joseph Goldberger, an officer of the US Public Health service. In the early twentieth century he and his co-worker Edgar Sydenstricker (by training an economist familiar with statistics who had previously studied the health effects of gradients in workers' wages) undertook studies of pellagra in the American South. Pellagra was at the time widely attributed to some infectious agent still to be discovered. In studies of cotton mill workers in South Carolina during 1916–18, Goldberger and Sydenstricker documented the relation of pellagra risk to low household income levels and subsequent deficient dietary intake (Goldberger *et al.* 1964).

Another body of work unbound by the predominant germ theory of the first half of the twentieth century followed the invention of cohort analysis. William O. Kermack, A. G. McKendrick, and W. L. McKinley (Kermack *et al.* 1934) devised an approach to gain a longitudinal view of the evolution of mortality, drawing on the work of at least one important predecessor, K. F. Andvord. The patterns of mortality within birth cohorts from Great Britain and Scandinavia in these analyses provided convincing evidence for the projection of effects of early life experience onto health in adulthood. Their analyses were persuasive with regard to socio-economic conditions and rural–urban variations in the subsequent mortality patterns. Over the next several decades several authors made use of the method to understand the changing effects of social conditions on health, including Susser and Stein in an analysis of the influence of socio-economic development on peptic ulcer morbidity and mortality (Susser and Stein 1962).

These works addressing societal factors in disease were well outside the mainstream of epidemiological and public health research during the first half of the twentieth century. However, the role of societal factors in mental health continued to be a focus within sociology and related disciplines during this period. In the USA, Robert Faris and H. Warren Dunham's ecological study of Chicago neighbourhoods reported an excess of new hospital admissions for psychotic mental illness within 'socially disorganized' areas of the city (Faris and Dunham 1939). Although later investigations showed that the association was largely a matter of 'social drift' of the afflicted to lower-class neighbourhoods, the idea that social contexts were potential determinants of health outcomes gave fresh impetus to social hypotheses among sociologists interested in understanding the population determinants of health.

Social epidemiology, 1950–80

In the aftermath of the Second World War, the changing health profile of industrialized nations spurred a general shift in the focus of epidemiology from infectious to 'chronic' diseases. Refinements during the post-war period in epidemiological methods for the study of chronic diseases propagated a focus on the role played by individual-level 'risk factors'—environmental exposures and behaviours—in disease aetiology. The increased focus of epidemiology on the search for risk factors generally led to a decreased emphasis on the societal determinants of population health. This effect was particularly marked in academic epidemiology in the USA from the 1950s through the 1980s.

Forerunners of social epidemiology in the social medicine movement

The social determinants of health remained prominent during the growth of epidemiological research in Europe during the post-war period. In British medical schools, newly created departments of social and preventive medicine displaced more narrowly defined departments of public health, many of which had undergone a degree of ossification since John Simon had given public health an academic presence during the late nineteenth century. In Britain the earliest departments of social and preventive medicine were established during the 1940s[1], beginning with John Ryle gaining a chair at Oxford in 1948. Other universities soon followed with notable heads

---

[1] An earlier initiative in Europe was the establishment of the School of Public Health at Zagreb University by Andrija Štampar in 1927. Despite Stampar's work, the public health and social medicine movement in Croatia was largely extinguished under oppressive political regimes, and Stampar himself was repeatedly imprisoned for his work. He later went on to play a seminal role in the international public health movement, including work with the Health Organization of the League of Nations and then the World Health Organization (established in 1948).

of newly formed departments of social and preventive medicine, including Francis Crew in Edinburgh, Thomas McKeown in Birmingham, C. Fraser Brockington in Manchester, A. C. Stephenson in Belfast, and W. J. E. Jessop in Dublin. These individuals were among the central figures in the development of epidemiology as a discipline in the UK.

Although the term 'social epidemiology' appeared rarely in British post-war social medicine, socio-economic factors had a prominent place in the thinking of epidemiologists and public health physicians. The expansion of social medicine in Britain and Ireland during the post-war period led to the establishment in 1956 of the academic and scientifically oriented British Society of Social Medicine, with a predominantly academic membership (Porter 1997). Paralleling the developments in social medicine, this period also saw the rise of social psychiatry under the leadership of Aubrey Lewis (Susser 1968). In addition to revolutionizing psychiatric services in England, Lewis led a team of researchers including Peter Sainsbury, John Wing, and Michael Shepherd whose approach to psychiatric epidemiology focused on the role of social factors in the aetiology and course of mental illness.

Perhaps more than any other individual in Britain during the post-war period, J. N. 'Jerry' Morris forged a central place for the role of social determinants in the study of health in populations. Early in his career, in collaboration with R. M. Titmuss he took a position that echoes many of the current themes in social epidemiology. Thus he wrote: 'Society largely determines health; ill-health is not a personal misfortune due often to personal inadequacy but a social misfortune due more commonly to social mismanagement and social failure' (Morris 1957). He carried forward and explored this view in the studies he launched as Director of the Social Medicine Research Unit of the Medical Research Council, which he founded in 1948. True to his broad vision of social medicine with epidemiology and social science as the core, he recruited a talented interdisciplinary staff that combined medically trained epidemiologists with psychologists, sociologists, and statisticians.

Morris generated ingenious and relatively inexpensive studies of the pressing health problems of the time. One such project, a comprehensive study of mortality in children in England and Wales, showed that death rates closely mirrored the gradient of social class among the mothers. Later, Morris focused on the role of chronic diseases underlying mortality in post-war Britain. Most notable was the seemingly new and growing epidemic phenomenon of coronary heart disease, in which he established the protective effect of physical exercise. In this work, Morris and his colleagues studied both social factors and individual behaviour as interrelated causes. His multi-disciplinary staff included Matilda Goldberg, a psychiatric social worker who explored psychological factors and the family relations of peptic ulcer patients. Much of this thinking is crystallized in successive editions of Morris's *Uses of epidemiology*, a lively text written in characteristic staccato style (Morris 1957).

Contemporaneously at the London School of Hygiene and Tropical Medicine, John Brotherston recruited to his department no fewer than three sociologists: Margot Jefferies, Ann Cartwright, and Fred Martin. All concerned themselves mainly with the study of health systems with particular settings, such as general practice and mental health services. The work of Morris, Brotherston, and others in British social medicine integrated what today we would describe as social epidemiology into a comprehensive understanding of the determinants of chronic disease and other health outcomes. Rather than viewing disease aetiology in solely behavioural, or environmental, or social terms, these post-war investigators extended epidemiological approaches to examine the full spectrum of health determinants. During this period, Susser and Watson's text, *Sociology in medicine* (Susser and Watson 1962), accomplished a first thorough melding of epidemiological and sociological thought in addressing the significant supporting role that the social sciences can play in the study of disease.

Another seminal contribution to contemporary social epidemiology during this period was made by Thomas McKeown and the talented team he recruited, among them Reginald Record, George Knox, Alwyn Smith, and Brian MacMahon. Much of the work of McKeown and his faculty at Birmingham University, including advances in case–control methodology, focused on the identification of risk factors for chronic diseases. But like many epidemiologists in Britain and Ireland during this period, his thinking regarding the determinants of population health was expansive enough to incorporate individual behaviour as well as socio-economic conditions. Building on a series of prior works, McKeown's 1976 book *The modern rise of population* examined mortality trends in England and Wales from the eighteenth century onwards to explain the increases of population during and after the Industrial Revolution (McKeown 1976). His provocative analysis suggested that the dramatic reductions in mortality during this period occurred independently of specific public health interventions; McKeown attributed these changes instead to improved socio-economic conditions and nutrition. While specific aspects of this analysis have been called into question, McKeown's overarching perspective on the determinants of population health has had a lasting impact on modern social epidemiology.

Sociology and social epidemiology in the USA

During the post-war period in the USA, social and economic determinants received little attention in mainstream epidemiological research. The researchers who gave the greatest attention to such factors were in the main social scientists and psychiatrists, and much of this work focused on mental health. However, the concept of social medicine did not take root in the USA to the same degree as in the UK. Attributable at least in part to a conservative post-war political climate, notable collaborations between epidemiologists (nearly all of whom were drawn from a medical background) and social scientists were relatively few.

Until the Second World War the main focus of American epidemiology was on infectious diseases. From the mid-1950s, however, Brian MacMahon at Harvard and Abraham Lilienfeld at Johns Hopkins shifted the emphasis to the search for individual risk factors as 'exposures' which predisposed to chronic conditions. Contemporaneously, most major developments in the epidemiological study of the societal determinants of health in America were based in the social sciences, primarily sociology. While American sociologists had studied biomedical practice for some time—thus creating a sociology *of* medicine—the post-war period marked new ventures in medical sociology which addressed the influence of social conditions on the causes of disease. Building on the work of Faris and Dunham, in 1958 sociologist August Hollingshead and psychiatrist Frederick Redlich at Yale University in New Haven published *Social class and mental illness* (Hollingshead and Redlich 1958) which demonstrated a gradient of mental disorders: lowest in the highest social class and rising with the descending class strata, which they attributed largely to a parallel decline in the quality of psychiatric care. Meanwhile the work of the physician Sidney Cobb and his student Stanislav Kasl at the University of Michigan centred on the psychological effects of stress, and Hollingshead's student Leonard Syme was among several sociologists who applied epidemiological methods to study the social determinants of cardiovascular disease. Syme and Leo Reeder (1967) (also a sociologist and colleague at the University of California at Berkeley) studied the role of stress in the aetiology of cardiovascular disease. Later, Syme and his student Michael Marmot (Marmot and Syme 1976), in a study of the incidence of cardiovascular disease among Japanese-Americans, showed that morbidity declined with the increasing degree of Western acculturation independently of known risk factors.

The work of Syme, Reeder, and their students gave rise to a contemporary area of research into how social connections affect the occurrence of disease and death, a particular focus within social epidemiology in the USA. Perhaps the best known of these is the work of Lisa Berkman and Syme in the Alameda County study (Berkman and Syme 1979). Between 1965 and 1974, individuals with reduced social integration (a measure based on marital status, community group membership, and contacts with family and friends) were two to three times more likely to die than individuals with increased social integration. The association persisted after adjustment for various self-reported high-risk health behaviours.

Beyond such contributions of sociologists, mainstream epidemiologists in the USA attended little to societal determinants during this period. One important exception to this was the career of John Cassel. After emigrating from South Africa to the USA in the 1950s, Cassel became an influential teacher as Chair of Epidemiology at the University of North Carolina. A student of Sidney Kark's, Cassel looked to the social sciences for insights into how social conditions shape health outcomes. True to Kark's concepts and practice, he turned to studies of rural migrants from the hills of North Carolina, then in transition as they sought work in urbanized environments. Much of this work was focused on psychological stress as well as physiological and psychological vulnerability manifesting in cardiovascular disease. Cassel's influential and widely cited paper, 'The contribution of the social environment to host resistance' (Cassel 1976), stimulated a body of work on how psychosocial responses induced by social and economic factors might influence health states. Of note, Cassel advocated an approach which viewed the health effects of social conditions in broad rather than disease-specific terms, a perspective which has had a lasting impact on social epidemiology. Other notable developments in social epidemiology in the USA during this period were driven by Milton Terris, Saxon Graham, and the group led by Zena Stein and Mervyn Susser.

Early social epidemiology in South Africa

As this discussion indicates, most of the developments in the epidemiological study of the health effects of social and economic conditions during the post-Second World War period took place in Europe and North America. One significant exception to this was the work of Sidney Kark in South Africa, where there was a strong thread of social medicine beginning in the mid-twentieth century. Working in rural African communities, Kark and his colleagues documented the social and economic structures which facilitated the spread of disease through impoverished populations. His 'Social pathology of syphilis' (Kark 1949) attributed the spread of sexually transmitted infections to migration patterns created by structural economic conditions, foreshadowing the devastating spread of the HIV/AIDS pandemic in recent times (Myer *et al.* 2004). Of particular note, Kark's followers during the 1950s, including Cassel, Stein and Susser, would go on to make significant contributions to the development of social epidemiology.

'Social' epidemiology in the later twentieth century, 1980–2000

Towards the end of the twentieth century, research attention to the societal determinants of health increased considerably, and with this social epidemiology grew into a discrete specialist area within epidemiology. This has been marked by the publication since 1990 of several notable texts integrating epidemiological and sociological perspectives on population health, as well as the first volume focused specifically on 'social epidemiology' (Berkman and Kawachi 2000). This period has also seen the evolution of social epidemiological research into new thematic areas beyond descriptions of the general association between increasing socio-economic status and improved health, to focus on better understanding of the disparities in health among ethnic groups, and of the effect of community characteristics on individual health.

Social epidemiology in the UK

The strong emphasis on socio-economic factors as health determinants within epidemiological research continued in the UK throughout the last quarter of the twentieth century. This sustained interested was accompanied by a series of government commissions investigating national inequalities in health, producing the 1980 Black Report and the 1998 Acheson Report, both highlighting the persistence of socio-economic gradients in morbidity and mortality in the UK despite economic growth. These inquiries drew heavily on epidemiological analyses showing how social class is inversely related to morbidity and mortality across a range of causes, and did much to maintain the prominence of social epidemiologists within public health.

In this period, Michael Marmot and Geoffrey Rose developed the Whitehall studies, a programme of socially oriented research within a cohort of British civil servants. The initial Whitehall study (Marmot *et al.* 1984) found a risk of death in the lowest grade of civil servants roughly three times that in the highest grade. Cause-specific mortality manifested the same gradients as reflected, for example, in cardiovascular death rates. Differences in smoking, blood pressure, and plasma cholesterol explained only part of these differences. On further follow-up, occupational factors, such as low job control, at the lower grades proved to be substantial predictors of their higher risk. Indeed, they were better predictors of increased risk of coronary heart disease than many established risk factors. The Whitehall studies are particularly important because they show marked gradations in health within a relatively homogeneous population of office workers, indicating that occupational and socio-economic factors affect health even within groups which are not exposed to frank poverty.

Lifecourse epidemiology

With some notable exceptions (Susser 1962), many epidemiologists viewed social and economic factors as relatively static phenomena that are temporally proximate to disease, with social inequalities during adulthood being of primary concern in understanding the causes of adult disease and death. However, some social epidemiologists have focused on the potential impact of socio-economic conditions in early life on disease during adulthood. Much of this work arose in the early social medicine era with the birth cohorts from England and Scotland established during the 1930s and 1940s. Several decades later, George Davey-Smith, Diana Kuh, and colleagues used these longitudinal data to demonstrate links between social class at different stages of life and different causes of adult morbidity and mortality, as well as with a number of markers for cardiovascular disease (Kuh and Ben-Shlomo 1997).

Modern social epidemiology in the USA

In the USA, social epidemiology since 1980 has had a distinctly different trajectory. Continuing previous trends, social epidemiology was a distinctly marginalized subspecialty during much of the 1980s. Social scientists continued to make important contributions to understandings of social determinants of health during this period, but with the vast majority of epidemiologists focused on the pursuit of individual behaviours or exposures as risk factors for disease, the concept that social and economic conditions were significant determinants of health received minimal attention. This regression reached its nadir when one prominent epidemiology textbook in the USA stated that the role of socio-economic position in epidemiology was confined to that of a confounder of exposure–disease associations (Rothman 1986)—a view which presented a clear obstacle to epidemiological thinking about societal conditions as causes of morbidity and mortality. However, since 1990 the study of socio-economic factors in disease aetiology has rapidly gained prominence within American epidemiology. Although the reasons for this are unclear, the rise of social epidemiology has been accompanied by new developments on a variety of fronts.

Ethnicity and health

Social epidemiologists have generated compelling evidence that mortality rates within the USA are higher among African-Americans and other minority groups. In many instances, these differences persist after adjusting for markers of socio-economic position such as employment, income, and education. Interestingly, epidemiological studies in this area provide one of the few examples from the USA of social epidemiology helping to influence public health policies. While ethnic differences in morbidity and mortality are widely acknowledged, the explanations for these differences are far more contentious. In explaining ethnic disadvantage in morbidity and mortality Nancy Krieger and others take a contextual view of racial differences in health (Krieger 1999). They posit ethnic discrimination—or more simply, racism—as the principal factor of interest. In this light, a sustained socio-economic differential is not merely a confounder requiring analytical adjustment, but the vehicle for the effects of race discrimination on health. Further epidemiological research into such ethnic disparities makes clear, however, that even persistent associations of adverse health outcomes with particular racial categories provide no more than indirect inferences of racial discrimination.

Multilevel research

Social epidemiologists in the USA have made significant advances in recent years in understanding how social and economic conditions at different levels of social organization (e.g. individual, household, community, or society) influence health outcomes. These and other epidemiological analyses of social determinants of health across different levels of organization echo the work of Durkheim a century before. Sampson and colleagues, for example, demonstrated in a seminal paper that the social features of social neighbourhoods helped to explain levels of violent crime, independent of the characteristics of the individuals living there (Sampson *et al.* 1997). This body of work helps to demonstrate that populations as entities may themselves have features that shape health outcomes beyond the aggregated characteristics of the individuals comprising them (Susser 1994). Nonetheless, as hazardous as it obviously is to attribute the social and economic properties of groups to individuals and vice versa, group-level variables serve as an important vehicle for social epidemiologists.

Both in research design and analysis, the differing properties of group- and individual-level variables demand alertness in maintaining the distinctions between them, and multilevel analysis has also presented new challenges to epidemiological thinking (Diez Roux 2000). 'Nested' data structures are inherent in multilevel analysis in which, for example, individuals may be nested within households and households nested within communities. Analysis of these data structures has required the application of such analytical approaches as hierarchical modelling, generalized estimating equations, and mixed effects modelling. In large part, these methods are adapted from statistical methods developed for the analytical needs of the social sciences. Such statistical tools have enabled a body of research showing that communities or neighbourhoods encapsulate a range of structural properties which influence individual health. Approaches to unravelling the associations between the character of social groupings and health are at the cutting edge of social epidemiology.

Social epidemiology outside of Europe and North America

Though the bulk of social epidemiology has focused on the USA and Europe, there have been important developments in social epidemiological research in other regions. Research involving aboriginal populations in Western Australia carried out by Fiona Stanley and colleagues has demonstrated both the impact of socio-economic conditions on child health, as well as the potential of community-based interventions to address socio-economic differentials. In South Africa through the 1970s and 1980s epidemiologists such as Cyril Wyndham and Derek Yach played an important role in highlighting the stark health inequalities that resulted from government policies of apartheid. Since the first democratic elections in 1994, epidemiologists and health economists have shifted their focus to understanding why the social and economic disparities in health persist (Myer *et al.* 2004). In addition, social medicine has a rich history in Brazil, Argentina, and other parts of Latin America, where the integration of social sciences alongside traditional epidemiological perspectives on population health has played an important role in public health thinking, often despite political opposition.

Contributions of social epidemiology to the general discipline

In addition to providing significant new insights into how socio-economic factors shape health outcomes, the explosion of social epidemiological research during the 1990s has been linked to important new conceptual directions in the discipline. Through much of the second half of the twentieth century, mainstream epidemiology focused almost exclusively on how individual behaviours or exposures contributed to the risk of disease or death, building on important methodological developments in cohort and case–control designs. But during the 1990s, a series of critiques from many of the leaders in the field noted that in modern epidemiology an exclusive focus on individual characteristics (so-called 'risk factor epidemiology') had neglected the investigation of societal conditions as significant causes of health and disease. These critiques called for a re-evaluation of conceptual underpinnings, leading to two important developments for social epidemiologists.

First, these discussions drew attention to the position of epidemiological research in the advancement of public health. Some epidemiologists felt that the discipline's function in elucidating the mechanisms of disease aetiology was of principal importance, regardless of the application of epidemiological research to public health. In taking issue with this position, others argued that epidemiology's value, both past and present, was defined largely through its contributions to public health. This tension between 'academic' and 'public health' approaches in epidemiology—which is by no means resolved—created an important space in which social epidemiologists could position their work. Secondly, the 1990s critique of mainstream epidemiology helped to point out that epidemiology as a discipline often operated as a set of methods applied to study specific exposure–disease associations, with few overarching theoretical perspectives to help develop new hypotheses or refine existing understandings of disease aetiology. In response to this, social epidemiologists at the beginning of the twenty-first century have been at the forefront of the discipline in developing novel theoretical perspectives on the determinants of population health, with significant implications for the broader discipline.

Conclusion

Although the study of the influence of social and economic conditions on health was far from the mainstream of epidemiology during much of the twentieth century, during the 1990s social epidemiology returned to a central position in the discipline. The social determinants of health received sustained attention from epidemiologists in the UK since the post-war period under the umbrella of social medicine; in the USA, sociologists and mental health researchers have driven research in this area which was seen to fall outside of the focus of infectious or chronic diseases epidemiology. In both settings, social epidemiological research—both historically and in the present—has been a fundamentally interdisciplinary undertaking balancing the inputs of medicine, sociology, economics, demography, and other social sciences.

Most recently, perspectives from social epidemiology have played a major role in pressing epidemiologists of all kinds to consider how social contexts influence all manner of health outcomes, and in turn the potential for societal interventions to reduce morbidity and mortality. However, this renaissance has raised important questions about how the study of societal determinants of health relates to the broader discipline. Is 'social epidemiology' best considered a subdiscipline within epidemiology, alongside 'genetic epidemiology', 'cancer epidemiology', or 'infectious disease epidemiology'? Or is understanding the ubiquity of social and economic conditions in shaping morbidity and mortality a concept with which all epidemiologists should be familiar, regardless of specialization? While the answer to this question remains unclear, the increased attention which various epidemiological specialties have paid to socio-economic determinants suggests that these perspectives are of cross-cutting relevance to the discipline rather than simply a speciality field.

References

Berkman LF and Kawachi I (ed.) (2000). *Social epidemiology*. Oxford University Press, New York.

Berkman LF and Syme SL (1979). Social networks, host resistance, and mortality: a nine-year follow-up study of Alameda County residents. *American Journal of Epidemiology*, **109**, 186–204.

Cassel J (1976). The contribution of the social environment to host resistance. *American Journal of Epidemiology*, **104**, 107–23.

Diez-Roux AV (2000). Multilevel analysis in public health research. *Annual Review of Public Health*, **21**, 171–92.

Faris RE and Dunham W (1939). *Mental disorders in urban areas: an ecological study of schizophrenia and other psychoses*. University of Chicago Press, Chicago, IL.

Goldberger J, Wheeler GA, and Sydenstricker E (1964) A study of the relation of family income and other economic factors to pellagra incidence in seven cotton-mill villages of South Carolina in 1916. In *Goldberger on pellagra* (ed. M Terris), pp. 225–67. Louisiana State University Press, Baton Rouge, LA.

Hollingshead A and Redlich F (1958). *Social class and mental illness*. John Wiley & Sons Inc., New York.

Kark SL (1949). The social pathology of syphilis in Africans. *South African Medical Journal*, **23**, 77–84.

Kermack WO, McKendrick AG, and McKinley PL (1934). Death rates in Great Britain and Sweden: some general regularities and their significance. *Lancet*, 31 March, 698–703. (Reprinted in *International Journal of Epidemiology* 2001, **30**, 678–83.)

Krieger N (1999). Embodying inequality: a review of concepts, measures, and methods for studying health consequences of discrimination. *International Journal of the Health Services*, **29**, 295–352.

Kuh D and Ben Shlomo Y (1997). *A life course approach to chronic disease epidemiology*. Oxford University Press, New York.

Marmot MG and Syme SL (1976). Acculturation and coronary heart disease in Japanese-Americans. *American Journal of Epidemiology*, **104**, 225–47.

Marmot MG, Shipley MJ, and Rose G (1984). Inequalities in death-specific explanations of a general pattern? *Lancet*, **1**, 1003–6.

McKeown T (1976). *The Modern Rise of Population*. Academic Press, New York, NY.

Morris JN (1957). *Uses of epidemiology*. Livingstone, Edinburgh.

Myer L, Ehrlich R, and Susser ES (2004). Social epidemiology in South Africa. *Epidemiologic Reviews*, **26**, 112–23.

Porter D (1997). *Social medicine and medical sociology in the twentieth century*, Wellcome Institute Seminars on the History of Medicine. Rodopi, Amsterdam.

Rothman K (1986). *Modern epidemiology*, 1st edn. Lippincott Williams & Wilkins, Philadelphia, PA.

Sampson RJ, Raudenbush SW, and Earls F (1997). Neighborhoods and violent crime: a multilevel study of collective efficacy. *Science*, **277**, 918–24.

Susser M (1968). *Community psychiatry: epidemiologic and social themes.* Random House Press, New York.

Susser M (1994). The logic in ecological: II. The logic of design. *American Journal of Public Health*, **84**, 830–5.

Susser M and Stein Z (1962). Civilization and peptic ulcer. *Lancet*, **1**, 115–19.

Susser M and Watson W (1962). *Sociology in medicine*, 1st edn. Oxford University Press, New York

19

Nutritional epidemiology

Basil S. Hetzel

Personal experiences

I first developed an interest in nutritional epidemiology in a developing country, Papua New Guinea. My concern was with the problem of goitre and brain damage as seen in Highland villages. This work was carried out in collaboration with the Public Health Department of the then Territory under Australian administration. It made use of injections of iodized oil as a depot source of iodine for 3 to 5 years.

The critical step was a controlled trial (1966–70) which demonstrated that injection of iodized oil prevented brain damage (cretinism) if given before pregnancy. Prior to this there was considerable doubt about the relation of iodine deficiency to brain damage.

These findings were confirmed by studies of the effect of iodine deficiency on brain development in animal models in the sheep and marmoset, which confirmed the aetiological role of iodine deficiency in causing brain damage in pregnancy (1976–84).

Subsequent visits to Indonesia (1976–81) and China (1981–84) revealed the massive problem of goitre and cretinism due to iodine deficiency in these countries. Subsequent WHO estimates indicated in excess of two billion at risk from 130 countries. This was a challenge that was not being met (Hetzel *et al.* 2004).

This chapter on nutritional epidemiology illustrates the application of epidemiology to two conditions. One is associated with undernutrition—the relation of iodine deficiency to fetal brain damage and the other associated with overnutrition—the fall in mortality due to coronary heart disease.

Iodine nutrition and the brain

Formerly there was dispute as to whether goitre (an enlarged thyroid gland) and the associated cretinism (a form of brain damage associated with goitre) were related to iodine deficiency. These conditions have been historically associated with mountainous regions, notably the European Alpine region. This work was carried out in the mountainous areas of Papua New Guinea situated in a large island bordering the Indonesian Archipelago and Australia.

An initial controlled trial by the Papua New Guinea Public Health Department (PHD) revealed that the injection of iodized oil (iodine in poppy seed oil, Lipiodol) would prevent goitre. However, the relation to iodine deficiency was questioned (McCullagh 1963).

A subsequent study in collaboration with the PHD revealed that there was severe iodine deficiency in the population of Papua New Guinea as indicated by low iodine excretion in the urine. This study also revealed that a single injection of iodized oil would correct this deficiency for over 4 years, depending on the dosage (Buttfield and Hetzel 1967).

There had been much uncertainty about the relation of brain damage (cretinism) to iodine deficiency. Cretinism is the name given to a clinical syndrome, usually characterized by brain damage, squint, and ataxia due to weakness or paralysis of the legs (neurological cretinism). A less common form of brain damage with dwarfism is due to hypothyroidism (hypothyroid cretinism).

Both conditions can coexist. Cretinism was originally described in the European Alpine region—Switzerland, with adjacent mountainous areas in Italy, Germany, and France also affected.

The geographical association with goitre was well established, but the apparent spontaneous decline of cretinism in mountainous areas in southern Europe—including Switzerland, Italy, and the former Yugoslavia without any formal iodized salt programme had raised the question of the relation to iodine deficiency.

I realized that the demonstration of the effect of a single dose of iodized oil in correcting iodine deficiency for over 4 years made possible a controlled trial to see whether the condition could be prevented. Such a controlled trial was not practicable with iodized salt.

In 1966 I put a proposal to the New Guinea Medical Research Advisory Committee and to the Director of the Public Health Department, Dr Roy Scragg, who agreed to cooperate in the trial. (As he pointed out, it was not possible to inject every iodine deficient individual in New Guinea at once. It was not inappropriate therefore to withhold the injection from a group to enable a scientifically controlled trial to be carried out.)

For this trial, the Jimi River District north of Mount Hagen in the Western Highlands was chosen. It was an area where cretinism was prevalent, particularly in younger age groups, access was available by air and the missions (both Anglican and Lutheran in this case) were cooperative. At my request Dr Peter Pharoah, an experienced New Guinea medical officer was released by Dr Scragg to carry out the follow-up study.

The task facing us was much more difficult than in the case of prevention of goitre. It was necessary to establish criteria for the diagnosis of cretinism in young infants. This had not been done before. For this purpose, Pharoah, with great skill, developed a clinical assessment based on motor milestones (sitting, standing, walking), evidence of deafness, and squint. These proved satisfactory for a survey of a large population of children.

The trial was set up at the time of the first census in New Guinea in September 1966. Alternate families were given injections of iodized oil or saline by Buttfield. Follow-up was then carried out by Pharoah by regular patrols over the succeeding four years. This involved extensive mountain climbing to reach remote villages. It was impossible to cover the whole population of 8000 originally injected. Instead he concentrated on a series of eight villages where good records could be kept. Pharoah made an assessment (double blind) of all children born to mothers without knowing who had received iodized oil or saline. This was most important, as the clinical diagnosis was not precise and bias could readily have occurred. Subsequent follow-up has confirmed diagnoses of cretinism in these cases (Pharoah and Connolly 1987).

The results of the follow-up became available when the code was broken. They are shown in Table 19.1 and Fig. 19.1. They indicated that cretins were greatly reduced in the offspring

Table 19. 1 Pregnancy outcome in the controlled trial of iodized oil in the Western Highlands of Papua New Guinea (Jimi River District)

	Births	Children examined	Normals	Deaths	Cretins[a]
Untreated	534	406	380	97**	26***
Iodized oil	498	412	405	66**	7***

Reproduced with permission from Pharoah POD, Buttfield IH, and Hetzel BS (1971). Neurological damage to the fetus resulting from severe iodine deficiency during pregnancy. *Lancet*, **1**, 308–10.

[a]Pregnancies were already established when mothers were injected with iodized oil (six cases) or with saline (five cases).

**P < 0.05.

***P < 0.001.

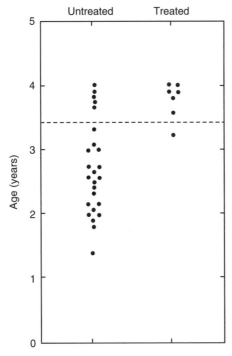

Fig. 19.1 Ages of infants born in the Papua New Guinea controlled trial (1966–70).

of mothers who had received iodized oil injections, but continued to appear in those who had received saline. Only six cretins had appeared following injection of iodized oil, but in all except one case the mother had been noted to be pregnant at the time of the injection. In this case, there was some doubt about the precise date of birth and she may well have also been pregnant when injected. It was concluded that the injection of iodized oil *before* pregnancy would prevent cretinism.

These findings were reported to the 6th International Thyroid Congress in Vienna in 1970. They created immediate interest and when published in *The Lancet* (Pharoah *et al.* 1971) were accepted as definitive at a symposium held at the Institute of Human Biology, Goroka, New Guinea. A subsequent editorial (*Lancet* 1972) pointed out that the long-standing controversy was now resolved. It could now be assumed that the apparent disappearance of cretinism in southern Europe could be attributed to an increase in dietary intake of iodine as a result of economic development leading to diversification of the food supply.

The elimination of cretinism following correction of iodine deficiency has been confirmed in other parts of the world, although no further controlled trials have been carried out. They would not be feasible and can no longer be ethically justified for this purpose.

Another result of the controlled trial was a reduction in fetal deaths in the treated group (Table 19.1). This indicates an effect of iodine deficiency on survival of the fetus. It expands the concept of iodine deficiency beyond that of goitre and cretinism to that of miscarriages and still-births. A subsequent follow-up study by Pharoah *et al.* (1976) has demonstrated the importance of the level of maternal thyroid hormone (T_4) to both the survival of the pregnancy and the occurrence of cretinism. The lowest range of T_4 (<25 µg/ml) was associated with a much higher rate of deaths and cretinism than levels of maternal T_4 of 25 µg/ml or more.

The above results therefore indicate the importance of maternal thyroid hormones to fetal brain development. These studies revealed prevention of a broad spectrum of effects on fetal development, ranging from mortality to cretinism and later psychomotor defects in apparently normal children. This means that a much higher proportion of the iodine-deficient population is affected than had previously been thought. This led to my proposal of the term 'iodine deficiency disorders' to refer the full spectrum of the effects of iodine deficiency in an iodine-deficient population (Hetzel 1983).

The control of severe iodine deficiency in Papua New Guinea was achieved with an iodized oil injection campaign in 1971 and 1972 shortly after completion of the controlled trial in the Western Highlands. Some 120,000 people living in the Highland villages were injected by Aid Post Orderlies (APO), the basic village health worker of the Papua New Guinea Public Health Department. A national iodized salt programme has been operating since that time.

Experimental studies

Subsequent studies in animal models (sheep and marmoset monkeys) confirmed the relation of iodine deficiency to brain damage (Hetzel and Mano 1989). In the sheep an iodine-deficient diet was administered for a year with the establishment of severe iodine deficiency as revealed by the lowered urine iodine levels before mating took place.

Large goitres always developed in the iodine-deficient ewes. There was some retardation of wool growth. The fetal lambs were removed before the end of pregnancy (150 days) by surgical means (hysterotomy) in order to avoid any loss during natural labour and delivery. A retrospective review of the sheep pregnancies showed a 21% loss to the iodine-deficient ewes compared to 4% in the controls. This parallels the predisposition to miscarriages and stillbirths of both iodine-deficient and hypothyroid human mothers.

Observations of the thyroid showed gross hyperplasia of the cells with loss of colloid. Observation of the brains from fetuses removed from 70 days' gestation revealed lowered brain weight. This was associated with a reduced number of cells as measured by deoxyribonucleic acid (DNA) content. There was a less striking reduction in brain cell size. This finding indicated that there was a slowing in the rate of early nerve cell (neuroblast) multiplication, a process known to occur over the period of 40–80 days' gestation in the sheep. These changes were first evident as early as 70 days, or before the end of the first half of pregnancy, the normal gestation period in the sheep being 150 days (Hetzel and Mano 1989).

Observations under the microscope revealed a denser brain than normal due to a failure of development (arborization) of the normal nerve cell branching (the axon and the dendrites). This was evident in the cerebral hemispheres and also in the cerebellum where retardation in the development of the special Purkinje cells resulted from failure of the normal migration of the granular cells from the external granular layer into the central medulla. (The cerebellum is involved in the smooth coordination of movements. The Purkinje cell acts as a storage cell.)

There was a major reduction in the level of both maternal and fetal thyroid hormones.

Proof that there was a causal relationship between the reduced thyroid hormone secretion and the effects on the brain and other organs was demonstrated through further surgical studies. Removal of the thyroid from the fetal lamb at 70 and 98 days' gestation and removal of the maternal thyroid 6 weeks before conception had an effect similar to that of iodine deficiency on fetal brain maturation. A combination of the two procedures produced the most striking effect similar to that of iodine deficiency.

It was concluded that the effect of the iodine deficiency on the brain was mediated through reduced maternal and fetal thyroid gland function (Hetzel and Mano 1989).

Similar findings have been demonstrated in the iodine-deficient marmoset monkey and in the iodine-deficient rat fed an iodine-deficient diet associated with severe goitre and cretinism in China (Hetzel and Mano 1989).

The animal studies indicate clearly the spectrum of effects of iodine deficiency including fetal death, stillbirths as well as brain damage covered by the concept of the iodine deficiency disorders (Hetzel 1983).

A full description of the iodine deficiency disorders is provided elsewhere (Hetzel *et al.* 1990).

Conclusion

The WHO recognizes that iodine deficiency is the most common preventable cause of brain damage in the world today with 2.2 billion at risk in 130 countries (WHO/UNICEF/ICCIDD 1999).

A global public health programme involving a global partnership between national governments, the WHO, UNICEF, and specialist agencies has been developed since the World Summit for Children in 1990 and has been directed to the elimination of brain damage due to iodine deficiency using iodized salt. By 2000 coverage of 66% of households had been reached (Hetzel *et al.* 2004; Hetzel 2005).

The rise and fall in coronary heart disease mortality

The rise and fall of mortality due to coronary heart disease in certain Western countries since 1950 has been well documented (World Health Statistics 1950–79; Havlik and Feinlieb 1979).

There were substantial international differences to be seen and these continued for a number of years with the USA and Australia showing much higher rates than England and Wales and many European countries. By 1968 the Australian rates had risen to that of the USA but since that time there has been a remarkable progressive fall in mortality in both countries so that by 1982 the rates had fallen by approximately 50% compared to 1967–68 (Fig. 19.2).

Analysis by age and sex revealed similar falls in both sexes in different age groups including those above 70 years (Table 19.2). These consistent changes across all age groups indicate a

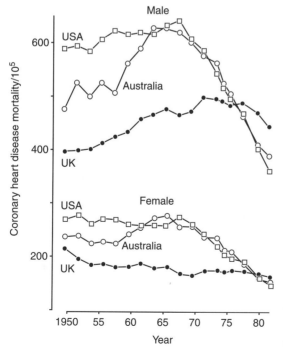

Fig. 19.2 Coronary heart disease mortality: Australia, USA, and UK (England and Wales only) 1950–85. Individual age-specific curves demonstrate similar trends in men and in women with the exception of younger women in England and Wales (data from *World Health Statistics Annuals*).

Table 19.2 Changes in age-specific mortality rates from 1967–71 to 1982–86 as percentages of 1967–71 rates, from ischaemic heart disease in Australia for men and women aged 30–84 years

Age(years)	Change from 1967–71 to 1972–76[a]		Change from 1967–71 to 1977–81[a]		Change from 1967–71 to 1982–86[a]	
	Men	Women	Men	Women	Men	Women
30–34	−1	−9	−18	−54	−27	−65
35–39	−8	+3	−31	−40	−46	−60
40–44	−9	+6	−30	−25	−46	−51
45–49	−9	−4	−30	−26	−49	−46
50–54	−11	−14	−28	−35	−46	−50
55–59	−14	−13	−32	−33	−46	−48
60–64	−11	−17	−28	−33	−44	−47
65–69	−12	−14	−26	−19	−41	−44
70–74	−8	+3	−24	−31	−35	−39
75–79	−10	+12	−24	−10	−32	−32
80–84	−4	−6	−25	−25	−27	−27

Reproduced with permission from Al-Romi KA, Dobson AJ, Hall E, Heller RF, and Magnus P (1989). Declining mortality from ischaemic heart disease and cerebrovascular disease in Australia. *American Journal of Epidemiology*, **129**, 503–10.

[a]As a percentage of the 1967–71 rate.

remarkable general effect on the whole population including the aged. Clearly the reasons for such a striking change were of great interest and importance.

Such a fall was not seen in England and Wales until after 1978 and the fall was much less striking than it has been in the USA and Australia (Dwyer and Hetzel 1980; Heller *et al.* 1983). The levels in England and Wales were some 20% higher than in the USA and Australia which contrasts greatly with the situation in 1950 (Fig. 19.2).

We began our epidemiological analysis by asking the question as to why such an international difference should have occurred (Dwyer and Hetzel 1980).

It seemed likely that there would be similar standards of medical care in all three countries so that any difference would be unlikely to be due to this factor. This was supported by the observation of similar falls in mortality related to hypertension in the three countries (Dwyer and Hetzel 1980), which would reflect the usage of hypotensive drugs as a significant factor in the fall in mortality from hypertension-related causes of stroke and renal failure.

Another major risk factor that might be important would be cigarette smoking. Similar changes occurred but initial levels were different with a greater proportion of smokers in the UK then in the USA but smokers in the USA smoked more than in the UK. A fall occurred in middle-aged males with some rise in women in younger age groups (Dwyer and Hetzel 1980).

Consideration of the other major risk factor of diet led to the careful collection of data available from apparent consumption statistics gathered regularly by the FAO (1949–77) from national sources. These apparent consumption data were admittedly crude—they simply estimate the disappearance of food by purchase across the shop counter. But the data for fat consumption has been supported by evidence from human adipose tissue biopsy which has been shown to reflect prior consumption over a period of some years (Hetzel *et al.* 1989).

Particular attention has been paid to the pattern of fat consumption because of extensive previous data indicating its relevance to coronary heart disease mortality (Havlik and Feinleib 1979). Estimates of fat consumption in the USA since 1908 reveal that total saturated fat has been fairly steady but there have been substantial increases in both oleic acid and linoleic acid with a rise in the ratio of linoleic acid to saturated fat from 0.29 in 1957–59 to 0.48 in 1981. This rise in consumption of linoleic acid is supported by evidence from adipose tissue biopsy which reveals a progressive rise in the USA over the period 1960–80. But there was no such rise in the UK over the same period 1960–80.

In Australia a similar change to that found in the USA was observed in the apparent consumption data which has shown since 1960 a progressive rise in vegetable fats generally high in polyunsaturated fatty acids (Dwyer and Hetzel 1980; Hetzel *et al.* 1989). This is indicated by a rise in margarine consumption from 1.5 kg per head per year in 1966–69 to 6.9 kg per head per year in 1985–86, with a fall in butter consumption from 9.8 kg per head per year in 1966–69 to 3.8 kg per head per year in 1985–86 (Thompson *et al.* 1988).

These data therefore suggested that there was some possible association between the progressive fall in CHD mortality in the USA and Australia with an increased consumption of polyunsaturated fat. The absence of any such change in the consumption of polyunsaturated fat in the UK, at least until 1978, associated with a much later fall in CHD mortality (Heller *et al.* 1983) was consistent with this observation (Fig. 19.2).

We then carried our epidemiological study to a further stage.

Death from coronary heart disease can be associated with three different pathological processes. These are atheroma, where there is deposition of fat in the wall of the coronary artery, thrombosis, where there is clot formation with or without blockage of the artery, and arrhythmia, where there is a rapid regular or irregular beat of the heart—ventricular tachycardia or ventricular fibrillation, which could cause sudden death.

Careful analyses in monitoring centres in the USA and Australia have revealed that the fall in mortality is due mainly to out of hospital acute deaths including sudden deaths which account for a large percentage of the increase in deaths from coronary heart disease (Gillum *et al.* 1984; Thompson *et al.* 1988) (see also Chapter 7).

The hypothesis therefore posed by the epidemiological analysis was that there may be a relation between the progressive fall in sudden deaths observed in both the USA and Australia with the rise in polyunsaturated fat consumption observed in both countries. We then proceeded to carry out a test of this hypothesis by an experimental approach in animal models in the rat and marmoset (Hetzel *et al.* 1989).

Experimental studies

Special attention was paid to the arrhythmia phenomenon in view of the importance of the fall in sudden death. Earlier experimental studies had suggested some relationship between linoleic acid and direct effects on myocardial contractility and the susceptibility of the heart to develop arrhythmia (Charnock *et al.* 1985).

In the present studies, it was found that longer-term feeding (18 months) than previously studied was associated with changes in contractility of the isolated papillary heart muscles. Using the stimulus of isoprenaline, a significantly greater incidence of dysrhythmia was observed in the papillary muscle (suspended in a pharmacological bath) from the hearts of mature rats fed a dietary supplement of saturated animal fat compared with that which could be induced in the muscles from animals that had received the dietary supplement of polyunsaturated fats. In addition it was significant that this dysrhythmia increased with age but was much less in the rats fed the polyunsaturated supplement than in the case of those fed either the saturated fat supplement or even the low-fat control diet.

Parallel studies were carried out *in vivo* by observation of the dysrhythmia produced by ligation of the anterior descending branch of the left coronary artery for 5 min or 15 min using a standard technique (McLennan *et al.* 1989).

There was a highly significant reduction in the incidence and duration of ventricular fibrillation and tachycardia in the animals that had received a dietary supplement of polyunsaturated fatty acids compared with the extent of fibrillation or duration of tachycardia which was observed in animals fed a saturated fat dietary supplement.

There was further evidence of the effect of age. The tendency to dysrhythmia increased with age but this was reduced in the polyunsaturated fed animals (Hetzel *et al.* 1989) and again was well below that found in the low-fat control group.

All changes in function of the heart muscle were accompanied by significant changes in the fatty acid composition of the heart membranes. These changes would be expected to underlie the mechanisms of the alterations and action of the prostaglandins and the availability of calcium ions (Charnock *et al.* 1985, McLennan *et al.* 1989).

Similar changes in relation to the two supplemented diets have been shown in the marmoset (Hetzel *et al.* 1989). There was a marked reduction of isoprenaline-induced dysrhythmia in both the isolated papillary muscle and the left atrial muscle from animals which had received a polyunsaturated fat increment for 20 months compared with those which had received a saturated animal fat intake.

Conclusions

The results of these experimental studies in both rat and marmoset provide strong support for the findings from the epidemiological analysis which suggest that changes in dietary fat with an increased consumption of polyunsaturates have been a major factor in the decline in mortality in the USA and Australia. These effects may be mediated not only by effects on atherogenesis and thrombogenesis but also by effects on the mechanical performance of the heart, particularly its susceptibility to develop dysrhythmias and so sudden death.

These findings support dietary modification by increasing the polyunsaturated fat (linoleic acid) composition of the diet in the prevention of deaths from coronary heart disease.

Acknowledgements

The author is indebted to a group of colleagues named in the text who have been team members in the work described in this paper. He acknowledges the special epidemiological contributions of Professor Peter Pharoah (a former editor of the *International Journal of Epidemiology*) and Professor Terry Dwyer.

References

Al-Roomi KA, Dobson AJ, Hall E, Heller RF, and Magnus P (1989). Declining mortality from ischaemic heart disease and cerebrovascular disease in Australia. *American Journal of Epidemiology*, **129**, 503–10.

Buttfield IH and Hetzel BS (1967). Endemic goitre in Eastern New Guinea with special reference to the use of iodized oil in prophylaxis and treatment. *Bulletin of the World Health Organization*, **36**, 243–62.

Charnock JS, McLennan PC, Abeywardena MY, and Dryden WF (1985). Diet and cardiac arrhythmia: effects of lipids on age-related changes in myocardial function in the rat. *Annals of Nutrition and Metabolism*, **29**, 306–18.

Dwyer T and Hetzel BS (1980). A comparison of trends of coronary heart disease mortality in Australia, USA and England and Wales with reference to three major risk factors – hypertension, cigarette smoking and diet. *International Journal of Epidemiology*, **9**, 65–71.

Gillum RF, Folson AR, and Blackburn H (1984). Decline in coronary heart disease mortality: old questions and new facts. *American Journal of Medicine*, **76**, 1055–65.

Havlik RJ and Feinleib M (1979). *Proceedings of the Conference on Decline in Coronary Heart Disease Mortality*, NIH Publication No 79–1610. US Department of Health, Education, and Welfare, Public Health Service, Washington, DC.

Heller RF, Hayward D, and Hobbs MST (1983). Decline in rate of death from ischaemic heart disease in the United Kingdom. *British Medical Journal*, **286**, 260–72.

Hetzel BS (1983). Iodine deficiency disorders (IDD) and their eradication. *Lancet*, **2**, 1126–9.

Hetzel BS (2005). Towards the global elimination of brain damage due to iodine deficiency—the role of the International Council for Control of Iodine Deficiency Disorders. *International Journal of Epidemiology*, **34**, 762–4.

Hetzel BS and Mano M (1989). A review of experimental studies of iodine deficiency during fetal development. *Journal of Nutrition*, **119**, 145–51.

Hetzel BS, Charnock JS, Dwyer T, and McLennan PL (1989). Fall in coronary heart disease mortality in USA and Australia due to sudden death: evidence for the role of polyunsaturated fat. *Journal of Clinical Epidemiology*, **42**, 885–93.

Hetzel BS, Potter BJ, and Dulberg EM (1990). The iodine deficiency disorders: nature, pathogenesis and epidemiology. *World Review of Nutrition and Dietetics*, **62**, 59–119.

Hetzel BS, Delange F, Dunn JT, Ling J, Mannar V, and Pandav CS (ed.) (2004). *Towards the global elimination of brain damage due to iodine deficiency*. Oxford University Press, New Delhi.

Lancet (1972). New light on endemic cretinism [Editorial]. **2**, 356–66.

McCullagh SF (1963). The Huon Peninsula endemic: I The effectiveness of an intramuscular depot of iodized oil in the control of endemic goitre. *Medical Journal of Australia*, **1**, 767–9.

McLennan PL, Abeywardena MY, and Charnock JS (1989). The influence of age and dietary fat in an animal model of sudden death. *Australian and New Zealand Journal of Medicine*, **19**, 1–5.

Pharoah POD and Connolly KJ (1987). A controlled trial of iodinated oil for the prevention of endemic cretinism: a longer term follow up. *International Journal of Epidemiology*, **16**, 68–73.

Pharoah POD, Buttfield IH, and Hetzel BS (1971). Neurological damage to the fetus resulting from severe iodine deficiency during pregnancy. *Lancet*, **1**, 308–10.

Pharoah POD, Ellis SM, Ekins RP, and Williams ES (1976). Maternal thyroid function, iodine deficiency and fetal development. *Clinical Endocrinology*, **5**, 159–66.

Thompson PL, Hobbs MST, and Martin CA (1988). The rise and fall of ischaemic heart disease in Australia. *Australian and New Zealand Journal of Medicine*, **18**, 327–37.

WHO/UNICEF/ICCIDED (1999). *Progress towards the elimination of iodine deficiency disorders*, WHO Document WHO/NHD/99.4. WHO, Geneva.

World Health Statistics Annual (1950–1976). WHO, Geneva.

Section 4

Methodology

20

Theoretical developments

Olli S. Miettinen

As a medical student in Helsinki, around 1960, I was involved in cardiological research and headed for an academic career in cardiology; but I became uncomfortable with the lack of any theoretical framework for the research. In particular, the data that were produced were sent out for statistical 'analysis' (synthesis, really) and select ones of the received results of this were incorporated into papers without express understanding of their meaning.

This treatment of statistical expertise as extrinsic to competence in medical research together with the implicit idea that the essence of medical research data can be understood from the vantage of statistics alone, without any familiarity with the subject matter, struck me as strange and unjustifiable, notably because of my study (for 1 year) of technological physics and electrical engineering before medicine and my consequent keen awareness that mastery of the requisite mathematics is expected of the technological researcher or engineer him- or herself. So I left behind my then career plan and decided to concern myself, upon graduation from medical school, with the theory of medical research, expressly inclusive of the requisite statistical theory.

I consulted my professor of physiology, Martti Karvonen, who was working with Ancel Keys on the famous Seven Countries Study on dietary aetiology of cardiovascular disease (see Chapter 7), and he advised me to study epidemiology and biostatistics as preparation for my intended career. He recommended study in the University of Minnesota where Keys was a professor. I heeded the advice and completed the course work for PhD in both epidemiology and biostatistics, following that for the MPH degree. Two courses were particularly gratifying in the Minnesota studies. The one by Keys himself on nutritional epidemiology was extraordinary and exemplary in its laying bare the genesis of knowledge, as it was, essentially, a virtual discourse between himself and his critics. And the two-semester course on mathematical statistics by Bernard Lindgren was admirably rigorous and also otherwise elegant. There was, notably, no course on epidemiological statistics. Three years in Minnesota were followed by a 1-year study of the coordination of collaborative clinical trials under Christian Klimt at the University of Maryland.

Approaching the end of these studies I accepted, enthusiastically, an invitation from Brian MacMahon to join the Department of Epidemiology at the Harvard School of Public Health, with joint appointment in the school's Department of Biostatistics, then headed by Robert Reed. This I took to be as good a setting as any for me to advance my understanding of the theory of epidemiological research; and as for clinical research, I valued my added appointment in paediatric cardiology, which was headed by its pioneer, Alexander Nadas.

In this setting there were no obstacles to my early, decade-long work as the coordinator of a national collaborative research programme in paediatric cardiology nor to my consultation on research by others, including as the long-term principal consultant to the Boston Collaborative Drug Surveillance Program and the Netherlands Heart Foundation. And as for theoretical work, there inherently was proximity to the then pioneer of epidemiological methods, Brian MacMahon himself, and to a towering mathematical and 'applied' statistician at Harvard, William Cochran. There also was access to the two then pre-eminent epidemiology-oriented biostatisticians,

Jerome Cornfield and Nathan Mantel, though at the distance of Washington. My theoretical work was essentially a hobby, conducted in my spare time.

In the early period at Harvard, 1966–70, when my teaching concerned genetics from the vantage of probability theory and statistics, my theoretical development interests focused on something that I subsequently became embarrassed about. For my PhD thesis I had chosen a topic that I thought was central to the theory of epidemiological research, typically addressing aetiological causality in non-experimental terms. The prevailing idea was that the non-experimental counterpart of randomization as the basis for causal inference is the pursuit of comparability through matching, and I meekly accepted this. So I went on to write my PhD thesis on statistical theory of studies with matching, publishing some of the developments in three *Biometrics* articles.

Recognition of the fundamental error in my early reverence for matching matured in full, I am embarrassed to have to say, only two decades later. When it did, I wrote a manuscript entitled 'Up from matching'. In it I posited, first, that while it remains commonplace to take the choice to be between unmatched and matched selection of the reference series, the fundamental choice actually is between 'indiscriminate' and 'discriminate' selection, matching being but a special case of discriminate selection. Regarding discriminate selection, I made two major points: first, that matching is always irrelevant for the attainment of validity, of freedom from confounding in the study result; and second, that the efficiency–optimal target distribution of the reference series—base/referent sample in an aetiological study—according to the identified confounders is determined not only by the corresponding distribution of the index series of cases, as in matching, but also by the pattern of the unit costs of the base probes and of the aetiological history distributions across the confounder-based strata of the study base. I also developed the efficiency–optimal target distribution for the base series and noted that matching never represents efficiency–optimal sampling, either.

I submitted the manuscript for publication in a leading journal of epidemiology; but it was rejected, without any critical commentary. Dejected by the rejection, I did not submit the manuscript to any other journal. Some echoes of it can, however, be found in a subsequent essay on the more general stagnancy in the theory of aetiological research (Miettinen 1999). Mantel, when learning about my paper's rejection, pointed out that he, too, was having frustrating difficulties in getting his papers published. To me this was a strong indication of the existence of a conservative establishment in the theory of epidemiological research.

My early concern for the statistical theory of non-experimental causal studies with matching had the salutary consequence of making me examine the relative merits of the two principal 1950s contributions to epidemiological statistics, two chi-squared test statistics for stratified 2×2 tables, one by Cochran (1954) and the other by Mantel and Haenszel (1959).

For a single 2×2 table the statistic can be formulated conditionally on both pairs of marginal frequencies or only one of these. In the former approach the use of the exact hypergeometric variance of a cell-specific frequency is customary, while in the latter it is customary to use the maximum-likelihood rather than the unbiased estimate of the null variance of the difference between the two proportions. The latter statistic is algebraically fully interchangeable with the meticulously formulated hypergeometric one only if the unbiased variance estimate is used; and in the extreme case of matched pairs the stratified chi-squared of the latter type and involving the maximum-likelihood estimates is too large by a factor of two.

Cochran's statistic was formulated conditionally on only one pair of marginal totals and, unfortunately, with maximum-likelihood estimates of the stratum-specific variances, while the Mantel–Haenszel statistic was conditional on both pairs of the stratum-specific marginal totals. Thus, only the latter applied even to individually matched series, and I therefore became a champion of it in preference to Cochran's statistic. In the early 1970s Mantel remarked to me, quite questionably, 'You are the only one who really understands the Mantel–Haenszel test'.

While a stratified test statistic inherently addresses association conditional on the characteristics on which the stratification is based, appreciation of the need for this conditionality in respect to all material confounders as the basis for causal inference still remained quite underdeveloped in the 1960s. The landmark textbook by MacMahon *et al.* (1962) posited three considerations for distinguishing between causal and 'secondary' associations: 'time sequence', 'strength of association', and 'consistency with existing knowledge'. In the epochal 'Smoking and health' report of the US Surgeon General's *ad hoc* committee in 1964, the criteria for an association's causality included its 'consistency', 'strength', 'specificity', 'temporal relationship', and 'coherence'. And Bradford Hill (1965) extended this set to nine elements, with 'biologic gradient' (dose–response pattern) being one of these. This pattern, however, is prone to characterize confounding-induced associations just the same.

Only subsequently has it become generally understood that an outcome's empirical association (descriptively correct) with a potentially causal antecedent has, in principle, two components: a causal one and a confounding-induced one (Miettinen 1972). Thus, for such an association's causality there now is only a single criterion: its unconfoundedness, due to its conditionality on all material confounders of the study base—extraneous determinants of the outcome's occurrence associated, by chance or otherwise, with the aetiological determinant in the study base.

On this subject of confounding in epidemiological research on causality, Albert Hofman urged me to here bring out a point I made around 1980, first informally to colleagues at Harvard and then in two publications: The successes of epidemiological research on causality have pertained to unintended effects, and in the study of these the attainment of practical unconfoundedness of results (by control of confounding) is commonly feasible, whereas dealing with potential confounding by indication in the study of intended effects (of interventions) commonly requires the experimental approach (with prevention of confounding by randomization). A poignant example of this has to do with the preventive effect of the use of aspirin on coronary heart disease. We discovered this, non-experimentally, in the 1970s as an unintended effect of the use of aspirin for other purposes. Given that the effect in the study experience was unintentional, experimental confirmation of its discovery could have been considered unnecessary; but it wasn't. And so, a very major randomized trial was mounted, under the leadership of my Harvard colleague Charles Hennekens.

In the 1960s the counterpart of the development the stratified tests of the 1950s, supplemented by the stratified point estimator of 'odds ratio' in the paper by Mantel and Haenszel, was the introduction of logistic regression. It was developed as an adaptation of the Fisher discriminant function involving least-squares fitting (Truett *et al.* 1967) and, separately, from first principles with maximum-likelihood fitting (Walker and Duncan 1967). The former development, in which Cornfield was involved, was inspired by requirements of the famous Framingham Heart Study and illustrated by application to data from that 'study' (actually a multipurpose research programme).

While 'binary' regression with least-squares fitting had been available before, it was unsatisfactory in that the fitted linear compound could take on realizations outside the 0–1 range of probabilities. The solution was replacement of the probability P—the 'expectation' of the Bernoulli dependent variate as the dependent parameter—by its 'logit' transform, $\log [P/(1 - P)]$, the range of which is boundless. The regression thus became 'nonlinear' and, later, 'generalized linear'.

In 1968, at the end of a congress session on cardiovascular epidemiology, I expressed surprise that logistic regression was not even mentioned in any of the many presentations. The chairman responded by saying that logistic regression does not apply to epidemiological studies—thus unwittingly providing an illustration of how even great innovations tend to be initially received by the scientific establishment.

I started my teaching of the theory of epidemiological research in 1970, responsible for the most advanced course in this area at Harvard at the time. While my predecessor in this was a very senior biostatistician, Jane Worcester, I brought to it my own education not only in epidemiology and statistics following that in medicine, but also in the paradigm for sciences generally, physics, and my quite extensive informal study of the philosophy of science besides.

The course notes, updated each year as I went along, got to be accessed and studied in a variety of places by the early 1970s. One of these was the School of Public Health of the University of North Carolina, where Hal Morgenstern, as a doctoral student, organized a study group. Morgenstern also got me invited to come and explain what had remained unclear in the notes. He subsequently became a co-author in 1982 with D. G. Kleinbaum and L. L. Kupper of quite a novel—statistically fully learned—textbook on epidemiological research, *Epidemiologic research. Principles and quantitative methods*.

Kenneth Rothman was my teaching assistant in 1970–75 and exported his learning to the international summer courses in the University of Minnesota in the late 1970s. He also operationalized, with John Boice, the epidemiological statistics he learned for application by the use of a programmable calculator.

Theory of epidemiological research is, first, a matter of concepts and their corresponding terms; and then it is a matter of principles, formulated on the basis of (reasoning involving) those concepts and expressed by the use of those terms. In physics, a sharp distinction is made between the concepts of mass and weight, for example; and in it, just as in its parent discipline, philosophy, there is no tolerance for terminological sloppiness, calling mass weight, for example.

In epidemiology, the most central one of all concepts concerning an illness is itself already a statistical one: the frequency of its occurrence, expressed as a rate of its occurrence, whether as a rate of its prevalence, as a state, or of its incidence, as an event (commonly its first rule-in diagnosis). A concept intimately related to rate, in epidemiology as in demography, is population, either closed—a cohort—or open/dynamic; for an empirical rate has a population involved in its referent.

In respect to these core concepts, remarkably, the development of epidemiology in recent decades has been regressive—while non-existent in the prevalence of the unjustifiable notion that all illnesses are diseases (Miettinen and Flegel 2003a).

True to the then history of epidemiology, MacMahon *et al.* (1962) wrote about rates of both prevalence and incidence; and my 1998 edition of *The New Oxford Dictionary of English* defines a rate as 'a measure, quantity, or frequency, typically one measured against some other quantity or measure'. It thus remains a matter of standard English to speak of, say, the unemployment rate, meaning the prevalence rate of the state of being unemployed, to put it in traditional epidemiological terms.

A mathematician in a 1975 paper of hers, however, taught that whereas the level of prevalence is expressed as a proportion, at issue is not a rate because, properly understood, a rate is the change in one quantity per unit change in another. She failed to appreciate that the level of prevalence can actually be thought of as the change in one quantity—the number of cases of an illness state encountered—per unit change in another—the number of person-moments covered. For example, a prevalence rate of 0.5% represents the change of five cases when moving across 1000 person-moments.

Even though there thus is no such reason to rebel against the English language, Kleinbaum *et al.* (1982) joined this rebellion, and many others have subsequently done the same. Most remarkably, *A dictionary of epidemiology*—a 'handbook' of the International Epidemiological Association—now declares use of the term rate in reference to a proportion-type quantity, whether expressing the level of prevalence or incidence, to be unacceptable usage in epidemiology!

As for population, then, in the early 1970s there was, still, quite generally a clear understanding of what one of the two fundamental types of population is: a cohort, an aggregate of people with entry into its membership based on experiencing a particular event, such as enrolment into the population constituting the framework of a 'cohort' study. It was understood that once one became a member, one remained a member in perpetuity. Hence the concern in the then 'cohort' studies for complete follow-up to the closing date of the study or until further follow-up became irrelevant because of, notably, death or the outcome event whose aetiology was at issue. A cohort was, thus, understood, implicitly at least, to be a closed population in the meaning of being closed for exit.

Given the clarity on this, in my teachings, at Harvard and internationally, I took it to be equally clear what the alternative to a cohort-type population is, namely a dynamic one in the meaning of having turnover of membership on account of membership being based on a state instead of an event, and for the duration of the state; it is an open population in the meaning of being open for exit, through the state's termination. The dynamic-population term thus entered into epidemiologists' consciousness, but the concept itself remained obscure, and with the consequence that even the concept of cohort got to be obfuscated.

In the 1982 textbook by Kleinbaum *et al.*, cohort in the meaning above got to be termed 'fixed cohort', and its alternative, while termed dynamic population, was defined as one that 'may gain and lose' members in its course over time. Any cohort, however, also gains members until its size is 'fixed', if ever; the cohort of Nobel prize winners, for example, just keeps on gaining members (albeit that most of them are deceased). The distinction thus got to be so unclear that in some instances, so Kleinbaum *et al.* themselves explained, the population may be viewed as being of either one of these two types.

This obfuscation, again, got to be widely adopted, so much so that the common idea now seems to be that all populations are cohorts, some fixed and others dynamic in the muddled meanings just described; and the IEA dictionary now defines a dynamic population as one that 'gains and loses' members.

Next to rates and populations, the core concepts of epidemiology are those of comparative measures based on rates; comparison of rates generally is inescapable in aetiological research, typical of epidemiological research.

In my teachings, from the beginning I termed the difference between two rates, simply, rate difference; and their ratio I termed rate ratio. MacMahon, however, remarked to me that the corresponding terms 'attributable risk' and 'relative risk' are so well established that they really are not subject to being replaced by what he agreed would indeed be preferable terms for conveying the meanings. I nevertheless took it to be important for everyone concerned to understand, for a start, that the epidemiological concept of rate is very different from that of risk: there is the difference between population and individual as the respective referents, and that between the commonly empirical nature of rates in contrast to the inherently theoretical essence of risk; a rate can be time-dimensioned while a risk measure is inherently dimensionless; a rate difference is not inherently 'attributable' (causally) to the determinant contrast; etc.

MacMahon was vindicated to the extent that the traditional terms were still used by Kleinbaum *et al.* (1982), though along with the difference and ratio elements in the terms I had adopted; but to those authors even the empirical measures expressed differences and ratios of 'risks', even though these same authors expressly, and correctly, defined risk as a type of probability. The IEA dictionary now perpetuates this duality in terminology, and thus the corresponding duality in the degree of rigour of concepts.

In respect to comparative measures in epidemiology, a remarkable 1950s development was the very simple yet generally well-performing stratified point estimator of 'odds ratio' that was adduced in the same paper that brought us the Mantel–Haenszel chi-squared test statistic for stratified 2×2 tables. However, two problems remained: generally applied in 'case–control' studies, this empirical measure was thought to represent an approximation to 'relative risk' in the framework of the familiar 'rare-disease assumption' in such studies (Cornfield 1951); and there was no associated interval estimator.

I then showed, for one, that in the ordinary type of 'case–control' study the 'odds ratio' point estimate actually is, if anything, an estimate of incidence-density ratio without any rare-disease assumption (Miettinen 1976). That idea got to be the subject of several articles by others, as though not obvious once set forth; but now it is recognized by the IEA dictionary, along with the associated incidence-density term also introduced in that article. Nevertheless, it remains commonplace to report results from 'case–control' studies in terms of 'relative risk' or 'odds ratio' instead of incidence-density ratio. In the same article—a citation classic—I also gave a very simple yet generally well-performing interval estimator corresponding to the stratified point estimator of rate ratio that Mantel and Haenszel had so ingeniously formulated, and for other measures besides—the respective 'test-based' interval estimators. This concept, however, does not appear in the IEA dictionary.

A comparative measure in aetiological research, generally a rate ratio in the meaning of incidence-density ratio, always pertains to a contrast between particular index and reference categories of the aetiological factor at issue; and the empirical rate ratio is always to be made conditional on all of the rate's material extraneous determinants whenever their distributions in the ratio's referent, the study base, are materially imbalanced; that is, it is to be made conditional on all material confounders, known or suspected, of the study base (cf. above), whether risk factors or mere risk indicators. All of the concepts and terms in this passage, fundamental to the theory of aetiological research, were part of my teachings, at Harvard and internationally, by the 1970s, and they were defined in the glossary of my 1985 textbook (Miettinen 1985).

The key concept in that passage is, of course, that of aetiology itself. This the IEA dictionary now defines as, 'Literally, the science of causes, causality; in common usage, cause', without the elementary understanding that by no means all 'logies' are sciences, and that there is no science with aetiology at large as its unique, defining object. Nor is the concept that of cause. Aetiology, correctly understood, is the medical concept—retrospective—of causal origin, aetiogenesis, of an illness, the aggregate of influences initiating and/or advancing pathogenesis (Miettinen and Flegel 2003b).

The other elements in that passage, too, the dictionary either misdefines or does not define at all. The idea in that dictionary that a determinant inherently 'brings about a change' in something, instead of merely being an entity on which that something depends, non-causally perhaps, is consistent with my dictionary of English; but I still like to say, for example, that if the magnitude of a rate of illness occurrence depends on age—a dependence which cannot be thought of as causal—then age is a determinant of the rate's magnitude. I know of no other term being used for this. My *Roget's International Thesaurus* (fourth edition) equates determinant with limiting factor and boundary condition.

Next to comparative measures pertaining to causal contrasts of interest, the epidemiological concern is commonly with the proportion of cases of a particular illness that have a particular antecedent involved in their aetiology in a particular place at a particular time. This is the proportion of cases in which that antecedent, present in lieu of a particular alternative, had/has the critical role of completing a sufficient cause.

The structure of this proportion—I term it the aetiological fraction—was first formulated in the 1950s. In the early 1970s I gave it a much simpler and thus much more commonly applicable formulation, so simple that textbook authors may commonly have failed to understand it, as they commonly have ignored it (Hanley 2001); and the IEA dictionary still gives only the 1950s formulation (and gratuitously at that, as only the concept belongs in a dictionary).

In the 1970s, the most consequential statistical development bearing on epidemiological research was, as it has subsequently turned out, the introduction of a type of regression intended for 'survival analysis' in clinical trials (Cox 1972, 1975). This 'Cox regression' has, by now, gained almost routine application in the study of 'hazard ratio'—the momentary risk ratio, identical to incidence-density ratio—in 'cohort' studies. The use of logistic regression—also developed to accommodate suitably conditional maximum-likelihood estimation from even pairwise matched sets (Breslow and Powers 1978)—has gained the corresponding status in 'case–control' studies.

The underlying duality in this, constituted by 'cohort' and 'case–control' studies, persists (Samet and Muñoz 1998; Armenian 1994) as the most fundamental idea concerning epidemiological methods in aetiological research. This persistence is, however, the prime example of the lack of necessary development in the theory of epidemiological research over the past half century.

The 'cohort' versus 'case–control' duality persists in the context of continuing failure to appreciate what the always necessary elements are in the structure of an aetiological study, specifically the necessary structure's singularity in the context of a given type of rate whose relation (causal) to an aetiological determinant is at issue. Typically an aetiological study addresses the incidence density of the occurrence of an event-type outcome, and in this situation the study structure necessarily involves these elements:

1. A defined study base—as the basis for learning and, thus, as the result's referent—constituted by the aggregate of population-time in the defined study population's movement over a defined span of time.

2. Data collected on the study base in terms of two series:
   ◆ a case series, representing the person-moments at which the outcome event occurred in the study base, and
   ◆ a base series, representing, as a sample, the study base *per se*, the infinite number of person-moments in it,
   ◆ the data, synchronic and retrospectively diachronic, pertaining to the person-moments in these 'numerator' and 'denominator' series.

3. The study result, derived from the data on those two series and representing the empirical incidence-density ratio (and its imprecision) for at least one aetiological contrast conditional on all of the identified material confounders of the study base, this ratio as a function—generally based on logistic regression—of whatever modifiers of it were designed into the object of the study, if any.

With this structure a given, study design concerns only the process by which this structure will be brought about. For this design, the point of departure is the rate-ratio function that had been designed as the object of study, inclusive of its referent domain (abstract).

The concepts 'cohort' and 'case–control' studies, then, should have been understood in the framework of this necessary structure. In a 'cohort' study, it should have been understood that it is the study population's source population that is a cohort, while the actual study population within it generally is a dynamic one. Characterization of an aetiological study as a 'cohort' study on the ground that it was constructed in the framework of a cohort-type source population is making a major point of what actually is inconsequential: with the source population dynamic, the resulting structure of the study itself, *ceteris paribus*, is the same.

'The central feature of a case–control design', in turn, 'is comparison of two groups, one with a specific outcome and the other without that outcome. The frequency of the hypothesized factor(s) suspected of being related to the outcome is compared in the two groups' (Armenian and Lilienfeld 1994). Whereas for the 'cohort' study, properly understood, the logical alternative is the 'dynamic-population' study, the 'case–control' study as the purported alternative is but a conceptual malformation, devoid of justification for its existence. Most notably, the concept of study base is missing in its just-cited definition; and related to this is replacement of the contrast between the index and reference segments of the study base by that between 'groups' based on the outcome— with the consequence that even the alternative to an association's causality, confounding, gets to be seriously misunderstood.

It should have been learned, decades ago, that when an aetiological study is constructed with primary commitment to the scheme of case identification, the corresponding source population is the catchment population, in its entirety, of this scheme; that the study population and study base again need to be defined in the framework of the source population; that the concept of 'control group' needs to be replaced by that of the base/referent series; etc.

The genuine duality thus is, as I explained in my textbook (Miettinen 1985), constituted by two ways of defining the source population: direct/primary definition versus indirect/secondary definition (given primary definition of the scheme of case identification). When, for validity assurance with the latter approach, the admissible cases are specified as ones that are severe and typical and occurring in residents of a defined metropolitan area or participants in a particular health insurance programme, say, and when all of the relevant care facilities in such a framework are canvassed for case identification, the indirectly defined source population becomes quite concrete. Indeed, in these terms even the genuine duality becomes moot.

While the persistence of the 'cohort' study versus 'case–control' study duality indeed is the prime example of the stagnancy of the theory of epidemiological research over the past half-century, its equivalent in a smaller but nevertheless important realm has surrounded screening for a cancer. Such has been the confusion of epidemiologists about the concept and potential implications of screening and, consequently, about screening research, that the end result of having involved half a million women in randomized trials on breast cancer screening has been nothing but controversy.

And now, with nothing learnt about the theory of screening or of research on screening, from that experience, even, a randomized trial at a cost of a quarter of a billion US dollars is under way to assess whether CT screening reduces mortality from lung cancer—again leaving largely undefined the regimen of pursuing early, latent-stage detection/diagnosis (rule-in) of the disease; again without distinguishing between the issues of early versus late, overt-stage diagnosis and those of early versus late intervention; etc.

The fundamental conceptual error in this is viewing the screening as merely the application of the initial test and not understanding what this testing actually is, namely the first step in the clinical pursuit of early diagnosis—taking this testing to be, instead, a matter of preventive intervention in community medicine! Screening research, properly understood, is a genre of diagnostic research, in which there is no proper place for randomized trials; but it may need to be supplemented by research contrasting early, latent-stage intervention with late, overt-stage intervention in the context of some subtypes of early diagnosis and/or some other prognosis-relevant subdomains.

Unjustifiable stagnancy of generally adopted theory intrinsic to epidemiology is one thing, general passivity in the face of encroaching extrinsic and utterly untenable theory quite another. The salient example of the latter has recently been epidemiologists' lack of resistance to the doctrines of David Sackett, as they have come to bear on epidemiological research and practice.

As I reflect on the past half century of theoretical developments in epidemiology overall, I am impressed with the statistical advances and, as has become evident above and elsewhere (Miettinen 2005), disappointed with the stagnancy and in some central contexts even the regressiveness of the rest. As for the latter, I quote arguably the greatest humanist scholar of the twentieth century (Berlin 1997): 'Where concepts are clear, firm and generally accepted, and the methods of reasoning and arriving at conclusions are agreed between men..., there and only there is it possible to construct a science, formal or empirical'. Concepts are a prerequisite for any thought, tenable concepts that for rational thought, including the development and adoption of principles for epidemiological research. A major obstacle for the advancement of epidemiological concepts in the last two decades I take to have been, as also is evident from the foregoing, the IEA *Dictionary of epidemiology*. It fails even to appreciate what the concept of a concept really is, and what the structure of a concept's proper definition is in principle.

Having here sketched—from a personal perspective, as requested—the theoretical developments in epidemiology (in epidemiological research, to be specific) in the past half century, I close by noting that the entire history of this topic has recently been more objectively delineated in a single volume (Morabia 2004) by a number of scholars on epidemiology.

References

Armenian HK (ed.) (1994). Applications of the case-control method [special issue]. *Epidemiologic Reviews*, **16**.

Armenian HK and Lilienfeld DE (1994). Overview and historical perspective. In Applications of the case-control method (ed. HK Armenian), *Epidemiologic Reviews*, **16**, 1–5.

Berlin I (1997). *The proper study of mankind*. Chatto and Windus, London.

Breslow NE and Powers W (1978). Are there two logistic regressions for retrospective studies? *Biometrika*, **34**, 100–5.

Cochran WG (1954). Some methods for strengthening the common chi-square tests. *Biometrics*, **10**, 417–51.

Cornfield J (1951). A method of estimating comparative rates from clinical data. Application to cancer of the lung, breast and cervix. *Journal of the National Cancer Institute*, **11**, 1269–75.

Cox DR (1972). Regression models and life tables. *Journal of the Royal Statistical Society, Series B*, **34**, 187–220.

Cox DR (1975). Partial likelihood. *Biometrika*, **62**, 269–76.

Hanley JA (2001). Heuristic approach to the formulas for population attributable fraction. *Journal of Epidemiology and Community Health*, **55**, 508–14.

Hill AB (1965). The environment and disease: association or causation? *Proceedings of the Royal Society of Medicine*, **58**, 295–300.

Kleinbaum DG, Kupper LL, and Morgenstern H (1982). *Epidemiologic research. Principles and quantitative methods*. Lifetime Learning Publications, London.

MacMahon B, Pugh TF, and Ipsen J (1962). *Epidemiologic Methods*. Little, Brown and Company, Boston.

Mantel N and Haenszel W (1959). Statistical aspects of the analysis of data from retrospective studies of disease. *Journal of the National Cancer Institute*, **22**, 719–48.

Miettinen OS (1972). Components of the crude risk ratio. *American Journal of Epidemiology*, **96**, 168–72.

Miettinen OS (1976). Estimability and estimation in case-referent studies. *American Journal of Epidemiology*, **103**, 226–35.

Miettinen OS (1985). *Theoretical Epidemiology. Principles of Occurrence, Research in Medicine*. John Wiley & Sons, New York.

Miettinen OS (1999). Etiologic research: needed revisions of concepts and principles. *Scandinavian Journal of Work, Environment & Health*, **25** (special issue), 484–90.

Miettinen OS (2005). Commentaries on 'Epidemiology: quo vadis?' *European Journal of Epidemiology*, **20**, 11–15.

Miettinen OS and Flegel KM (2003a). Elementary concepts of medicine: V. Disease: one of the main subtypes of illness. *Journal of Evaluation in Clinical Practice*, **9**, 321–3.

Miettinen OS and Flegel KM (2003b). Elementary concepts of medicine: VI. Genesis of illness: pathogenesis, aetiogenesis. *Journal of Evaluation in Clinical Practice*, **9**, 325–7.

Morabia A (ed.) (2004). *History of epidemiologic methods and concepts*. Birkhäuser Verlag, Basel.

Samet JM and Muñoz A (ed.) (1998). Cohort studies [special issue]. *Epidemiologic Reviews*, **20**, 1–136.

Truett J, Cornfield J, and Kannel W (1967). A multivariate analysis of the risk of coronary heart disease in Framingham. *Journal of Chronic Disease*, **20**, 511–24.

Walker SH and Duncan DB (1967). Estimation of the probability of an event as a function of several independent variables. *Biometrika*, **54**, 167–79.

21

Outbreak investigations

Kenrad E. Nelson

Personal experiences

My interest in epidemiology and public health increased during my residency in internal medicine at Cook County Hospital in Chicago in the early 1960s. Cook County Hospital, at that time, had about 3000 inpatient beds and mostly served the large indigent population of Chicago. Patient care at the hospital was managed by interns, residents, and subspeciality fellows along with a small full-time faculty and many visiting volunteer physicians.

One of the most important medical problems at that time was tuberculosis. Patients who developed tuberculosis often had other conditions, especially alcoholism, addiction to illicit drugs, malnutrition, or mental health problems. Indeed, these were common health problems in the entire hospital patient population, but they were particularly common in patients with tuberculosis.

When I was a medical resident on the chest service, I became frustrated by the frequent problem of relapsing tuberculosis after patients discontinued their therapy soon after they were discharged from hospital care when their acute symptoms had subsided. It seemed obvious to me that relapsing tuberculosis, often with antibiotic-resistant organisms, was a major public health problem that required more than hospital-based medical care to resolve.

So, when I was the Chief Resident in Internal Medicine on the Northwestern University Service at the hospital, I decided to do a research project to determine the extent of the problem and the epidemiology and primary reasons for relapse and treatment failure. In order to evaluate the outcome of treatment after a diagnosis of tuberculosis had been confirmed, I compiled a list of all 140 patients who had *Mycobacterium tuberculosis*-positive cultures during 1 month 2 years earlier. I then searched for their subsequent hospitalizations, Municipal Tuberculosis Clinic records, death records, and, in some cases, contacted the patients or their families to determine their follow-up history.

The results of this study were very disturbing. Nearly 40% of the patients had died, commonly with active tuberculosis. Only about 35% had been followed regularly by the Municipal Tuberculosis Clinic and had been cured after receiving appropriate therapy. Many patients had been readmitted to the hospital multiple times before they received effective treatment. The study documented the incredibly poor communication and interaction between the hospital laboratory, the ward physicians, and the public health system that had adversely affected patient care.

At that time the reporting of tuberculosis cases to the Public Health Department was believed to be the responsibility of the treating physician, not the laboratory, and there was no Hospital Infection Control Service. It wasn't unusual for a laboratory report of a positive *M. tuberculosis* culture never to reach the physician who submitted the culture, when he or she was on a different service when the report arrived on the ward 6–8 weeks later!

This experience motivated me to become interested in epidemiology and public health, as well as clinical medicine. It seemed obvious that tuberculosis was a public health problem that involved the community, not only the ill patient. Control of tuberculosis would require a system to ensure that each tuberculosis patient actually received and took their medication, that their contacts were screened and that their other health and social problems were dealt with as well. This problem still persists today to some extent but has resulted in the development of a DOTS (directly observed therapy) strategy and its promotion by the Centers for Disease Control and the World Health Organization, as a part of the programme to control tuberculosis.

The Centers for Disease Control (CDC)

Largely because of my interest in public health and epidemiology I decided to join the Epidemic Intelligence Service (EIS) at the Centers for Disease Control after I finished my residency in internal medicine. The EIS is a 2-year programme, which emphasizes field epidemiology, including outbreak investigation, as well as epidemiological analysis of public health morbidity and mortality data in order to develop and implement strategies to control infectious and non-infectious diseases.

When I joined the EIS programme in 1963 the programme provided a very dynamic and exciting experience. My group in EIS included about 50 physicians with a few biostatisticians, veterinarians, and trained epidemiologists. Most subsequently entered a career in academic medicine and public health or epidemiology after they left the CDC. I selected an assignment with the Washington State Health Department. This was a fascinating experience that was very different from my previous clinical experience. My first field experience was to investigate the house and barn of a girl who had been bitten by a bat that proved to be rabid. Subsequent investigations included cases of type E botulism from consumption of fermented salmon eggs by a Native American on his reservation, an outbreak of diphtheria during a Native American 'powwow', several food borne outbreaks, an outbreak of leptospirosis, and polio associated with the Sabin polio vaccine.

Clostridium perfringens food poisoning

The first major outbreak I investigated was of *C. perfringens* food poisoning in a college population (Nelson *et al.* 1966). This involved 314 ill students who were living on campus in a college in eastern Washington. The vehicle was contaminated and reheated lamb stew, which had been served in the college cafeteria. At the time the American literature on food-borne *C. perfringens* was very sparse. However, several reports had been published from the UK. This reflected, I think, both a difference in culinary habits and a greater interest in defining the nature of food-borne illnesses in the UK compared to the USA at the time. This outbreak had the characteristics more of an intoxication than an infection. The illness was short lived, with a short incubation period of about 6–12 hours and involved diarrhoea, cramps, and headache, but rarely fever. There was no secondary spread to the contacts of the ill students. Subsequently several enterotoxins have been isolated from *C. perfringens* that are implicated in food-borne disease from this organism (Cliver 1990).

Outbreaks of *C. perfringens* food poisoning occur most commonly from consumption of reheated meats in which the sauces are contaminated with the organism and are kept with the meat, with growth of the organism occurring upon reheating. The contaminated meat is usually stored at temperatures which allow replication of *C. perfringens* prior to reheating. Symptoms require ingestion of *C. perfringens* which produce enterotoxins in the intestine. This continues to be a common problem in the USA and Europe with several dozen outbreaks reported each year.

Salmonella food poisoning

A large outbreak of *Salmonella* infections occurred in 1963, originally identified as a food-borne outbreak among students at a college in western Washington (Ager *et al.* 1967). This outbreak illustrated the common epidemiological observation that outbreaks in defined populations may be more easily recognized and therefore reported but sometimes may represent a much more extensive epidemic in the community and their investigation may uncover a significant public health problem.

Investigation of this outbreak, which involved about 45% of the 1300 students at the college, was found to be related to consumption of lemon meringue pies in the school cafeteria that were contaminated with *Salmonalla heidelburg*. Subsequently, other persons outside the college population were identified who had become ill with the same organism after consumption of meringue pies prepared by the same bakery in western Washington. Cases were eventually identified from the two surrounding states as well. A similar outbreak had occurred a year earlier of *Salmonella typhimurium* infections after consumption of pies from this same bakery. Upon investigation, we determined that the bakery had prepared about 400 pies per day using a variety of ingredients, including frozen egg whites, which had been purchased from a local creamery. When we visited this creamery with scientists from the FDA, with a court order to permit our investigation, we found that the eggs to be sold to the bakery were commonly of low quality, i.e. cracked, checked, or soiled with chicken faecal material. The yolks and whites were separated by hand and the whites were put into 30 pound cans and stored frozen until they were sold. The creamery had about 15,000 cans of frozen egg whites in their walk-in freezers. We obtained core samples from 1131 cans for culture using an electric drill, which was sterilized with a blow torch between samples. Overall, 235 (20.8%) of the cans were found to be contaminated with one of seven different serotypes of Salmonellae. The creamery was subsequently closed. However, the numbers of human illnesses that could have been caused by these frozen egg whites, if they were consumed without cooking, as in meringue pies, custards, eggnog, cake mixes, and other such products would have been enormous.

This outbreak was not an isolated event. It was one of several that had occurred in the USA in the 1960s and earlier related to eggs and poultry products (Philbrook *et al.* 1960; Sanders *et al.* 1963). In fact, during the Second World War powdered eggs were sent from the USA, Canada, and Argentina to the UK for food supplementation. However, about 10% of those eggs products were contaminated with pathogenic Salmonellae and 33 new serotypes of Salmonellae were introduced into the UK that had not been isolated previously.

Although there has been some improvement, the problem of human salmonellosis transmitted from eggs, poultry, and other animal foods has continued to the present (Smith and Fratamico 1995). The potential for large outbreaks of human illness has increased with the advent of 'industrialized farming' and massive production and distribution of foods, contaminated animal feed, use of antibiotics in agriculture, and other common practices. Certainly, the problem of foodborne infection is not limited to salmonellosis but now includes other pathogens as well, such as *Campylobacter*, *Escherichia coli* O157:H7, variant Creutzfeldt–Jakob disease and other pathogens (Smith and Fratamico 1995). In a sense, the results of this investigation opened up a Pandora's box!

Leptospirosis

During the summer of 1964 the Washington State Health Department received a call from the local health authorities asking for assistance in evaluating and controlling an outbreak of a febrile illness among adolescents in three rural communities in central Washington. When I arrived at the site it was apparent that the illness was unusual, consisting of fever, shaking chills, and severe headache. Stiff neck was reported by about half the cases. I was not aware, until years later, that there was some official and secret concern about this epidemic, since it was located near the Hanford atomic works plant, which had recently detected some leaks of radioactive material from their plant into the environment near where the cases occurred.

In any event, the high school and junior high school students who had been ill had a theory as to the cause of their illness. The region where it occurred was very hot and dry with a semi-desert climate. That summer the temperature had been quite high, reaching 110°F (43°C) in mid-July. Since there were no public swimming pools available, the students had utilized an irrigation ditch as a swimming hole. They named this location 'The Bubbles', since the water bubbled up as it was pumped in a different direction through the field. Diving into the water at 'The Bubbles' caused a person to swirl around and career into the concrete walls of the irrigation canal. Since the area was heavily farmed, a herd of cattle had grazed several hundred yards upstream from 'The Bubbles'. They also used the irrigation ditch as a swimming hole as it traversed their farm to cool off.

We found that the students had infections with *Leptospira pomona*, which had entered through their often scraped skin and mucosa from colliding with the concrete walls of 'The Bubbles' after they jumped into the water. We isolated *L. pomona* from the ill adolescents, the urine from the cattle, and standing water in the field where the cattle had grazed (Nelson *et al.* 1973).

This outbreak illustrated another significant public health problem, namely infections acquired during recreational swimming. A number of other infectious agents have been acquired by similar exposures, including *E. coli* O157:H7, legionellosis, and Norovirus among others (Bruce *et al.* 1999). Also, the transmission of animal pathogens to humans, i.e. zoonoses, has become very common recently. They have accounted for about half of the emerging infectious diseases in the last decade. It is increasingly necessary for modern infectious disease epidemiologists to be aware of the animal reservoir of many infectious diseases and the potential for non-species transmission of pathogens.

Epidemiological issues at CDC in the 1960s

The 1960s were a dynamic and interesting time at CDC. All of the EIS officers and many visiting scientists from CDC and academia generally attended the Annual EIS held at the CDC in April each year.

At the EIS meeting there was great interest and intense discussion about important infectious disease issues of the time.

Polio

One of the important problems was the control, prevention, and even eventual elimination of poliomyelitis using the recently developed inactivated and oral vaccines. The incidence of polio had decreased dramatically after the licensing and widespread use of the inactivated Salk polio vaccine. Nevertheless, the 'Cutter incident', in which 82 people developed polio from an inadequately inactivated vaccine preparation, detracted from the otherwise spectacular success story of this vaccine.

However, the potential for the more recently licensed Sabin attenuated polio vaccine to better control, possibly even eliminate, polio seemed possible. This vaccine was simple to administer and provided intestinal immunity, which was believed to provide long-term, probably permanent, immunity to effectively prevent spread of the virus. The oral vaccine was soon incorporated into the routine paediatric immunization schedule. This was supplemented with periodic mass campaigns targeted at young children. Consequently, the incidence of polio dropped dramatically, even below the rates achieved with the inactivated vaccine. However, soon reports emerged of 'vaccine-associated polio' among persons who had received the oral vaccine (Nathanson and Langmuir 1963).

Initially the scientists who had developed the oral vaccine were sceptical that these cases were caused by the vaccine. When wild poliovirus is still circulating in a population, without genetic studies of viruses isolated from the cerebrospinal fluid (CSF) it may be difficult to differentiate vaccine-associated polio from disease caused by wild polio. Also, other enterovirus infections were soon shown to cause occasional cases of acute flaccid paralysis, simulating polio. Nevertheless, with more experience it became clear that vaccine-associated paralytic polio was a real entity, which occurred at a rate of about 1 per 1,000,000 vaccines (WHO Collaborative Study Group 1976). Indeed, one of the major potential benefits of the eradication of polio is that immunization can then be stopped and the risk of vaccine-associated polio can be avoided. Between 1980 and 1997 about 8–10 cases of vaccine-associated polio were reported each year in the USA in the absence of endemic polio. The current prospects for the global eradication of polio are very promising. Successful eradication has become especially urgent, since in the last few years unimpeded transmission of vaccine virus in several communities with low population immunity to polio has resulted in reversion to virulence of vaccine virus with outbreaks of paralysis due to vaccine-associated polio (Kew *et al*. 2002, 2004). This is a recent and very troubling development.

Rubella

The association of rubella infection in early pregnancy with congenital malformations in the infant was originally described by Norman Gregg following an outbreak of rubella in Australia in 1941 (Gregg 1941). Gregg reported that ocular defects and cardiac abnormalities occurred in the infants of women who had rubella infections in the first trimester of pregnancy. Subsequently, these findings have been confirmed during outbreaks in other countries. These studies defined the congenital rubella syndrome (CRS) among infants whose mother had been infected with rubella virus in the first trimester of pregnancy to include cataracts and other ocular abnormalities, cardiac defects, deafness, microcephaly, and mental retardation. Infants exposed during the first trimester had a risk of developing CRS of 90% or more. However, among infants exposed during the second trimester 20–40% developed isolated deafness.

These observations emphasized the importance of developing a rubella vaccine to prevent infections among pregnant women. In 1962 two groups of researchers, one at Harvard and the other at the Walter Reed Army Institute of Research, independently isolated the rubella virus in cell culture.

In 1964 a very large outbreak of rubella occurred in the USA with an estimate of over 30,000 cases of CRS and possibly five times that number of intrauterine infections leading to abortions. In 1969 three live attenuated vaccines were licensed in the United States: the HPV-77 (DE5 and DE12) vaccines and the Cendehill vaccine. In 1997 the RA22/3 vaccine was licensed. It is currently the only vaccine used in the USA.

The licensing of these rubella vaccines was critical for the eventual control and prevention of rubella. However, deciding on the most appropriate strategy for the use of these vaccines was complex and controversial. In the USA the decision was made to use the vaccine in all children as part of the routine immunization schedule. However, in several European countries and Israel the vaccine was targeted only to adolescent, pre-pubescent girls. The most important value of the vaccine was in preventing infections among pregnant women, since childhood rubella is usually a benign and self-limited disease. Immunizing girls before they begin sexual activity was believed to target the critical population. However, since the virus is primarily spread by school-aged children, targeting the younger population would indirectly decrease the risks of exposure of pregnant women by increasing the immunity among children and decreasing viral circulation in the population. In Europe and Israel epidemics of rubella continued during the period when only adolescent girls were immunized. In the USA epidemics of rubella were prevented but the proportion of pregnant women who remained susceptible was not affected initially. Furthermore, the development of an optimal strategy for the use of rubella vaccine was complicated by several factors. Since the rubella vaccines contained attenuated live virus, there was the theoretical concern that giving the vaccine to a woman who was in early pregnancy could lead to CRS. Therefore, the vaccine had to be used cautiously in adult women. Secondly, the immune response following the administration of the first vaccines that were licensed appeared to be inferior to that following natural rubella.

This raised concerns that immunized young children could become susceptible again to infection several years later when they were older after their immunity waned. Several mathematical models were reported to evaluate the short-term and long-term consequences of the various strategies for the use of rubella vaccine to prevent CRS (Knox 1980; Cooper 1985). These models helped evaluate the various vaccine strategies. Currently, rubella and CRS are rare in the USA and Europe. Between 1990 and 1999, 117 cases of CRS were reported. However, one-third of these cases occurred in two clusters in unimmunized religious communities (Mellinger *et al.* 1995; Robertson 2003). However, rubella and CRS are still common in developing countries that have not implemented rubella immunization programmes. These developing countries should now implement rubella immunization.

Measles

The measles virus was first isolated and propagated in cell culture by Enders and Peebles in 1954. Soon thereafter vaccines were developed, tested, and licensed. The initial measles vaccine was developed from a virus that had been passed in primary kidney cells followed by passage in primary human amnion cells and then adapted to chicken embryos. This vaccine was named the Edmonston B vaccine after the patient from whom the virus was originally isolated. This vaccine, along with another vaccine, which was adapted to dog kidney cells, were licensed in 1963. At about the same time a killed measles vaccine was licensed.

These vaccines were quite effective in producing immunity to infection with wild measles virus. However, the Edmonston B vaccine was associated with fever of 39.4°C (103°F) or greater in about 20–40% of recipients and a mild measles rash in 40–50% of recipients. However, the simultaneous administration of small dose of human immunoglobulin (0.02 ml/kg) reduced these reactions by 50% or more.

Another strategy for measles immunization involved the use of the formalin-inactivated killed measles vaccine (K), either in three doses (KKK) or as two does of killed vaccine followed by one dose of live vaccine (L), i.e. KKL. However, the use of killed measles vaccine was abandoned in 1967, after it was discovered that the use of this vaccine produced short-lived immunity. Even more troublesome was the occurrence of atypical measles from an exaggerated delayed hypersensitivity reaction upon exposure to wild measles a few years after immunization with the killed measles vaccine. The killed vaccine primed the immune system but failed to produce complete lasting immunity to the measles virus.

Subsequently the Edmonston B measles vaccine has been further attenuated by additional passages in various cell cultures to develop the Schwartz and Moraten vaccines. These vaccines are associated with much lower reaction rates and are widely used throughout the world at present in the global measles eradication campaign.

The experience with the various measles vaccines illustrated that post-licensing surveillance for adverse reactions and efficacy of new vaccines together with continued development of modified vaccines to improve safety and efficacy is often needed to develop an optimal vaccine strategy to prevent infections.

Analytical methods in outbreak investigation case–control studies

During the last several decades new techniques of data collection and analysis have been utilized frequently in the investigation and control of infectious disease outbreaks. In order to effectively control an outbreak of infectious disease detailed knowledge is needed concerning the important risk factors and exposures associated with infection. The information needed may not be evident initially but often becomes more apparent as the field investigation proceeds. Some outbreaks can be investigated using a retrospective cohort approach, if the entire population at risk is known. But often this information is not apparent initially, so a case–control method is used.

Case–control methods were initially utilized to study chronic diseases in order to efficiently determine aetiological factors when the disease was rare in the population. Sometimes, but not always, outbreaks of infectious diseases involve a small proportion of the population. Nevertheless, case–control methods often are useful in identifying the critical exposures associated with outbreaks of infectious diseases as well. Two examples of acute outbreaks in which multiple case–control studies were done to identify causal factors and control acute disease outbreaks will be discussed briefly, staphylococcal toxic shock syndrome and Reye syndrome:

Toxic shock syndrome

Staphylococcal toxic shock syndrome (TSS) was originally described in 1978 by Todd and colleagues in seven adolescents (Todd *et al.* 1978). The syndrome consisted of an acute febrile illness, with hypotension or shock, a scarlatiniform rash, and a multisystem illness with gastrointestinal, muscular, renal, and/or hepatic involvement. The rash desquamated 1–2 weeks after the acute illness. The patients had a localized infection with a phage group 1 *Staphylococcus aureus* and no other infection to explain the symptoms.

Subsequently, in early 1980, several young otherwise healthy women were seen at emergency rooms in Wisconsin and Minnesota with similar symptoms to those described by Todd that had onset during an otherwise normal menstrual period. Because cases of TSS continued to occur in menstruating women, a case definition was developed and cases were reported to the Health Department and CDC, so that case–control studies were done.

The first case–control study done by the Wisconsin State Health Department enrolled 35 cases of TSS who had onset during a menstrual period (Davis *et al.* 1980). Three controls per case (total = 105) were selected from the medical practice of several local physicians. Controls were females who had normal menses and were matched with the TSS cases by age ±2 years. Telephone interviews collected data on marital status, sexual activity, evidence of genital or sexually transmitted infection, duration and intensity of menses, use of contraceptives, patterns of tampon use, including the brand and duration of use of tampons.

The study found that TSS cases had used tampons more often (97%) than controls (76%) and more cases than controls had used oral contraceptives (*P* < 0.01). However, the types or brands of tampons used by TSS cases and controls weren't different; both cases and controls frequently used a 'highly absorbent' brand of tampons named 'Rely'.

Subsequent case–control studies were done by the CDC, since additional TSS cases were reported from these states and nationwide. The first CDC case–control study was done by telephone interviews from Atlanta. This study confirmed the Wisconsin data in that 100% of TSS cases and 80% of controls had used tampons, but in contrast with the Wisconsin study fewer cases than controls had used oral contraceptives.

A second CDC study was done between 1 July and 5 September 1980. This study enrolled 50 cases and 150 controls, who were nominated by the cases to participate in a telephone interview. Since this study only included cases who had occurred within an interval of a few months, the interviewers asked the women to check the label of the box from which tampons had been used most recently. The investigators were able to determine the brand of product and the lot and serial number. This study clearly implicated 'Rely' tampons, since 100% of cases used tampons and 83% of them used the 'Rely' brand. In contrast 75% of controls had used tampons but only 26% had used the 'Rely' brand. No particular lot number was involved in the outbreak.

Rely tampons had been introduced into the market in 1977 as 'super tampons' which were highly absorbent and more convenient to use, since they could remain in place for a longer

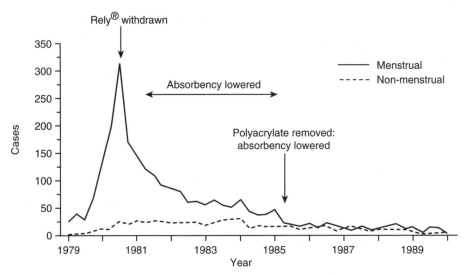

Fig. 21.1 Reported cases of toxic shock syndrome (includes only cases meeting the CDC case definition) by quarter—USA, 1 January 1979 to 31 March 1990. (Note that the use of trade names is for identification only and does not imply endorsement by the Public Health Service or the US Department of Health and Human Services.) Reproduced with permission from Belay *et al.* (1999). Copyright 1999 Massachusetts Medical Society.

period of time. They were made of more absorbent synthetic materials, including polyacrylate fibre, carboxymethyl cellulose, high-absorbency rayon-cellulose and polyester foam.

While these new tampons could absorb more menstrual blood, they also more frequently caused mucosal abrasions. Furthermore, they probably allowed growth of a larger number of microorganisms when they were left in place for a longer period of time. Women who were colonized with *S. aureus* containing the TSS plasmid were likely to develop symptoms if they used the highly absorbent tampons.

On 22 September the manufacturer removed these tampons from the market. During the next few years the absorbency of tampons were reduced and the syndrome of menses-related toxic shock syndrome virtually disappeared as a clinical entity (Fig. 21.1) (Centers for Disease Control 1990). However, occasional cases of TSS have been reported from wound infection, or infections at other sites with toxin-producing *S. aureus*. The control of these outbreaks of a new emerging disease, TSS, depended on the data from a series of case–control studies.

Reye syndrome

In 1963 Reye and colleagues from Australia described a clinical pathological condition consisting of acute encephalopathy and fatty degeneration of several visceral organs, especially the liver, following an acute febrile illness (Reye *et al.* 1963). These patients did not have inflammatory involvement of the brain or liver. Cerebral oedema and fatty changes in the liver were the major findings. The patients had elevated liver enzymes and ammonia levels and some had low blood glucose. There were no cells in the CSF but some had increased CSF pressure.

Subsequently, in 1963, an outbreak of Reye syndrome was reported following an outbreak of influenza B virus infection in North Carolina. In the decade following this outbreak increasing numbers of cases of Reye syndrome were reported in the USA, usually following outbreaks of influenza but occasionally associated with varicella outbreaks.

The CDC developed an epidemiological definition of Reye syndrome for surveillance purposes and the disease became officially reportable. The definition included acute non-inflammatory encephalopathy with microvesicular changes in the liver confirmed by biopsy or autopsy, or an elevation (three or more times the upper limit of normal) of liver enzymes (ALT, AST) or ammonia, they could not have CSF with elevated leucocytes (i.e. <8 WBCs/mm^3) and there were no other explanation for the symptoms.

The disease primarily occurred among adolescents who had been in normal health. Typically, an influenza illness occurred and 3–7 days after the illness the patient became obtunded, stuporous, or comatose and had evidence of fatty liver. Between 1974 and 1980, 400–500 cases were reported each year in the USA in association with influenza epidemics. This prompted several investigations to detect exposures among the Reye syndrome cases that differed from similar aged controls who were infected during the same influenza epidemic but had recovered without sequelae. The initial positive finding was reported by Starko *et al.* (1980) after an influenza outbreak in Arizona in 1978. Seven cases of Reye syndrome had all consumed aspirin for their influenza in comparison with only 50% of controls. The Reye syndrome in the cases was more severe among those who had taken more aspirin prior to their symptoms of Reye syndrome. However, the influenza did not appear to be more severe in the Reye syndrome cases than the controls.

This initial report evoked a great deal of scepticism, since aspirin had been available and used for febrile illnesses, including influenza, for nearly a century. Why should Reye syndrome suddenly appear to complicate the use of aspirin in 1978?

Nevertheless, several subsequent case–control studies were done among cluster of Reye syndrome cases following influenza epidemics in Michigan in 1979–80 and 1980–81, in Ohio in 1978–80 and by the Centers for Disease Control in 1985–86 (Hurwitz *et al.* 1985). All of these studies found a similar strong association between aspirin use for symptoms during outbreaks of influenza and Reye syndrome.

Consequently, the American Academy of Pediatrics recommended that their members advise their patients against the use of aspirin during influenza outbreaks and the Food and Drug Administration required aspirin manufacturers to add warning labels to their product about the dangers of the use aspirin for influenza symptoms among children and adolescents.

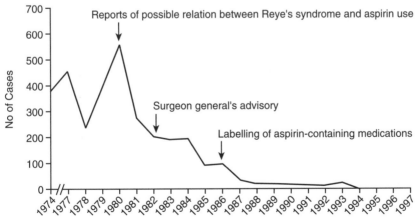

Fig. 21.2 Number of reported cases of Reye's syndrome in relation to the timing of public announcements of the epidemiological association of Reye's syndrome with aspirin ingestion and the labelling of aspirin-containing medications. Reproduced with permission from Belay *et al.* (1999). Copyright 1999 Massachusetts Medical Society.

Subsequently, there has been a dramatic reduction in the frequency of Reye syndrome cases in the USA in the last decade (Fig. 21.2; Belay *et al.* 1999). The pathogenesis of Reye syndrome is still unclear. Why the syndrome emerged as a health problem in the 1970s when aspirin had been used commonly for many decades before that is not apparent. Nevertheless, the use of aspirin for influenza does satisfy several of the Bradford Hill criteria for causality, namely (1) temporality, the exposure preceded the outcome, (2) the relative risk was high, (3) the association was consistently found in many studies and most important (4) reducing the exposure to aspirin has resulted in a dramatic reduction in the incidence of RS (Fig. 21.2).

The finding of a consistently strong association between Reye syndrome and aspirin in several case–control studies led to the successful efforts to prevent Reye syndrome in the USA, despite the fact that the exact pathogenesis of this condition remains obscure.

Recent advances in the recognition and investigation of outbreaks

Many advances have occurred in the investigation and control of outbreaks of infectious diseases in the past 10–15 years. Among these are improvements in surveillance so that infectious disease outbreaks can be recognized more quickly and quantified, evaluated, and controlled.

Surveillance

There are many examples of improved and integrated surveillance systems in the USA, Europe, and globally:

- ARBONET is a CDC surveillance system that contains all data on vector-borne viral infections in humans and animals and infected mosquitoes and birds. It was developed in 1999 to monitor the West Nile virus epidemic.

- FLUNET is a CDC surveillance system that monitors influenza activity, including respiratory morbidity, mortality, absenteeism, and virological data. It is linked with the Global Influenza Monitoring System of the World Health Organization.

- FoodNet is a collaborative surveillance project of CDC, seven state health departments, the US Department of Agriculture and the US Food and Drug Administration (FDA). It supports active surveillance and epidemiological investigation of food-borne illnesses in a catchment population of about 20 million persons in the USA.

- PulseNet is a laboratory-based programme of the CDC that supports the DNA fingerprint analysis, using pulse-field gel electrophoresis (PFGE), of pathogens associated with food-borne illness outbreaks in the FoodNet outbreaks.

- WHO-directed surveillance of influenza and other acute outbreaks of emerging infectious diseases has allowed the monitoring of outbreaks of infectious diseases, such as H5/N1 influenza, SARS coronavirus, Ebola, monkey pox, yellow fever, and many other emerging infections. The success of the WHO Infectious Diseases Surveillance System in identifying and monitoring outbreaks of infectious diseases has led to effective control efforts. The WHO surveillance system is now critically important in international health.

Molecular epidemiology

The use of molecular genetic studies to characterize microbial pathogens has increased dramatically since the mid-1990s. These methods have allowed the identification of pathogens, such as hepatitis C virus (Choo *et al.* 1989) and human herpes virus-8 (HHV-8) (Chang *et al.* 1994) which could not be readily grown in tissue culture.

Also the use of molecular methods to study outbreaks of disease has established the identity of organisms involved in an outbreak and a possible source. An example is an outbreak of diarrhoea from a chloramphenicol-resistant strain of *Salmonella newport* that contained a plasmid which could be traced from ill persons to hamburgers, contaminated beef, and ultimately to the farm, which had added chloramphenicol to the cattle feed as a growth stimulant (Spika *et al.* 1987). Restriction enzymes are now commonly used to study outbreaks and identify genetically related organisms from ill patients and environmental sources (Riley 2004).

Molecular epidemiology based methods were used to rapidly identify a unique Coronavirus (SARS-CO-V) as the aetiological agent of the SARS pandemic (Ksiazek *et al.* 2003). DNA finger-printing of *M. tuberculosis* isolates has been used to help link index and secondary cases and to distinguish active disease resulting from reactivation of a latent infection from recent transmission (Small *et al.* 1994). These studies have indicated that the proportion of active tuberculosis cases among adults that are from recent transmission is higher than was believed prior to the use of these molecular methods.

Likely developments of outbreak epidemiology in the future

It is probable that the frequency and diversity of infectious disease outbreaks will continue to grow in the future. The term 'emerging infectious diseases' has become a commonly used label for the growing diversity of infectious diseases. These new emerging diseases have arisen because of several factors including increased human travel, more frequent human–animal contact, AIDS, urban crowding, global warming, bioterrorism, and others.

In response it is likely that surveillance and communication will improve and the use of molecular methods to identify pathogens and host susceptibility will become more effective as well.

References

Ager EA, Nelson KE, Galton MN, Boring JR, and Jernigan JR (1967). Two outbreaks of egg-borne salmonellosis and implications for their prevention. *Journal of the American Medical Association*, **199**, 372–8.

Belay ED, Bresee JS, Holman RC, Khan AS, Shabriari A, and Schonberger LB (1999). Reye's syndrome in the United States from 1981 through 1997. *New England Journal of Medicine*, **340**, 1377–82.

Bruce Mg, Curtis MB, Payae MM, *et al.* (1999). Lake-associated outbreak of *Eschericia coli* O157:H7 in Clark County, Washington August 1999. *Archives of Pediatrics and Adolescent Medicine*, **157**, 1016–21.

Centers for Disease Control (1990). Reduced incidence of menstrual toxic-shock syndrome—United States, 1980–1990. *Morbidity and Mortality Weekly Report*, **39**, 421–3.

Chang Y, Cesarinam E, Pessin MS, *et al.* (1994). Identification of herpes-like DNA sequences in AIDS-associated Kaposi's sarcoma. *Science*, **266**, 1864–5.

Choo QL, Koo G, Weiner AJ, Overby CR, Bradley DW, and Houghten M (1989). Isolation of a cDNA clone derived from a blood borne non-A non-B viral hepatitis genome. *Science*, **244**, 351–62.

Cliver DO (1990). *Foodborne diseases*. Marcel Dekker, San Diego, CA.

Cooper LZ (1985). The history and medical consequences of rubella. *Reviews of Infectious Diseases*, **7**, S2–S10.

Davis JP, Chesney PJ, Wand PJ, and LaVenture M (1980). Toxic-shock syndrome: epidemiologic features, recurrence, risk factors and prevention. *New England Journal of Medicine*, **303**, 1429–35.

Gregg NM (1941). Congenital cataract following German measles in the mother. *Transactions of the Ophthalmological Society of Australia*, **3**, 35–46.

Hurwitz ES, Barrett MJ, Bregman D, *et al.* (1985). Public Health Service Study on Reye's syndrome and medication use. *New England Journal of Medicine*, **313**, 849–57.

Kew O, Morris-Glasgow V, Landavorde M, *et al.* (2002). Outbreak of poliomyelitis in Hispaniola associated with circulating type 1 vaccine-derived poliovirus. *Science*, **296**, 356–9.

Kew O, Wright P, Agol V, *et al.* (2004). Circulating vaccine-derived poliovirus: current state of knowledge. *Bulletin of the World Health Organization*, **82**, 16–23.

Knox EG (1980). Strategy for rubella vaccination. *International Journal of Epidemiology*, **9**, 13–23.

Ksiazek TG, Erdman D, Goldsmith CS, *et al.* (2003). A novel coronavirus associated with severe acute respiratory syndrome. *New England Journal of Medicine*, **348**, 1953–66.

Mellinger A, Cargan J, Akinson W, *et al.* (1995). High incidence of congenital rubella syndrome after a rubella outbreak. *Pediatric Infect. Dis Journal*, **14**, 573–8.

Nathanson N and Langmuir A (1963). The Cutter incident: poliomyelitis following formaldehyde-inactivated poliovirus vaccination in the United States during the spring of 1955. *American Journal of Epidemiology*, **78**, 27–81.

Nelson KE, Ager EA, Galton MM, Gillespie RNH, and Sulzer CR (1973). An outbreak of leptospirosis in Washington State. *American Journal of Epidemiology*, **98**, 336–47.

Nelson KE, Ager EA, Marks JR, and Emanuel I (1966). *Clostridium perfringens* food poisoning: report of an outbreak. *American Journal of Epidemiology*, **83**, 86–95.

Philbrook FR, MacCready R, van Rockel H, *et al.* (1960). Salmonellosis spread by a dietary supplement of avian source. *New England Journal of Medicine*, **263**, 713–18.

Reye RDK, Morgan G, and Baral J (1963). Encephalopathy and fatty degeneration of the viscera: a disease entity in childhood. *Lancet*, **2**, 749–52.

Riley LW (2004). *Molecular epidemiology of infectious diseases: principles and practice.* ASM Press. Washington, DC.

Robertson S (2003). Rubella and congenital rubella syndrome: global update. *Pan-American Journal of Public Health*, **14**, 306–15.

Sanders E, Sweeney FJ Jr, Friedman EA, Boring JR, Randall EL, and Polk LD (1963). An outbreak of hospital-association infections due to *Salmonella derby*. *Journal of the American Medical Association*, **186**, 984–6.

Small P, Hopewell P, Singh S, *et al.* (1994). The epidemiology of tuberculosis in San Francisco. *New England Journal of Medicine*, **330**, 1703–9.

Smith JL and Fratamico PM (1995). Factors involved in the emergence and persistence of food-borne diseases. *Journal of Food Protection*, **58**, 696–716.

Spika J, Waterman S, Soo Hoo G, *et al.* (1987). Chloramphenicol-resistant *Salmonella newport* traced through hamburger to dairy farms. *New England Journal of Medicine*, **31**, 565–70.

Starko KM, Ray CG, Dominguez CB, Stromberg WL, and Woodall DF (1980). Reye's syndrome and salicylate use. *Pediatrics*, **66**, 859–64.

Todd J, Fishant M, Kapral F, and Welch T (1978). Toxic-shock syndrome associated with phage-group 1 staphylococci. *Lancet*, **2**, 1116–18.

WHO Collaborative Study Group (1976). The relationship between persisting spinal paralysis and poliomyelitis vaccine (oral): result of a WHO inquiry. *Bulletin of the World Health Organization*, **53**, 319–31.

22

Data sources and their utilization

Manolis Kogevinas

Personal experiences

The 1970s were turbulent years for Greece. During my very first months in medical school, in 1973, I participated in the student revolt that was brutally suppressed by the Greek military junta. The years that followed the collapse of the totalitarian regime in 1974 were extremely creative and promoted solidarity and social consciousness, but were disastrous for our medical training: there is little opportunity for study at revolution time! As the situation became more normal, we had to seek solutions to our own lives rather than only finding solutions for society. Surprisingly, public health was not an option at that time, although for many of us this would have been a natural choice. There was no public health tradition in post-war Greece and modern epidemiology had only recently started through the work of Dimitri Trichopoulos. I started my training in oncology/radiotherapy knowing that that was not my world. During a short visit to a colleague at the London School of Hygiene, I discovered a new world of social determinants of disease. On my return I contacted Dimitri and worked mainly using routine statistics in Greece. I decided I needed formal training in epidemiology and went to the London School. After my MSc I did my doctoral thesis with Michael Marmot and John Fox on social inequalities in cancer. I frequently feel I started the wrong way round, examining general factors that affect disease as my first steps as an epidemiologist rather than starting from specific factors. Be that as it may, I still feel that this period of my first contact with epidemiology has marked my views and helped me preserve a wider perspective on health, society, and disease even at times when I am deeply engaged with molecular and genetic determinants of disease. I strongly believe that population-based research is the basis of our work and still enjoy giving lectures to my students on 'persons, times, and place'.

Mortality statistics remain the most widely available health data sources. The availability of adequate mortality data in more than 100 countries is without doubt the most important achievement of that last 50 years in the area of data sources. The second transforming achievement is linked to the development of the World Wide Web that signified the public availability of a rich variety of health-related information in populations. Connected to the latter is an extremely positive change among researchers in the last 10 years regarding the public availability of information and a willingness to share data. In this chapter I will first discuss the availability of diverse data sources and their use, and then discuss limitations, mistakes, and challenges for the future.

Availability and use of data sources

Mortality statistics are the most widely available health data and have increasingly become available to the World Health Organization (WHO). In 1970, 65 countries provided useable mortality data to the WHO, in 1999, 90 countries and in 2003, 115 countries (Mathers *et al.* 2005). This is a major achievement that allows an evaluation of global health and for many countries also time trends in disease. Even so, at the end of 2003 data on death registration were not available for 77 countries and less systematic health data sources have to be used to estimate disease occurrence over wide parts of the world. Currently most of the countries in Europe have adequate mortality data, while only 10% of the countries in Africa provide these data. An analysis by WHO researchers found that among the 115 countries with recent mortality data, only 64 were considered as having essentially complete registration. Although death registration is still not complete in major countries such as China and India, enough partial data are available to derive valid estimates of the total number of deaths and of the distribution by cause. A second problem is the quality of registration and the use of ill-defined codes. These are widely used even in European countries with well-developed death certification systems. Finally the use of different coding systems may accentuate differences in registration between countries. Approximately 40 countries are coding death certificates using the ICD9 system that is considerably different from ICD10 that was implemented in 1993 and that is currently used by about 75 countries (see Chapter 5).

There exist a wide variety of systematic data sources on morbidity. Cancer registries are the most complete data source on morbidity at the international level (Terracini and Zanetti 2003). The International Agency for Research on Cancer (IARC) has systematically collected and published information from cancer registries applying specific quality criteria and regularly publishes data in the series 'Cancer incidence in five continents' (Parkin *et al.* 2002). The eighth edition of 'Cancer incidence in five continents' includes information from approximately 200 cancer registries (www-dep.iarc.fr/). The distribution by continent is unequal. While North America, Oceania, and Western and Central Europe have excellent coverage, there are large areas of the world with no population-based registries. In Africa, for example, there are 13 registries in nine countries covering a small part of the population. Twenty countries, mostly in Europe, have national registries. Most cancer registries are regional but the combination of incidence data, national mortality data, and modelling allows the estimation of valid figures on national cancer incidence rates (GLOBOCAN 2002, Ferlay 2004). The basic information collected in all registries includes demographics and tumour information.

Numerous other systematic data sources on morbidity data include congenital malformations registers, registers of respiratory or other specific diseases, general household surveys, etc. EUROCAT is among the largest international initiatives and is a European network of population-based registries for the epidemiological surveillance of congenital anomalies that started in 1979 (Fig. 22.1). More than 1.5 million births (29% of the European birth population) are surveyed per year in Europe from 43 registries in 20 countries (www.eurocat.ulster.ac.uk/index.html). Several countries have developed random population surveys such as the General Household Survey in England and Wales. Probably the largest population survey is the National Health and Nutrition Examination Survey (NHANES) in the USA (www.cdc.gov/nchs/nhanes.htm). NHANES has been in existence since the early 1960s and has surveyed over 130,000 people. Similar to other surveys it has developed and includes the collection of biological samples determining, for example, levels of lead, apart from collecting questionnaire information. Apart from the main research instruments and objectives, information on specific items, for example a vision exam, is requested in different surveys. The availability of subsequent surveys allows the evaluation of time trends using comparable methods. Figure 22.2 shows the development of obesity in children of different ages in three consecutive NHANES surveys. An extremely important characteristic of most of these surveys is the free access to the data that has permitted multiple uses.

The WHO and other international organizations have done an impressive effort to compile health-related data on the web. A wide variety of data are available on all type of diseases, such as the WHO's Communicable Disease Global Atlas that brings together standardized data and statistics for infectious diseases at country, regional, and global levels (www.who.int/globalatlas/default.asp). The Cochrane Collaboration (www.cochrane.org/index0.htm) produces and disseminates systematic reviews of health-care interventions and promotes the search for evidence in the form of clinical trials and other studies of interventions. The major product of the

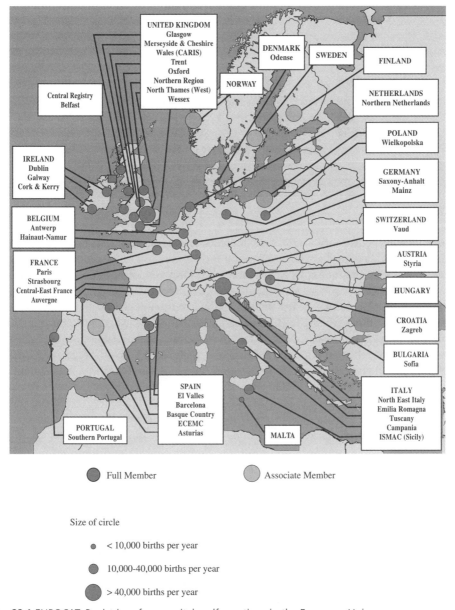

Fig. 22.1 EUROCAT. Registries of congenital malformations in the European Union.

collaboration is the Cochrane Database of Systematic Reviews which is published quarterly. Extensive information is available on health indicators and health services in all areas of the world such as data provided for developing countries on population, health, and nutrition programmes by 'MEASURE DHS' (www.measuredhs.com/countries/start.cfm). Finally there exists a whole universe of information on lifestyle, environment, and any potential risk factor such as air-pollution registers (www.emep.int/index.html), contraceptive use, and more generally sexual behaviour (www.un.org/esa/population/publications/contraceptive2003/wcu2003.htm),

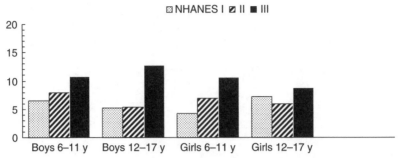

Fig. 22.2 Age-adjusted prevalence (per cent) of overweight boys and girls (>95th percentile body mass index (BMI)-for-age) by age from three consecutive surveys (NHANES I to III, USA) (www.cdc.gov/nchs/products/pubs/pubd/hestats/overwght99.htm).

use of swimming pools (www.swimmersguide.com/), disasters such as fires (Fig. 22.3) and innumerable others. Many of these data sources on the web contain unique information but are frequently lacking a report on completeness and validity of the reported information.

The late 1990s, and particularly the twenty-first, century brought the revolution in genetic research and the establishment of vast publicly available sources of genetic data. The largest data sources are by far those relating to DNA sequence variation. Following the publication of the Human Genome Project the scientific community has witnessed the establishment of numerous Web resources for genetic and medical information. Websites with genetic information include generic ones such as OMIM (Online Mendelian Inheritance in Man) that is a catalogue of human genes and genetic disorders. Similar to other related sites it contains textual information and references and multiple links (www.ncbi.nlm.nih.gov/entrez/query.fcgi?db=OMIM). There exist numerous specific databases on nearly every single disease such as the SNP500Cancer of the NCI that is specifically designed to generate resources for the identification and characterization

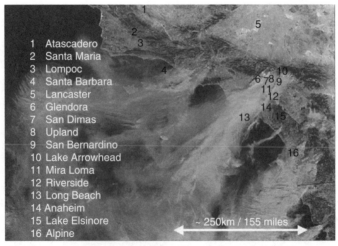

Fig. 22.3 Satellite image of south California taken on 24 October 2003 showing the smoke plumes from numerous fires. Locations of the 16 communities participating in the fire study are highlighted (Kuenzli, 2006) University of Southern California Children's Health Study).

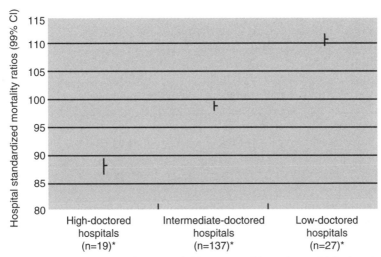

Fig. 22.4 Hospital standardized mortality ratios (with 99% confidence intervals) for hospitals and areas in England and Wales with low, medium, and high staffing levels of doctors (from Jarman *et al.* 1999. *British Medical Journal*, **318**, 1515–20).

of genetic variation in genes important in cancer (snp500cancer.nci.nih.gov/home_1.cfm) or the p53 mutations register at IARC (www-p53.iarc.fr/index.html).

Vast data sets of hospital in- or outpatient data are available in many industrialized countries. Even though these data are mainly concerned with administration they have been extensively used for health services research and to a lesser extent for aetiological research. For example, hospital inpatient mortality in England (www.hesonline.nhs.uk) was examined to determine which factors best explain the variation in hospital death ratios (Jarman *et al.* 1999). It was found that among the best predictors of hospital death rates were the number of hospital doctors per bed and of general practitioners per head of population (Fig. 22.4). In this analysis eight million discharges from NHS hospitals were used together with other routine statistics. The hospital episode statistics database form includes information on every inpatient spell in NHS hospitals in England. Each spell includes information on a patient's age, sex, postcode of residence, primary diagnosis, and up to six additional coded subdiagnoses, type of admission (emergency or elective), and length of stay. General practitioner (GP) data, for example in the UK, or prescription data, as for Medicare in the USA (www.medicare.gov/) are computerized and constitute large, population-based, data sets that are available over time. Information in these data sets is publicly available and has multiple applications such as free use by the public to evaluate performance indicators, use for health services research such as evaluating the costs and effectiveness of medical interventions (Dubinsky and Ferguson 1990), or use in aetiological research to evaluate, for example, cardiac failure. The availability of these population rosters, such as those provided by the Centers for Medicare & Medicaid Services, allows them to be used to select random population samples for cohort and cross-sectional studies or to selection of population controls in case–control studies. Similar to other data sources that are not primarily collected for research purposes, these data need critical scrutiny but their availability in computerized form makes them attractive. Users of these data should take particular care to carefully examine changes in data collection protocols such as organizational changes in GP data, the adoption of new coding schemes, and data quality problems that are often year specific.

A related issue is the availability of public data sources that include descriptions, data, and results from specific studies such as the birth cohorts website (www.birthcohorts.net) or the database from the Survey of Health, Ageing and Retirement in Europe (SHARE). This latter is a large cross-national database on health, socio-economic status, and social and family networks and, similar to an increasing number of studies, the organizers have a free access policy regarding use of their data (www.share-project.org/index.php?page=Home&menue=1&sub=). Among the largest data sources with results from specific studies are those associating DNA sequence variation with disease or with specific traits. This type of evidence is growing exponentially and there are serious problems with availability (due to selective reporting) and systematic accessibility to these data. Several initiatives have been taken to systematically report results from genetic association studies. The most well known initiative in epidemiology is the Human Genome Epidemiology Network (HuGENet), a global collaboration of individuals and organizations committed to the assessment of the impact of variation of the human genome on population health and how genetic information can be used to improve health and prevent disease which intends to systematize information on genetics and health (http://www.cdc.gov/genomics/hugenet/). Aware of the acute problem of systematic access to evidence, HuGENet is sponsoring a network of Investigator Networks that will publish guidelines and develop literature databases with published and unpublished data including negative studies etc.

Epidemiological and statistical methodology: their development and application in the analysis of routine statistics

The analysis of routine statistics was based for several decades on the application of standard approaches such as direct and indirect standardization, or proportional mortality. For a long period these methods were also applied in aetiological research and particularly occupational epidemiology or studies examining social inequalities (Registrar General 1978) (see Chapter 16). Retrospective cohort studies, particularly in occupational epidemiology, made extensive use of mortality statistics and the calculation of standardized mortality ratios (SMRs) was the standard approach in studies on occupational cancer. The 1970s was also a time of extensive use of ecological studies and the development of studies on migrant populations. These studies provided clues on disease causation, for example the causes of stomach and colon cancer or the effects of cultural factors on myocardial infarction. The 1980s brought the development, and with the availability of computer power, the wide use of more elaborate statistical methods such as Poisson regression. Mortality and population statistics were still used to calculate SMRs and direct standardized rates but more advanced techniques allowed modelling of data. Among the most influential books in the development of statistical analysis have been the ones by Breslow and Day (1980, 1987). The 1980s also saw the development of new methods for examining time trends, and specifically the age–period–cohort methods for evaluation of temporal trends (Osmond and Gardner 1982). An evaluation of time trends by age, period, or cohort was not new. The publication of Wade Hampton Frost in 1939 on age and time trends for tuberculosis mortality was probably the first that directed attention to the analysis of cohort effects. However, the age–period–cohort models combined the three variables in one single model. These models are now accepted as a standard tool and their limitations, particularly the problems of identification (produced by the fact that two of the time variables may predict the third one), have been well discussed (Clayton and Schifflers 1987).

The uses of routine statistics to evaluate geographical differences have developed with regard to both graphical representation (mapping) and the statistical approach for the analysis of these differences. More information has become available, and maps with the geographical distribution

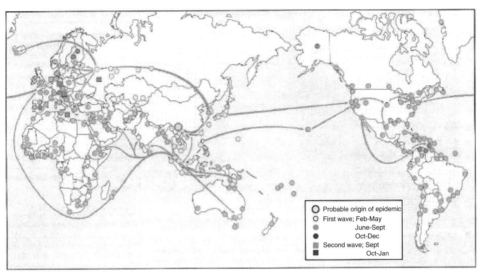

Fig. 22.5 Origin and spread of the 'Asian flu' pandemic. Global sequence of spread of the 1957–58 pandemic is shown by vectors indicating the month when the first cases appeared in each location. (Source: WHO archives; Cliff A, Haggett P, and Smallman-Raynor M (2004). *World atlas of epidemic diseases*. Hodder Arnold, London.)

of disease for wide areas of the world and for many distinct diseases have been produced. Among the most cited ones are the maps produced by the National Institutes of Health (NIH)/National Cancer Institute (NCI) on cancer mortality in the USA and those produced by the IARC on cancer mortality in Europe. Extensive maps are available of the distribution of infectious diseases and epidemics (Fig. 22.5; Cliff *et al.* 2004). The discussion about how to represent rates resulted in a more comprehensive approach that took into account the size of the differences and statistical significance. The problem of small numbers due to mapping of smaller areas led to the application of techniques that deal with random variation. Bayesian approaches were applied taking into account the proximity of different areas when modelling disease (Best *et al.* 2005; Viik-Kajander *et al.* 2003).

A significant development in comparing health and disease between regions of the world and different countries was the use of disability adjusted life years (DALYs). Alternative measures of disease estimated from mortality data such as person years of life lost (PYLL) have been used since the early years. PYLL measures the occurrence of a death taking into account the age when death occurred. More weight is put on deaths occurring at young ages than those occurring at older ages. DALYs are the sum of life years lost due to premature mortality and years lived with disability adjusted for severity. They are therefore time-based health outcome measures that include weights for years of life lost and time spent in less than perfect health. The value choices incorporated into DALYs are arbitrary. For example in the Global Burden of Disease (GBD) study (Murray and Lopez 1997), severity weights on a scale of 0 (perfect health) to 1 (death) were assigned to each of the 483 disabling sequelae examined. The application of DALYs allowed the evaluation of the importance of diseases that are not necessarily fatal. In the GBD study, communicable, maternal, perinatal, and nutritional disorders explained 44% of DALYs worldwide; the remainder were non-communicable causes 41%, of which injuries 15%, malignant neoplasms 5%, neuropsychiatric conditions 11%, and cardiovascular conditions 10%. The application of this methodology allowed the recognition of the substantial burden of neuropsychiatric disorders and injuries worldwide. However, their use has also significant limitations, mainly due to their subjective nature and the arbitrary value choices they incorporate.

The 1990s saw a promotion of use of ecological data (Susser 1994) and, connected to this, of multilevel modelling (Diez-Roux 2004). This responded to the evaluation of the importance of societal values for the occurrence of disease that could not be explained just by the analysis of individual characteristics. The idea that community variables are important for the occurrence of disease in individuals was not new. It had been presented in another context by Geoffrey Rose when discussing the concepts of sick individuals and sick populations. The new interest in eco-logical or group-level variables has been applied in several fields including studies on income inequality and neighbourhood characteristics. The availability of accessible statistical techniques allowed the simultaneous evaluation of both group-level and individual-level predictors of health. This type of analysis is now regularly applied.

Finally a recent development is the new statistical techniques necessary to analyse population-based genetics. Concepts that had been discussed extensively in the past, such as the occurrence of chance findings in epidemiological studies and the use of P-values (Rothman 1990) had to be discussed again. The identification of a high proportion of false positive findings in genetic asso-ciation studies (Ioannidis *et al.* 2001) led to the application of techniques that were not new, such as Bayesian approaches, but that had not been mainstream in the past. The availability of huge amounts of genetic data that lead to multiple comparisons and evaluation of even more interac-tions leads to totally new approaches aimed at overcoming the limitations of classical statistical methods such as logistic regression (Thornton-Wells *et al.* 2004). These types of analyses (non-parametric or other) are still under development and include an important graphical component to visualize results.

Mistakes and missed opportunities

One of the classical 'mistakes' when examining descriptive statistics such as geographical data is the temptation to over-interpret the data and identify specific causes for small deviations in disease risk. In most diseases we do not understand and cannot predict geographical or temporal variations of disease rates, unless the exposure is a major determinant of the disease (such as socio-economic status and mortality or tobacco and lung cancer) or if exposure, even if not prevalent, is associated with a specific disease entity (such as wood dust and adenocarcinomas of sinuses or asbestos and mesothelioma or Epstein–Barr virus and Burkitt's lymphoma in Africa). At best, some risk factors can be shown to contribute to the geographical distribution of disease, but rarely can we explain population patterns of diseases through specific factors. 'Minor' devia-tions are frequently attributed to environmental exposures that can rarely be identified. A recent example comes from the studies evaluating breast cancer in Long Island, New York. Increased breast cancer incidence in that area was attributed to environmental exposures such as pesticides. Despite extensive research efforts, the specific causes of the increased breast cancer risk in that area were not identified (Winn 2005). It is frequently perceived that presentation of descriptive statistics should be accompanied by an explanation of the deviances observed. Descriptive statistics, however, have their own value and are useful for monitoring disease, planning health services or other interventions, and producing new hypotheses.

The extensive use of SMRs for aetiological research should be considered among the 'mistakes' associated with the use of routine statistics. The use of SMRs has several advantages concern-ing availability of rates and, hence, facility of application, and statistical advantages (Breslow and Day 1987). However, SMRs were adequate methods in the past since many of the risks evalu-ated were high and 'minor' biases associated with the use of SMRs were not important.

However, inherent problems of bias when using routine mortality data become important when examining smaller risks.

Public health authorities in some countries consider the frequent and substantive modifications of the codes of the International Classification of Diseases (ICD) to be a mistake. The use of the ICD intends to provide a standard way of recording underlying cause of death and comparing cause of death data over time and across countries. Several revisions have had substantive changes and comparisons should be done with caution. For example, ICD10 includes about 10,000 conditions for classifying causes of death compared to around 5100 in ICD9. In addition the rules for selecting the underlying cause of death have been re-evaluated. An example of the influence of changes in coding when examining time trends in mortality from pneumonia and influenza is shown in Fig. 22.6 (Dushoff *et al.* 2006). In 2003, 75 countries used ICD10 while around 40 countries still reported data using the ninth revision of ICD. Biases when doing time or place comparisons do not depend, however, solely in the use of different codes. Accuracy in diagnosing causes of death varies by country, and differences also occur in the process of coding underlying causes of death. A particular problem is the significant variations in the use of coding categories for unknown and ill-defined causes.

Current preoccupations are probably associated with one of the major missed opportunities in the use of descriptive statistics and of population-based research. Recent developments in genetics and molecular techniques have had a negative 'collateral' effect on public health research including the development and use of population-based research. Without much scrutiny of what we may gain from their massive application—the gains are not immediate—much attention and money

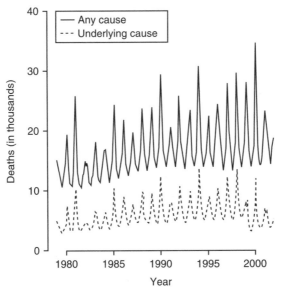

Fig. 22.6 Reported pneumonia and influenza deaths (deaths in thousands), by underlying cause and by multiple causes, USA, 1979–2001.The sharp drop in underlying pneumonia and influenza deaths in 1999 is due to the change in coding under the International Classification of Diseases system from the ninth revision to the tenth revision. In general, the series that consider multiple causes are expected to be less sensitive to changes in coding methodologies. (Reproduced with permission from: Dushoff J, Plotkin JB, Viboud C, Earn DJD, and Simonsen L (2006). Mortality due to influenza in the United States: An annualized regression approach using multiple-cause mortality data. *American Journal of Epidemiology*, **163**, 181–7.)

nevertheless go to genetics and molecular biology, which results in the abandonment of crucial areas of research including public health research. The examination of, for example, migrant populations was popular in the past but has fallen into disuse in recent years. Early studies examined migrants from populations from the large migratory movements from the Indian subcontinent to the UK, south Europeans to Australia, and Japanese to the USA. The loss of interest in this field is ironic since recent decades have seen massive migration from Africa to Europe, South and Central America to North America and Europe, and Southeast Asia to Australia and also massive migrations within the continents and within countries.

The applications of findings from routine statistics to prevention and disease control

Analysis of data sources such as geographical and temporal differences in disease rates has led to the development of new hypotheses, for example the decrease of mortality from stomach cancer, the association of air pollution and asthma in east–west Germany, and studies of Epstein–Barr virus and Burkitt's lymphoma in Africa. However, with a few exceptions of major risk factors (e.g. tobacco and lung cancer) or very specific associations (e.g. asbestos and mesothelioma), established risk factors do not adequately explain most geographical or temporal differences in disease rates (e.g. differences in atopy and asthma within and between countries). The analysis of temporal trends such as the increasing incidence but decreasing mortality of breast cancer or decreasing mortality from myocardial infarction have led to a better evaluation of the efficiency of preventive and therapeutic interventions and to a better understanding of the causes of diseases. Surveillance systems such as SWORD (McDonald *et al.* 2005) or large population-based surveys such as NHANES have led to better control of selected occupational diseases or led to a better understanding of modern epidemics such as childhood and adult obesity.

Major 'drivers' of epidemiological endeavours in the development and use of routine statistics and other data sources (Table 22.1)

The systematic collection and analysis of routine mortality records was first done in England and Wales about 150 years ago by pioneering medical statisticians such as Farr, Ogle, and Tatham. The expansion of the collection of mortality statistics and of disease registers, and particularly cancer registries, in the post-Second World War era should probably be regarded as the major drivers of epidemiological endeavours of the last 50 years. The availability of a wide variety of information on health-related issues on the Web has been without any doubt the most important development during the last decade regarding the availability and use of data sources.

Table 22.1 Major 'drivers' of epidemiological endeavours in the development and use of routine statistics and other data sources

Expansion of mortality statistics worldwide and improvement in quality of certification
Development of disease registers
Development of statistical and graphical techniques
Development of record linkage studies including small-area statistics
Availability of a wide variety of data on the Web, including genetic information
Change in attitude among researchers concerning public availability and sharing of data

The most important development of the last 50 years has been the development of valid population and mortality statistics in all industrialized countries and in most developing countries. These statistics existed and were (more or less) valid from the beginning of the twentieth century in several countries, but we frequently forget that valid mortality data were not available as late as the 1950s or 1960s even in many European countries. For example in Greece, in the late 1950s, about a quarter of death certificates did not have an underlying cause of death. When examining long-term time trends in mortality spanning a period of around 100 years it is not surprising to see that the figures quoted are actually very few: the classical cancer mortality trends in the USA showing the dramatic increase in lung cancer and decrease in stomach cancer, or the time trends in overall mortality in England and Wales some Scandinavian and a few more countries.

A major development of disease registers for cancer, congenital malformations, asthma, and others took place in many countries in the 1970s and even more so in the 1980s. Until quite recently, knowledge of patterns of disease in many parts of the world was based mainly on the work of clinicians. Clinical and pathological case series frequently constituted the only available data source in the 1950s and 1960s, but comparisons based upon relative frequency of different diseases in case series can be biased. Incidence rates derived from population-based registries were necessary to evaluate differences in risk between populations. These, together with the development of the mortality statistics that occurred earlier, provided an extensive body of information that had not previously existed. Most of these statistics became available in industrialized countries first, but data also started being collected in newly developed countries and some developing countries. There is still, however, a lack of morbidity statistics in large parts of the world. Characteristically IARC's eighth edition of 'Cancer incidence in five continents' includes data from nearly all industrialized countries. In Africa there are eight regional registries in the last edition of IARC's publication (Fig. 22.7) but only data for three of them have been available for a fairly long period of time.

The lack of routinely collected data to evaluate efficiently and quickly the occurrence of clusters or epidemics became evident following television reports of a cluster of childhood leukaemia near the Sellafield nuclear plant in northwest England. An extensive application of small-area statistics was first proposed as a proactive measure following the leukaemia cluster observed in Seascale, a village close to the plant (the Black Report 1984). This approach has been very important and influential in promoting the need for adequate surveillance and quick response systems but has probably been less successful in generating plausible new hypotheses (Kogevinas and Pearce 2005). There are several reasons why few, if any, risk factors have been identified by applying such approaches. Firstly, many of the environmental exposures examined in relation to cancers and reproductive outcomes such as congenital malformations are probably not associated with high risks at common environmental levels of exposure. Secondly, such studies involve a relatively high misclassification of the risk factor(s) of interest and of potential confounders. Finally, many of the hypotheses examined are frequently based on weak *a priori* evidence and are unlikely to be correct. Nevertheless, small-area-based approaches are becoming more attractive, as methods evolve, both with regard to the availability of records and methods of statistical analysis. The availability through the Web of a wide spectrum of exposure and health information has allowed the wide application of geographic information system (GIS) methodology. GIS allows the analysis of large volumes of spatially referenced information. It is still too early to examine the validity of many of the findings based on GIS but undoubtedly these data together with individually based records will help promote more complete studies, at least concerning environmental exposures.

An important development that is limited to a few countries has been linkage of records that allows the combination of individual information linking several registers such as birth, migration, death, hospitalizations, or cancer incidence. Among the pioneering studies is the

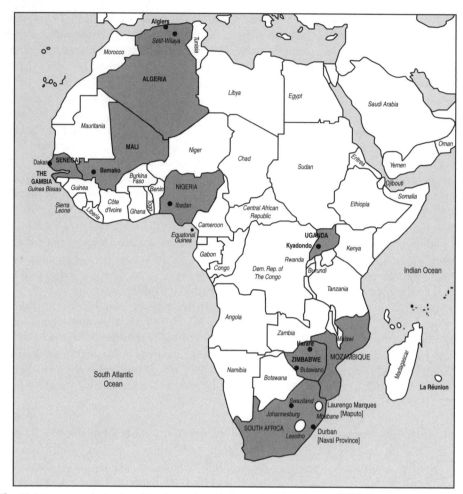

Fig. 22.7 Cancer registries in Africa (www.iarc.fr). Reproduced with permission from IARC.

Longitudinal Study in England and Wales (Fox and Goldblatt 1982) that linked records of half a million people and provided extensive information on health inequalities using a wealth of information on socio-economic status such as education, house ownership, house amenities, and others. Further development of record linkage has been carried out in Nordic countries in Europe opening up possibilities for the conduct of prospective analyses such as those based on the Swedish Cancer-Environment Register (Wiklund and Eklund 1986) used for studies on occupational cancer. Follow-up for mortality and other outcomes such as cancer incidence is close to 100% and linkage involves a wide variety of registers. Health-related registers include a wealth of information such as cancer registries, hospital in-patient registers, data on birth outcomes, and even specialized information such as data on cerebral palsy or infantile autism (Olsen *et al.* 2001). The difference between the Nordic countries and most other countries is not only the availability of the registers but also the possibility of reliable linkage between them.

In the last decade, the two most important developments regarding data sources and their use are the availability of public information on the World Wide Web and the change in attitude among researchers concerning the public availability of data. This latter change in attitude follows closely the development of the Web but also the increasing understanding among epidemiologists of the need for collaborative research to achieve solid conclusions. The promotion by the European Union of funds for collaborative biomedical research has undoubtedly contributed to this. The need for collaborative research has become even more obvious in the areas of genetics, and several innovative and ambitious initiatives have been in this field. The development of the web has created new needs concerning the identification of data sources and their use. Among the main challenges today is not so much the public availability of data but rather the high degree of heterogeneity of the information available in any specific area. This is particularly the case for genetic resources, and the difficulties in summarizing information have been extensively discussed. Finally, an important issue when examining Web-based data sources is the frequent lack of explicit reports on the methods followed for the collection of the data, the completeness of this information, and a discussion of limitations of the data source. The twenty-first century undoubtedly provides new horizons regarding the availability and use of data sources. Our knowledge of health and disease will certainly be greatly enhanced if use of this immense amount of information is made through the application of solid epidemiological principles.

References

Best N, Richardson S, and Thomson A (2005). A comparison of Bayesian spatial models for disease mapping. *Australian and New Zealand Journal of Medicine*, **14**, 35–59.

Black D (1984). *Investigation of the possible increased incidence of cancer in West Cumbria. Report of the Independent Advisory Group*. HMSO, London.

Breslow NE and Day NE (1980). *Statistical methods in cancer research. Volume I: The analysis of case–control studies*, IARC Scientific Publications No 32. IARC, Lyon.

Breslow NE and Day NE (1987). *Statistical methods in cancer research. Volume II: The design and analysis of cohort studies*, IARC Scientific Publications No 82. IARC, Lyon.

Clayton D and Schifflers E (1987). Models for temporal variation in cancer rates. II: Age-period-cohort models. *Statistics in Medicine*, **6**, 469–81.

Cliff A, Haggett P, and Smallman-Raynor M (2004). *World atlas of epidemic diseases*. Hodder Arnold, London.

Cordell HJ and Clayton DG (2005). Genetic association studies. *Lancet*, **366**, 1121–31.

Diez Roux AV (2004). The study of group-level factors in epidemiology: rethinking variables, study designs, and analytical approaches. *Epidemiologic Reviews*, **26**, 104–11.

Dubinsky M and Ferguson JH (1990). Analysis of the National Institutes of Health Medicare coverage assessment. *International Journal of Technology Assessment in Health Care*, **6**, 480–8.

Dushoff J, Plotkin JB, Viboud C, Earn DJD, and Simonsen L (2006). Mortality due to influenza in the United States: An annualized regression approach using multiple-cause mortality data. *American Journal of Epidemiology*, **163**, 181–7.

Ferlay J, Bray F, Pisani P, and Parkin DM (2004). *GLOBOCAN 2002: cancer incidence, mortality and prevalence worldwide*, IARC Cancerbase No 5, version 2.0. IARC Press, Lyon.

Fox AJ and Goldblatt PO (1982). *1971–1975 Longitudinal Study: socio-demographic mortality differentials*, LS Series 1. The Stationery Office, London.

Frost WH (1939). The age selection of mortality from tuberculosis in successive decades. *American Journal of Hygiene*, **30**, 91–6.

Ioannidis JP, Ntzani EE, Trikalinos TA, and Contopoulos-Ioannidis DG (2001). Replication validity of genetic association studies. *Nature Genetics*, **29**, 306–9.

Jarman B, Gault S, Alves B, et al. (1999). Explaining differences in English hospital death rates using routinely collected data. BMJ, **318**, 515–20.

Kogevinas M and Pearce N (2005). Geographically based approaches can identify environmental causes of disease. *Journal of Epidemiology and Community Health*, **59**, 717–18.

Kunzli N, Arol E, Wu J, *et al.* (2006). Health effects of the 2003 Southern California wildfires on children. *Americal Journal of Respiratory Critical Care Medicine*, **174**, 1221–8.

Mathers CD, Fat DM, Inoue M, Rao C, and Lopez AD (2005). Counting the dead and what they died from: an assessment of the global status of cause of death data. *Bulletin of the World Health Organization*, **83**, 171–7.

McDonald JC, Chen Y, Zekveld C, and Cherry NM (2005). Incidence by occupation and industry of acute work related respiratory diseases in the UK, 1992–2001. *Clinics in Occupational and Environmental Medicine*, **62**, 836–42.

Murray CJ and Lopez AD (1997). Global mortality, disability, and the contribution of risk factors: Global Burden of Disease Study. *Lancet*, **349**, 1436–42.

Olsen J, Melbye M, Olsen SF, *et al.* (2001). The Danish National Birth Cohort–its background, structure and aim. *Scandinavian Journal of Public Health*, **29**, 300–7.

Osmond C and Gardner MJ (1982). Age, period and cohort models applied to cancer mortality rates. *Statistics in Medicine*, **1**, 245–59.

Parkin DM, Whelan SL, Ferlay J, Teppo L, and Thomas DB (2002). *Cancer incidence in five continents*, Vol. VIII, IARC Scientific Publications No 155. IARC, Lyon.

Registrar General (1978). *Occupational mortality, the Registrar General's Decennial Supplement for England and Wales, 1970–72*, Series DS 1. The Stationery Office, London.

Rothman KJ (1990). No adjustments are needed for multiple comparisons. *Epidemiology*, **1**, 43–6.

Susser M (1994). The logic in ecological: I. The logic of analysis. *American Journal of Public Health*, **84**, 825–9.

Terracini B and Zanetti R (2003). A short history of pathology registries, with emphasis on cancer registries. *Sozial- und Präventivmedizin*, **48**, 3–10.

Thornton-Wells TA, Moore JH, and Haines JL (2004). Genetics, statistics and human disease: analytical retooling for complexity. *Trends in Genetics*, **20**, 640–7.

Viik-Kajander M, Moltchanova E, Salomaa V, *et al.* and the FINMONICA AMI Register Study Group (2003). Geographical variation in the incidence of acute myocardial infarction in eastern Finland—a Bayesian perspective. *Nature Reviews Cancer*, **35**, 43–50.

Wiklund K and Eklund G (1986). Reliability of record linkage in the Swedish Cancer-Environment Register. *Acta Radiologica Oncology*, **25**, 11–14.

Winn DM (2005). Science and society: the Long Island Breast Cancer Study Project. *Nature Reviews Cancer*, **5**, 986–94.

23

Development of modern epidemiology: clinical epidemiology

Richard F. Heller

Personal experiences

In days long ago, you could be a pre-medical medical student. At Charing Cross Hospital Medical School in London, we had some special lectures to keep us interested in our ultimate goal of becoming doctors. Sidney Chave inspired me about the importance of the population approach, I can't exactly remember how, but I guess it was the Broad Street pump. My father was a chest physician, and I thought to do a research project in my spare time on the uptake of smoking by schoolchildren (of which I had only recent been one—a schoolchild, not a smoker!). Jerry Morris and his colleague Martin Gardner advised me, and I was lucky enough to get a non-randomized before/after study published as a medical student (as well as a not very systematic literature review). Inspired by them and the subject, I planned an epidemiological career.

On graduation, I found that I really enjoyed clinical practice. It was not something learned as a medical student, I just liked talking to people, being part of a team that attempted to understand the cause of a clinical problem, and to help find some way of making the person feel better. The cut and thrust of clinical practice attracted me, and the appeal of the immediacy has never left me (nor has its fear).

When I explained this to my early mentors, they put me in touch with Geoffrey Rose who was advertising a job. This allowed me to have epidemiological training while continuing clinical skills development. Both Geoffrey and Stan Peart at St Mary's Hospital in London encouraged me to maintain this dual approach, which I could continue throughout my training. Walter Holland, with whom I then worked, was sceptical about the advisability of combining the clinical and population approaches, but was always supportive and has done much to build bridges between clinical and public health professionals. The combination of epidemiology and clinical practice which I was able to maintain has allowed a fantastically interesting and varied career in the UK, Australia, and a number of international settings.

As a wise clinician once said to me, many years ago, 'When the epidemiologist gets involved in therapeutics, the wise man takes to the hills'. I have used this as a theme previously, in an attempt to show how misguided was this statement from an otherwise intelligent individual. Now I think further, maybe he was not so wrong! In fact, he misjudged the contribution that epidemiology was later to make to clinical practice, which has been substantial. What he did get right, is that this emphasis by the epidemiologist on clinical practice has had deleterious consequences—it has allowed both the clinician and the epidemiologist to focus on the patient, and ignore the population.

Clinical epidemiology was a term that was not understood by most people, and around 1992 it became translated to 'evidence-based medicine' (EBM; JAMA 1992). Suddenly the clinician could understand that epidemiology allowed the application of a scientific approach to the practice of medicine.

Sackett, who should really be writing this piece as he has made by far the most important contribution to concepts of clinical epidemiology of anyone, has defined clinical epidemiology/EBM

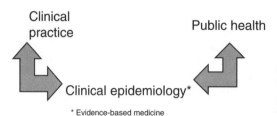

Fig. 23.1 Clinical epidemiology bridges clinical practice and public health: but have we got the balance right?

as 'the conscientious, explicit and judicious use of current best evidence in making decisions about individual patients' (Sackett *et al.* 1996). My own definition of clinical epidemiology (Heller 1991) was rather longer, but was clearly labelled as a tactic to improve public health, and included: ' ... clinicians are better prepared in ... turning their thoughts towards the prevention of major diseases of importance in the community ... designed to encourage the clinician to develop skills in research...tackle health problems of real importance in the community'. While the population health sciences have contributed to clinical practice through clinical epidemiology, have we got the balance right (Fig. 23.1)? Unfortunately, the acceptance of EBM as a phrase has lost us the opportunity to use the clinician to help improve the health of the community. This, together with the emphasis of epidemiologists on 'risk factorology', where we get better at predicting the outcome of individuals rather than populations, focuses us to heavily on individuals and loses the population approach. But let's start at the beginning.

Clinical epidemiology research in the early days: obstacles?

Geoffrey Rose told the story of how he went to the Department of Health with the idea of a trial to prevent heart disease among industrial workers. Of course, was the reply, how much do you want? Good ideas could be funded, and competition was less intense. In view of some of the problems faced in the conduct and interpretation of the results of that trial, maybe more extensive peer review has its place. It is to the credit of the pioneers of epidemiology that they managed to get research funding for this area, so even if it was less competitive, a good case still had to be made.

Other barriers to research were also less obvious. Confidentiality was vitally important, as was consent and an ethical approach to research. However, the obstacles of political correctness in research governance were not in evidence. A good research proposal, with appropriate ethical safeguards, would be allowed to proceed.

It was the advent of EBM as a research area which provided access to major funding for clinical epidemiology. Funding opportunities took off when epidemiology became mainstream through the linkage to clinical practice, in the form of clinical trails. EBM has been defined as PBM, or pharmaceutical-based medicine. The pharmaceutical industry has sponsored a great deal of research. This has led to important advances. We now know about methods for improving survival of a large number of conditions, both clinical and pre-clinical. The converse of this is the dominance of pharmaceutical research in EBM. There is much less research into diagnosis and natural history and non-pharmaceutical interventions than into drug treatments.

What has clinical epidemiology become?

I think we can divide clinical epidemiology/EBM into two major methodological themes: 'statistical' and 'implementation' (Heller and Page 2002). The use and analysis of large trials, meta-analyses, systematic reviews, evidence hierarchies, cost-effectiveness analyses, and number needed to treat would come under the 'statistical' while the improved access to evidence through literature searching, library and critical appraisal tools, guideline development, risk framing, etc. would be 'implementation'. Each of these is well served by journals, websites, training programmes, academic positions, etc. and there is a whole movement of 'true believers'. This is best exemplified by the Cochrane Collaboration (www.cochrane.org), which started with a few enthusiasts who wanted to make systematic reviews widely available to clinicians, and has spread to many countries and thousands of people who contribute to the ever-growing body of evidence.

Number needed to treat (NNT) merits a special section. In a blazingly simple insight, Sackett and colleagues realized that taking the inverse of the absolute risk reduction, gives the numbers of individuals who are to be subjected to an intervention in order for one to benefit (Laupacis *et al.* 1988). Immediately, the clinician can appreciate the chance that an intervention has of leading to a favourable outcome for the patient. More important in many ways than the actual appreciation of risk and benefit to an individual, is the appreciation that the data to produce such estimates comes from research. The research is population research, usually the randomized controlled trial, underpinned by epidemiological methods. The other insight, now appreciated by the clinician as well as the epidemiologist, is that small changes applied to large numbers can both be measured and can have a large impact on populations (if a small impact on individuals). Say we are to compare the benefits of aspirin and thrombolysis on secondary prevention after non-haemorrhagic stroke. While only seven patients have to be treated (the NNT) with thrombolysis to prevent one adverse outcome (death or disability 6 months later), 33 patients have to be given aspirin to achieve the same outcome as the risk reduction in treated individuals is smaller. Unfortunately, only 4% of the stroke population are eligible for thrombolysis (due to the time window and other aspects) while 70% are eligible for aspirin. The population benefit of a policy of using aspirin works out as being nearly six times greater than that of using thrombolysis, despite the greater clinical benefit for those actually treated (Heller 2005). Large differences such as these are easy to distinguish. Smaller differences require estimates from large trials, or the combination of trial results through systematic review techniques.

Much of my own research has been in the field of cardiovascular clinical epidemiology, which was one of the first to develop. This partly reflects the clinical interests of the early protagonists and the educational initiatives of international short courses through which, over the years, many hundreds of cardiologists have passed. It is a delight to see clinical epidemiology extending to mental illness, rheumatic diseases, and a number of other important chronic disease states.

Clinical epidemiology has also spawned an interest in health economics. Cost-effectiveness is the rage currently (although I hope only transiently). In order to assess the cost-effectiveness of an intervention, an estimate of effectiveness is essential. Measures of effectiveness come largely from intervention trials, and it is the clinical epidemiologists who have identified the need to use outcome measures that are of relevance to clinicians and their patients. (I have inserted a note of caution about the value of cost-effectiveness, as I would have preferred policy-makers to have focused more on the population impact of interventions than the economic benefit, but I realize that this is swimming against the current tide.)

The methods of clinical epidemiology also help with the interpretation of diagnostic tests. It comes as a revelation to many medical students (and perhaps graduates as well) that the result of a diagnostic test does not necessarily imply the presence or absence of disease. The basis for the understanding of this is probability. Epidemiologists talked about sensitivity and specificity for years in relation to screening (probability of a positive or negative test reflecting true positives or negatives), but its application to clinical practice resulted in the development of other measures that were of clinical relevance, such as the positive and negative predictive value and receiver operating characteristic curves. The link between the different sets is the reliance on prevalence for the clinical measures. Thus a test with good 'epidemiological' characteristics (sensitivity and specificity) may not have such good 'clinical' characteristics in conditions of varying prevalence. In this way, while epidemiological methods are of use in the clinical setting, clinical insights are also of use in the population setting in the interpretation of the outcomes of population screening. As can be seen in Fig. 23.1, clinical epidemiology finds itself at the interface of clinical practice and public health—here is an example of 'traffic' in both ways, the population sciences and clinical practice influencing each other.

Partly as a result of the methods now available to help with various levels of policy-making, EBM has now become one of the basic sciences of clinical practice, as foreshadowed by the Fletchers for clinical epidemiology (Fletcher *et al.* 1996). It is practised ubiquitously at the clinical coalface. NNT is used in clinical decision-making, and clinical decision support aids used to help introduce evidence into practice (O'Connor *et al.* 2003). Clinical meetings are not complete without some discussion about evidence. Research is performed to build the evidence base. EBM is talked about and practised.

A Google search in November 2006, using exact terms 'clinical epidemiology' and 'evidence-based medicine' revealed 703,000 and 1,020,000 hits respectively.

Interaction—between the individual and the population

Interaction is the key to clinical epidemiology. Some have felt that 'clinical', which is to do with individuals, and 'epidemiology', which is to do with groups, are unlikely partners. However, it is this interaction between the individual and the population which has led to the success of the field. The population approach gained credibility when applied to individual patient care. How can we understand natural history unless we see it in the context of large numbers of patients? How can we understand the performance of a diagnostic test unless we know about group probability? How can we understand the efficacy of a therapy unless we compare groups who are exposed with groups who are not exposed? How can we understand cause unless we compare group exposures?

Paradoxically, it is currently (at least in the UK) more difficult to develop interaction between the public health practitioner and the epidemiologist. Both have the population at heart, but so much public health policy is conceived and carried out without an epidemiological evidence base that it is not funny. It is no longer possible to introduce a new drug without good evidence of efficacy, but quite possible to introduce public health interventions (such as the current UK threat of health trainers to deal with obesity and cardiovascular risk) without any epidemiological (or other) evidence base. I don't think that the UK is alone in having politicians dominate the health agenda with attempts to shorten waiting lists—without evidence of the population health benefits of such an intervention.

The interaction between epidemiology, clinical practice, and health policy is strong in a number of international settings. The International Clinical Epidemiology Network (INCLEN) has been responsible for capacity building in many low- to middle-income countries (www.inclentrust.org). Not only have many clinicians been trained in epidemiology, but much valuable research has been performed and has influenced health policy. Many examples of policy-related research can be given—they include findings which have influenced policy at the 'micro' level, such as descriptions of antibiotic prescribing patterns in local health-care environments and descriptions of international differences in patterns of care for chronic disease. Broader policy-related research such as that of family violence in international settings, and the socio-cultural understanding of prescribing and immunization patterns in different settings have been performed. Research networks have been created, where interventions have been planned and evaluated. The development of clinical prediction rules for pharyngitis and improvements in the treatment of depression in primary care and in neonatal care are all examples of work by networks formed by combinations of clinicians and other research areas across disciplines and countries. The incorporation of economic and social science theory into clinical and population research has been a special feature of much of the research. Numerous projects into the major health problems of developing countries have been planned and executed, underpinned by the research excellence introduced by a carefully monitored and benchmarked education programme.

INCLEN originally trained a core unit in each of 26 medical schools in developing countries, through Masters degree programmes in Canada, Australia, and the USA. Many of these units then developed their own Masters courses, and they then taught others in their institutions and created secondary units within their own and neighbouring countries—an excellent example of translation of research capacity from 'north' to 'south'. Within the institutions involved, EBM has been incorporated into the medical school curricula and new clinical epidemiology post-graduate courses have been established. A number of graduates of the programme are now in leadership roles in their own institutions and international organizations. The Rockefeller Foundation, in setting up INCLEN, insisted on institutional capacity building. I would term this the population approach, and contrast it with much capacity building which is lost as individuals who have been trained move on and their expertise is lost to the setting for which it was intended. Lessons about the international population approach to capacity building in epidemiology could well be applied to other areas of geography and speciality.

The future of clinical epidemiology

I can see nothing but a secure future for this subject. Despite some reported initial reluctance among some clinicians to the introduction of clinical epidemiology, methods are continually developing (McDonald and Daly 2000; Daly 2005). In the UK, there are organizational changes which currently place public health and primary care together. This has the potential to improve the links between clinical epidemiology and primary care—secondary care (hospital-based medicine) has been quicker to embrace an evidence-based approach than has primary care. Because of the new structure, which includes service commissioning as part of the role of the primary care organization, a population perspective might be added to a clinical perspective as a potential way of using epidemiology and the population approach to have an impact on health policy.

Other organizational approaches include the attempts to introduce systematic reviews to clinical practice, and these are becoming increasingly well established. The obvious example of this is the Cochrane Collaboration, which is now expanding to more countries and conditions. A number of Cochrane Collaboration activities are funded by national government departments. Governments are also funding systematic approaches to reviewing evidence and introducing clinical practice guidelines. The Agency for Healthcare Research and Quality in the USA produces clinical guidelines and sponsors research (www.ahrq.gov). In England, clinical guidelines are produced by the National Institute for Health and Clinical Excellence (NICE) (www.nice.org.uk). The methods of clinical epidemiology have underpinned the evidence reviews (although there are some of us who feel that the health economists have had too much sway in the guidance being produced). NICE has incorporated the organization previously funded to produce public health guidelines, and this should have two positive results. First, public health interventions can be assessed using the NICE rigour, and second a public health focus might be able to be turned to clinical guidelines. In Canada, which had a head start on others through Sackett and colleagues at McMaster University and the Fletchers originally at McGill University, EBM is particularly well established, although the need to develop from EBM to public health evidence has been recognized (Kiefer *et al.* 2005). Australia can also boast a number of government-supported initiatives in the field, such as the insistence on cost-effectiveness evaluations being part of the approval process for pharmaceutical agents (Henry and Hill 1999). Many other countries have all sorts of initiatives, all of which indicate that epidemiology is firmly established as a key plank in decision-making, now and into the future.

Conclusion

I have tried to show that the population approach, through epidemiological theory and practice, has found a ready and sustained application in clinical practice through clinical epidemiology and evidence-based medicine. Our challenge as epidemiologists is to build on the success of clinical epidemiology, and build and institutionalize epidemiology as key to the development and implementation of an evidence base for population health.

References

Daly J (2005). *Evidence-based medicine and the search for a science of clinical care.* University of California Press and Milbank Memorial Fund, Berkely, CA.

Fletcher RH, Fletcher SW, and Wagner E (1996). *Clinical epidemiology: the essentials.* Williams and Wilkins, Baltimore.

Heller R (1991). Centre for Clinical Epidemiology and Biostatistics. *Annals of Community Oriented Education,* **4**, 99–102.

Heller RF (2005). *Evidence for population health.* Oxford University Press, Oxford.

Heller RF and Page JH (2002). A population perspective to evidence based medicine: 'evidence for population health'. *Journal of Epidemiology and Community Health,* **56**, 45–7.

Henry DA and Hill SR (1999). Assessing new health technologies: lessons to be learned from drugs. *The Medical Journal of Australia,* **171**, 554–6.

JAMA (1992). Evidence-based medicine. A new approach to teaching the practice of medicine. Evidence-Based Medicine Working Group. *Journal of the American Medical Association,* **268**, 2420–5.

Kiefer L, Frank J, Di Ruggiero E, *et al.* (2005). Fostering evidence-based decision-making in Canada. *Canadian Journal of Public Health,* **I**, 1–40.

Laupacis A, Sackett DL, and Roberts RS (1988). An assessment of clinically useful measures of the consequences of treatment. *New England Journal of Medicine,* **318**, 1728–33.

McDonald IG and Daly JM (2000). The anatomy and relations of evidence-based medicine. *Australian and New Zealand Journal of Medicine,* **30**, 385–92.

O'Connor AM, Legare F, and Stacey D (2003). Risk communication in practice: the contribution of decision aids. *British Medical Journal,* **327**, 736–40.

Sackett DL, Rosenberg WM, Gray JA, Haynes RB, and Richardson WS (1996). Evidence based medicine: what it is and what it isn't. *British Medical Journal,* **312**, 71–2.

Section 5

Regions and countries

24

Epidemiological methods: a view from the Americas

Eduardo L. Franco, Salaheddin M. Mahmud, and Andrew G. Dean

Personal experiences

Epidemiological practice tends to attract public health workers with a strong interest in studying health outcomes that cross international boundaries. This chapter was written by three such epidemiologists who began their careers in places as distinct as Brazil (ELF), Libya (SM), and the USA (AGD) but who always had an international orientation in the substantive focus of their work. ELF and SM spent much of their careers as cancer epidemiologists, whereas AGD developed Epi Info, the most widely used database and statistical software program for the study of disease outbreaks by surveillance epidemiologists. How their paths crossed and strong intellectual bonds were permanently formed illustrates the cross-fertilization of ideas that create synergy and open new doors in the scientific world. Telling how they came to know each other would require more premium space in a textbook such as this than the publisher would care to allow. It suffices to say that the three co-authors' joint productivity over the years improved substantially because their professional lives intersected at the right moments.

Writing a chapter that describes the history of epidemiological methods from the perspective of the American continent is a daunting task in any context. As others have written in this tome, there is no pedagogically correct way of compartmentalizing by geography the intellectual contributions of so many people who interacted across continents in producing the scientific framework that shaped the profession as we experience it today. Key concepts, such as measuring descriptive rates of health-related events and confounding, had their intellectual roots in the contributions of British statisticians. Over time, epidemiological concepts have been re-examined by different authors and become more or less harmonized as common accepted knowledge with uniform terminology. Some of today's epidemiology textbooks provide the historical perspective that helps those entering the profession. As examples, the reader is referred to the excellent compilations of Alfredo Morabia, from the Division of Clinical Epidemiology, University Hospital, Geneva (Morabia 2004), and of Sander Greenland, University of California, Los Angeles (Greenland 1987).

This chapter provides a personal account of how the three authors view the evolution of study designs, statistical methodology, and the development of epidemiological computer software that aided progress in the field. Whenever appropriate, emphasis is given to the view from the Americas. However, as justified above and in the interest of providing a seamless historical perspective, we have included key scientific developments from other continents as well. Because of editorial guidelines, the account that follows is rather selective in providing references. On the other hand, the names of prominent epidemiologists and biostatisticians are given throughout the chapter, which will assist the reader to make specific bibliographic searches for the collective opus of any of the names mentioned below.

The development of study design

Scientific cogency in probing for cause–effect relationships was the driving force for the development of study designs that forms the mainstay of substantive findings in epidemiology. There is nothing particularly intrinsic about epidemiology that makes it more or less concerned about demonstrating a phenomenon or testing a hypothesis than other areas of science. Nearly all empirical disciplines require strong reasoning in laying out the basis for why an experiment should be interpreted in a certain way. Use of control groups that provide the necessary contrast between a target condition whose effect must be quantified and the expectation of the same effect in its absence is central to all lines of scientific enquiry that can afford to use experimentation or controlled observation. What is particularly relevant about epidemiology is the fact that more often than not experimentation is not possible, and thus insights about causation must come from judicious observation of the joint distribution in the population of putative causal factors, potential confounding variables, and the outcome of interest. Being judicious, however, does not provide a safe passage to a valid conclusion. Any observational study must contend with the difficulty of making choices about empirically 'capturing' in study samples the above relations at the population level and dealing with unmeasured or unobservable confounders and measurement errors in one or several key variables. Even when the work goes according to plan, sometimes regrettable choices about subject selection and analytical approaches may become known only at the end of the study after the findings have reached the public domain. In the last 10 years, a general theory of counterfactuals in epidemiology has become increasingly popular because it reconciles causal thinking in other disciplines, such as sociology, behavioural sciences, psychology, and education, with that practised in public health. Work by Sander Greenland, UCLA, Jay Kaufman and Charles Poole, from the University of North Carolina at Chapel Hill, Douglas Weed, from the US National Cancer Institute, and others have provided much of the impetus for a common statistical framework that entertains the seemingly intractable complexity in the pursuit of understanding causal relations in population health.

The typology of study designs described in epidemiology textbooks evolved in response to the need for ever more cogent approaches to empirically probing for causal relations in a manner in which biases and alternative explanations could be more easily dismissed in the pursuit of understanding a possible aetiological effect attributable to a factor of interest. It was not only scientific cogency that helped this progress. Pragmatic considerations about the cost of epidemiological investigations became a reality in the last three decades, particularly with the emergence of molecular and genetic epidemiology. The advent of subsampling-based designs, such as the nested case–control and case–cohort studies, came in response not only to the demonstration that they are scientifically valid but to a large extent also because of the reduced costs in measuring exposure and confounders in only a sample of the study participants to obtain the counterfactual contrasts for exploring cause–effect relations. In the interest of pedagogy, we briefly describe below the progress and the reasoning behind each study design even though for theoretical reasons the distinction is not so important given the unified framework described above. Because of space considerations we also restricted the overview to observational study designs, but we hasten to add that intervention studies form a rich history of contributions to North American public health.

Case–control studies

The scientific approach of comparing patients with a given illness with a suitable group of individuals without the condition was used only occasionally in the first half of the twentieth century. Interest in understanding the aetiology of cancer was the driving force for the development of the first historically prominent case–control studies. Three such studies targeted lung cancer and smoking and appeared in print in 1950. They belong to any anthology of cancer prevention. Two of them were conducted in the USA, by Ernst Wynder and Evarts Graham (Wynder and Graham 1950) of Washington University, and by Morton Levin and colleagues (Levin *et al.* 1950) from the Roswell Park Memorial Institute. The third study, by Richard Doll and Bradford Hill (Doll and Hill 1950), was conducted in London, UK, and has enjoyed more of the historical lime-light of cancer prevention perhaps because it had many of the ingredients of today's case–control studies and devoted much attention to ascertaining exposure. These studies ushered a landmark period in medicine as a new era in disease prevention which officially opened in the USA with the 1964 report on smoking and health (Advisory Committee to the Surgeon General of the Public Health Service 1964). This comprehensive report and others that followed by the US Department of Health, Education, and Welfare (later reorganized as Department of Health and Human Services) provided the basis in North America for all actions aimed at promoting smoking cessation and policies restricting smoking in public places.

The impact of these studies' findings went far beyond the intended public health consequence of placing tobacco smoking among society's ills. These studies elicited an enormous scientific confrontation between two camps of thinkers of that era, one in favour of the findings as implying a causal effect for smoking and the other preoccupied with alternative explanations for the observed statistical relations. Much of the debate that ensued between camps, from the early 1950s until the 1980s, around the topic of active smoking and risk, and then from the 1980s until the mid-1990s, on the effects of environmental tobacco smoke, can be viewed as extremely positive to the practice of epidemiology and public health. The criticisms of many of the opponents of an aetiological relation between smoking (or passive smoking) and lung cancer (and other neoplasms), such as R. A. Fisher, J. Berkson, P. R. Burch, T. Sterling, A. Feinstein, N. Mantel, and other prominent epidemiologists and biostatisticians, are now viewed as necessary challenges that raised the bar for scientific standards in epidemiological research. Our understanding of concepts such as the need for entertaining temporality in assessing putative causal relations, the impact of selection biases, confounding, and measurement error was considerably advanced as epidemiological methods evolved to face these challenges. These critics' views not only helped strengthen the practice of epidemiology but also brought a healthy dose of scientific conservatism in considering evidence for setting permissible thresholds of occupational exposures and for accepting the putative efficacy of public health interventions.

One of the initial challenges to the approach of retrospectively investigating exposure–disease relationships via case–control studies was the fact that it did not consider latency in the design. The need for accommodating temporality (which emerged as the most unequivocally necessary causal criterion in public health) led to much of the subsequent impetus for using prospective cohort studies of smoking and health effects. Findings from case–control studies served, nonetheless, as the primary knowledge base for most of the chronic disease prevention initiatives in the past half century. The proof that the exposure odds ratio had the attractive feature of empirically replicating the underlying risk ratio for the exposure–disease relation (see below, under statistical developments) provided the necessary theoretical foundation that sustained the case–control study over the years as a valid tool in epidemiology. Subsequent work in the 1970s by Olli Miettinen, then at Harvard University, and others that further refined his thinking led to the concepts of study base and incidence-density sampling and helped establish the modern case–control study as a sampling exercise in an underlying dynamic cohort in which the exposure–disease relationship of interest is operative. The investigator is thus concerned with efficiently and validly capturing, via a case–control sampling strategy, the person–time experience and joint distributions of exposure, outcome, and any confounders and modifiers that exist in the underlying cohort structure. The relations of interest are then measured via regression modelling (e.g. logistic regression) and depicted as per the original hypotheses that spawned the need for the study. Among those who championed the theoretical developments surrounding design and analysis of case–control studies were Norman Breslow, at the University of Washington, Sander Greenland, at UCLA, and Kenneth Rothman, then at Harvard and later at Boston University, and their disciples. Much of this knowledge has been crystallized in now classical textbooks of epidemiology: Breslow and Day's (1980) *Statistical methods in cancer research, Vol. 1: The analysis of case–control studies*, Schlesselman's (1982) tome *Case–control studies: design, conduct, and analysis*, and Rothman's (1986) *Modern epidemiology* (now in its second edition (1998) with Greenland).

Cohort studies

The very early controversy surrounding the association of smoking and lung cancer that stemmed from the aforementioned case–control studies led almost immediately to the formulation of prospectively designed cohort investigations. The main criticism was related to the fact that data on both exposure and outcome were known to the investigators at the time the studies began. Also of concern was the then prevalent view that selection and recall biases invalidated many of the findings from such retrospective investigations. Fortunately, the problem had been recognized at the outset by Doll and Hill and by the American Cancer Society's epidemiologists Hammond and Horn, who conducted prospective cohort investigations that became widely known for elegantly corroborating the findings from the early case–control studies of smoking and lung cancer. The two studies were based on clever use of existing resources available to both sets of investigators, in the UK and in the USA.

Cohort studies also formed the basis for much of the early progress on occupational health. Efficient use of record linkage using company records and mortality or cancer registry databases permitted the identification of many environmental and occupational exposures. The theoretical work that ran in parallel with these studies also provided dividends by introducing the principles of indirect standardization in computing risk ratios of disease in the absence of suitably comparable unexposed groups. Some of the prominent prospective cohort studies have spanned periods of decades and have also made major contributions to our understanding of risk factors for a variety of chronic diseases. The interested reader is referred to the abundant literature on the Framingham Heart Study, the Tecumseh Community Health Study, the Alameda County Study, and the Nurses' Health Study as salient examples of the enormous contribution of cohort studies to public health.

Causal thinking

As mentioned above, the dispute that placed mainstream epidemiologists in opposition to a minority of illustrious public health scientists and biostatisticians (with some help from tobacco industry advocates) during most of the 1950s and 1960s provided much of the foundation for a theory of causality for chronic diseases. The most important development in this area was a position paper by A. Bradford Hill, the aforementioned British co-author with Richard Doll of the most prominent of the case–control studies implicating tobacco smoking in the genesis of lung cancer. This key contribution, published in 1965 in the *Proceedings of the Royal Society of Medicine*, contained a most lucid account of the different ways that scientific reasoning can help establish causality. It is by far the most cited reference in the medical literature in the area of causal thinking. The list of arguments he provided to assist in the discussion of causality became known as Hill's criteria and can be found in any mainstream textbook of epidemiology and public health. Oddly enough, Hill stated at the opening of the article's fourth paragraph 'I have no wish, nor the skill, to embark upon a philosophical discussion of the meaning of "causation". Little did he know that with this article he set in motion the intellectual foundation for the entire discussion on epidemiology and causality that would ensue quite vigorously over the next four decades and continues unabated to this day.

Many prominent North American epidemiologists have made scholarly contributions to the evolution of causal thinking in public health. Hill's views in 1965 augmented his own previous work and that of Jerome Cornfield (US National Institutes of Health) on the use of statistical inference as proof in medicine in the early 1950s. It also expanded considerably on those of J. Yerushalmy (University of California, Berkeley) and Carroll Palmer (US Public Health Service) and subsequent commentaries on that work by Abraham Lilienfeld and Philip Sartwell, both at Johns Hopkins University. With the subsequent growth of epidemiology and the ongoing tobacco–cancer debate subsequent writers adopted bolder, theoretically more inclusive and sometimes philosophical postures to define the role of epidemiology in establishing cause–effect relations in public health. Of note are the writings of Brian MacMahon (Harvard) in 1970, Rothman (also Harvard) in 1976, and anthological exchanges on the application of Popper's philosophy that took place in 1975–76 in the *International Journal of Epidemiology* in response to an initial commentary by Carol Buck (University of Western Ontario). Douglas Weed (US National Cancer Institute) also contributed quite eclectically to this most important aspect of epidemiology by bringing together the philosophical foundations to the historical perspective of the scientific criteria to infer causal relations.

Another giant of the era, Mervyn Susser from Columbia University, brought a tinge of controversy to the debate in 1977 by arguing against over-reliance on statistics, particularly significance testing. The latter in fact triggered a debate on the use of confidence intervals versus P values that to this day has not yet subsided. Key to this debate is the tenet, mostly held by Rothman and Charles Poole, that in observational studies one is concerned with measuring relations as free of biases and as precisely as possible given the constraints of instrumental error and funding limitations. Rothman (1986) argued that decision-making, which is the implied next step after one conducts tests of significance, is not the goal of observational studies.

It is of note that over the years the role of epidemiology has gained considerable ground in medicine as a discipline to assist policy decisions concerning preventive actions. Such decisions are taken by agencies, such as the World Health Organization's International Agency for Research on Cancer and the US Environmental Protection Agency, on a variety of perceived environmental and biological hazards that may increase cancer risk. Evidence from epidemiological studies is held in high esteem by these agencies in the overall process of sifting through reams of published studies on any suspected carcinogen.

The development of statistical methodology

Statistical methods are essential to the practice of epidemiology. Over the years, the collaboration between epidemiologists and statisticians has led to the development of many epidemiological and statistical methods that transformed the practice of epidemiology. One could think of the history of modern (twentieth century) statistics as spanning two distinctive eras: the era of mathematical statistics before the Second World War, and the era of applied statistics afterwards. The first half of the twentieth century saw the formulation of a mathematical theory of probability and the consolidation of a wide range of *ad hoc* statistical techniques into a coherent and robust theory of statistics. Many of these developments took place in Britain and continental Europe and were motivated to a great extent by contemporary problems in biology. Examples of this can be found in the work of Francis Galton (1822–1911) and Karl Pearson (1857–1936), which was originally aimed at providing empirical support for Darwin's theory of evolution, and in Fisher's work in genetics. In particular, Sir Ronald Fisher (1890–1962) is credited with the conceptualization of the ideas (e.g. maximum likelihood inference, randomization, and design of experiments) that formed the core of statistical theory and the basis for many developments in biostatistics and epidemiology after the Second World War.

The Second World War heralded a big change in direction that led to the widespread application of statistical methods in all fields of scientific inquiry including economics, sociology, medicine, and epidemiology. In epidemiology, as in many other fields, many of these developments took place in North America and particularly in the USA. Not only because political instability and war atrocities drove many European statisticians to North America but also because the war effort had stimulated research and training in statistics and its applications. Before the Second World War there were few academic departments of biostatistics; the first was founded in 1918 at Johns Hopkins University as the Department of Biometry and Vital Statistics. Its first head was Raymond Pearl (1879–1940) who studied statistics and biology in Britain under Karl Pearson and is famous for the rediscovery, with the help of his deputy and successor Lowell Reed (1886–1966), of the logistic function. (The logistic function was first described by the Belgian mathematician Verhulst in the nineteenth century.) Following the Second World War, biostatistics became a recognized academic discipline and several academic and research departments were established in many American universities and government agencies. However, the most influential development was perhaps the establishment of the Division of Statistical Methods at the National Cancer Institute (between 1946 and 1948). The new department was chaired by Harold Dorn (1906–63) who managed in just a few years to recruit some of the most influential figures in the history of epidemiology including Jerome Cornfield, Nathan Mantel, Sam Greenhouse, and William Haenszel. In the 1950s and 1960s the new department, and similar departments in other National Institutes of Health (NIH) institutes, were the source of several breakthroughs in epidemiology and applied statistics. The stimulus for many of these developments was the appearance of new and complex epidemiological studies such as the Framingham Heart Study and other prominent cohort studies.

During the1950s and 1960s statistical applications in epidemiology grew rapidly in response to the shift in emphasis to the vastly complex topic of chronic disease epidemiology and the introduction of complex study designs that required more efficient and sophisticated approaches for the analysis of their data. In particular, case–control studies were increasingly being used to investigate the aetiology of chronic diseases such as lung cancer and heart disease.

In the following section we enumerate a few of the landmark developments in the application of statistics in epidemiology. The list is by no means complete and the choice of topics necessarily reflects the areas with which we are most familiar.

Analysis of case–control studies

Data from the early case–control studies were analysed and presented in a simple straightforward fashion. Causal association between a risk factor or exposure and the condition under study was inferred by contrasting the proportion of exposed cases with that of exposed controls. There was no easy way of judging the strength of the association in a case–control study because disease rates, and therefore the relative risk, could not be calculated since the number of cases and controls were fixed by design. In a seminal paper, Jerome Cornfield (1912–79) showed that exposure odds ratios obtained from case–control studies estimate the disease relative risk (Cornfield 1951). Cornfield predicated his analysis on the assumption that the disease is rare, hence the famous rare disease assumption. Later he would also propose a method to compute confidence intervals around the odds ratio. Cornfield was a self-taught mathematician. He majored in history though it appears that he did some graduate studies in statistics at the US Department of Agriculture Graduate School during the Second World War.

Another breakthrough came when William Haenszel and Nathan Mantel (Mantel and Haenszel 1959) introduced in a famous paper their procedure to calculate a common or pooled odds ratio from several 2×2 contingency tables generated by stratification of the data to control for confounding. In addition, they proposed a slightly modified version of a chi-squared test first introduced by the famous statistician William Cochran (1909–80). The Cochran–Mantel–Haenszel test assumes a common odds ratio (no three-way interaction) and tests the null hypothesis that two nominal variables are conditionally independent given a third variable (a confounder). The same paper introduced a method for calculating confidence intervals around the common odds ratio. This paper remains one of the most commonly cited papers in the field. Mantel later published other papers to generalize the application of the Mantel–Haenszel procedure to stratified data from cohort studies and laboratory experiments and to the analysis of survival curves.

Adjustment for confounding by several factors provided the motivation for another monumental development; the introduction by Cornfield (1962) of logistic regression for the analysis of case–control data. Cornfield recognized the link between discriminant analysis and the logistic model and suggested the use of the multiple logistic risk function to smooth sparse data resulting from cross-classification by multiple confounding factors. He also showed how the parameters from the model could be interpreted as odds ratios. The method became the mainstay in the analysis of case–control studies when it was later recognized as a special case within the framework of generalized linear models (as formulated by Nelder and Wedderburn (1972)) and was incorporated in many statistical software packages.

Analysis of cohort and time to event data

The method of analysis now known as age–period–cohort analysis (or simply cohort analysis) was developed by Wade Hampton Frost (1880–1938) who used it to study historical data on mortality from tuberculosis in the USA.

In 1958, Paul Meier and Edward Kaplan introduced their method to estimate cumulative survival probabilities from censored time to event data. The paper that described their method is the most frequently cited statistical paper and among the most cited papers in science.

The increased popularity of longitudinal studies with repeated measurements provided the impetus for the development of new statistical methods to account for the correlation between observations and to best utilize all the information collected by such studies. Generalized estimating equations (GEE) models developed by Zeger and Liang (1986) at Johns Hopkins to extend generalized linear models to correlated data are increasingly being used in the analysis of epidemiological studies, especially in relation to the study of HIV/AIDS. There was also a surge in the popularity of multilevel (hierarchical) models in epidemiology. Multilevel models are a class of models that can be used to analyse data that are naturally hierarchical (a common example arises in the context of health services research where patients are clustered by surgeons who are in turn clustered by hospitals) or by design (the results of clustered multistage sampling schemes used in many surveys). Multilevel models explicitly model the effect of explanatory variables on the variance as estimated for each level. Multilevel models, also known as hierarchical models, random effect models, and variance component models, were always very popular in the social sciences but recently they have found their way into epidemiology where they are now being used to solve a wide range of problems from accounting for contextual levels in classic epidemiological studies to meta-analysis and the estimation of generalized linear models with covariates measurement error.

Other important developments

Measurement error

Measurement errors are always a source of concern for epidemiologists. Improvements in the design of case–control and cohort studies and the adoption of improved questionnaires and laboratory-based approaches to ascertain lifestyle and environmental exposures have greatly enhanced the validity of inferences from epidemiological investigations. Advances in the quality of study design notwithstanding, a new field of statistical methodology also came to the rescue. The new trend has been for qualitative assessment of the impact of measurement errors to be replaced or enhanced by quantitative methods that aim to reduce bias (or at least assess its magnitude). Some are validation methods such as regression calibration and the simulation extrapolation method. Other approaches include semi-parametric and Bayesian methods.

Missing data

Missing data abound in epidemiological studies. Recently, there has been significant progress in this area. Rubin provided the original ideas of dealing with missing data and he and others developed the expectation-maximization algorithm for maximum likelihood estimation from incomplete data.

Causal models

The 1990s witnessed a plethora of activities in this area. Rubin proposed the counterfactual model for causal inference but the idea could be traced back to Neyman. More recently, Pearl introduced the method of causal graphs for drawing causal inferences from observational studies. Given a fully constructed causal diagram that links all pertinent covariates, Pearl illustrated conditions for confounding and gave several rules for identifying confounders and causal effects.

Meta-analysis

This is a formal statistical procedure for combining data from independent studies. Interest in meta-analysis has surged in response to the demand of the evidence-based medicine movement in the 1990s. The method which was originally introduced to combine results from clinical trials is now widely used, not without controversy, to summarize the findings of observational studies.

The development of computer software

One historical component that must not be forgotten in the contributions from North America is the advent of computing to assist data processing. For roughly 100 years after John Snow's cholera investigations of 1854, epidemiology depended on pencil and paper for data capture and processing. The history of computing and epidemiology since the 1960s is one of transformation of both epidemiological data and the biomedical literature from paper to digital formats, and the creation of analytical programs for all levels of public health professionals. At the same time, with the help of the Internet and its search engines, data, tools, and literature are increasingly available in the remotest corners of the world, rather than being confined to large academic or government centres.

At the beginning of the era, essentially all public health observations were made by transferring data manually to a paper format. Before the 1960s, edge-punched cards and knitting needles were used to look for associations between two or more study characteristics. As mainframe computers became available in the 1960s and 1970s, paper information was then transferred by keyboard entry to IBM punch cards or into computer files where statistical software could be used for analysis. In recent years, increasing numbers of data for analysis are available in digital format from large clinical databases, online surveillance systems, and vital statistics sources.

Communication and searching and retrieval of information, using computers and the Internet, have blossomed since the early 1990s. In the 1960s, access to current research information and the epidemiological literature was limited to major centres in developed countries; those outside the medical library network depended on books and paper copies by mail. In the twenty-first century, an epidemiologist can search, share data, and communicate with colleagues anywhere in the world where there is Internet access.

The advent of epidemiological computing

With the availability of statistical regression methods in the late 1970s the work of a typical epidemiologist broadened tremendously. In those early days, data analyses of complex data sets required punching coded instructions in IBM cards for processing in a mainframe computer somewhere on campus. Centralized computing was the norm but the process was largely inefficient when examined by today's standards. With the first regression programs for case–control and cohort data analysis came the opportunity to examine associations in multivariate models in ways that were never thought possible. As card punchers were replaced by computer terminals one could simply dispatch the instruction set by pressing a button. Yet epidemiological computing was far from being a personal experience.

This state of affairs changed dramatically with the advent of personal programmable calculators and computers in the late 1970s and early 1980s, which created the impetus for epidemiologists to write specialized software to accomplish tasks that up until that point required centralized computing resources. The history of personal computing in epidemiology has produced many unsung heroes. Probably the first landmark contribution was the compilation by Kenneth Rothman and John Boice (1979) (US National Cancer Institute) in the late 1970s of a series of programs they had written for the HP-67 calculator. These programs performed analysis of crude and stratified data from case–control and cohort studies, sample size calculations, binomial confidence intervals, and life table analysis. They became the methodology staple of Epidemic Intelligence Service (EIS) officers-in-training at the Centers for Disease Control (CDC) in Atlanta, Georgia. The initial compilation was expanded in 1982 with the adaptation of all the original programs to the legendary HP-41C programmable calculator. Rothman and Boice's formulae and algorithms inspired many epidemiologists throughout the world to write their own code and macros for different computing platforms. The early 1980s also saw the advent of spreadsheet programs for the then nascent IBM personal computer.

Software for multivariate analysis began to appear in the late 1970s. An important early development was PECAN, a FORTRAN program written by J. Lubin for the analysis of case–control data using conditional maximum likelihood techniques. PECAN was subsequently modified by Barry Storer at the Fred Hutchison Cancer Research Center, who added an interactive routine and options for linear and user-defined risk models. Also implemented by Storer were the ability to compute Cox proportional hazard models and algorithms for regression diagnostics. The source code of PECAN and Storer's subsequent modifications inspired many statisticians and epidemiologists (including one of the present authors (Campos-Filho and Franco 1989)) to write their own software for regression analysis of case–control and cohort studies that could be executed in personal computers. Nowadays, epidemiologists enjoy a vast array of resources in this area, including some robust commercial programs, such as SAS, SPSS, BMDP (the mainstay of advanced data analysis in the early 1980s), STATA, and the more specialized epidemiological software EGRET.

Three attributes have served as the driving force behind so many useful epidemiological programming contributions in the past 25 years: talent, altruism, and passion for the hobby of writing computing code. Many epidemiology programmers derive their satisfaction by placing their software in the public domain and by learning that others have found it useful, validated it, and perhaps even improved on their algorithms. Epi Info, the most well known of these software programs, is the best example of a product of this generous attitude, particularly that of one of the co-authors, Andrew Dean, then at the CDC. His first-person narrative below is a wonderful example of how these attributes helped advance epidemiological computing over the years.

Examples through four decades

I [Andrew Dean] have been fortunate enough to participate in epidemiological informatics both as an epidemiologist and as a software developer since the mid-1960s. My first job after medical school and internship was as Peace Corps Physician for Somalia in 1965 and 1966, and my first epidemiological study was a survey of tuberculin positivity in northern Somalia, using pencil and paper for tabulating the data, and purple copies from a ditto machine for 'publication'. In 1967, the NIH sent me to the EIS course at CDC under Alex Langmuir, where we were issued slide rules for rate calculations and simple statistics. Shortly afterward there was an earnest discussion in our laboratory about the purchase of an electronic calculator to replace a mechanical model. Square root capability, now available in a two-dollar calculator, was an option that raised the price to more than $1000!

In 1968, I led an investigation of annually recurring diarrhoea epidemics in the Philippines that produced 18,000 IBM cards. Although mainframe computers were coming into general use with the release of the IBM 360 in 1965, I did not have access to one at our Honolulu base. I used a card sorter to analyse frequency distributions for a single variable and cross-tabulation could be done painstakingly by sorting and counting stacks of cards.

As Acting State Epidemiologist of Arkansas in 1975–76 and State Epidemiologist of Minnesota from 1978 to 1984, I found that access to computer facilities required much planning and the cooperation of programmers through contracts. I employed a pre-medical student, who was able to use SPSS on the university mainframe to produce the analyses I wanted.

Our colleagues in the Minnesota Heart Health project had a large NIH grant, and I was impressed by their limitless data storage capacity of 900 Mbytes in three or four washing-machine-sized hard disks in a large room. Today an average laptop has at least 50 times more storage capacity than the entire complex. I spent the evenings learning computing by first soldering together an IMSAI computer kit, and then learning to program in assembly language and later in BASIC and Pascal.

A CDC experiment in 1976 during the swine flu emergency allowed epidemiologists to access a minicomputer from terminals. A FORTRAN program called SOCRATES, written by Rick Curtis, allowed an epidemiologist to define questions, enter data, and summarize the results without the aid of a programmer. The Epidemiologic Analysis System (EAS), a more flexible version of SOCRATES, was written in BASIC by CDC's Anthony Burton and set up on a minicomputer for remote access by the Georgia State Health Department in the early 1980s.

The Conference (now Council) of State and Territorial Epidemiologists (CSTE) formed a Computer Working Group, which I chaired, and, together with Keewhan Choi and Stephen Thacker of CDC, developed a plan for the development of epidemiological computing. This contained ideas for a system to transmit state surveillance data to CDC in Atlanta by modem, using a data standard, later known as the National Electronic Telecommunications System for Surveillance (NETSS).

After several years of encouraging the state epidemiologists and CDC to join the microcomputer revolution, I served as president of CSTE and then was offered a CDC position where I spent the next 18 years leading the Epi Info development effort. At first, I set about developing a program called EpiAid which was an ambitious effort to develop an epidemiologist's assistant for epidemic investigation. Later, this work evolved into programming tools to create and analyse questionnaire data defined by the epidemiologist.

Development of Epi Info—free software for epidemiology

The DOS version of Epi Info

My son, Jeffrey Dean, then a junior in high school, came to CDC as an intern in March 1985 and wrote the first version of Epi Info's ENTER. Tony Burton provided ideas for the first version of ANALYSIS, programmed by Jeff during the summer of 1986. Several years later, Tony moved to the Global Programme on AIDS, World Health Organization, Geneva, and he and Jeff continued to collaborate on later versions of Epi Info™ as Jeff travelled to Geneva during college vacations, and then wrote Epi Map for DOS in Geneva in the year after graduation.

Many individuals contributed to the development of Epi Info. Richard Dicker, author of the 'Epidemiology in action' training manual and coordinator of the EIS course at CDC, provided advice on the statistics that were included in Epi Info. Kevin Sullivan, then with the Division of Nutrition at CDC, helped in incorporating the WHO/CDC growth curves into Epi Info. He also provided input into additions and improvements to EpiCalc and Analysis. He developed the concept of the Complex Sample Analysis module, produced by William Kalsbeek and Mario Chen, and further documented by Ralph Freirichs. Denis Columbier, designed and programmed Nutstat, the nutritional anthropometry module, and Epi Table, a statistical calculator for Epi Info for DOS. He and Leroy Hathcock of the Delaware State Health Department developed the idea of providing a programmable menu to serve as the unifying factor ('EpiGlue') for permanent applications such as surveillance systems. Nelson Campos and Eduardo Franco in Brazil provided an efficient algorithm for the Fisher exact test, based on work by Cyrus Mehta, and DOS programs for logistic and Cox proportional hazards regression and Kaplan–Meier survival analysis.

Epi Info for Microsoft Windows

Using ideas from a workshop on 'Microcomputers and the future of epidemiology' held in 1993 (Dean 1994) and experience with Epi Info 6, I began to develop Epi Info 2000, the Windows version, in Visual Basic and using the Microsoft Access database format. It could read and write in 20 other file formats, web page (HTML) output, and included a mapping program. Statistics in Epi Info for Windows included programs for logistic and Cox proportional hazards regression and Kaplan–Meier, analysis, written by Chris Smith based on the DOS programs. These were later rewritten by Nicholas Fontaine during a summer internship. Kevin Sullivan, David Gu, and Ray Simons wrote the statistical module for frequencies, tables, means, and linear regression, including exact statistics for 2×2 tables based on source code by David Martin. During subsequent years, Epi Info was improved by user feedback and careful debugging. The current version can be found on the CDC/Epi Info web pages, and tutorials are available there and from many other sites.

Epi Info's availability in the public domain made the product especially popular in developing countries, and several epidemiologists in other countries volunteered to translate the programs or the manual. Translations of the DOS and Windows versions are available in Spanish, French, Chinese, Arabic, Russian, Italian, and Czech and other languages.

The Internet

The Internet swept the world in the early 1990s. Prior to that time, Epi Info for DOS had gone through six successive versions, and now had a 600-page printed manual available from distributors for $50 as shipping and handling cost. After the programs and manual became available on the CDC website (with the help of Greg Fegan, a summer graduate student who programmed the first Epi Info website) sales of the manuals dropped off, but the program became freely available in the most remote corners of the world. Internet distribution continued with Epi Info 2000, and more than a million and a half copies have been downloaded.

I retired from CDC in 2002, and spent the next couple of years producing an Internet-based calculator system called OpenEpi (www.openepi.com) with fellow developers Kevin Sullivan, Minn Minn Soe, and Roger Mir, designed as a Windows replacement for the DOS Statcalc, and a foray into the popular area of open source software. I also produced teaching materials for two Master in Public Health courses on Epi Info, and programmed an Epi Info data entry and verification system for a multi-drug resistant tuberculosis project in Peru. Currently I am Director of Information Systems for an HIV/AIDS clinic in La Romana, Dominican Republic, where I develop Epi Info applications for clinical use, and experience the problems of local health agencies and clinics first hand, with the added spice of frequent power outages and operating in Spanish. In contrast to epidemiological computing, clinical informatics copes with the complexity of patient management and the challenge of serving medical professionals whose knowledge of computers often does not parallel their medical skills.

References

Advisory Committee to the Surgeon General of the Public Health Service (1964). *Smoking and health: report of the Advisory Committee to the Surgeon General of the Public Health Service*. US Department of Health, Education and Welfare, Washington, DC.

Breslow NE and Day NE (1980). *Statistical methods in cancer research. Volume I: The analysis of case–control studies*, IARC Scientific Publications No 32. IARC, Lyon.

Campos-Filho N and Franco EL (1989). Epidemiologic programs for computers and calculators. A microcomputer program for multiple logistic regression by unconditional and conditional maximum likelihood methods. *American Journal of Epidemiology*, **129**, 439–44.

Cornfield J (1951). A method of estimating comparative rates from clinical data; applications to cancer of the lung, breast, and cervix. *Journal of the National Cancer Institute*, **11**, 1269–75.

Cornfield J (1962). Joint dependence of risk of coronary heart disease on serum cholesterol and systolic blood pressure: a discriminant function analysis. *Federation Proceedings*, **21**, 58–61.

Dean AG (1994). Microcomputers and the future of epidemiology. *Public Health Reports*, **109**, 439–41.

Doll R and Hill AB (1950). Smoking and carcinoma of the lung; preliminary report. *British Medical Journal*, **2**, 739–48.

Greenland S (ed.) (1987). *Evolution of epidemiologic ideas: annotated readings on concepts and methods*. Epidemiology Resources Inc., Chestnut Hill, MA.

Hill AB (1965). The environment and disease: association or causation? *Proceedings of the Royal Society of Medicine*, **58**, 295–300.

Kaplan EL and Meier P (1958). Nonparametric estimation from incomplete observations. *Journal of the American Statistical Association*, **53**, 457–81.

Levin ML, Goldstein H, and Gerhardt PR (1950). Cancer and tobacco smoking; a preliminary report. *Journal of the American Medical Association*, **143**, 336–8.

Mantel N and Haenszel W (1959). Statistical aspects of the analysis of data from retrospective studies of disease. *Journal of the National Cancer Institute*, **22**, 719–48.

Morabia A (ed.) (2004). *A history of epidemiologic methods and concepts*. Birkhäser Verlag, Basel.

Nelder J and Wedderburn R (1972). Generalized linear models. *Journal of the Royal Statistical Society*, **132**, 107–20.

Rothman KJ (1986). Significance questing. *Annals of Internal Medicine*, **105**, 445–7.

Rothman KJ and Boice JD (1979). *Epidemiologic analysis with a programmable calculator*, NIH Publication 79-1649. US Government Printing Office, Washington, DC.

Rothman KJ and Greenland S (1998). *Modern epidemiology*, 2nd edn. Lippincott-Raven, Philadelphia, PA.

Schlesselman JJ (1982). *Case–control studies: design, conduct, and analysis.* Oxford University Press, New York.

Wynder EL and Graham EA (1950). Tobacco smoking as a possible etiologic factor in bronchiogenic carcinoma; a study of 684 proved cases. *Journal of the American Medical Association*, **143**, 329–36.

Zeger SL and Liang KY (1986). Longitudinal analysis using generalized linear models. *Biometrika*, **73**, 13–22.

25

Epidemiology as a common European endeavour

Jørn Olsen and Rodolfo Saracci

The European countries have a plurisecular tradition in scientific research, often bearing the mark of a country's individual history, social and cultural as well as political. Collaboration across frontiers has also been coeval to modern science. Harvey, the English discoverer of blood circulation and founder of physiology, worked from 1598 to 1602 at Padua University, where Sanctorius was at that very time measuring the weight of water lost by perspiration and where Galileo was laying the foundations of physics. At the population level comparisons of frequency of occurrence of diseases had been done in the past, a classical example being the work of the French sociologist Durkheim on suicide. However, the history of true collaborative transnational studies investigating different population groups in European countries is much more recent and has acquired momentum only in the last three decades. A not negligible factor for this 'late' start has been the speed at which modern epidemiology has been developing in the European countries, particularly marked differences occurring between four zones, namely the UK, the Nordic area, West continental Europe and East continental Europe, as highlighted in several chapters of this book.

The role of the World Health Organization

An important role in the shaping of modern epidemiology within Europe has been played by the World Health Organization (WHO). Structured, since its establishment in 1948, in geographical regions, the WHO has its European Office in Copenhagen and its headquarters in Geneva, an element facilitating contacts with European researchers. The role of the WHO has materialized in several ways.

Firstly, it has encouraged the development of epidemiology, from data collection and descriptive statistics to more or less sophisticated analytical studies, through the establishment of reference and collaborating centres at national and academic institutions (though inevitably in a minor proportion of cases they became mere labels). In recent years a few WHO centres, branches of the European office, have been established, e.g. the European Centre for Environment and Health in Rome.

Secondly, a large number of technical reports have been prepared, throughout the years, which represented the occasion for a two-way reinforcement of epidemiology: the WHO benefited from the input by experts and the experts benefited from the opportunity of spending time in discussion and actual work with colleagues from other countries, a particularly valuable circumstance for epidemiologists of many countries in continental Europe who were working (at least until the 1980s) in relative isolation.

Thirdly, the WHO promoted several large-scale epidemiological studies in Europe: in a number of studies the role of the WHO went beyond promotion into actual coordinating aspects in close collaboration with national research institutions. Perhaps the best known and most valuable of these investigations is the MONICA study, 'the world's largest study of heart disease, stroke, risk factors, and population trends', aimed at monitoring the evolution in time of myocardial infarction and stroke incidence and mortality in relation to the evolving prevalence of risk factors in different populations. The study was carried out worldwide, but three-quarters of the centres actually came from Europe: many are currently following prospectively the subjects examined cross-sectionally during the successive MONICA surveys. The study has contributed a substantial amount of information, for instance on the relative contribution of falling incidence and falling fatality in the decline of myocardial infarction.

Fourthly, the WHO established in 1965, on the initiative of a small number of European and extra-European countries, the International Agency for Research on Cancer (IARC), located in Lyon and entirely devoted to research, in particular epidemiological with interdisciplinary collaborations at an international level. IARC has played, since the beginning, a worldwide role, with initial epidemiological studies in such countries as Singapore, Iran, and Uganda. European collaborations came later but developed extensively, particularly when the European Community started to become involved—by virtue of its successive treaties—in matters of health: at this stage the experience of IARC staff in designing, conducting in the field, and analysing epidemiological investigations proved a most valuable technical resource for epidemiological projects in areas such as cancer screening, occupational and environmental hazards, and nutritional factors and cancer. Although obviously targeted on the cancer endpoints these studies contributed substantially to the development of expertise in Europe on the conduct of multicentre studies, including such aspects as dealing with variable ethical and legal requirements. The IARC has also actively promoted, since its beginning, the creation of good quality cancer registries in Europe, later grouped in the network of European Cancer Registries, and, particularly during the 1980s, developed and systematized methods for statistical analysis of both case–control and cohort studies, neatly presented in two now classic volumes—still best sellers—by N. Breslow and N. Day.

Last but not least, the contribution of the WHO materialized in promoting training and educational activities: for instance, the first course on modern epidemiological methods carried out in Pisa, Italy, in April 1974 was under the joint sponsorship of the WHO European Office and the International Epidemiological Association. A very substantial role in the educational endeavour was played by the IARC through 1–2 week courses on methodology in many European countries and through its fellowship programme that permitted a good number of young graduates to be trained in cancer epidemiology research, usually for 1 year, mostly in centres in the UK and USA.

The role of the European Union

Health and biomedical research had no place, as such, in the initial treaties of the European Community (which became the European Union in 1992). They came in rather obliquely as very restricted areas of research within the 'Coal and Steel' treaty and the 'Euratom' (nuclear energy) treaty. The former supported studies on occupational hazards, particularly in miners, and the latter projects in radiobiology and radioprotection of workers and the general public. One may confidently state that at the beginning of the 1970s epidemiology was totally new in the milieu of the European Commission, the propositional and executive organ of the Community. One of us remembers being dispatched by his boss—who had contracts for research in radiobiology and nuclear medicine—in late spring 1972 to Brussels to help a puzzled engineer, employed at the Commission, who had been ordered from above to find out what epidemiology was and whether it could have any real relevance to health.

Some work started to be developed with the support of the Social Affairs Directorate, which led to the formation of the 'Panel of Social Medicine and Epidemiology in the European Community', grouping the scientific societies of a number of countries. The Panel was instrumental in promoting the constitution of epidemiological associations in some countries and organized meetings, focused in particular on the publication of epidemiology books pertinent to public health analyses and health services evaluation in the European context. Albeit on a modest scale, this work had an important catalytic function, developing a nucleus of epidemiologists with a genuine European outlook and helping to sensitize the European Commission (EC) and national politicians to the need to include health and health research within the EC areas of competence (on this wider issue there was of course convergence from the biomedical world at large).

By the end of the 1970s a small-scale programme on topics in biomedicine was implemented within the Directorate of Research of the European Commission, with only three projects supported for the equivalent of about 1 million Euros. The critical expansion occurred in the 1980s, when research in general was reorganized, starting in 1984, in the form of 'Framework Programmes', intended to deal only with projects which could be carried out more rationally, effectively, and efficiently at the European level than nationally. A further important element in this development was the passing of the 'Single European Act' in 1987 which recognized research as having the same status as economic and social policy. Within this frame biomedical research gained formal recognition and momentum so that in the first half of the 1990s the biomedical and health research programme had reached a budget of 133 million Euros supporting more than 200 projects. Epidemiology was one of the beneficiaries of this development, with projects supported within the 'BIOMED' programmes in environmental epidemiology, occupational epidemiology, health services research, chronic disease epidemiology, perinatal and paediatric epidemiology. Projects received support essentially in the form of 'concerted actions' targeted to cover only the expenses for the coordination of work (including some staff time and laboratory expenses for standardization purposes) of the different participating groups. Typically a project would receive a sum of less than 1 million Euros, usually a half or a third of it, over 3 years. Support for the actual running expenses of an epidemiological, or, more generally, a biomedical research project, was not covered under the 'concerted action' formula, a serious hurdle to the development of large collaborative projects on the European scale. The EPIC project, the largest study worldwide on nutrition, cancer, and health, involving more than half a million people (and a repository of biological samples for more than 400 of them) in 10 European countries, started in the late 1980s and for years obtained substantial EU funds only thanks to the special programme 'Europe against Cancer'. In fact this programme had been designed not for research but for projects geared to public health actions, and as such it was administered by the Directorate on Social Affairs. Towards the end of the century the all pervasive shift of biomedical research towards molecular biology and genetics involved a shift of priorities within the 'Framework Programme(s)', of which epidemiology fell partially victim, as will be briefly mentioned in the final section of this chapter.

In the successive EU programmes the identification of research priority areas open to epidemiology has been subject to the intricacies of the decision-making processes in force at the EU level, not always mixing in a rational sequence scientific, political, and pure lobbying elements. As a result, every 5 years or so, important priority changes have occurred, as well as changes in the procedures to translate them into actual themes for project calls, funding applications, and project implementation. Rather than follow the fragmented outline of these numerous changes we prefer to try and sketch our view on at least some of the more permanent priorities for collaborative epidemiological research, their support, and training needs in Europe.

Collaborative epidemiological research

In recent years EU research has often been applied and tightly linked to specific and very detailed research programmes, probably developed to meet the interest of powerful lobbying groups (Saracci *et al.* 2005). Although many of these programmes have core epidemiological elements, they appear to be written and formulated by people with a limited knowledge of epidemiology. As a first priority these programmes would look different if they were to take inspiration from population-oriented health documents such as the World Bank's 'millennium development goals and epidemiology'. Although health problems are much worse in many places outside the EU, many of the targets mentioned by the World Bank are important for Europe as well.

Secondly, epidemiologists should also be able to, at least partly, explain the distribution of disease occurrence and mortality. It is important that not all epidemiologists become so fascinated with studying disease mechanisms at the molecular level that they lose the ability to see what are the true important determinants of public health. If epidemiologists do not take an interest in 'the big picture', they neglect one of their traditional roles in public health. Even within the European region we see a large variation in death and disease that probably reflects differences in lifestyles, income distribution, environmental exposures, and differences in health care much more than genetic differences. In fact, we have no reason to believe that differences in life expectancies, for example, between countries can be explained by genetic differences within the European region, although genetic differences may explain differences between countries for specific diseases. The large variety in lifestyles and environmental exposures provides excellent research opportunities for collaborative research across the European borders. So far, not enough effort has been put into studies that try to describe the consequences of differences in diet, climate, and occupational exposures. Health services epidemiologists have in like manner plenty of opportunities to compare the health consequences of the vast differences in European health care provision.

Health care systems have a different mix of private and public components, a different emphasis on primary and secondary health care, differences in diagnostic facilities, treatment option, screening practices, etc. We have differences in our training and educational systems and there are different procedures for most preventive programmes. These methods or procedures cannot all be 'the best', and we should at least make use of these 'man-made experiments' to try to understand more about their strengths and weaknesses. The European project on producing statistics on 'avoidable deaths'(the *European Community atlas of avoidable death* (Holland 1991)) and the present development of monitoring programmes are steps in the right direction, but much more could be done if we had the resources or used the resources available in a better way.

Thirdly, emerging diseases, like bird flu or monkey pox, illustrate that increasing travel activity can start a pandemic outbreak that may get out of control before effective preventive measures are available. Surprisingly little research funding is devoted to monitoring the evolution of infectious pathogens in terms of both genotyping and their disease characteristics on site by using updated technology for both genotyping and outbreak characterization. HIV and SARS have illustrated that the threats are real and may be multiplied by the biological sophistication posed by terrorists. Considering the amount of money devoted to military budgets, this biological threat to humankind has been grossly neglected. It would require a coordinated research action as well as a coordinated action plan implementing both new and well-established public health actions.

Fourth, not all of this can be done by merely analysing existing data, or even by new observational data, as observational epidemiology has its limits. There are many things we can do to improve the methods we apply, but results still come with substantial uncertainties. Randomized trials will not eliminate these uncertainties but will, in most cases where possible to conduct, produce results with fewer methodological reservations. The European Union should be prepared to invest in large-scale trials that are outside the area of pharmacoepidemiology. It is paradoxical that all countries insist on randomized trials before new drugs are introduced on the market but have no such requirements when governments manipulate health care, taxation, educational programmes, etc. Everybody would agree that decisions on how to manage health are political by nature, but if democracy is to work the public needs to know something about the health consequences of the decisions.

Support for collaborative research

The EU's earlier focus upon 'concerted actions' was in fact very successful in bringing European epidemiologists together, and these programmes facilitated much new research at a relatively low cost. In recent years much larger grants have been given to research by the EU; however, these grants are often large because they combine many smaller sub-studies on different related topics and are distributed in an increasing number of countries, so that the result may be not doing big science on a small set of problems, but rather doing small science on many problems. In physics it is accepted that large investments are needed to carry out important experiments, and the same may be needed in epidemiology at the European scale. For instance the preventive trials already mentioned will be generally expensive with costs typically adding up to several million Euros for a single study. At present, there seems to be no way of financing these large trials outside the private sector.

Health care is in most European countries regarded as a public responsibility, as part of being a member of society, even as a moral obligation for citizens of a democracy. In other countries, outside Europe, this responsibility may be left for people to organize themselves or as a responsibility for the employer. While the practice of heath promotion and preventive medicine involves both personal and public components, public health research is predominantly a public matter. What are the health consequences of our lifestyles, our working conditions, our environment, our social conditions, the nutrition we get, the health treatment we receive? That type of research usually has to be paid for by the public with a few exceptions. The most important of these exceptions is related to research that is part of the legal conditions for introducing a medicine on the market (e.g. pharmacoepidemiology). The other important exception concerns epidemiological research on diseases like cancer and other serious diseases (e.g. neurological, genetic) where private donations have provided important funding sources. One of the main reasons for the strong position of cancer epidemiology is without a doubt the private cancer foundations. With the support of these foundations (and other sources) epidemiologists have demonstrated how we can reduce the burden of cancer substantially by making changes in our personal life and by reducing the environmental carcinogenic load.

To a large extent, epidemiological research has to rely on public funding, unlike clinical research. Curing a wealthy patient may generate a grateful patient donor who may leave his or her fortune to research. Preventing a disease from developing does not have the same visible effect. Effective smoking cessation policies, implemented in many countries, and banning asbestos prevent thousands of lung cancer cases, but we will never know who they are. Prevention of occupational cancers and other occupational diseases, has been in many respects, a successful enterprise in Europe. Although cases are still accumulating because of past poorly controlled exposures and some occupational diseases have been 'exported' to developing countries, others have been almost eradicated by legislation supported by research.

European taxpayers should appreciate that this type of research actually leads to reduced costs, not only for those who remain healthy, but also to a downsizing of research needs (prevention is one of the few areas where you may lose your job if you do well). Public financing of epidemiological research requires that the governments are genuinely interested in the health of the people and are willing to accept research results that may be unpleasant or even embarrassing for the government. Low life expectancies or large social inequalities in health are not good news for governments that have the opposite political aims. For that reason, epidemiological research plays a limited role in non-democratic societies. Public support of epidemiology is a sign of democratic well-being, and it is probably more than a coincidence that the strongest epidemiological roots in Europe are found in the UK, the country with the longest uninterrupted democratic track. As one of the uncontroversial merits of the European Union is to aggregate, on a democratic basis, an increasing number of countries, public EU support to epidemiological research appears consistent with EU ideals and should rank high as a specific chapter in the funding agenda. It should be articulated, much better than hitherto, over a spectrum of different categories of projects, ranging from large and long-term single-purpose studies (e.g. large population trials), to studies involving epidemiological and other research groups in a substantial number of European countries, to smaller-scale studies developing novel ideas in a limited number of countries.

Teaching and training needs

Epidemiology has a place in most medical faculties in Europe, but not in all. In addition in some countries epidemiology has also moved out of the core medical disciplines to schools of public health.

A main argument for keeping epidemiology within medical faculties is that epidemiology is largely a medical scientific discipline and benefits from the biological thinking that underpins medical research. A second argument is that if epidemiology is taken out of the medical faculties it will become even more difficult to combine treatment and prevention. Doctors will become much less interested in prevention if they never had any training in public health epidemiology. Those who want to practice evidence-based prevention will find themselves amateurs in the field and will stop doing what they are not educated to do. A further and related argument is that clinical and public health epidemiology share a common set of methods although they focus upon different segments of the population. Public health epidemiologists study the transition from health to disease, and clinical epidemiologists study the transition from disease back to health or to disease progression and death. Public health epidemiology is about the aetiology and prevention of diseases. Clinical epidemiology is about prognosis and therapy. Both types of epidemiologist do, however, have much in common (see Chapter 23). Studying the unwanted side effects of drugs falls, for example, under the domain of both public health epidemiology and clinical epidemiology. These two areas of epidemiology should not be separated in different departments. A serious threat to epidemiology is, in fact, that the many epidemiologists are spread in many different departments, leaving only a few to develop the methodology and making it difficult for epidemiologists to feel a common responsibility for the discipline.

On the other hand, it could be argued that keeping epidemiology within medical faculties may prevent epidemiology departments from expanding to any large extent. Also it will not be possible to fully develop a curriculum for professionals in public health epidemiology if it has to be essentially based upon support from clinical medicine. Prevention may be better than cure, but it is not always without problems, especially not if it is invasive, like many screening programmes. Long-lasting medical treatment of risk factors like high blood pressure or high cholesterol also has the risk of side-effects that may even outweigh the benefits of the drugs for some. These activities require specific professional skills largely founded on epidemiology. In the USA, a number of very successful schools of public health have been established that graduate a large number of highly qualified professionals to work in prevention and health administration. Europe should probably try to follow a similar route, strengthening the resources to train these professionals, but without losing a formal training programme in epidemiology for all doctors and nurses within the medical faculties.

Research training is not yet fully developed in Europe as compared to the USA. Only some European countries have specialized, strongly research-based PhD programmes in epidemiology. Often the programmes are small in size and focused exclusively upon learning by doing rather than by being exposed to updated research methodology. Many large-scale studies take years to conduct, making learning exclusively by doing a slow and restrictive method. Epidemiology, on the other hand, is a discipline that is well suited to formal education, which is also a good way to present up-to-date methodology, integrating lectures and practical sessions, computer supported. This is especially relevant for an international audience of young European epidemiologists who need to know each other and acquire a common set of methodological references to carry joint projects. A number of such educational opportunities are available in the form of doctoral programmes, particularly at universities in the UK and the Netherlands or, at the level of short, targeted courses, in summer schools such as the IEA-sponsored EEPE summer school in Florence.

Current trends

At the time of writing, in spring 2006, the seventh 'Framework Programme' of research of the European Union is in preparation. The allocation of funds to biomedical and health research is, not yet, been defined, but should increase with respect to the sixth 'Framework Programme' (2002–06). While the latter had substantial funds, close to 3000 millions Euros available for the sector of health sciences (in real value about 15 times the funds available in the period 1990–94), these were assigned to two large priority themes; 'Genomics and biotechnologies' and 'Food quality and safety'. The formulation of topics under these two headings was dominated by a purely biomedical and technological approach to health and health research, pushed to the forefront by the impetuous development of molecular genetics on the one hand and by the interests of European industries competing on the international markets on the other: although epidemiological and public health studies were not excluded, the viewpoint of population-based research was clearly absent. This represented a net regression with respect to all preceding programmes, each of which had provided specific room for epidemiological and public health research. Since the sixth 'Framework Programme' went into implementation some corrections to this basic orientation have taken place, favourable to epidemiology. The current outline of the seventh 'Framework Programme', covering the period 2006–13, should mark a return to a more correct view of what the 'health by European citizen' is and which types of research are needed to maintain and improve it. Although still largely inspired by a concept in which health is seen as the end of a one-way linear path starting with basic research and translating its results into applications, it recognizes the need for specific research to evaluate and optimize these applications. More generally the population dimension of research is not absent and could hopefully be made more clearly explicit in the development of the programme.

A second positive step is the recent creation of the European Centre for Disease Control, located in Stockholm, which, besides its mandate in the coordination of public health practices in the EU, has at least the potential for some population-based research activities.

Epidemiological research as a collaborative European endeavour has come a long way between the early steps in the 1960s and 1970s and the dozens of projects which are currently under way.

Yet the backward, hopefully reversible, movement that occurred with the sixth 'Framework Programme' clearly shows that the equation 'health = medicine = biological and technological sciences' still largely dominates professional circles as well as the public's consciousness and that the population-based concept of health and health research needs continuous reaffirmation. This is a permanent challenge, at a scientific and political level, for epidemiologists within each country and within the European Union.

References

Holland WW (ed.) (1991). *European Community atlas of avoidable death*, 2nd edn, Vol. 1, Commission of the European Communities Health Services Research Series No 6. Oxford University Press, Oxford.

Saracci R, Olsen J, and Hofman A (2005). Health research policy in the European Union. *British Medical Journal*, **330**, 1459–60.

26

Epidemiological methods: a view from Africa

Adetokunbo O. Lucas

Personal experiences

Strongly influenced by two uncles, I had decided to become a doctor before entering secondary school. My maternal uncle, Dr I. Ladipo Oluwole, DPH, a Glasgow graduate, worked as a general practitioner before moving to the health office in Lagos, where he later become the first Nigerian Medical Officer of Health. My uncle-in-law, Sir Samuel Manuwa, MD, FRCS, FRSE, the first Nigerian Director of Medical Services, graduated from Edinburgh and trained as a surgeon. I sought to emulate my role models by first practising clinical medicine before switching to public health. But a series of fortunate accidents accelerated the change in career. In 1957, shortage of space in the Department of Medicine at Queen's University, Belfast where I was training in internal medicine, led to my being lodged in an office in the Department of Preventive Medicine. There I met Ken Newell and a year later, John Pemberton, both of whom exerted a strong influence on me, showing me some of the fascinations of epidemiological tools in problem solving. At first, I audited courses in epidemiology and statistics but later enrolled for the Diploma in Public Health course. Back home in Nigeria in 1960, I pursued my career in internal medicine at the teaching hospital in Ibadan, and planned to switch to public health after a decade or more in clinical medicine. Meanwhile, at John Pemberton's invitation, I had my first contact with the International Epidemiological Association (IEA) at the conference in Korcula in 1961. In 1962, when the Professor of Preventive and Social Medicine at the University of Ibadan left to head a newly established university, I was invited to become his designated successor. From then on I became more deeply involved with epidemiology, deriving much inspiration and knowledge from participating in IEA activities at different levels including organizing the first regional conference in 1970 and serving as the chair of the Council, 1971–74.

In no part of the world has health and disease had such a great impact on the lives and fortunes of the people as in Africa. Portuguese settlement in the fifteenth century foundered mainly because of disease but lasted long enough for the coastal 'Eko' to be renamed 'Lagos' after a lagoon-sited town in Portugal. In other parts of the world, the political map was drawn by the outcomes of wars of conquest, treaties, and migrations. In Africa, however, the political map was largely determined by the ability of early European explorers and other invaders to survive and settle in various parts of the continent. Under pressure from tropical diseases, Africa's geopolitical map evolved into three zones: the north with its strong Arab influence; East and southern Africa with history of substantial European settlements; and West and Central Africa which remained almost exclusively African. In the specific case of a country like Nigeria, the health effects on Europeans who approached from the south and Moslem conquerors, who invaded from the north, determined the political map of the country. Whilst malaria, yellow fever, and other infections limited the European push from the south, the invaders from the north lost their horses through vector-borne infections in the wet savanna and so their influence was mainly confined to the northern region of the country. These historical movements resulted in the present situation

Table 26.1 Mortality among European explorers in West Africa

Expedition	Year	Europeans	No of deaths
Mungo Park	1805	44	39
Tuckey	1816	44	21
Clapperton	1825–7	5	4
MacGregot-Laird	1832–4	41	32
Trotter	1841	145	42

in which the northern areas of the country are largely Moslem and the south has a higher proportion of Christians. Warfare, trade, and treaties determined the political fortunes of other countries, the anopheles mosquito, *Aedes aegypti*, the tsetse fly, and other vectors tipped the scales in Africa! As shown in Table 26.1, European explorers suffered massive death rates and this gave the region its nickname of 'the white man's grave' (Sabben-Clarke *et al*. 1971).

The historical development of the northern part of Africa, bordering the Mediterranean Sea, was strongly influenced by its Arab and European neighbours and was therefore not typical of the rest of the continent. This chapter will mainly deal with the events in sub-Saharan Africa, a region that shares many characteristic features, especially with regard to its pattern of health and disease.

The development of epidemiology in Africa can be viewed in three broad historical dimensions:

◆ the age of discovery, largely dominated by work on communicable diseases;

◆ wider applications of epidemiology to chronic diseases and accidents;

◆ modern epidemiology including sophisticated applications of epidemiological tools including mathematical modelling.

I also discuss:

◆ cross-national studies and

◆ epidemiological research capacity in Africa.

The age of discovery

Early contacts of Europeans with tropical Africa from the fifteenth century initially involved trade but later followed centuries in which the slave trade was the dominant feature of the interaction. Following the abolition of the slave trade in the nineteenth century, the new relationship was through colonial conquest and European settlement in parts of Africa. Quite predictably, the earliest applications of epidemiology in colonial Africa related largely to description and analysis of communicable diseases. These infections constituted major challenges to the European traders and settlers but also affected indigenous populations, especially children, pregnant women, and other vulnerable groups. The medical teams accompanying the early explorers to Africa encountered a variety of communicable diseases that were largely unknown in Europe and other parts of the world. Descriptive and analytical epidemiology featured prominently in the identification and classification of the strange syndromes that the early explorers encountered. The application of classical epidemiological methods helped to characterize these infections as well as providing clues as to the risk factors and determinants.

Epidemiological studies aided the analysis of the variety of febrile illnesses that occurred in the region. The study of yellow fever in West Africa complemented the research undertaken by scientists in the Western Hemisphere and culminated in the development of an effective vaccine for controlling the disease. Dr B. B. Waddy's work on the study of a strange blinding illness in Ghana (formerly known as the Gold Coast) is an illustration of the successful use of classical 'shoe-leather' epidemiology. Waddy's maps showed that the prevalence of blindness in the Ghanaian villages was highest near the rivers and declined as one moved to more distant communities. In association with Sir John Wilson of the Commonwealth Institute for the Blind, they coined the term 'river blindness' to describe the disease. Subsequent work led to the discovery of the causative agent, the worm *Onchocerca volvulus* and the vector, the black fly, *Simulium damnosum*. Similarly, work on African sleeping sickness led Castellani to identify the protozoa, *Trypanosome rhodesiensis* as the causative agent. This was complemented by the identification of the tsetse fly as the vector of both the human and animal disease. Epidemiological studies made significant contributions to knowledge of the distribution and determinants of these and other tropical infections as well as assessing the dimensions of the burden of disease that resulted from the endemic and epidemic diseases (Sabben-Clarke *et al.* 1971).

In addition to its contribution to the understanding of specific tropical infections, epidemiological studies in Africa provided many useful illustrations of the ecological basis for the occurrence and distribution of diseases. Thus, for example, onchocerciasis was shown to be a disease of people living near the river basin of fast-moving streams, whilst the distribution of schistosomiasis is largely determined by the pattern of water contact in slow-moving streams, lakes, and ponds. Furthermore, epidemiological studies showed the impact of large-scale agro-engineering works like artificial lakes in altering the intensity of these water associated infections.

Epidemiological studies in Africa also stimulated the development of multidisciplinary approaches to health problems. The study of vector-borne diseases recruited the interests of biologists in defining the ecology of arthropod vectors in the study of malaria, sleeping sickness, and other insect-borne diseases. Malacologists contributed to the study of schistosomiasis, paragonomiasis, and other mollusc-related diseases. Social scientists provided tools that were used to study the role of human behaviour in the prevalence and distribution of tropical infections, as for example in the relation between water contact and schistosomiasis.

Studies in Africa also drew attention to the influence of climate and season on the epidemiology of certain diseases. The classical studies of Lapeysonnie on cerebrospinal meningitis in Africa produced evidence of a strong correlation between epidemics of the disease and geographical factors. In West Africa, the epidemics occur within a defined geographical zone characterized by the level of rainfall; the southern boundary is limited by the 1100 mm isobar and the northern limit by the 300 mm isobar. Furthermore, the epidemics start during the dry season and end abruptly as soon as humidity rises and the rains begin (Lapeyssonnie 1963).

These ecological assessments provided useful clues for disease control. For example, applying epidemiological and ecological information, the health authorities dealt with a persistent focus of epidemic sleeping sickness in the Zaria area of Nigeria; the local population 'had become so attenuated and the survivors so weakened and demoralized that farms, wells, market places, and dwellings fell into decrepitude under the very eyes of the inhabitants'. The colonial medical service tackled this challenge by developing an ambitious but successful resettlement scheme—known widely as the Anchau scheme—which included extensive clearance of the riverine vegetation that supported the breeding of the tsetse fly (Duggan 1980). Intensive effort over a decade from 1936 eventually led to the elimination of the infection over an area of 700 square miles in Zaria province.

HIV/AIDS in Africa

In recent decades, the pandemic of HIV/AIDS has severely affected populations in sub-Saharan Africa. Epidemiological research in the region has been effectively used in designing and monitoring control measures. In addition to medical studies, there has been great interest in behavioural studies to analyse patterns of sexual networking. For example, Orubuloye and his collaborators in Nigeria and abroad have produced a massive collection of research results on the sociology of sexual behaviour that are of particular relevance to the current epidemic of HIV/AIDS (Orubuloye *et al.* 1991, 1994; Orubuloye 1993). There has been considerable interest in the epidemiological finding that a small proportion of prostitutes who are highly exposed apparently have a natural immunity that protects them from being infected with the HIV virus. It is hoped that the natural mechanism can be adapted to develop an effective vaccine (Fowke *et al.* 1996; Iqbal *et al.* 2005). Immunologists are following up a similar observation among commercial sex workers in the Gambia (Rowland-Jones *et al.* 1998).

Broader application of epidemiology in Africa

The tropical diseases that severely affected European explorers, especially in West Africa, were tamed but not completely eliminated. The further progress of epidemiology in tropical Africa extended to the study of chronic, non-communicable diseases. Many myths had developed about the occurrence of chronic diseases among the indigenous populations of tropical Africa but the steady accumulation of epidemiological data provided more reliable information. Some of the early observers had the impression that cancers did not occur among Africans but this myth was abolished with the steady accumulation of clinical and epidemiological information about the occurrence of various cancers in African populations. Denis Burkitt, working in East Africa, described the tumour that bears his name—Burkitt's lymphoma. Mapping the distribution of cases, Burkitt showed that the geographical boundaries of the cancer suggested a vector-borne infection, a clue that led to the identification of the Epstein–Barr virus as the probable aetiological agent of this cancer. Other cancers that have been studied in great detail include cancer of the bladder and its probable relationship to infection with *Schistosoma haematobium*, primary hepatoma and its association with the ingestion of mycotoxins and chronic infection with the hepatitis B virus; and oesophageal cancer in parts of Central and southern Africa (Bababunmi *et al.* 1978; McGlashan *et al.* 1982, 2003).

Diseases of civilization

Burkitt and his co-worker, Trowell, adduced convincing evidence about the role of dietary fibre in preventing certain cancers and chronic diseases, notably colonic–rectal cancer, diverticulosis, and varicose veins. Their observations showed that indigenous populations with traditional lifestyles were at lower risk of acquiring these diseases of civilization (Burkitt 1973, 1978, 1982; Trowell and Burkitt 1979). These authors helped to set the foundation of the current concept that lifestyles are important risk factors in the genesis of cancers, cardiovascular diseases, and non-insulin dependent diabetes mellitus. Their observations dispelled the view that chronic diseases were merely degenerative processes that were inevitable concomitants of advancing age (Osuntokun 1988).

Cardiovascular diseases have also attracted the attention of epidemiologists in Africa. Some of the studies related to the definition of unusual cardiovascular diseases like endomyocardial fibrosis, idiopathic cardiomyopathy, and multiple non-luetic arterial aneurysm, but of greater interest has been the epidemiology of cosmopolitan cardiovascular diseases (World Health Organization 1966). Earlier records showed that ischaemic heart disease occurred infrequently in many African populations. The rarity of ischaemic heart disease was confirmed by autopsy studies that showed a low prevalence of atherosclerosis. However, the situation has changed dramatically in the past few decades with rapid increase in the frequency of ischaemic heart disease as Africans adopt foreign lifestyles in diet, smoking, and sedentary habits (Falase *et al.* 1973; Akinboboye *et al.* 2003).

Unusual diseases and syndromes

The epidemiological picture in Africa shows wide diversity. Some of these differences are clearly associated with recognizable climatic and other geographical differences but some are related to peculiar local behavioural factors. For example, chronic cyanide intoxication of dietary origin was identified as the cause of a tropical ataxic neuropathy that occurs in Nigeria and in other African countries in communities that rely on cassava as a staple food. Recurrent epidemics of a neurological disease were traced to a seasonal intake of a larva of the fly *Anaphe venata* (see Box 26.1).

Epidemiological surveys

The lack of reliable morbidity and mortality statistics from routinely collected data is a major constraint on planning, implementing, and evaluating health services in Africa. Public health practitioners and scientists have used epidemiological surveys to fill some of this information gap. An expedition from Harvard University journeyed from Liberia to the Belgian Congo, collecting plant and animal specimens and studying disease (Strong 1930). Epidemiological surveys have been extensively used in Africa to define the distribution of specific diseases or groups of diseases but also more broadly to assess community health and the pattern of diseases. Some cross-sectional studies have assessed chronic disease on a national scale (Akinkugbe 1971). Long-term longitudinal studies provide a powerful tool for the gathering of information,

---

Box 26.1

Two distinct ataxic neuropathies linked to local dietary habits have been identified in southwestern Nigeria:

- Tropical ataxic neuropathy. This neurological problem affected communities in the coastal lagoon area of southwestern Nigeria. In the worst affected communities in the Epe and Ososa districts, in some age groups, up to 8–10% of the adults walked with a staggering gait. More severely affected persons were crippled and bed-ridden. Because of evidence of vitamin B deficiency in the affected communities, previous workers had attributed the neurological problem to malnutrition, specifically to vitamin B deficiency. Clinical, biochemical, and epidemiological studies by Osuntokun linked the occurrence of the disease to chronic cyanide intoxication from the local cassava diet (Money 1958; Osuntokun 1971)

- Seasonal epidemic ataxic 'the Ijesha shakes' occurs around the town of Ilesha, an inland area some 200 miles from the Epe district. Clinically, the disease presented with acute cerebellar ataxia in all patients, and with ophthalmoplegias and encephalopathy in the more severe cases. These features are remarkably similar to those of acute thiamine deficiency. The aetiology was eventually traced to the consumption of a stew containing the roasted larvae of *Anaphe venata*, a seasonal protein supplement peculiar to the area (Adamolekun 1993; Adamolekun and Ndububa 1994; Adamolekun *et al.* 1997). A double-blind placebo-controlled study, demonstrating the efficacy of thiamine hydrochloride in relieving the symptoms of the disease, further strengthened the theory of the pathogenesis of the disease (Adamolekun *et al.* 1997)

especially on chronic diseases. In Tanzania, local scientists in collaboration with colleagues from Newcastle University, UK, carried out extensive studies on adult mortality. This collaboration generated data about the patterns of morbidity and mortality as well as information on specific diseases like diabetes (Kitange *et al.* 1996; Ramaiya *et al.* 1990; Setel *et al.* 2000; Swai *et al.* 1990).

Modern epidemiological methods

African epidemiologists and their partners have applied modern epidemiological methods to the study of both communicable and chronic diseases. Mathematical models of malaria transmission, first introduced by Ronald Ross and George MacDonald, were further developed and tested in a field project in Garki, Nigeria. The Garki models give insights into the importance of quantitative aspects of the dynamics of malaria transmission in this area of hyper-endemic malaria (MacDonald *et al.* 1968; Molineaux and Gramicca 1980).

Quantitative methods were widely applied in the assessment of the epidemiology of onchocerciasis using such indicators like community microfilarial load (CMFL) and entomological data (annual biting rate (ABR) and crude annual transmission potential (ATP)) (Basanez *et al.* 2002).

Geographical information systems are being used to generate risk assessment models for diseases such as malaria, onchocerciasis, and schistosomiasis (Gebre-Michael *et al.* 2005; Rogers *et al.* 2002; Stensgaard *et al.* 2002)

Cross-national comparative studies

Cross-national comparative studies have yielded valuable epidemiological information and provide useful clues for unravelling the complex web of risk factors and determinants of health and disease. International comparisons provide opportunities for examining key variables in high-prevalence and in low-prevalence groups; and also in situations where the disease is newly emerging or rapidly declining. Such studies enable scientists to examine hypotheses that seem valid in one country or geographical area, by testing them at other sites and in other settings. International comparative studies can be used to develop and test new or modified technologies for prevention, diagnosis, and the management of diseases. Such studies have helped to adapt some expensive, complicated technologies into affordable cost-effective interventions. Not only do such modified techniques benefit developing countries but they have, in turn, been adopted by developed countries. Cross-national studies involving African populations have examined cardiovascular diseases (Williams and Resch 1968; Williams *et al.*1969, 1971; Resch *et al.*1970), senile dementias (Ogunniyi and Osuntokun 1991; Ogunniyi *et al.* 1992, 1997; Osuntokun *et al.* 1992; Baldereschi *et al.* 1994; Hendrie *et al.* 1995; see also the 10/66 Dementia Research Group website at www.alz.co.uk/1066/), various neurological disorders (Schoenberg *et al.* 1988), and some cancers (Jackson *et al.* 1975, 1977).

Epidemiological research capacity

Several international agencies such as the World Health Organization and private charitable foundations like the Rockefeller Foundation and the Carnegie Corporation of New York have contributed to the training of African epidemiologists and the strengthening of national institutions. The International Epidemiological Association has influenced the development of epidemiology in the continent; it held its first Regional Conference in April 1970 in Ibadan, Nigeria. The Council for Health Research and Development (COHRED) is another organization that is promoting health research in developing countries (COHRED; cohred.org/cohred/Home.action). The African chapter of the International Clinical Epidemiological Network (INCLEN) is similarly promoting and coordinating epidemiological research. An increasing number of African institutions and networks are making useful contributions to epidemiological research. For example, INDEPTH, a major research network of field sites, undertakes continuous demographic evaluation of populations and their health in developing countries (www.indepth-network.org/).

References

Abrahams DG and Cockshott WP (1962). Multiple non-luetic aneurysms in young Nigerians. *British Heart Journal*, **24**, 83–91.

Adamolekun B (1993). *Anaphe venata* entomophagy and seasonal ataxic syndrome in southwest Nigeria. *Lancet*, **341**, 629.

Adamolekun B and Ndububa DA (1994). Epidemiology and clinical presentation of a seasonal ataxia in western Nigeria. *Journal of the Neurological Sciences*, **124**, 95–8.

Adamolekun B, Adamolekun WE, Sonibare AD, and Sofowora G (1994). A double-blind, placebo-controlled study of the efficacy of thiamine hydrochloride in a seasonal ataxia in Nigerians. *Neurology*, **44**, 549–51.

Adamolekun B, McCandless DW, and Butterworth RF (1997). Epidemic of seasonal ataxia in Nigeria following ingestion of the African silkworm *Anaphe venata*: role of thiamine deficiency? *Metabolic Brain Disease*, **12**, 251–8.

Akinboboye O, Idris O, Akinboboye O, and Akinkugbe O (2003). Trends in coronary artery disease and associated risk factors in sub-Saharan Africans. *Journal of Human Hypertension*, **17**, 381–7.

Akinkugbe OO (1971). National Expert Committee on Non-Communicable Disease, final report of a national survey, series 4. OO Akinkugbe (ed.) *Federal Ministry of Health and Social Services*.

Bababunmi EA, Uwaifo AO, and Bassir O (1978). Hepatocarcinogens in Nigerian foodstuffs. *World Review of Nutrition and Dietetics*, **28**, 188–209.

Baldereschi M, Amato MP, Nencini P, *et al.* (1994). Cross-national inter-rater agreement on the clinical diagnostic criteria for dementia: WHO-PRA Age-Associated Dementia Working Group, WHO Program for Research on Aging, Health of Elderly Program. *Neurology*, **44**, 239–42.

Basanez M, Collins RC, Porter CH, Little MP, and Brandling-Bennett D (2002). Transmission intensity and the patterns of *Onchocerca volvulus* infection in human communities. *American Journal of Tropical Medicine and Hygiene*, **67**, 669–79.

Burkitt DP (1973). Some diseases characteristic of modern Western civilization. *British Medical Journal*, **3**, 274–8.

Burkitt DP (1978). Colonic-rectal cancer: fiber and other dietary factors. *American Journal of Clinical Nutrition*, **31**, S58–S64.

Burkitt DP (1982). Western diseases and their emergence related to diet. *South African Medical Journal*, **61**, 1013–15.

Duggan AJ (1980). Sleeping sickness epidemics in health in tropical Africa during the colonial period. In *Health in tropical Africa during the colonial period* (ed. EE Sabben-Clare, DJ Bradley and K Kirkwood). Clarendon, Oxford.

Falase AO, Basile O, and Osuntokun BO (1973). Myocardial infarction in Nigerians. *Tropical and Geographical Medicine*, **25**, 147–50.

Fowke KR, Nagelkerke NJ, Kimani J, *et al.* (1996).Resistance to HIV-1 infection among persistently seronegative prostitutes in Nairobi, Kenya. *Lancet*, **348**, 1347–50.

Gebre-Michael T, Malone JB, and McNally K (2005). Use of geographic information systems in the development of prediction models for onchocerciasis control in Ethiopia. *Parassitologia*, **47**, 135–44.

Hendrie HC, Osuntokun BO, Hall KS, *et al.* (1995). Prevalence of Alzheimer's disease and dementia in two communities: Nigerian Africans and African Americans. *American Journal of Psychiatry*, **152**, 1485–92.

Iqbal SM, Ball TB, Kimani J, *et al.* (2005). Elevated T cell counts and RANTES expression in the genital mucosa of HIV-1-resistant Kenyan commercial sex workers. *Journal of Infectious Diseases*, **192**, 728–38.

Jackson MA, Ahluwalia BS, Attah EB, *et al.* (1975). Characterization of prostatic carcinoma among blacks: a preliminary report. *Cancer Chemotherapy Reports*, **59**, 3–7.

Jackson MA, Ahluwalia BS, Herson J, *et al.* (1977). Characterization of prostatic carcinoma among blacks: a continuation report. *Cancer Chemotherapy Reports*, **61**, 167–72.

Kitange HM, Machibya H, Black J, *et al.* on behalf of the Adult Morbidity and Mortality Project (1996). Outlook for survivors of childhood in sub-Saharan Africa: adult mortality in Tanzania. *British Medical Journal*, **312**, 216–20.

Lapeyssonnie L (1963). La menigite cerebro-spinale en Afrique. *Bulletin of the World Health Organization*, **28**(Suppl. 1), 3–114.

MacDonald G, Cuellar CB, and Foll CV (1968). The dynamics of malaria, *Bulletin of the World Health Organization*, **38**, 743–55.

McGlashan ND, Bradshaw E, and Harington JS (1982). Cancer of the oesophagus and the use of tobacco and alcoholic beverages in Transkei, 1975–6. *International Journal of Cancer*, **29**, 249–56.

McGlashan ND, Harington JS, and Chelkowska E (2003). Changes in the geographical and temporal patterns of cancer incidence among black gold miners working in South Africa, 1964–1996. *British Journal of Cancer*, **88**, 1361–9.

Molineaux L and Gramicca G (1980). *The Garki Project: research on the epidemiology and control of malaria in the Sudan savanna in West Africa.* WHO, Geneva.

Money G (1958). Endemic neuropathies in the Epe district of southern Nigeria. *West African Medical Journal*, **7**, 58–62.

Ogunniyi AO and Osuntokun BO (1991). Relatively low prevalence of Alzheimer's disease in developing countries and the racial factors in dementia research. *Ethnicity and Disease*, **1**, 394–5.

Ogunniyi A, Osuntokun BO, Lekwauwa UG, and Falope ZF (1992). Rarity of dementia (by DSM-III-R) in an urban community in Nigeria. *East African Medical Journal*, **69**, 10–14.

Ogunniyi A, Gureje O, Baiyewu O, *et al.* (1997). Profile of dementia in a Nigerian community – types, pattern of impairment, and severity rating. *Journal of the National Medical Association*, **89**, 392–6.

Orubuloye IO (1993). Sexual abstinence patterns in rural Western Nigeria: evidence from a survey of Yoruba women. *Social Science and Medicine*, **37**, 859–72.

Orubuloye IO, Caldwell JC, and Caldwell P (1991). African women's control over their sexuality in an era of AIDS. A study of the Yoruba of Nigeria. *Studies in Family Planning*, **22**, 61–73.

Orubuloye IO, Caldwell JC, Caldwell P, and Santow G (ed.) (1994). *Sexual networking and HIV/AIDS in sub-Saharan Africa: behavioural studies in the social context.* Health Transition Series No.4. Health Transition Centre, The Australian National University, Canberra.

Osuntokun BO (1971). Epidemiology of tropical neuropathy in Nigeria. *Transactions of the Royal Society of Tropical Medicine and Hygiene*, **65**, 454–79.

Osuntokun BO (1988). Lifestyles and changes in patterns of non-communicable diseases in developing countries. *Nigerian Journal of Basic and Applied Psychology*, **1**, 165–81.

Osuntokun BO, Ogunniyi AO, and Lekwauwa UG (1992). Alzheimer's disease in Nigerians. *African Journal of Medical Science*, **21**, 71–7.

Ramaiya KL, Kodaii VRR, and Alberti KGMM (1990). Epidemiology of diabetes in Asians of the Indian Subcontinent. *Diabetes Metabolism Reviews*, **6**, 125–46.

Resch JA, Williams AO, Lemercier G, and Loewenson RB (1970). Comparative autopsy studies on cerebral atherosclerosis in Nigerian and Senegal Negroes, American Negroes and Caucasians. *Atherosclerosis*, **12**, 401–7.

Rogers DJ, Randolph SE, Snow RW, and Hay SI (2002). Satellite imagery in the study and forecast of malaria. *Nature*, **415**, 710–15.

Rowland-Jones S, Dong T, Krausa P, *et al.* (1998). The role of cytotoxic T-cells in HIV infection. *Developments in Biological Standardization*, **92**, 209–14.

Sabben-Clare EE, Bradley DJ, and Kirkwood K (ed.) (1971). *Health in tropical Africa during the colonial period*. Clarendon, Oxford.

Schoenberg BS, Osuntokun BO, Adeuja AOG, and Bademosi O (1988). Prevalence of Parkinson's disease in Black populations in rural US and in rural Nigeria: door-to-door community studies. *Neurology*, **38**, 645–6.

Setel P, Whiting D, Hemed Y, and Alberti KG (2000). Educational status is related to mortality at the community level in three areas of Tanzania, 1992–1998. *Journal of Epidemiology and Community Health*, **54**, 936–7.

Stensgaard A, Jorgensen A, Kabatereine NB, Malone JB, and Kristensen TK (2005). Modeling the distribution of *Schistosoma mansoni* and host snails in Uganda using satellite sensor data and Geographical Information Systems. *Parassitologia*, **47**, 115–25.

Strong RP (ed.) (1930). *The African republic of Liberia and the Belgian Congo; based on the observations made and material collected during the Harvard African expedition 1926–1927*. Harvard University Press, Cambridge, MA.

Swai ABM, Lutate J, and Melarty DG (1990). Diabetes in tropical Africa: a prospective study, 1981–1987. 1 Characteristics of newly presenting patients in Dar es Salaam, Tanzania, 1981–7. *British Medical Journal*, **300**, 1103–6.

Trowell HC and Burkitt DP (1979). Diverticular disease in urban Kenyans. *British Medical Journal*, **1**, 1795.

Williams AO and Resch JA (1968). Cerebral atherosclerosis: a comparative study between an African and a Minnesota autopsy population. *Neurology*, **18**, 287.

Williams AO, Resch JA, and Loewenson RB (1969). Cerebral atherosclerosis–a comparative autopsy study between Nigerian Negroes and American Negroes and Caucasians. *Neurology*, **19**, 205–10.

Williams AO, Resch JA, and Loewenson RB (1971). Comparative study on cerebral atherosclerosis between an African (Nigerian) and American population groups (caucasian and negroes). *East African Medical Journal*, **48**, 152–62.

World Health Organization (1966). Cardiomyopathies. *Bulletin of the World Health Organization*, **33**, 257–66.

27

The development of epidemiology in New Zealand and the South Pacific

Ian Prior and Robert Beaglehole

Introduction

The beginnings of epidemiology in New Zealand date back to the 1920s with the work of Charles Hercus on iodine deficiency diseases. This research contributed directly to the addition of iodine to salt with immediate public health impact. It remains a noteworthy example of the potential of epidemiological research to influence public policy with positive benefits for the health of the whole population and, in this case, particularly to the health of the most disadvantaged (see Chapter 19). In the 1930s and 1940s detailed epidemiological studies were made of the impact of tuberculosis on Maori. Again this research had direct policy applications with positive health impacts.

This chapter describes the development of epidemiology in New Zealand with a focus on the last 50 years and on cardiovascular diseases, which by about 1950 had become the leading cause of death in New Zealand. The story is told from the perspective of the first author who was instrumental in ensuring that epidemiology took hold and eventually flourished in New Zealand as it responded to the challenges of the health transition and the growing epidemics of chronic diseases.

There are important lessons to be learnt from our story even though the Pacific populations are for the most part relatively small (Fig. 27.1). A feature of the New Zealand and Pacific studies conducted by the Epidemiology Unit of the Wellington Hospital has been the recognition that our teams have been involved not only in epidemiological studies but also in providing ongoing advice on medical care and public health measures with strong links with the local medical services. At the same time these studies have been conducted with a high degree of community participation. This approach is a far cry from the major epidemiological studies that were being developed at around this time where data were collected, mainly from middle-aged men, on risk factors for coronary heart diseases, particularly cholesterol and high blood pressure.

This story may have interest in its own right. Of more importance are the lessons learned that can inform the development of epidemiology and public health more generally in low-resource settings today. These lessons are important, given the relatively weak state of epidemiology in almost all countries except some of the wealthiest.

Personal influences

In retrospect, several distinct influences ensured that both authors moved from clinical medicine into epidemiology and then public health. Ian Prior can trace his epidemiological antecedents back to his paternal great grandfather, who as a missionary in Fiji convinced his parishioners to give up cannibalism—a very successful public health intervention with immediate effects. Critical influences on his early career development were a Fulbright Research Scholarship which allowed him to work in Boston, a key centre for cardiological research, which also marked the

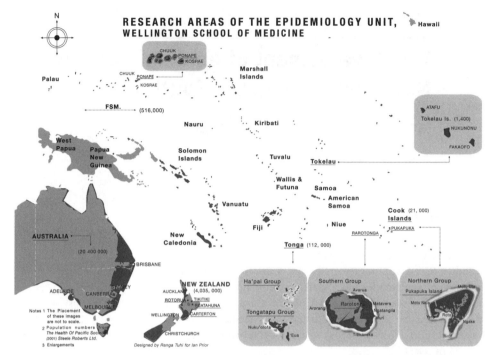

Fig. 27.1 Map of Oceania (underlined countries and areas, current populations as at 2005). The current population numbers are: Melanesia, 6,475,900; Micronesia, 516,000; Polynesia, 613,100; Australia, 20,400,000; New Zealand, 4,035,000; Tokelau, 1400; Samoa, 177,000; and Cook Islands, 21,000.

beginning of his close friendship with Bernard Lown who went on to found International Physicians for the Prevention of Nuclear War (IPPNW).

In 1959 as a well-trained physician and cardiologist Ian Prior became the Director of the Medical Unit at Wellington Hospital and increasingly focused his research on the health of New Zealand Maori. In 1962 Ian responded to a government report calling for population-based research into ethnic inequalities in health. The report, written by Richard Rose from the Department of Health, was entitled 'Maori and European comparisons of mortality 1962'. The document used routinely available mortality and hospital statistics to highlight the high risk of coronary heart disease and diabetes experienced by Maori.

Ian Prior realized that the routine statistics required confirmation by population-based research and he was able to secure modest funding from the Medical Research Council for studies of the health of Maori in urban and rural settings in New Zealand and of a contrasting 'European' population. Before this research began, extensive discussions were held with Maori elders and the isolated Maori communities which seemed suitable for testing hypotheses about the potential influence of the 'modern' way of life on Maori.

In the late 1960s this epidemiological interest expanded to include the health of Pacific peoples undergoing a rapid health transition under the influence of changing patterns of living in Polynesia and, especially, of migration to New Zealand. In 1970, in recognition of the importance of the epidemiological research, the Epidemiology Unit of Wellington Hospital was established and Ian Prior now had the liberty to expand the epidemiological research.

The trajectory of Robert Beaglehole was directly influenced by the first author and was much more straightforward. Parental influences were also important, given their social anthropological research interests in the South Pacific and New Zealand and especially their 9 month stay in 1935 on Pukapuka, a northern Cook Island atoll. This atoll was later chosen for an epidemiological study of Polynesians as yet unexposed to 'Western' styles of living. An elective as a medical student in the academic unit at Wellington Hospital developed his interest in epidemiology. He was firmly instructed to become an established clinician before entering epidemiology, on the expectation that an MRCP diploma—and the associated clinical training—would confer respectability on his interests in the still rather dubious field of epidemiology. It is hard to assess now the importance of a clinical training in addition to the epidemiological and public health training. However, in retrospect it does seem to have given a modest amount of credibility to the evidence-based advocacy which became such an important aspect of the public health work in New Zealand. Without doubt, the biological training associated with a medical degree remains an important aspect of public health practice.

Overcoming the obstacles

The initial epidemiological studies were undertaken in time taken from clinical duties and holidays. Inevitably this led to concerns expressed by senior colleagues who did not appreciate the value of epidemiology or approve of time being taken from clinical and academic responsibilities. Fortunately, the Director General of Health and the Medical Research Council of New Zealand saw the merit of the proposed studies and supported the establishment of the Wellington Hospital Epidemiology Unit. This support included the secondment of staff from the Department of Health as well as critical, if modest, financial support.

A major early difficulty was the lack of critical mass of experienced staff for field work and, especially, the lack of quantitative skills so essential for a successful epidemiological team. An Australian clinical colleague volunteered to help with field work and the research funding agencies eventually appreciated the importance of providing financial support for fulltime epidemiological and analytical staff.

Support from the Department of Health, especially Dr Douglas Kennedy, Director General of the department, and the Medical Research Council provided legitimacy for this new venture. Of equal importance in ensuring the successful development of epidemiology were the links established with the World Health Organization in Geneva and with internationally recognized overseas epidemiologists, particularly in the USA, who were intrigued with the data from the early studies in New Zealand and the Pacific. Strong support was provided by Dr Fred Epstein of Ann Arbor University and director of the Tecumseh Study, Dr John Cassel from the University of North Carolina and director of the Evans County Study, and Dr Kenneth Newell, Director of the WHO Division of Research in Epidemiology and Communication and Science.

The conceptual and practical help provided from overseas was of importance in ensuring the New Zealand studies were methodologically sound and that they contributed to the growing evidence on the health impacts of 'modernization'. Of great interest was the impact of migration on the cardiovascular health of people moving from relatively isolated South Pacific communities to urban areas in New Zealand with very rapid changes in eating and habits of physical activity; this interest led to the Tokelau Island Migrant Study.

One of the outstanding contributions of the Tokelau Island Migrant Study has been the crucial engagement by behavioural scientists such as Tony Hooper, Judith Huntsman, and Al Wessen who developed an extraordinary knowledge of the Tokelauan communities both in their home islands and also in New Zealand. There is no doubt that this study could not have developed in an effective scientific way without the strong partnership between the social scientists and Ian Prior heading the epidemiological part of the team. It has been a major collaborative study and outputs include the papers that were published and also the more definitive studies on the anthropology of Tokelau published by Hooper and Huntsman; very little could have been achieved without the financial and material support given to the project by the Medical Research Council of New Zealand, the Wellington Hospital Board, and the WHO.

Interactions and partnerships

The initiation of modern epidemiology in New Zealand by a clinician helped to ensure the close connection between the epidemiological studies and the health needs of the participating communities. The decision by Maori and Pacific communities to participate in an epidemiological study could only be taken after extensive discussion by all concerned. This had multiple benefits, for example in ensuring high participation rates. It also imposed constraints, for example it limited the applicability of random sampling of the population and necessitated the use of chunk or convenience sampling. The close engagement with the community from the beginning led to a strong and enduring two-way relationships which on the part of the investigators required the provision of long-term medical management and advice from many individuals.

The long-standing engagement of the epidemiologists with the Department of Health encouraged the relatively smooth translation of the results of the studies into the policy-making process. The relatively early and successful response, both formal and informal, to the cardiovascular disease epidemics in New Zealand can be attributed to the availability of population-based risk factor data. Similar data are only now becoming available from many low- and middle-income countries, much of this stimulated by the WHO STEPwise approach to surveillance.

The data on the health needs of Pacific communities in urban environments contributed to efforts to improve basic needs such as access to health services, especially primary health care, and to improved housing. More generally, it is probable that the community partnership in this health project also contributed to improving the sense of well-being of the migrant communities.

The further development of epidemiology in New Zealand and the South Pacific

Following the pioneering work in Wellington, epidemiological research groups were established by Robert Beaglehole in the early 1980s at the University of Auckland with a focus on cardiovascular disease and, to a lesser extent, asthma and injuries. At the University of Otago, Dunedin a major focus of research was on cancer. The leader of this cancer research group, Professor David Skegg, trained under Sir Richard Doll in Oxford. This cancer research has contributed to the development and implementation of a national cancer control strategy and the group has had a major input into many difficult and controversial issues related to screening for cervical and breast cancer. Later in the 1980s epidemiological research expanded in Wellington to focus on asthma and the environmental determinants of health, especially housing and climate change.

The development of epidemiology in the South Pacific has been in two phases. Epidemiologists, many from New Zealand and Australia, conducted the initial work. More recently, there has been a welcome strengthening of Pacific epidemiology, much of it based on the Fiji School of Medicine, although external epidemiologists are still active.

Lessons learnt

Many lessons arise from the New Zealand experience in building epidemiological research and public health practice. The origin of much of the New Zealand research can be traced to the leadership of an individual who was driven by academic curiosity and a strong and sustained sense of social justice. The importance of mentoring is apparent. Perhaps this was more important in the early phases of epidemiological development, but even today it seems important to guide and support the next generation of epidemiologists.

It takes time to build a critical mass of epidemiologists. Even now after almost four decades, the number of practising epidemiologists is small and prone to losses to more attractive working conditions overseas. Supporting the existing workforce remains a priority and the responsibility lies with all stakeholders—universities, the Ministry of Health, and, above all, research funding organizations.

The Department of Health and then the Ministry of Health have always been supportive of, and interested in the results of, epidemiological research. Without the support of the department in the 1960s it is unlikely that the initial research would have started. The Ministry of Health has recognized the importance of epidemiology and has systematically engaged researchers in a wide variety of advisory bodies.

The Medical Research Council, which became the Health Research Council in the late 1980s, provided research funding for the initial studies and continued to give priority to public health research more generally. Of course, the public health community has never been happy with the relatively low level of funding and the competition for the limited funding remains intense.

It is noteworthy that the early epidemiological research received strong support from a hospital board, testifying to the important leadership role of a respected clinician. Subsequently, most of the epidemiological work has been based within universities, usually in a department of public health since, until recently, no schools of public health existed in New Zealand. Without this university base epidemiology in New Zealand would long since have withered.

An important and enduring feature of epidemiology in this region, beginning with Hercus, has been its close connection with public health practice. Epidemiologists have been involved in the full range of public health activities: aetiological research, surveillance, advocacy, policy formulation, implementation, and evaluation. An example of the advocacy role was the establishment of Action on Smoking and Health by an academic epidemiologist in the early 1980s. The engagement beginning in the early 1970s of cardiovascular epidemiologist with the national prevention and control policy stimulated a more comprehensive government-led approach and probably contributed to the continuing decline in cardiovascular mortality rates. Much of this policy engagement has been through national non-governmental organizations such as the National Heart Foundation and the New Zealand Cancer Society.

Engagement with communities, especially Maori and Pacific communities, has been a strong feature of epidemiology in the South Pacific and New Zealand, beginning with the work in the 1960s. However, it remains true that one of the most enduring features of the epidemiological scene in New Zealand is the entrenched inequalities in health status among ethnic groups. From this perspective, although the overall health of all population groups continues to improve, there has been very little reduction in the ethnic health inequalities. Health inequalities remain one of the major public health challenges in the region, as elsewhere.

The final lesson from this experience is the importance of international networks for research, training, and more general support and collaboration. In the early twenty-first century global networking is an everyday occurrence. However, without the early international support, the epidemiological take-off in the region would have been seriously delayed, perhaps by up to two decades.

Recruitment into epidemiology—a personal note by Ian Prior

It is important to attract bright individuals into epidemiology and to show that it can be as stimulating as the provision of services to patients. We give here some examples of how we have succeeded in this task.

This next section outlines some of the pathways to epidemiology and public health taken by people who had their interest aroused by the work we were doing, the way we were doing it, and the rewards that could come from well-conducted scientific epidemiological work. The rewards for clinical cardiology were certainly very real and often immediate. The rewards from working in public health and epidemiology are less immediate and some come from working in a multidisciplinary team. Certainly our unit based at Wellington Hospital has been fortunate in that direction.

Neil Pearce

Neil had a good science degree with a first-class knowledge of theory and application of statistics. He was working as a bus driver and on one of his lunch breaks came and saw me in my office asking me if there was a possibility of working as a statistician. We already had Clare Salmond and at that stage did not have a second position. I referred him down the corridor to Professor Ken Newell, the first Professor of Public Health in the Wellington School of Medicine. Ken recognized Neil's desires to get a first-class training in biostatistics and epidemiology and got MRC support to work in his group. Neil has done some outstanding work including cancer epidemiology. He has built up an active unit at Massey University in Wellington.

Paul Zimmet

In 1966 my wife Elespie and I went to Brisbane for an Australasian College of Physicians meeting where I presented a paper setting out the problem of diabetes in the Pacific and the wide gradients of this condition in different populations. In the audience was a young Australian physician well trained and interested in internal medicine. His name was Paul Zimmet. Paul told me later that my presentation opened up his mind and eyes about how he could see a career ahead in diabetes. Over the years he has worked in Nauru and many other countries helping them develop programmes for diabetes research and effective prevention and control. His founding and leadership of the International Diabetes Institute has been of importance not only to Australia and the Pacific, but also globally.

John Grimley Evans

John is an Oxford graduate with considerable skills in mathematics, who became interested in epidemiology. I had persuaded the MRC in 1967 that I had to recruit and help train a really good epidemiologist as part of our team. They accepted a 3 year fellowship with the first 3 months being at Ann Arbor with Fred Epstein and then with several other key groups. John took up that position and did it extremely well. He came with our team to Tokelau in 1968 and helped carry out the medical examinations as well as supervising the data collection. At this stage we worked from field sheets that we filled in onto work sheets that we completed each night. John's important contribution was coming back to Wellington where he helped analyse our Cook Island, Rarotonga, and Pukapuka studies. He was the key person writing this up for publication. He continued his training at the London School of Hygiene and Tropical Medicine and developed major interests in the health of the elderly. He went to Newcastle and implemented a landmark decision that the elderly should not be sequestered from the rest of the medical world. He came back to Oxford as professor, has been knighted for his work and is still making an important contribution to the health of the elderly.

John Stanhope

John Stanhope is an Australian graduate who came from a family where mathematical skills were deeply ingrained. We were working in Guam on curious neurological disorders. Elespie and I stopped off in Guam and met John and his wife and encouraged him to come and join our team in Wellington. He proved to be a major asset with his public health knowledge developed with 5 years working in Papua New Guinea and very real analytical skills and biostatistical knowledge. He helped greatly in the fieldwork and publications, particularly the Rotorua Lakes high school study, of Maori and young European in the 4th form. We showed that that young Maori did in fact have higher uric acid levels, supporting our hypothesis that there were genetic factors contributing to the gout problem facing young Maori men. Since leaving our unit John has worked in Sydney with people with alcohol problems.

Michael Marmot

On the occasion of the major WHO-sponsored meeting based on our unit in the early 1970s a good friend of mine, Peter Harvey, came. He was the other physician who came to Pukapuka. After the WHO meeting he went back to Sydney and had as his house physician a young well trained man—Michael Marmot. Michael was already thinking through an idea about community problems. He immediately thought that he would like to move into the public health field and get some further training. John Cassel said he would be glad for him to come on a fellowship to Chapel Hill. Michael was also attracted by issues on social health being investigated in California. He chose to go there and found himself involved in a very important study on risk factors and social health. He subsequently went to London and continued studying the impact of the social environment on health. He has since been knighted and is the director of the International Centre for Health and Society in the Department of Epidemiology and Public Health, University College London.

John and Sonja McKinlay

The McKinlays received their undergraduate education in Wellington before heading to Scotland for doctoral studies in the social sciences and statistics, respectively. In the mid-1970s they spent a sabbatical year from Boston University in Wellington and become engaged in the work of the Epidemiology Unit. They then went on to establish the New England Research Institutes which have made a huge contribution to a full range of public health research issues, from controlled clinical trials to basic public health research. They have maintained their contacts with New Zealand colleagues and continue to support public health research and practice in New Zealand.

A tribute

The pattern of epidemiological studies that our unit has been involved with over the years requires at times quite long periods away from families, and as such can pose some difficulties. The rewards are considerable and in some of the studies my wife Elespie and other family members were able to visit the scenes of action. This was enjoyable to them and certainly to the people we were working with. Many of our collaborators, such as the Rangihau family, remain strong friends and support us in some of our ongoing joint activities.

Conclusion

It has been very rewarding to see how younger people that have had some exposure to the discipline and excitement of epidemiology and public health may have been helped by their involvement with the Wellington Hospital Unit. There is no doubt that epidemiology and public health are coming of age. When I qualified cardiology was the glamour field. The situation is now different and public health is attracting a small number of high achievers who will contribute to the improvement of population health in the coming decades.

Some of Ian Prior's key references

Other references can be found in *The health of Pacific societies: Ian Prior's life and work*. Steele Roberts, Aotearoa, New Zealand (2000).

Ostbye T, Welby TJ, Prior IAM, Salmond CE, and Stokes YM (1989). Type 2 diabetes mellitus, migration and westernisation: the Tokelau Island Migrant study. *Diabetologia*, **32**, 585–90.

Prior IAM (1962). A health survey in a rural Maori community with particular emphasis on cardiovascular, nutritional and metabolic findings. *New Zealand Medical Journal*, **61**, 333–48.

Prior IAM (1975). Migration and health in New Zealand and the Pacific. In *The Tokelau Island Migrant Study* (ed. JM Stanhope), pp. 95–8. Epidemiology Unit, Wellington Hospital.

Prior IAM (1977) The Tokelau Island migrant study. In *Migration & Health – New Zealand & the Pacific* (ed. JM Stanhope), pp. 95–7. Epidemiology Unit, Wellington Hospital.

Prior IAM and Davidson F (1966). The epidemiology of diabetes in Polynesians and Europeans in New Zealand and the Pacific. *New Zealand Medical Journal*, **65**, 375–83.

Prior IAM and Rose BS (1966). Uric acid, gout and public health in the south pacific. *New Zealand Medical Journal*, **65**, 295–300.

Prior IAM and Tasman-Jones C (1981). New Zealand Maori and Pacific Polynesians. In *Western Diseases, Their Emergence & Prevention*, (ed. HC Trowell and DP Burkitt), pp. 227–67. Edmond Arnold Publishers Ltd., London.

Prior IAM, Davidson F, and Evans JG (1964). Gout and diabetes in Polynesia. *Lancet*, **2**, 1258.

Prior IAM, Rose BS, and Davidson F (1964). Metabolic maladies in New Zealand Maoris. *British Medical Journal*, **1**, 1065–9.

Prior IAM, Evans JG, Harvey HP, Davidson F, and Lindsey M (1968). Sodium intake and blood pressure in two Polynesian populations. *New England Journal of Medicine*, **279**, 515–20.

Stanhope JM and Prior IAM (1980). The Tokelau Island Migrant Study: prevalence and incidence of diabetes mellitus. *New Zealand Medical Journal*, **92**, 417–21.

Trowell HC and Burkitt DP (ed.) (1981). *Western disease: their emergence and prevention*, pp. 227–67. Edwards Arnold, London.

Wessen A, Hooper A, Huntsman J, Prior I, and Salmond C (1992). *Migration and health in a small society: the case of Tokelau*. Clarendon, Oxford.

28

Epidemiological methods: a view from the East Mediterranean

Mohamed H. Wahdan and Ahmed Mandil

Mohamed H. Wahdan

Factors influencing me to start epidemiology, and my training

Several factors influenced me to work in epidemiology, namely:

1. The epidemics of communicable diseases that occurred in my country, Egypt, during my childhood, have always been in the back of my mind, leaving me to wonder why they occurred. When I was in primary school, in the early 1940s, the image of tens of deaths in my village, from typhus and relapsing fever, was engraved in my memory. My school was on the road leading to the cemeteries, and I was watching these funerals every day. Again, when I was 14 years old (1947), a severe cholera epidemic occurred and I volunteered for the control operation. I tried to convince people to allow their relatives to be taken to the hospital. A most difficult job, as very few of the patients returned cured, and the majority died (20,000 deaths out of 30,000 cases admitted to hospitals). Families were not allowed to have the bodies to bury them.

2. In the medical school I was greatly influenced by the professor of public health, who was a real reformer in the sense that he modified the course in public health from basically sanitation and individual study of communicable diseases to epidemiological principles, as it was called at the time. It was the first time we had heard terms such as 'social diseases', under which the group of TB, typhus, relapsing fever, etc. were lumped. We were introduced to the importance of 'personal characteristics' in the occurrence of diseases and to the importance of studying the 'geographic distribution of diseases'. We went into the field and saw the linkage between diseases and social and environmental factors.

3. After graduation from medical school, I was offered a fellowship and without hesitation I chose to study epidemiology. I was lucky to be accepted at the London School of Hygiene and Tropical Medicine. Under the supervision of Professors Sir Austin Bradford Hill, Dr Richard Doll, Professor Donald Reid, Professor Armitage, and together with Professor Walter Holland, I learned the basics of epidemiology and epidemiological research. During my time in London I joined in a number of studies on hypertension and on blood pressure measurement which were being carried out by the Department of Epidemiology. The subject of my doctoral thesis was on the relation between atmospheric pollution and upper respiratory infection in children.

4. I returned to Egypt in February 1963 and served as a lecturer at the Faculty of Medicine, Alexandria University. During my first years of work my main efforts were to develop the rather neglected discipline of public health. I managed with one of my colleagues to introduce the principles of epidemiology into various topics and disciplines.

5. My membership of the International Epidemiological Association (IEA) was another important landmark in my career. Later on, when I was elected as Regional Councillor for the Eastern Mediterranean Region (EMR) in 1976. I felt increasingly the obligation to serve the principles of epidemiology. When I joined the World Health Organization (WHO) as a staff member in 1979, I had to give up membership of the Council of the IEA. My memberships of the Global Expert Advisory Panel on Communicable Diseases, from 1968 until I joined the WHO as a staff member, and of the Committee for Control of Communicable Diseases of Egypt, from 1964 to the early 1980s, in addition to giving me professional satisfaction were important learning experiences. They also gave me a chance to influence decisions taken in this field, although my efforts were not always met with success.

Major obstacles to undertaking epidemiological research

When I returned to Egypt in 1963, I faced several problems in undertaking research. The first and most important was the resentment of Ministry of Health officials, who did not want any research on communicable diseases, probably because they did not want anyone to disclose the real magnitude of these diseases in Egypt. What helped me most is that I was working in the university, and some of the senior officials, including some ministers of health, were personal friends, who gave me permission to undertake epidemiological research. The road was not that easy, and on several occasions my research was stopped by orders from Ministry of Health officials. I was lucky to get the studies back again on track through persistence.

The reasons for the resentment of Ministry of Health officials were multiple. They included hiding facts, such as for example the epidemic of cholera in Egypt in 1969 with more than 80,000 cases which was even denied its proper name, being given a new name 'summer diarrhoea'. I should put on record that the Minister of Health and the Governor of Alexandria, at that time, gave me full authority to investigate the epidemic and were very receptive to my advice on control measures and facilitated their implementation. However, they were overruled by senior politicians who decided not to declare cholera and hid the way it was introduced to Egypt. It was not possible to publish data on this epidemic, which was officially denied.

A very interesting outbreak of bubonic plague, that occurred in one of the border provinces of Egypt, was also hidden upon instruction from the Under Secretary of the Ministry of Health. I failed to convince him to declare it in respect of international health regulations and also because of the important observations made in its investigation. The outbreak started when a military contingent was stationed near a well known zoonotic plague focus in the Western Desert, and because of the refuse wild rodents probably came near to the domestic rodents and infected them. Cases appeared among the inhabitants of a nearby civilian population living near the camp who were breeding rabbits in their dwellings. The rabbits died in large numbers and then over 30 cases of bubonic plague were identified in the population. It was also not possible to publish data on this outbreak.

Another reason for Ministry of Health resentment about research is probably the fact that research would show the deficiencies in official data. As an example, in 1975, an epidemiological study carried out on cases of fever of unknown aetiology admitted to the communicable disease hospital in Alexandria revealed over 5000 cases of laboratory-confirmed typhoid fever while official data were just over 100 cases in the same period.

More recently, up to 2000, a senior Ministry of Health official was not declaring all cases of poliomyelitis although there was much evidence pointing to a large number of cases, simply because he had previously notified politicians that polio was eradicated in Egypt. It was, however, possible to introduce an additional epidemiological surveillance method for poliomyelitis, to look for wild polioviruses in the environment and publish a paper to demonstrate continued circulation (El Bassioni *et al.* 2003). Another paper was published to highlight shortfalls and failures in the National Immunization Days as an explanation for the reasons for continued viral circulation in Egypt (Reichler *et al.* 1998). At present the position of the responsible officials in the Ministry of Health is completely different, with total transparency, which has been very helpful in directing efforts and hence the successful cessation of transmission of the wild poliovirus since 2004.

I believe now that the previous resentment of the Ministry of Health officials to epidemiological research is no longer the major obstacle to epidemiological research it used to be in the last decades. Another example of this change is the publication of studies indicating weaknesses in the delivery of some health-care interventions, such as the study of the spread of human immunodeficiency virus in renal dialysis centres in Egypt (El Sayed *et al.* 2000).

The second major obstacle to epidemiological research was a lack of financial resources. This was eventually solved through a few research grants from the WHO for clinical trials of some vaccines and grants given for the conduct of training courses on epidemiology. In the 1970s, US agencies supported some of our epidemiological studies from the surplus of Egyptian Pounds available from the price of wheat exported to Egypt. There are now more resources available for epidemiological studies from UN agencies and private enterprise as they feel more and more the value of epidemiological research.

The third constraint was the fact that preventive medicine, in general, was not as attractive to talented graduates as clinical medicine. It was, however, possible for me to attract a number of very promising young graduates to join the Department of Epidemiology and I exerted every possible effort to maintain their interest and they became a very valuable support. Some of them are now leading figures not only in Egypt but in many countries of the region. This previous constraint is no longer a major one in many countries where clinical practice no longer exerts the same degree of attraction as in the past and more attention and priority are given by national authorities to preventive services and epidemiological activities.

Interaction/coordination between epidemiology and the public health service

One of the main achievements introduced during my work in the Faculty of Medicine from 1963–69, was the introduction of epidemiological principles in the design of research carried out in many disciplines in the Faculty of Medicine. This was facilitated through giving general lectures in the university in which basic principles were introduced, and also through supporting some investigators in the design and analysis of data. The word 'epidemiology' started to be seen in the titles of papers, such as epidemiology of peptic ulcer, epidemiology of smoking, etc. Research during this period was mostly directed towards assessing the occurrence of certain diseases and their epidemiological characteristics, for example a serological survey in rural areas on viral haemorrhagic fevers (Mayer *et al.* 1967). Another field was in clinical trials. The WHO, having been convinced of the technical capabilities developed at the Department of Epidemiology, commissioned the department to conduct clinical trials, the most important of which was the trial of meningococcal meningitis vaccine type A (Wahdan *et al.* 1973, 1977) and the clinical trial on ty21 oral typhoid vaccine (Wahdan *et al.* 1975, 1980, 1982). Giving evidence through epidemiological research, it has been possible to influence the development of health policies; for example publishing data on a lameness survey made it possible to influence decisions to make polio vaccination compulsory all over Egypt. Also, the publication of a number of studies carried out in Egypt on hepatitis B infection made it possible to influence the decision to introduce hepatitis B vaccination as a national policy. The same goes for the introduction of meningitis AC vaccination, after proving its effectiveness and safety.

It was unfortunate that some of these initiatives faced some unfounded rejections from some of the people occupying senior scientific positions in Egypt, whom I shall refrain from calling scientists. They include those who were either unaware of scientific advances, for example new vaccines, or who tried to twist facts to please Ministry of Health officials and rationalize their past wrong decisions. The WHO recommendation that 'by 1995 all countries should be vaccinating children with hepatitis B vaccine' was argued by one of them to mean that no vaccination should begin before 1995 in Egypt. These were the same persons who did not agree to stop smallpox vaccination after its eradication and also continued to convince the Ministry of Health of the importance of requesting cholera vaccination certificates from international travellers. At a time of shortage of meningitis vaccine one of them was behind the statement made by the Minister of Health at that time that meningitis vaccination increases the carrier state! He twisted the fact that the carrier to case ratio among vaccinees is higher than among non-vaccinees to say that the vaccine causes more carriage, although the absolute carriage rate among vaccinees is much lower than among non-vaccinees.

Highlighting weaknesses in certain aspects of public health practice, such as in the early detection of epidemics, made it possible to convince national health authorities to ensure that all their medical officers, working in health offices, be trained in epidemiology. It was only in the early 1970s that priority for fellowships offered by the Egyptian Ministry of Health to its staff was made for the study of epidemiology.

International support was also obtained to train epidemiologists from various WHO regions, and annually between 15 and 25 public health staff were trained in epidemiology. Some of them were from Egypt. This training continued for 10 years from 1969–79.

During my work as the Head of Epidemiology at the High Institute of Public Health, it was possible to convince the Ministry of Health to designate a number of health facilities in Alexandria to be field training sites and to make public health training and the academic studies for the Diploma of Public Health, Master of Public Health, and Doctorate of Public Health more practical and relevant to the problems of Egypt. Thirteen such facilities, including health offices, mother and child health (MCH) centres, rural health units, a communicable disease hospital, and a centre for tuberculosis control and another for control of sexually transmitted diseases were used for practical training and for field studies. It was further agreed with the Ministry of Health to have joint management of these centres between the university and the Ministry of Health to allow for development and improvement in their functions. These centres served as pilot projects for such developments.

In public health practice the 16 years of my university work had its main impact in Egypt. But it has also influenced development in other regional countries, where a substantial sector of the workforce was from Egypt or trained in Egyptian institutes, and also since most countries of the region followed the system and public health practices of Egypt.

My real contribution in epidemiology in other countries of the EMR was during my work at the WHO, starting in 1979, where I served in several capacities as Regional Advisor on Communicable Diseases, then Director of Communicable Diseases, and then Assistant Regional Director.

During this period, it was possible to influence developments in epidemiology in countries of the WHO/EMR through several means:

1. Working with the ministries of health to arrange for workforce development through encouraging and supporting the conduct of training courses and provision of fellowships.

2. Facilitating research through the provision of research grants. One field which benefited most was research in tropical diseases. Through reaching an agreement with the WHO Tropical Diseases Research Programme to provide funds which were matched from regional

funds small research grants were extended to tens of scientists every year. This initiative is still continuing and has been of great value in helping and encouraging young scientists.

3. Publishing an epidemiological bulletin which was eventually developed to become the *Eastern Mediterranean Health Journal*. Through this journal it was possible to publish analytical and promotional papers on epidemiological surveillance in the region (Wahdan 1999).

4. Making presentations to the Regional Committee for the WHO Eastern Mediterranean Region, which is the governing body for health in the region, on priority aspects to promote general epidemiological surveillance and on specific disease conditions and their prevention and control.

5. The occurrence of epidemics was utilized to introduce basic principles and approaches to strengthen work in epidemiology. For example, realizing there were weaknesses in the investigation and control of communicable diseases in Syria, the WHO/EMRO responded positively to the initiative of the Minister of Health in Syria to develop a national team in the field of public health, particularly in epidemiology. As a result, the Ministry of Health decided to establish a training course in public health for their medical officers, and in a matter of 10 years all the Ministry of Health's services became staffed with qualified public health experts. The impact of this training on the improvement of Public Health in Syria has been significant. Similar efforts were made in Yemen and are under way in Pakistan to ensure that each health district has an epidemiologist among its staff to direct efforts for disease control after they have felt the value of such a contribution in the polio eradication programme.

6. Introduction of the concept of anticipation of the epidemiological situation, through regular analysis of routinely collected data, and data in neighbouring countries, and taking any necessary preventive measures. Through this approach it has been possible to prevent or at least limit the spread of epidemics. This started with cholera and meningococcal meningitis. Preparedness for potential cholera epidemics meant enhancing sanitation and ensuring that oral rehydration salts (ORS) and antibiotics are available in sufficient quantities. This has been very instrumental in reducing fatalities. The same is also the case for meningitis by beginning vaccination in high-risk areas before the expected time of occurrence of epidemics, which was helpful to abort epidemics or limit their extent. Recently this approach has been applied to a large extent in the field of eradication of polio. Through regular analysis of the immunity profile of children, from the history of vaccination and the number of doses received, it was possible to highlight the potential danger of spread of the wild virus in the susceptible population if the virus is introduced into a polio-free population.

Possible future

The future is much brighter now that epidemiology is well accepted as the basis for most public health work. There is a need, however, to continue to ensure that influential officials give epidemiology the importance it deserves. There are obvious examples of the significant role that can be played by senior officials in promoting epidemiological thinking, for example in Kuwait, the role played by the Minister of Public Health in the 1980s on the development of public health services was a very clear example of how much an epidemiologist can influence public health in his or her country.

There is a need for epidemiologists to make themselves part of the solution to any health problem. They should engage themselves in planning for health-care services under normal and unusual circumstances and ensure that they are part of the decision-making process. The modern technical developments in handling information, in modelling, and in the use of computers have made it very easy for epidemiologists to be involved in the process of designing the services and in anticipating the needs as well as in evaluating the impact of decisions.

The IEA also has a role to play by working with regional councillors in organizing meetings for IEA members and by encouraging and facilitating participation of regional members in regional meetings and consultations. This can be done through the WHO and other UN agencies and by offering assistance to member states at times of need, such as during epidemics.

Ahmed Mandil

Factors influencing me to start in epidemiology and the nature of my training

Having lived in many Arab nations during the years of my basic education (1963–75)—Egypt, the Sudan, and Saudi Arabia—I closely witnessed the transition from a health burden mainly attributable to communicable diseases to a double burden attributable to both communicable and non-communicable (chronic) diseases.

I was very intrigued to understand how and why young children in such nations suffered multiple childhood diseases, such as measles, mumps, chickenpox, and rubella (having been a victim of most of these myself!) which appeared in widespread school-based epidemics, mainly during the 1960s, 1970s, and early 1980s. Such a pattern was observed to change afterwards to fewer and less severe outbreaks with loss of past periodicity (it was years before I discovered that such changes were mainly attributed to wide-scale use of national immunization programmes against vaccine-preventable diseases, better known as the WHO/UNICEF Global Programme of Immunization or GPI).

I also yearned to understand why many young and middle-aged adults, my relatives, friends, or colleagues, at school, university, or the community at large, suffered or died prematurely from a new group of diseases with which our societies were not familiar. All I was told at that time was that they mostly died of cancer, and that many of them were heavy smokers. This did not explain why a school colleague died at 12 years (leukaemia) and a relative died at 40 (spinal cord cancer).

In an attempt to find answers to such questions, I gave lots of attention and care, during my medical education (at the Alexandria University Faculty of Medicine), to two disciplines: public health/community medicine and paediatrics. Fortunately, the professors who taught me these subjects were so efficient that I decided subsequently to start by specializing in clinical medicine—paediatrics (1985)—and ended up specializing in preventive medicine—epidemiology at the University of California, Los Angeles (UCLA) School of Public Health (1991).

During my studies at UCLA, Professor Roger Detels invited me to join the IEA, while Professor and Mrs Lester Breslow as well as Professor Ralph Frerichs asked me to be part of the Organizing Committee of the IEA International Scientific Meeting which took place in Los Angeles during 1990. Since then, I became interested in perpetuating the mission of the IEA by spreading the discipline of epidemiology, networking with those working in the field, helping young professionals receive better training, presenting the results of their research, and exchanging experience with fellow epidemiologists and contributing to the epidemiology literature. At first, I contributed by virtue of my work as IEA Councillor for the EMR for three consecutive terms, 1993–2002. During this period, I fully supported the establishment and work of national societies of epidemiology, including the Lebanese Epidemiological Association and the Tunisian Society of Preventive Medicine and Epidemiology. I also coordinated the organization of four regional IEA meetings, covering the North African (Alexandria, Egypt 1995 and Tunis, Tunisia 1998) and the West Asian (Beirut, Lebanon 1997 and Manama, Bahrain 2000) nations of the EMR, along with national ministries of health, local societies of public health/epidemiology, and the WHO. During this period, IEA/EMR membership increased threefold, many professionals went global with their research experiences, and training in epidemiology became more and more popular in the region. Consequently, I was elected Secretary of the IEA for two terms: the first (2002–05) was in Montreal during the IEA World Congress of Epidemiology (WCE) 2002, while the second (2005–08) was in Bangkok during the WCE 2005. Taking after Professor Haroutune Armenian, IEA Secretary (1996–2002), and through the efforts of the IEA Secretariat in Alexandria, Egypt, I am working hard towards achievement of the same IEA goals, but on a global scale, in coordination with the IEA Council and the seven regional councillors, who cooperate with a network of some 1200 epidemiologists worldwide. This includes close coopera- tion with the current IEA/EMR councillor Dr Hassan El-Bushra, which resulted in holding the 6th IEA/EMR Regional Meeting in Ahwaz, Iran, during December 2003, which witnessed 40 new members joining the IEA. The 7th meeting is planned to be held in Riyadh, Saudi Arabia, during November 2007. It will be organized by the Epidemiology & Biostatistics Department, King Faisal Hospital & Research Center. It is expected to witness the birth of the Saudi Epidemiological Association.

Research opportunities were made available to me through my work and experience at the different universities I served: Alexandria University High Institute of Public Health (Egypt), King Faisal University College of Medicine (Saudi Arabia), and the University of Sharjah College of Health Sciences (United Arab Emirates). My research work reflected the double burden of disease the EMR currently suffers from, i.e. from communicable disease research (schistosomiasis, poliomyelitis, TB, brucellosis) to non-communicable disease research (risk factors such as tobacco consumption, obesity or outcomes such as diabetes, hypertension, injuries).

Major obstacles to undertaking epidemiological research

An environment conducive to epidemiological research is always important for the development and birth of major research projects which have a significant impact on the decision-making process of the health-care delivery systems. Such an environment includes: characteristics of the place (the presence of important health problems which need epidemiological tools to suggest the best control measures; public and non-governmental sectors supporting research) and per- sonal characteristics (experienced research teams who can plan, operate, and evaluate useful community-based research; communities receptive to and cooperative with research operations; and decision-makers who are willing to take research results seriously).

Research in the EMR seems to have many obstacles relating to one or more of the place or personal characteristics conducive to research, as described above. Although major problems of significant morbidity and mortality burdens exist (malaria and TB are major communicable dis- ease problems in many EMR nations, while obesity, diabetes, and hypertension are showing increasing public health importance), the public sector, represented by the ministries of health, does not seem to be constructed to fund/operate/implement research results in many such nations and health-care delivery systems (Iran may be the only exception). This is partially com- pensated for by publicly owned research and training centres, such as the National Institute of Public Health (Tunis, Tunisia), the High Institute of Public Health (Alexandria, Egypt), and the Pasteur Institute (Casa Blanca, Morocco). Other educational institutions which carry out signifi- cant public health and epidemiological research include the American University of Beirut Faculty of Health Sciences (Beirut, Lebanon), the Tehran University of Medical Sciences (Tehran, Iran), the King Saud University College of Medicine (Riyadh, Saudi Arabia), the Agha Khan University (Pakistan), and the Arabian Gulf University College of Medicine and Medical Sciences (Manama, Bahrain).

Some public and private establishments fund research in the EMR. Examples are the King Abdul-Aziz City for Science and Technology (Riyadh, Saudi Arabia), the Academy of Scientific Research and Technology (Cairo, Egypt), the Kuwait Foundation for Advancement of Science (Safat, Kuwait), and the AG-Fund (Riyadh, Saudi Arabia). In addition, some UN organizations operating in the EMR fund public health research, including WHO/EMRO (through its Research Policy and Coordination (RPC), Women and Reproductive Health (WRH), and Tobacco Free Initiative (TFI) units), UNAIDS, UNICEF, UNFPA, and the World Bank. Moreover, some aid/research programmes of some nations such as the US Agency for International Development (USAID, USA), the Canadian International Development Agency (CIDA, Canada), the Overseas Development Agency (ODA, UK), the Japan International Cooperation Agency (JICA, Japan), and the Institut national de la santé et de la recherche medicalé (INSERM, France) fund research carried out in some EMR nations, such as Egypt, Sudan, Pakistan, Tunisia, and Morocco.

Major epidemiological research projects which have been carried out in the EMR include: the Global Youth Tobacco Survey EMR (seven EMR states coordinated by WHO/EMR/TFI), the Saudi Family Health Survey, nutritional assessment surveys in the Gulf States of Kuwait, Bahrain, Qatar, and the United Arab Emirates, and national capacity assessment for prevention and control of non-communicable diseases (NCD) (coordinated by WHO/EMR/NCD).

In Egypt, major projects during the period 1960–2004 include: oral rehydration for management of diarrhoeal disorders in children, serogroup A meningococcal polysaccharide vaccine (Wahdan *et al.* 1977), oral live *Salmonella typhi* oral vaccine Ty21a (Wahdan *et al.* 1980), azithromycin in trachoma management in children (Schachter *et al.*1999), universal salt iodization (USI), iodine supplementation for prevention and control of iodine deficiency disorders (IDD), a schistosoma research project, Health Profile of Egypt (HPE), and the Demographic and Health Surveys (DHS) carried out on a bi-annual basis.

On a personal level, I have been involved with several research projects as principal investigator or as co-investigator. Examples are:

◆ 2005—tobacco consumption among University of Sharjah students: prevalence and risk factors;

◆ 2003–04—a study of national health research systems in selected countries of the WHO Eastern Mediterranean Region: Egypt section (WHO/EMRO, 2004);

◆ 2002—country profiles on tobacco control in the Eastern Mediterranean Region (WHO/EMRO, 2002);

◆ 2000–01—assessment of national capacity for non-communicable disease prevention and control (this was a global survey carried out by WHO headquarters in coordination with WHO regional offices (Alwan *et al.* 2001));

◆ 1995–98—Adolescent Health and Nutrition in Egypt Survey (funded by CIDA and UNICEF): a community-based nationwide study with general health assessment and in-depth analysis of the problem of nutritional anemia in Egypt (El-Sahn *et al.* 2000);

◆ 1993–96—an epidemiologic and communication/education strategy for prevention of schistosomiasis in childhood funded by USAID (Sallam *et al.* 1997–98);

◆ 1993–96—an epidemiological study on burn injuries and their influence on patients' emotional adjustment (Attia *et al.* 2000);

◆ 1992–96—epidemiology of rheumatic fever and rheumatic heart disease among school children in Alexandria (Abdel-Moula 1998; Zaher and Mandil 1999).

Although a good number of epidemiologists graduate annually from public health institutions in Egypt, Lebanon, Iran, and Pakistan there is an acute shortage of epidemiologists in most nations of the EMR.

Interaction/coordination between epidemiology, public health, and the development of health policies

Being a university professor since 1991, I have tried to make a positive contribution to the training and capacity building of professionals in public health epidemiology, especially in the principles of research methodology and applications in different EMR nations. This was either through regular undergraduate programmes (as in Saudi Arabia and the United Arab Emirates), post-graduate programmes (as in Egypt), and training workshops (as in Libya, Iran, and the United Arab Emirates). Graduates of these programmes used such training in their work in ministries of health, municipalities, health insurance organizations, and health-related sectors of the armed forces in addition to providing consultation or becoming members of the regular staff of national, regional, and international organizations, including UN organizations (such as the WHO, UNAIDS, UNICEF), or others such as the Population Council, Family Health International, and the Social Fund for Development. Most such professionals now occupy leading roles in these organizations, playing important roles in shaping public health policies.

Leading epidemiological studies and surveys carried out in EMR nations, for example Morocco, Tunisia, Egypt, Lebanon, Saudi Arabia, Yemen, Pakistan, Sudan, Djibouti, and Oman, have played pivotal roles in decision-making processes concerning specific public health problems. Examples are:

♦ Health assessment surveys asking villagers about their priorities/important health problems led the authorities to begin providing the necessary sanitary services, such as a clean water supply, sanitary refuse disposal, and sanitary sewage disposal (primary preventive measures) as priority health-related services *before* providing anti-helminthic medications and antibiotics (secondary preventive measures). This reflected the importance of people's perceptions of their health problems and what they consider to be health priorities. This was a very important lesson to learn, for the researchers, health-care providers, and decision-makers alike.

♦ Surveys of iodine deficiency disorders (IDD), reflected in the high prevalence of goitre among school-children in oases of the Western Desert of Egypt, resulted in the adoption of a national policy of salt iodination, as a cost-effective measure, which was shown to result in a rapid drop in the prevalence of IDD in the same area within a few years.

♦ Promising results of the leading clinical trials of the utility and cost-effectiveness of oral rehydration therapy (ORT) in the secondary prevention of diarrhoeal diseases resulted in the wide-scale adoption of ORT as a standard management scheme for diarrhoea in most EMR nations.

Many of these studies were carried out by specialized teams at leading research institutions such as the Alexandria University High Institute of Public Health, in coordination with UNICEF (health assessment; IDD), JAICA (ORT), and CIDA/UNICEF/Population Council (the Adolescent Health and Nutrition in Egypt Survey), thus following international standards.

Examples pf the importance of surveillance of communicable diseases include:

♦ Poliomyelitis: there have been relentless efforts to eradicate polio from EMR nations. There were important lessons learnt from the recent resurgence of polio in some EMR states subsequent to declaring them polio-free.

♦ HIV/AIDS: to select the best prevention and control methods which could be culturally acceptable and hence effective in the region.

♦ Malaria: to assist in efforts for local / regional control.

♦ Measles: to assist in efforts to eliminate the disease.

◆ Rift Valley fever: important recommendations of field investigations of epidemics of Rift Valley fever in Saudi Arabia, Egypt, and Yemen emphasized the importance of surveillance, outbreak alert, and warning systems in forecasting such epidemics and their early control.

Most EMR states follow the recommended standards of the WHO for surveillance of communicable diseases in general. In addition, each state has developed its own list of reportable communicable diseases, using the method of passive surveillance. Nevertheless, each nation has chosen a much shorter list for active surveillance, for example HIV/AIDS, polio, meningitis, hepatitis.

Specifically, the rules and regulations for surveillance of acute flaccid paralysis (AFP) were widely implemented for use in polio surveillance in different EMR states, especially for eradication efforts are coordinated by WHO/EMR, with country-specific surveillance teams stationed in each state where polio is still reported, for example Pakistan, Sudan, and Egypt.

In addition, sentinel surveillance has been used for HIV/AIDS surveillance in several EMR states such as Djibouti, Sudan, Morocco, and Egypt, with special emphasis on high-risk groups, including intravenous drug users, bar girls, TB patients, patients with sexually transmitted infections, and prisoners.

Recently, surveillance of non-communicable diseases, as well as of their risk factors, is gaining more and more attention in many EMR nations following the emergence of a new epidemic of such diseases, especially diabetes, hypertension, cardiac disease, and cancers, and tobacco consumption, lack of physical exercise, an unbalanced diet, and obesity as their leading risk factors. Efforts are currently being initiated in some EMR states, especially in the Gulf nations.

Possible future

Decision-makers and health-care providers need to take epidemiology more seriously, and further consider the utilization of epidemiological evidence in all, not just a few, decisions which shape health policies in EMR nations. Epidemiologists should not shy from making their voice louder, and fight to convince health authorities of the importance of epidemiological training, evidence, and applications in public health and the decision-making process.

The IEA has played some role in furthering the discipline of epidemiology in the EMR through its regional and global meetings, but a lot still needs to be done to attract more professionals for training in epidemiology and to employ them to improve the health of the public.

Educational institutions like universities (at undergraduate and graduate levels) which have health-related programmes have an important role to play by making the study of epidemiology and its research methods an integral and indispensable part of the health curriculum without which a candidate would not graduate from such programmes. They should also fund and conduct research, disseminating its results to the decision-making authorities.

In addition, health-care providers (governmental and non-governmental) should facilitate well-planned research, carried out by credible epidemiologists and take its results into serious consideration.

It is expected that progress will occur, but at a rather slow pace, as public health/epidemiology research is not yet among the priorities of many stakeholders in the community.

References

Abdel-Moula A, Sherif A, Sallam S, *et al.* (1998). Prevealence of rheumatic heart disease among school children in Alexandria, Egypt. *Journal of the Egyption Public Health Association*, **LXXIII**, 233–54.

Alwan A, Maclean D, and Mandil A (2001). *Assessment of national capacity for noncommunicable disease prevention and control; the report of a global survey*, WHO/MNC/01.2. WHO, Geneva.

Attia A, Sherif A, Mandil A, *et al.* (1997). An epidemiologic and socio-cultural study of burnt patients in Alexandria, Egypt. *Eastern Mediterranean Health Journal*, **3**, 452–61.

El Bassioni L, Barakat I, Nasr E, *et al.* (2003). Prolonged detection of indigenous wild polioviruses in sewage from communities in Egypt. *American Journal of Epidemiology*, **158**, 807–15.

El-Sahn F, Sallam S, Mandil A, and Galal O (2000). Anemia among Egyptian adolescents: Prevalence and determinants. *Eastern Mediterranean Health Journal*, **6**, 1017–25.

El Sayed NM, Gomatos PJ, Beck-Sague CM, *et al.* (2000). Epidemic transmission of human immunodeficiency virus in renal dialysis centers in Egypt. *Journal of Infectious Diseases*, **181**, 91–7.

Mayer V, Hanna AT, Wahdan MH, Mohamed JS, and el-Dawla K (1967). Prevalence of Sindbis virus antibodies in an Egyptian rural community. *Journal of Hygiene Epidemiology Microbiology and Immunology*, **11**, 1–4.

Reichler MR, Darwish A, Stroh G, *et al.* (1998). Cluster survey evaluation of coverage and risk factors for failure to be immunized during the 1995 National Immunization Days in Egypt. *International Journal of Epidemiology*, **27**, 1083–9.

Sallam S, Glik D, Sherif A, *et al.* (1997–98). Sociocultural considerations in schistosomiasis control: focus group data from 3 Egyptian villages. *International Quarterly of Community Health Education*, **17**, 147–59.

Schachter J, West SK, Mabey D, *et al.* (1999). Azithromycin in control of trachoma. *Lancet*, **354**, 630–5.

Wahdan MH (1999). Epidemiological surveillance and its prospects in the region. *East Mediterranean Health Journal*, **5**, 878–9.

Wahdan MH, Rizk F, el-Akkad AM, *et al.* (1973). A controlled field trial of a serogroup A meningococcal polysaccharide vaccine. *Bulletin of the World Health Organization*, **48**, 667–73.

Wahdan MH, Sippel JE, Mikhail IA, *et al.* (1975). Controlled field trial of a typhoid vaccine prepared with a nonmotile mutant of *Salmonella typhi* Ty2. *Bulletin of the World Health Organization*, **52**, 69–73.

Wahdan MH, Sallam SA, Hassan MN, *et al.* (1977). A second controlled field trial of a serogroup A meningococcal polysaccharide vaccine in Alexandria. *Bulletin of the World Health Organization*, **55**, 645–51.

Wahdan MH, Serie C, Germanier R, *et al.* (1980). A controlled field trial of liver oral typhoid vaccine Ty21a. *Bulletin of the World Health Organization*, **58**, 469–74.

Wahdan MH, Serie C, Cerisier Y, Sallam S, and Germanier R (1982). A controlled field trial of live *Salmonella typhi* strain Ty 21a oral vaccine against typhoid: three-year results. *Journal of Infectious Diseases*, **145**, 292–5.

WHO/EMRO (2002). Country profiles on tobacco control in the Eastern Mediterranean region. WHO-EM/TFI/008/E/L/07.02. WHO, Cairo

WHO/ENRO (2004). A study of national health research systems in selected countries of the WHO Eastern region: Egypt Iran, Morocco, Pakistan and Sudan.

Zahar S and Mandil A (1999). Rheumatic heart disease in Eqypt: Situation analysis and prospects for prevention. *Egyptian Heart Journal*, **51**, 416–24.

Epidemiological methods: a view from China

Yu Shun-Zhang

Introduction

Epidemiology has had a long history in China. Emperor Huangdi (*Neijing Shuwen*) (BC 207–AD 24) recorded five epidemics and infections in the population. The Sui Dynasty implemented Li Ren Fang law (AD 181–68)for the isolation of leprosy patients. In the eleventh century there was a smallpox epidemic. A person from Omei Mountain developed human smallpox vaccination to prevent smallpox epidemics. In 1736 Shi Daonan wrote a poem 'March of the death rodents' describing a plague epidemic in Yunnan province. In 1910–20 Dr Wu Lienthe organized and controlled plague epidemics in northeastern and northern China. In each epidemic there were 60,000–100,000 deaths. He found the places where plague originated, in infected marmot, and discovered an epidemic of pneumonic plague. Dr Wu was also the founder of the Chinese Medical Association.

After the establishment of New China, Dr. Su Delong (1906–85) contributed to the control of schistosomiasis and cholera. He investigated an epidemic of dermatitis in Shanghai and identified it as due to an outbreak of *Euproctis similis*; he also hypothesized that contamination of drinking water was the reason for primary liver cancers. Another pioneer of Chinese epidemiology was Dr He Guanqing (1911–95), who found the vector for kala-azar in China, showed that phage was ineffective in preventing diarrhoea and suggested cessation of the use of mouse brain as a B-type encephalitis vaccine. He created a disease surveillance system in China.

Patterns of disease and death during recent years
Infectious diseases

China has changed remarkably since the mid-1950s. The incidence rate of infectious diseases was 2139.69 per 100,000 in 1955 and has reduced to about 200 per 100,000 since the mid-1990s. The mortality of infectious diseases was from 18.43 per 100,000 in 1955, it is now less than 0.21 (Fig. 29.1). Respiratory, digestive, vector-borne, and other disease foci have decreased by more than 80%. However, diseases carried by infected blood and sexual diseases have increased quickly. The top ten infectious diseases during the period 1999–2003 were viral hepatitis, pulmonary TB, diarrhoea, gonococcal infection, measles, typhoid fever, syphilis, haemorrhagic fever, malaria, and scarlet fever (Fig. 29.2). The number one cause of death was rabies.

The main reason for the decrease in infectious diseases is the national vaccination programme. Since 1978 China has adopted a policy of free vaccination with four vaccines to prevent six diseases (BCG, polio, pertussis, diphtheria, tetanus, measles). Since 1998, type B hepatitis has become part of the programme. The programme covers about 85% of the Chinese population. Some large cities have their own list of vaccinations to be given which may include vaccines for up to 10 diseases.

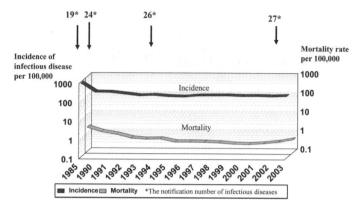

Fig. 29.1 Rates of infectious diseases and death in China.

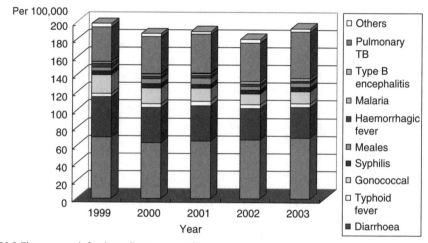

Fig. 29.2 The top ten infectious diseases: trend.

Infectious diseases have reduced from 3309.49 in the 1950s to 226.48 per 100,000 in 1998 and the mortality from 64.55 per 100,000 to 0.44 per 100,000. After vaccination was introduced, the incidence of infectious diseases reduced by more than 95%. For example, the prevalence rate of pulmonary TB reduced from 7500 per 100,000 in the 1950s to 80 per 100,000 in 1990s; the incidence of measles and pertussis were respectively 1 and 0.3 per 100,000 in 1990. Poliomyelitis and diphtheria have been eliminated. The prevalence of HBsAg carriers was reduced from 15% to 5%. Other reasons for the reduction in these diseases were economic development, an increase the availability of clean drinking water, and an improvement in living conditions. But there has been an increase in HIV/AIDS and sexually transmitted diseases and now TB is becoming more common.

It has been estimated that there are about 650,000 (range from 540,000 to 760,000) people infected with HIV, of whom 75,000 have developed AIDS. The prevalence averages 0.055% (range 0.04–0.06%). There are approximately 288,000 drug users living with HIV/AIDS, accounting for 44.3% of the total number of estimated HIV cases. Approximately 69,000 former blood and plasma donors and recipients are infected with HIV/AIDS (10.7%). Approximately

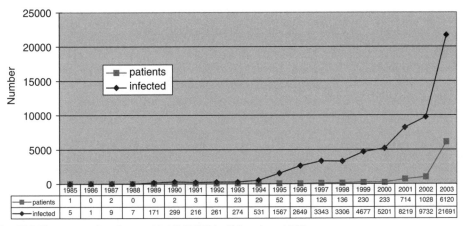

	1985	1986	1987	1988	1989	1990	1991	1992	1993	1994	1995	1996	1997	1998	1999	2000	2001	2002	2003
patients	1	0	2	0	0	2	3	5	23	29	52	38	126	136	230	233	714	1028	6120
infected	5	1	9	7	171	299	216	261	274	531	1567	2649	3343	3306	4677	5201	8219	9732	21691

Fig. 29.3 The reported patients with HIV/AIDS in China since 1985.

127,000 sex workers and their clients are living with HIV/AIDS (19.6%). It is estimated that there are 109,000 commercial sexual partners (16.7%), 47,000 gay men (7.35%), and 9000 cases of mother-to-child transmission (1.4%) who are living with HIV/AIDS. Among the estimated 75,000 AIDS deaths in 2005, 10,000 were of commercial blood and plasma donors and recipients. The most serious HIV epidemics in China to date have been clustered among specific population groups (such as injecting drug users, sex workers, former plasma donors, and partners) and in certain areas in the south and west of the country. There has been a warning of the spread of HIV from high-risk groups to the general population. However, there are only 21,690 reported patients with positive HIV and 6120 AIDS patients (Fig. 29.3).

According to 33 sentinel surveillance systems for sexually transmitted disease, the incidence rate in 1997 was 167.42 per 100,000. The Chinese Center for Disease Control and Prevention (CDC) has estimated that there are 1.8 million cases of sexually transmitted disease each year, including gonorrhoea, syphilis, and congenital syphilis.

China has the second highest burden of tuberculosis (TB) worldwide. With 1.4 million new cases of TB annually, 650,000 are smear-positive. In China the prevalence of TB is high because of a large mobile population, poor living conditions, high labour burden, nutritional deficiencies, and the lack of a system directly observed therapy (DOTS) care. The fourth national survey of TB in 2000 showed that the prevalence of active TB was 367 per 100,000 (4.5 million cases). The modern TB control strategy has, since 1992, been adopted by the National TB Control Programme (NTP) using funding from a World Bank loan and from the Chinese Ministry of Public Health (MOH). By the end of 2000, the NTP covered 59% of rural counties. The NTP follows the DOTS strategy and provides free or subsided TB care to smear-positive TB patients. The reduction in prevalence of pulmonary and smear-positive TB of 32% was attributed to the World Bank funded DOTS programme. The MOH-funded NTP also greatly improved notification of infectious cases with a cure rate of more than 90%.

In China before the use of vaccine for hepatitis A virus (HAV) and hepatitis B virus (HBV), hepatitis infection was a major public health problem. The incidence rate was about 100 per 100,000, including 50% HAV, 25% HBV, 5% HCV, 10% HEV, and 10% others. The prevalence of hepatitis was 80.2% HAV, 57.6% HBV, 3.2% HCV, and 18% HEV. The proportion of chronic HBV carriers was as high as 9.8%. There were almost 12 million chronic hepatitis carriers and 300,000 deaths from hepatic diseases, half of them hepatic cancer. The development of hepatitis

A and B vaccines was a landmark in the control and elimination of HAV and HBV infection, especially in infants and young children. After vaccination, the carriage rate has been reduced to 1–2%, and to 0.53% in Shanghai. In Longan, Guangxi after 15 years of HBV vaccination, the prevalence of HBsAg has reduced to 0.7–2.9% (average 1.5%), and the mortality from primary liver cancer in young people between the ages of 10 and 19 years was reduced from 5.7 per 100,000 in 1969 to only 0.4 in 1996.

Another problem in China is *Schistosomiasis japonica*. There were 11.6 million patients in 12 provinces in 1950. By 1989, in four provinces and Shanghai (nine counties) the disease had been eliminated. The main measures for control were the elimination of snails (*Oncomelania hupensis*) by chemical molluscicides and the removal of mammals, treatment of all patients and infected cattle, improvement of the drinking water, and night soil treatment. However, schitosomiasis is still common in the middle and lower reaches of the Yangtze River, the marshlands adjacent to the great lakes of central China, and certain mountainous areas in the provinces of Sichuan and Yunnan. There are still 433 counties which have the disease, with an estimated 65 million patients. The Three Gorges dam has been built. Changes to the ecological system in relation to the building and operation of Three Gorges dam may change the incidence of schistosomiasis.

The control of infectious diseases in China is still a priority. Some emergent diseases are still epidemic, such as type E and C hepatitis, *Escherichia coli* O:157 in Jiangsu, Anhui, and Henan, Type O139 cholera, and recently SARS, *Streptococcus suis*, and avian influenza.

Non-infectious disease

In 2005, chronic diseases were projected to account for 79% of all deaths (total deaths 9,427,000 with 7,471,000 due to chronic diseases) in China. The main non-infectious diseases are cancer, stroke, cardiovascular disease, and diabetes (Figs 29.4–29.6).

The estimated incidence of cancer was 117.2 per 100,000 (126 for males and 109 for females) in 1980 and 213.6 per 100,000 (174 for males, 120.5 for females) in 2000. Comparing cancer mortality between the two periods 1973–75 and 1990–92, stomach and oesophageal cancer have

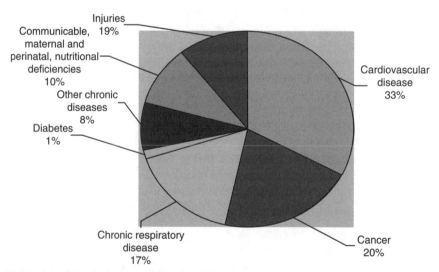

Fig. 29.4 Projected deaths by cause (all ages), China, 2005.

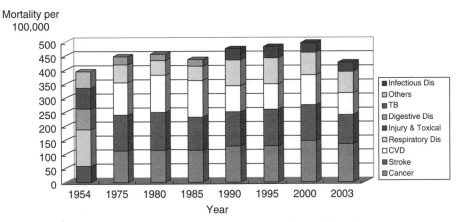

Fig. 29.5 Mortality from the top five chronic diseases in urban China during the past 30 years.

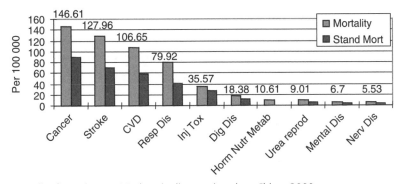

Fig. 29.6 Mortality from the top 10 chronic diseases in urban China, 2000.

decreased, cervical cancer has reduced by about 78% in urban areas and 64% in rural areas, and nasopharyngeal cancer has reduced by about 38% and 32%, respectively. Lung and liver cancer are still increasing remarkably, due to smoking, eating mouldy food, and drinking polluted water. The main reasons for the reduction in digestive cancers are improvements in living conditions and the environment, for example drinking tea, consuming less salt and eating more fruit and vegetables, especially garlic and onions.

The 'new' diseases—cerebrovascular and cardiovascular diseases—cause more than 5 million and 3 million deaths, respectively, each year. Economic losses are more than 10 million RMB yuan. The main risk factors are hypertension, hypercholesterolaemia, smoking, and physical inactivity. There are more than 50 million patients with hypertension with a prevalence of about 15% for urban adults aged more than 35 years. The intake of salt averages 12 g per person in the Shanghai area. Excess body weight is becoming another important risk factor; in 2005 34% of men and 30% of women aged 30 or more were overweight.

According to a national survey, the prevalence of diabetes in those aged over 20 was 0.67% in 1979, 3.21% in 1995–97 and 6.4% in 2001. In Shanghai, in 2000 the prevalence of diabetes in those aged more than 15 years was 7.3% in the urban area and 3.8% in rural areas after a 2-h post 75 g glucose tolerance test. The main risk factors are eating more (more than 31% of energy from fat intake), less exercise (physical inactivity in more than 60% of people), overweight (body mass index (BMI) 24–27.9; 15.9%) and obesity (BMI ≥ 28; 4.9%).

Maternal and child health

In China there are 3200 maternal and child health-care hospitals. Since 1986, the country has established three networks for the surveillance of birth defects and maternal and under 5-year child mortality. The main achievements are as shown in Table 29.1.

Maternal and child health is a concern for every family and for the government. Now more then 80% of pregnant women are delivered in hospitals or health-care centres. As a result, infant and maternal mortality has decreased remarkably; the surveillance data are shown in Figs 29.7 and 29.8.

Disabilities due to birth defects are common in China, and are a serious social issue. Congenitally disabled children make up 4–6% of the total birth population. This means there are 0.8 to 1.2 million congenitally disabled children born annually. They should be a high priority for maternal and child health institutions.

Because of overcrowding in Chinese cities the authorities decided upon the one child per family policy. In 2000 the population was 1.29533 billion (1.26583 billion on the mainland). The proportion of males to females was 106.74:100. The age distribution was 22.89% for 0–14 years, 70.15% for 15–64 years, and 6.96% for over 65 years of age. Thirty-six per cent of the population lived in urban areas and 64% in rural areas. To induce a change in the population structure, because of the pressure of child care with two working parents and the high cost of raising children,

Table 29.1 Improvement in population health status in China

Index	1949	2003
Life expectancy	35	71.8 (2000)
Maternal mortality rate (per 100,000)	1500	51.3
Infant mortality rate (per 1000)	200	25.5
Infectious disease incidence (per 100,000)	20,000	192.2

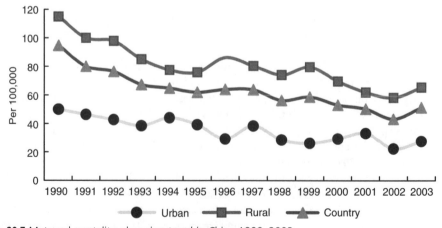

Fig. 29.7 Maternal mortality: changing trend in China 1990–2003.

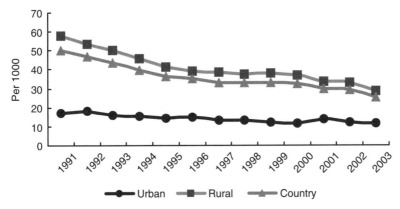

Fig. 29.8 Infant mortality: changing trend in China 1991–2003.

the total fertility (lifetime average number of deliveries per woman) needs to be kept to 1.5–1.8. This means that some families have more than one child.

Several disease epidemics in Shanghai

Hepatitis A epidemic

On 19 January 1988 there were 134 cases of hepatitis A reported in Shanghai, which was higher than on 18 January (an increase of 183.6%). During that week the notification of cases of hepatitis increased remarkably (Figs 29.9 and 29.10). Up to 18 March, the total number of cases was 292,301 with a prevalence of 4082 per 100,000. This was two to four times more cases than in an ordinary season in Shanghai. The inpatients were isolated at all hospitals, schools, and even new department stores. The clinical data showed this was a hepatitis A epidemic with 95.5% positive for HAV-IgM and anti-HAV. The clinical symptoms were fever in 92% of cases, jaundice in 90%, and aminotransferase activity >1000 U in 92.4%. There were only 11.5% who were HBsAg positive (just like the ordinary population in Shanghai and other cities). The distribution of this disease was found all over the city, including 12 districts, and prevalence varied from 2112.6 to 5729.1 per 100,000. Cluster cases (more than two cases per family) were only 8.03% of the total and followed a binomial distribution. There were three epidemic peaks on 20 and 25 January and 1 February. Before and during the period of the epidemic no water contamination was reported and no notable climate change, but it was noticed that people ate a lot of clams during the period. The results of 1208 matched cases and controls showed that the more clams eaten, the higher the prevalence of hepatitis A, with an odds ratio of 10.02 (95%CI 8.13–12.35). A cross-sectional survey (22,271 families and 77,065 persons) showed the prevalence in people who ate clams was 11,920 per 100,000 and in people who did not eat was 520 per 100,000. The relative risk was 22.92. Also the dates on which people consumed clams and the amount consumed were correlated with disease occurrence. We visited the place where the clams originated, and collected clams direct by from the bottom of the sea. The HAV virus was detected, with a positive RNA match. The Shanghai municipal authorities prohibited the eating of clams, and after that the HAV epidemic disappeared within a month.

Dermatitis and Euproctis similis outbreak

In July–August 1972 Shanghai was subject to an epidemic of dermatitis. More than 100,000 cases (because it was not a notifiable disease, the real number of cases is not known) were recorded in

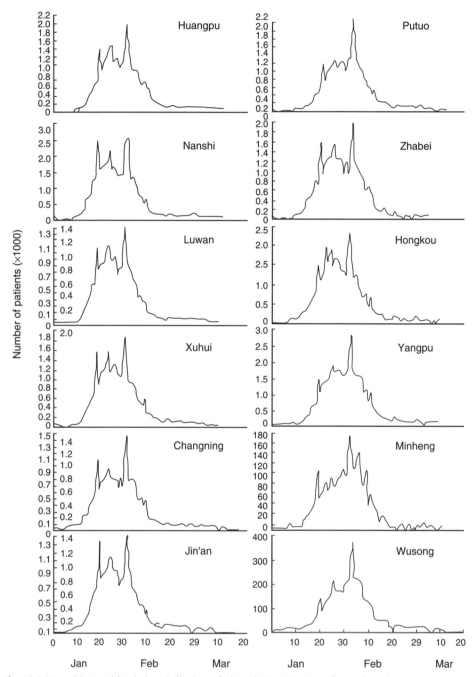

Fig. 29.9 Hepatitis A epidemic in 10 districts of Shanghai, 1988. Data from Shanghai CDC. Reproduced with permission from Professor Zhou Ting-gui.

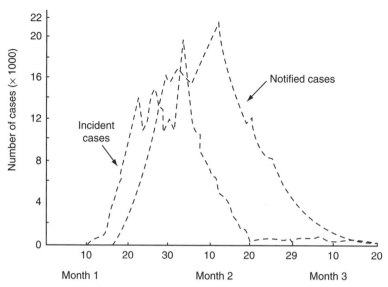

Fig. 29.10 Hepatitis A epidemic in Shanghai during January 1988. Data from Shanghai CDC. Reproduced with permission from Professor Zhou Ting-gui.

different hospitals in Shanghai, especially in the suburbs. The main symptoms were dermatitis on both forearms, chest and back, abdomen, and thighs. The itching affected work and required rest for several days. Most patients were workers and peasants, but some seamen from trading ships developed the disease before they entered the harbour. Professor Su Delong led a group of experts, visiting ship-yards and other high infection areas to investigate the cause of epidemic. They found that all patients worked outdoors although no cases were seen in welders. They found that the wind direction related to the high prevalence of dermatitis, people on the windward side (or those who wore no protective clothing, like the welders) being more affected than those where there was no wind. The only exception was in places with trees. So they considered out-door work, wind and trees together and exposed their forearms in places outdoors near trees. Similar symptoms were seen. The cause of dermatitis was found to be the hair of *Euproctis* (*E. flara*, *E. pseudoconspersa*, and *E. similis*), not air pollution or flower and plant dust. The epidemic was stopped after spraying outdoor areas with pesticides.

SARS in Shanghai

SARS is regarded as a milestone in the history of global public health. We had information about the outbreak of an unknown respiratory disease in early March 2003. At that time the Chinese CDC and MOH (Ministry of Public Health) invited two of our professors to research the cause of this disease in Guangdong. When they came back to Shanghai, they said it was a terrible infectious disease, it might be a virus infection but probably not Chlamydia. Shanghai CDC and the School of Public Health decided to cooperate in laboratory work and to prepare an epidemiological study. Every sample from a suspected case was separated into two parts, one of which was sent to the School of Public Health. On 27 March 2003 the first case (a woman who came from Guangdong and Hong Kong for business) was reported to the Shanghai CDC and we obtained viral evidence by the end of April in both laboratories. She transmitted the disease to her father on 4 April; we found her father by temperature surveillance and sent him to the Infectious Hospital. The Bureau of Public Health decided to isolate all suspected and probable cases in four

Table 29.2 The test results of eight SARS patients (data from Shanghai CDC)

Case no	Virus culture	PCR	SARS Ig-M	SARS Ig-G
1	+	+	+	+
2	+	+	+	+
3	−	−	+	+
4	+	−	+	+
5	+	−	+	+
6	+	−	+	+
7	+	−	+	+
8	−	−	−	−

hospitals (Infectious, Children, and Pulmonary Hospitals, and the Children's Center). The third case (6 April) had returned from Hong Kong, his clinical symptoms seemed like influenza and SARS, we had the antibody result after 2 weeks; during that time he was isolated in the Pulmonary Hospital until confirmed as a SARS patient. The fourth to seventh cases (26 and 28 April) were two couples who came from Beijing who were isolated in the Infectious Hospital, The last one was a rail worker, his symptoms were SARS-like but all laboratory tests were negative. Also during that time we examined 80 suspected cases, all of which were found to be other respiratory diseases (Table 29.2). Our experiment with early preparation detected all fever cases in a fever outpatient department, and isolated every suspected and probable case in the four hospitals or centres, quarantined epidemic areas, and repeated propaganda for establishing healthy habits and used respirators and ventilation in rooms.

Epidemiology in China is just beginning. China is still a developing country and the people suffer not only from acute infectious diseases but also chronic diseases. The epidemiological methods used in China are mostly descriptive epidemiology; analytical epidemiology and mathematical models rare. There are few epidemiologists, most of them are young. The Chinese Epidemiological Association and the Chinese Clinical Epidemiological Association have existed for a few decades and are trying to train people and exchange scientific information. We hope to cooperate with foreign scientists and epidemiologists to do more work on disease control and the elimination of serious diseases in China.

References

China Ministry of Health (2003). *2003 annual statistics for public health*. China Peking Union Medical University Press, Beijing.

Delong S (1981). *Epidemiology*, 1st edn. People's Health Publishing Ltd, Beijing.

Li Limin (1999). *Epidemiology*, 4th edn. People's Health Publishing Ltd, Beijing.

Xu Dezhong (1998). *Molecular epidemiology*. People's Military Press, Beijing.

Xu B, Jiang QW, Xiu Y, *et al.* (2005). Diagnostic delays in access to tuberculosis care in countries with or without the National Tuberculosis Control Programme in rural China. *International Journal of Tuberculosis and Lung Disorders*, **9**, 784–90.

Zhao Gen-ming, Zhao Qi, Jiang QW, *et al.* (2005). Surveillance for *Schitosomiasis japonica* in China from 2000 to 2003. *Acta Tropica*, **96**, 288–95.

Zhao SJ, Xu ZY, and Lu Y (2000). A mathematical model of hepatitis B virus transmission and its application for vaccination strategy in China. *International Journal of Epidemiology*, **29**, 744–52.

30

The development of modern epidemiology in the East

Chitr Sitthi-amorn

Personal experiences

Professor Chitr Sitthi-amorn has a very diverse background. He started his career as a neuroscientist, then became a clinician, and a clinical epidemiologist. His interest in epidemiology began when he became frustrated that his research into the function of the nervous system as well as his clinical experiences had limited value for solving the problems of drug dependency in Thailand. This frustration motivated him to understand the dynamics of the problem of drug dependency in communities. He applied and was accepted into the Department of Clinical Epidemiology and Biostatistics at McMaster University. He started to publish and became involved in strengthening human resources for epidemiology and was elected as the Southeast Asia Council member for the International Epidemiology Association, a position he held for three consecutive terms. He later became Head of the Clinical Epidemiology Unit and then the founding Dean of the College of Public Health. The programmes he helped establish have offered training for international students. These academic positions have given him the opportunity to influence the expansion of epidemiology in Thailand, Southeast Asia, and China. Thus, he has moved from the recording of single neurons via epidemiology to public health. He has enjoyed every bit of his experience and each experience has given him important insights for better subsequent work. As the Dean of the College of Public Health and President of the International Epidemiology Association, he has had opportunities to meet with scientists from various disciplines worldwide and become involved in big and small international activities in fields related to public health and epidemiology. He recently organized the XVII IEA World Congress of Epidemiology in 2005, attended by 800 individuals from around the world. The plenary and keynote sessions highlighted the need for multidisciplinary and multisector approaches to solve important public health problems and enhance equity in health for development. He believes in the development of a strong partnership and participative management between disciplines to solve difficult problems. As the second IEA president from a developing country, he might have brought a different but complementary background, experiences, struggles, perspectives, and viewpoints to human resource development for epidemiology and public health. It is hoped that such viewpoints may have added value for refining the existing strength of epidemiology worldwide.

The ecological approach to disease was very strong in Europe during the social and political reforms of the nineteenth century. Descriptions of the distributions of diseases and death among different social classes and groups were undertaken to highlight social injustices. In Asia, attempts by communities to prevent and limit the spread of disease go back to antiquity. There have been many beliefs about effective practices, such as avoiding eating inadequately preserved food, without a modern understanding of the aetiology of diseases. Some of the earliest systematic epidemiological investigations concerned the control of parasitic diseases in China in the 1870s. In 1877 the mosquito was reported to be the intermediate host and vector of *Wuchereria bancrofti*. Later, overseas doctors from missionary hospitals, set up mainly in the trading ports, turned to the study of pathogenic parasites. The outstanding scientist was Maxwell, who published a book giving a full account of the state of parasitic diseases in China at that time. After 1920, Faust and other foreign parasitologists came to China and continued epidemiological and basic scientific investigations of parasitic diseases involving filariasis, schistosomiasis, clonorchiasis, fascioliasis, and some protozoan infections. Around 1930, a small number of Chinese epidemiologists and researchers made very important contributions to the early development of strategies for the control of parasitic diseases in China. After 1930, Chinese investigators gradually replaced foreign doctors and scholars. Unfortunately, further development in this field was retarded until the mid-twentieth century, owing to the absence of funding and of professionals as a result of neglect by the government of pre-revolutionary China and the chaos caused by war (Mao 1989).

Although scientific investigations of distribution of diseases in the population had occurred in the past, the theory of epidemiology was little known in developing countries until the late 1970s and early 1980s. Notable key international collaborations have been the Tropical Disease Research Program (TDR) and the Human Reproductive Program (HRP) of the World Health Organization, the Field Epidemiology Training Program (FETP) of the Centers for Disease Control, and the International Clinical Epidemiology Network (INCLEN) initiated by the Rockefeller Foundation. The TDR has been instrumental in research for the control of tropical diseases such as malaria and leprosy. The HRP has assisted developing countries in capacity development for family planning and reproductive health using a multidisciplinary approach from laboratory sciences to health problems in population subgroups. Several mechanisms and capacities were developed and used to link research into policy and practices. International donors have also contributed to the development of epidemiological capacity such as the Sasakawa Foundation, the Regional Networking Group for Strengthening Surveillance, and Control of Asian Schistosomiasis. Many programmes have been supported by the National Institutes of Health (NIH) in the USA, the European Community, private foundations, and grants from foreign collaborators. Under the leadership of Kerr White and Scott Halstead, the Rockefeller Foundation has contributed to the establishment of the National Epidemiology Board in many countries of Southeast Asia and several clinical epidemiology units in the regions, most notably in the Philippines, Indonesia, and Thailand (Halstead *et al.* 1991; White 1991). Many clinical epidemiology units are having important multiplicative effects, have contributed to strengthening epidemiological capacity in the region, and have been instrumental in improving epidemiological capacity globally (Macfarlane *et al.* 1999). These capacities have been used for policy development at the national and facility levels. Multidisciplinary competencies (i.e. epidemiology, biostatistics, medical economics, and behavioural sciences) have been the crux of research of the clinical epidemiology units and training.

The FETP serves many disease surveillance and control functions and has been effective in recent epidemics of SARS, avian flu, and prevention of infections immediately after the tsunami natural disaster. The FETP was modelled after the Epidemic Intelligence Service created by the Centers for Disease Control (CDC) in 1951 to provide training and epidemiological services on the model of a clinical residency programme, the so-called applied epidemiology training programmes (AETPs). Many AETPs have been implemented around the world. Field Epidemiology Training Programs were complemented by the Public Health Schools Without Walls supported by the Rockefeller Foundation and implemented with the help of the CDC. AETPs use science as the basis for intervention programmes designed to improve public health. They train people by providing them with competencies in epidemiology, programme planning, and implementation of public health interventions, and therefore help strengthen health systems. The Training Programs in Epidemiology for Public Health Interventions Network was organized in 1997 to provide support, peer review, and quality assurance for AETPs (White *et al.* 2001).

The International Epidemiological Association (IEA) has also contributed to the development and strengthening of regional activities (Breslow 2005) as shown by the record of regional meetings and international publications coming from Southeast Asia. These regional meetings have taken place regularly since the 1987 meeting in Pattaya, Thailand. With support from the IEA, INCLEN, and FETP, the growth and interest in epidemiology and the enormous improvement in the quality, as well as the quantity, of epidemiological research has been particularly notable in Southeast Asia. Many countries had but a few epidemiologists in the late 1970s. There are now (2005) flourishing national associations and societies with their own publications in English and local languages. Thailand was the host for the IEA World Congress of Epidemiology (WCE) in 2005. The number of participants, 322 out of 800 participants in the WCE 2005, from China, India, Indonesia, Malaysia, the Philippines, Vietnam, Lao PDR, Cambodia, Bangladesh, Singapore, and Thailand illustrates the increasing penetration of our discipline.

As a result of these capacity strengthening efforts, the number and quality of epidemiological investigations in developing countries have grown constantly. Early papers reported anecdotal cases and case series. Descriptive and population-based studies prevailed in the 1960s. More analytical studies were reported in the 1970s. It was not until the 1980s and the 1990s that many more experimental, clinical, field, and health system studies were documented (e.g. Cheah *et al.* 1985; Sitthi-amorn *et al.* 2002).

In addition to increasing the quality of studies, epidemiological capacity has also generated critical, valid, and timely information that has guided planning and decision-making for effective disease control. In this chapter, the role of epidemiology in the control of malaria, tuberculosis, HIV/AIDS, and emerging infections such as SARS and avian flu in Asia and Thailand will be discussed.

Malaria

In Thailand, the occurrence of diseases with enlarged liver and spleen was recorded more than 220 years ago. In 1930, when Thailand started to record cases of confirmed malaria, more than 40,000 from a total population of 11.3 million died from the disease. The Thai government requested the assistance of the League of Nations, who recommended that the government give free quinine treatment to the affected and encourage people to avoid mosquito bites. In 1932, the first systematic malaria surveillance units were developed and tested in Chiangmai to give input for planning for disease control (Timasarn 1997).

After the Second World War, through the assistance of the Tropical Disease Research (TDR) programmes of the World Health Organization, Thailand was able to strengthen epidemiological and research capacity for the control of tropical disease. At one point, the TDR budget to Thailand exceeded 50% of the total TDR budget to Southeast Asia. TDR contributed significantly to strategic and applied research, clinical trails, and field trials as well as the development of research capacity. Technical support from TDR, with the development of infrastructure and human resources in diseases investigation and control, led to a continuous reduction in malaria in Thailand. Due mainly to political impediments at the local and national government levels, multidrug resistance has been a continuing problem associated mainly with migration, the use and sale of substandard drugs, poor quality use of medicines, and changes in the behavior of mosquitoes. This emphasizes that while continued epidemiological surveillance is important for monitoring the changing nature and extent of endemic malaria and the nature of drug resistance, effective control will require an understanding of human behaviour related to the use of medicines and the sale of substandard products as well as the ecological changes resulting from development which lead to the changes in the behaviour of the vector.

Similar to Thailand, epidemiology and other research for the control of parasitic diseases in China started with work in the 1870s carried out by foreign doctors and scholars. Subsequently, Chinese epidemiologists began their own investigations in this field. The Hangzhou Institute of Tropical Diseases, set up in 1928, was the first research institute in China for tropical diseases with emphasis on parasitic diseases. The Central Program for Hygiene followed in 1932–33, consisting of nine departments. Among them was a department of parasitology dealing with surveys and control of parasitic diseases. Later, several local research institutes were established. Since the 1950s, many research programmes for the control of tropical diseases in China have been highly productive and have led to numerous publications in journals. According to incomplete statistics, there were more than 20,000 articles and reports on the control of tropical diseases published in China in a variety of journals from 1949 to 1986. Some of these were published in international journals and local journals with English abstracts. These publications showed that successful control of tropical diseases in China required the application of epidemiological principles to basic scientific discoveries, including the development and application of diagnostic tools, mechanisms of pathogenesis, and modulation of the host's immune responses with special attention to vaccine development and application (Mao 1989; Wu 2005).

Tuberculosis (TB)

Tuberculosis or the 'white plague' was the second major killer after malaria in Thailand in the 1940s (TB Division, personal communication). In 1966, the World Health Organization recommended that Thailand establish the National Program for TB Control. Specialized TB clinics and TB zonal centres were established to provide curative services in the early years. It was not until 1982 that TB services were integrated into public health and general clinical services at district level and above (Sriyabhaya et al. 1993).

In addition to curative services, prevalence surveys by the TB Division of the Ministry of Health using mass miniature X-ray (MMX) and sputum examinations were carried out in 1962, 1977, and 1991, which showed a progressive decline of positive X-rays (2.1%, 1.4%, and 0.92%, respectively), and of positive sputum smear/culture (0.5%, 0.3%, and 0.23% respectively; Payanandana et al. 1992). The tuberculin skin test was thought to be unreliable for estimating the true nature and extent of TB infection. However, due mainly to the HIV/AIDS epidemic, the burden from TB has risen. Thus, the mortality rate per 100,000 was estimated at 35.2 in 1960, 21.4 in 1970, 14.3 in 1980, 6.8 in 1990, and 7.7 in 1996 (Payanandana et al. 1999). The prevalence was particularly high in north Thailand where the HIV epidemic has been rife. Early case findings, case holding, and treatment of smear-positive cases that have been the cornerstone of effective TB control have now been complicated by co-infection with HIV (Dye et al. 1999) and with increase in multidrug resistant TB (Dye et al. 2002). Therefore, the World Health Organization recommended that a two-pronged approach directing interventions against TB as well as against HIV is needed for effective control of TB in HIV epidemic settings. Measures to control TB are early intensified TB case finding and treatment, TB treatment prophylaxis (e.g. Isoniazid) to decrease the likelihood of a first episode of TB, and BCG immunization. Interventions to reduce HIV transmission include antiretroviral (ARV) therapy, early diagnosis and treatment of sexually transmitted infection, prevention of mother to child transmission, and condom use (World Health Organization 2002). Epidemiological surveillance and monitoring are of paramount importance in advising planning and financing policy and programmes.

The epidemic of human immunodeficiency virus

The control of AIDS/HIV in Thailand is one classic example of the power of epidemiology in informing policy and action programmes. The AIDS/HIV epidemic in Thailand began at a point when the epidemic was already well-established in parts of sub-Saharan Africa and North America. The first case of AIDS was diagnosed in Thailand in 1985. The patient was a homosexual Thai who returned to Thailand after becoming infected abroad. The serious consequences were not recognized and the report was received as an incident. Nevertheless the occurrence was reported in a local newspaper. Soon several more people were proven to have the disease and concern was raised among hospital personnel who were afraid of getting the disease from direct contact. Government officials responsible for promoting tourism in the country warned against publicizing the finding. The Thai government thus had a policy of suppressing or ignoring the information.

As in the rest of Southeast Asia, the spread of HIV in Thailand was rapid. As of the mid-1980s intravenous drug users rapidly fell victim to the disease. By 1992 an estimated 675,000 or more of the 11.8 million people living with HIV/AIDS were in Southeast Asia, of whom the majority were Thais. Thailand's initial encounter with the AIDS epidemic was marked by stern denial. Part of the difficulty was the credibility of the available evidence for making a case for stronger action, sufficient to overcome the threat of economic loss from tourism. To some, the projections at this stage seemed fanciful. The early official response was therefore negligible, with the execution of a few public health measures such as ensuring the safety of Thailand's blood supply and mandating that health establishments report all AIDS cases. The necessary protective measures in health-care settings and at the National Blood Bank led to large additional expense. Moreover, it was first considered at that time that a negative image of the country would lead to fewer tourists and a weaker economy. Over-reaction was thought to be costly and unjustified. Thus, it was not surprising to hear government officials playing down the significance of the epidemic with claims that it would not affect society at large. Only a few years later, more than a million people had been infected since the beginning of the epidemic with about 600,000 living with the virus today. This is making HIV/AIDS a frightening reality, with large numbers of people requiring treatment, care, and support. HIV/AIDS is now the leading cause of death among young adults and in 2003 accounted for twice the number of deaths as from road traffic accidents (Ministry of Public Health, 2003; United Nations Development Programme 2004).

The disclosure of epidemic—the U-turn of national policy

In 1990, the Thai Government made a U-turn on the disclosure policy. Information regarding the situation, the nature of the disease, and the threat as well as necessary measures were publicized. Advertisements, education programmes and campaigns as well as different types of services were initiated. Non-governmental organizations (NGOs) and community programmes were supported.

Thailand and South Africa had similar rates of HIV in late 1980s and early 1990s. However, Thailand adopted sentinel surveillance and reported the surveillance results to the public early on. This led to many policy changes, including universal condom use, targeting different social groups with different vulnerability, and avoidance of stigmatization. In the case of HIV, Thailand now believes that failure to disclose and the quest for secrecy promoted destructive silence. Thailand's comprehensive national response to the HIV/AIDS epidemic has been extensively documented. Substantial progress in the fight against HIV/AIDS has been made through raising awareness of the problem. The massive public education and information campaign was successful because the vast majority of the population could be reached through electronic media. With increased democracy and tolerance came more critical views, especially in the print media, which helped maintain public debate.

Top-level political commitment and multisectoral strategies mobilized funds and human resources to implement the control programme at all levels. Increased condom use in brothels on a national scale rose from virtually nil to more than 95%. This was accompanied by a 90% reduction in the rate of sexually transmitted diseases. In parallel, the rate of new HIV infections dropped by 80%; the yearly new HIV infections which had increased gradually since 1986 began to drop rapidly from a peak of nearly 150,000 in 1991 to less than 20,000 in 2003 (Punpanich *et al.* 2004).

The subsequent disparity

The rate of HIV/AIDS infection in South Africa is at least five times higher than the rate in Thailand. According to the results of a national community-based survey of HIV in South Africa, the infection rate was 11.4–12.8% in females and 9.5% in male (Connolly 2004). Until very recently, South Africa did not admit the full nature and extent of HIV/AIDS infection and thus deprived the country of systematic adoption of effective interventions, including peer education, condom promotion, STD management among sex workers, the improvement of STD management through syndrome recognition, interventions among high-risk men, and reduction of mother to child transmission using antiretroviral treatment and breast milk substitutes (Campbell *et al.* 2002).

The most important lesson learned over the past two decades is that there is nothing inevitable about HIV epidemics. Those individuals, communities, regions, and nations that have had the wisdom to recognize the threats posed by HIV and that have had the courage to confront those threats have greatly reduced risk behaviours, HIV infections, and the trauma and hardship the epidemic generates. None of these can be achieved without the 'timely disclosure' of the deadly epidemic.

The role of epidemiology: SARS and avian influenza

SARS

Similar to HIV/AIDS, failure to use epidemiology for timely disclosure of epidemics to guide responses to the outbreak of SARS and influenza A (H5N1) has resulted in some unwanted consequences.

The epidemic of 'severe acute respiratory syndrome' or SARS starting in China and alarmingly spreading to many countries in the world provides a good example for studying disclosure policies. The high fatality and infective rates led to a rapid sequence of events. At the beginning when a strange disease occurred in the south Chinese province of Quangsi there was limited recognition of the threat. The Chinese Government banned the media from covering the outbreak for fear of an adverse impact on the Chinese economy. The authorities worried that word of a mysterious new disease spreading on the mainland would crush commerce. In his first comments on the disease some 5 months after the initial signs of the illness, Minister of Health Zhang Wenkang on 3 April 2003 scoffed at the WHO's warnings to avoid travel in southern China, believed to be the source of SARS. 'It is perfectly safe to come to China to work, travel and hold business meetings' he insisted (Bird 2003). It was when the virus was carried to Hong Kong and rapidly spread to many contacts that the alarm was raised and intensive investigation as well as measures were initiated. In Hong Kong, on 12 March, 20 health-care workers developed influenza-like symptoms (high fever and lower respiratory symptoms). A number of people who had contacted the initial case carried the virus to countries of Southeast Asia and beyond.

The first case in Thailand was imported from Hanoi, Vietnam. An expert health professional of the World Health Organization travelled to Thailand on the 11 March from Hanoi. He personally informed the authorities in Thailand of the possibility of his being infected by a contagious disease. He was isolated and the authorities were made aware of the danger. Tight screening of incoming passengers at Bangkok Airport was immediately instituted. Other cases had, however, entered Thailand and the raised awareness at hospitals prompted surveillance of contacts. Hospitals were strengthened to handle suspected cases in the hope of containing the infection within hospitals. A system of notification and referral of suspected cases was set up. Technical guidelines for case management were provided to all hospitals whose staff were trained in personnel protection and patient care. The first patient unfortunately died. All detected cases were infected from contact abroad. There was no evidence of transmission of SARS inside Thailand.

Initial reluctance to deal openly with SARS also happened in Thailand. In an attempt to downplay the threat, the Prime Minister said that the situation would be contained in 1 month. Later, speaking to reporters outside a conference, attended by officials from 11 Asian countries, the United States, the European Union, and international agencies, he 'rephrased' his earlier assurances, estimating the effort would take 6 months.

The Ministry of Public Health had full cooperation from other relevant agencies. International agencies, in particular the World Health Organization, were in close collaboration with the Thai authorities. Technical guidelines for diagnosis, case management, laboratory investigation, surveillance, and control were developed. Global networks for technical collaboration in epidemiological, clinical, and laboratory work were organized. The ASEAN Summit, at which heads of state from ASEAN plus three countries met in Bangkok on 29 April 2003. This was instrumental in harmonizing efforts in the region. Thailand with its Field Epidemiology Training Program (FETP) was given the responsibility for capacity building in epidemiological surveillance.

During the initial phase of the epidemic, the public was confused due to inadequate information and uncertainty. Opinions and responses were many, and some were completely groundless. Some hospitals were closed for fear of infection affecting care-providing personnel, in part exacerbated by distrust arising from earlier lack of transparency and information dissemination. Some potentially infected persons and certain sectors of the public did not observe the quarantine rules, avoiding formal treatment due to its high cost and scepticism about its efficacy. This in turn increased the likelihood of infecting others. The impact on the health sector was expected to rise as the magnitude of the epidemic increased (Asian Development Bank 2003). With open debate in public and media coverage, the public in general understood the problem and cooperated with the necessary measures. Within 115 days from 11 March to 5 June 2003, 314 cases were investigated. They were from 52 of Thailand's 76 provinces. Fortunately, all 9 probable and 31 suspected SARS cases were those travelling into Thailand from China, Taiwan, Singapore, Vietnam, and the UK. No one was infected inside Thailand. When the epidemic subsided in late 2003, it was estimated that throughout the world, about 8000 people were infected and one-tenth of them had died. As a consequence, the number of tourists in Thailand from 1 to 21 April 2003 dropped by 41% compared to the same period in 2002. Restriction of tourists and visitors from China, Hong Kong, and Singapore was intentional to prevent possibly infected persons from coming to the country. Tourists from unaffected countries such as Japan and Korea were deterred by fear of the unknown. It was said that the epidemic had caused a reduction of about 1% in Thailand's GDP growth (Asian Market Research News 2003).

After China changed her Minister of Health and disclosed the full nature and extent of the SARS epidemics, integrated efforts were mounted as emergency responses to address immediate needs and long-term preparedness with the help of technical and financial partners like the World Health Organization, the World Bank, the Asian Development Bank (ADB) and NGOs from the Asian region. The SARS epidemic highlighted the importance of surveillance and disclosure in mounting effective responses by national and international stakeholders. Once disclosure was in place, integrated efforts to mount effective emergency responses and seek the cooperation of the public and international communities were possible. The control of SARS was a success for integrated global efforts and highlighted the importance of epidemiological surveillance information for effective control.

Avian influenza

In Thailand, researchers from the Faculty of Veterinary Science, Chulalongkorn University had noted and studied an unusual outbreak of a serious disease causing massive and rapid death of chickens in Nakorn Sawan province, about 200 km north of Bangkok, in early November 2003. From the clinical evidence they suspected bird flu to be the cause. The Livestock Department of the Ministry of Agriculture was informed and warned of a possible serious bird flu epidemic. While the BBC and Associated Press reported massive numbers of chicken deaths in Thailand in November 2003, Thai newspapers picked it up later. However, the Director-General of the Livestock Department, Ministry of Agriculture and Cooperatives was quoted as saying that over 100,000 chickens had died or were culled in order to control the unknown disease. A number of Thai newspapers and periodicals ran articles and editorials on the performance of actors in the development of the bird flu epidemic. Many in the press and general public said that the government had conducted an intentional, disingenuous, and systematic cover-up. Aside from its devastating economic impact, avian flu evolved into a month-long political crisis. The Thai Government supported the big agribusiness so blatantly that Thai consumers and small producers felt cheated. Not only were they reluctant to eat Thai chicken, but they also doubted what their officials said. This crisis of confidence was shared by some of Thailand's major commercial partners, including the European Union and Japan. Fifteen countries including the EU banned the importation of chicken from Thailand.

Following the disclosure, measures were put in place to control the epidemic. A National Avian Influenza Response Committee was established supported by an Avian Influenza Operation Center. Nationwide surveys of the nature and extent of animal and human infection were launched. More intensive and supervised activities in the control of spread of the disease among domestic and wild fowl were undertaken. Elimination of all fowl was carried out within a 5-km radius of the focus where infected chickens, ducks, or geese were identified. Surveillance was intensive within a 50-km radius. Compensation was given to farmers to facilitate cooperation and for the relief of hardship. Facts and risks about bird flu were openly distributed. Guidelines for handling of chickens, ducks, geese, and wild birds as well as for those exposed and those affected were made and publicized. Nevertheless there were failures to observe the guidelines, such as for fighting cocks which were of considerable monetary value. The practice of keeping free-range ducks in rice fields across the central plain by at least 3000 small-scale duck producers posed a social problem. After the discovery of the H5N1 virus in free-range ducks, 2.7 million ducks were culled as a drastic measure to stem the spread of avian influenza.

On the human side, the results of nationwide surveillance were made public. All confirmed cases resided in villages that experienced abnormal chicken deaths. Most lived in households whose backyard chickens had died, and many reported direct contact with dead chickens (Chotpitayasunondh 2005). During the second wave in June to September 2004 there were five confirmed human cases. There was no new human case in the following 10 months. Continuing education for doctors, nurses, veterinarians, and laboratory technicians was put in place. Research and capacity development for research was planned and executed. Intensive studies were carried out by teams of epidemiological and laboratory experts. A probable case of human-to-human transmission (Ungchusak 2005) and spread to tigers and leopards were reported (Keawcharoen *et al.* 2004).

After the disclosure, the Thai health authorities sought WHO's technical support and collaboration and a team of technical experts constituted at WHO HQ in Geneva was dispatched to work closely with Thais in the field. Collaboration with the CDC, which had had close links with the Ministry of Public Health, was enhanced.

Thus, the application of epidemiology in developing countries has come a long way despite tremendous odds. Bright young epidemiologists, through the support of international linkages, have recognized the importance of context, the value of local knowledge, and a problem-based approach in addressing major public health problems. By empowering developing countries to use epidemiology as a tool to solve local problems, we encourage the development of a truly global epidemiology, which not only better addresses the public health problems in non-Western populations but can also shed light on the limitations of epidemiology in addressing the major public health problems in the West (Mustaffa 1985; Cheah *et al.* 1985; White *et al.* 2001; Pearce 2004).

Gaps and requirements

For health system issues, epidemiology as well as other disciplines will be needed to optimize the linkage between various levels of policies such as public policy, system policy (public and private), facility policy, and practice policy. Optimization of the linkage between different policy levels is relevant during the current technological imbalances because developing countries are still dependent on imported medicines and technology. Special attention is needed for a health system coping with chronic and lifestyle diseases. A comprehensive health system linking multi-level interventions to deal effectively with multilevel causations is needed. Interventions include clinical care, clinical preventive services, modification of individual behaviour and lifestyle, changes in social norms, and adapting government infrastructure and public policy. These require innovative methodologies as well as classic methods to study the distribution of diseases and risks (Dawber *et al.* 1963; Morris *et al.* 1966; Cheah *et al.* 1985; Doll *et al.* 1994a,b; Ramsay 2001; Drancourt and Raoult 2002)

We also need to develop epidemiological and other capacities to understand the short- and long-term consequences on equity and health of globalization and protection of intellectual property rights. We need to develop strategies to cope with the powerful forces of foreign indus-tries and requirements of the World Trade Organization. This will require linking such disci-plines as international trade and law, international economics, population health, and epidemiology to the analysis of health equity. New tools may also be needed to understand and control the problem. Monitoring the performance of health systems using recently developed methods will also be important in linking information with the ethics of resource allocation (Larkins 1996; Berman 2000; Mannion and Davies 2002).

The way forward

Past successes have resulted from partnerships between developing countries and those with technical know-how. There is a continuing need for intelligent solidarity between countries to strengthen collaboration, optimize the use of resources for research, and develop appropriate infrastructure for relevant disciplines and innovative planning for capacity strengthening. Schemes will be needed to promote research as a viable career. New programmes may need scaling up to make local problems an important entry point to education and actions, such as the School of Public Health Without Walls. A consensual validation through Kalayanamitra or the friends-helping-friends philosophy will be essential if we are to fulfil our commitment towards epidemiology and research as an important link to equity in health for development.

Epidemiology as a means for providing information for action will be increasingly important in influencing policy and practices both nationally and internationally because of new threats from emerging diseases, ethnic conflicts, environmental pollution, and other risks including trade in agricultural products. Lessons learned from the epidemics of HIV/AIDS, SARS, and avian influenza A (H5N1) in Asia, and in particular in Thailand, have shown that epidemiology informing policy and practices can be effective despite the complexity. The recognition of the occurrence of epidemics is relative rather than absolute. Acute suspicion based on clinical syndromes is an important step, but early declaration, though desirable, can lead to over-reaction and panic. The rapidity of having definitive confirmation depends on the availability of laboratory facilities and capabilities. In general these are inadequate in developing countries. In such cases the time lapse depends on international assistance.

The rights of the citizen to be informed, educated, protected from avoidable risks, and protected from danger must be honoured by the government. Outbreaks of emerging infectious diseases, environmental pollution, exports of contaminated products (e.g. during mad cow disease and avian flu) as well as disasters from ethnic conflicts underscore these rights. The right to freedom of speech, freedom of the press, and academic freedom represent the necessary elements for a citizen's right in a democratic society. Disclosure is a basic principle; the whole truth and nothing but the truth must be given to the public. In situations of uncertainty, the best available options based on evidence should be given for everyone to make their own choice, so long as it does not endanger others. Rules, regulations, and practices following accepted standards should target the well-being of the majority, while protecting the minority. A failure to disclose delays appropriate responses, such as mobilization of community participation and inviting international collaboration. Academics including epidemiologists, the media, and the participation of all key and diverse stakeholder groups at community, national, and international levels of society can be key mechanisms to guard against failure to disclose and eventual effective control of threats from infection, ethnic conflicts, environmental disasters, international transfer of risks, and trade liberalization. When nations are interdependent, epidemiologists can be a key to social justice and global harmony. History has shown that partnerships to develop the capacity to tackle common problems can benefit all involved.

References

Andresen EM and Meyers AR (2000). Health-related quality of life outcomes measures. *Archives of Physical Medicine and Rehabilitation*, **81**, S30–S45.

Asian Development Bank (2003). *Action plan to address outbreak of severe acute respiratory syndrome (SARS) in Asia and the Pacific*. Asian Development Bank, Manila (available at http://www.adb.org/Documents/Others/SARS/SARS_Action_Plan.pdf).

Asian Market Research News (2003). SARS, Thailand, tourism and business travel: How fast for recovery. www.asiamarketresearch.com/nws/000305.htm (30 April).

Berman P (2000). Organization of ambulatory care provision: a critical determinant of health system performance in developing countries. *Bulletin of the World Health Organization*, **78**, 791–802.

Bird M (2003). World's doctor is taking down her shingle. *Time Europe*, 27 May 2003 (www.time.com/time/europe/eu/article/0,13716,454667,00.html).

Bobb Aj, Castellanos FX, Addington AM, and Rapoport JL (2005). Molecular genetic studies of ADHD: 1991 to 2004. *American Journal of Medical Genetics B Neuropsychiatric Genetics*, **132**, 109–25.

Breslow L (2005). Origins and development of the International Epidemiological Association. *International Journal of Epidemiology*, **34**, 725–9.

Campbell C and Mzaidume Y (2002). How can HIV be prevented in South Africa? A social perspective. *British Medical Journal*, **324**, 229–32.

Cheah JS, Yeo PP, Thai AC, *et al.* (1985). Epidemiology of diabetes mellitus in Singapore: comparison with other ASEAN countries. *Annals of the Academy of Medicine Singapore*, **14**, 232–9.

Chotpitayasunondh T (2005). Human disease from influenza A (H5N1), Thailand, 2004. *Emerging Infectious Diseases*, **11**, 201–9.

Connolly C, Colvin M, Shishana O, and Stoker D (2004). Epidemiology of HIV in South Africa—results of a national, community-based survey. *South African Medical Journal*, **94**, 776–81.

Dawber TR, Kannel WB, and Lyell LP (1963). An approach to longitudinal studies in a community: The Framingham Study. *Annals of the New York Academy of Sciences*, **107**, 539–56.

Doll R, Peto R, Hall E, *et al.* (1994a). Mortality in relation to consumption of alcohol: 13 years' observations on male British doctors. *British Medical Journal*, **309**, 911–18.

Doll R, Peto R, Hall E, *et al.* (1994b). Mortality in relation to smoking: 40 years' observations on male British doctors. *British Medical Journal*, **309**, 901–10.

Dye C, Scheele S, Dolin P, Pathania V, and Rariglione MC (1999). Consensus statement. Global burden of tuberculosis: estimated incidence, prevalence, and mortality by country. WHO Global Surveillance and Monitoring Project. *Journal of the American Medical Association*, **282**, 677–86.

Dye C, Williams BG, Espinal MA, and Raviglione MC (2002). Erasing the world's slow stain: strategies to beat multidrug-resistant tuberculosis. *Science*, **295**, 2042–6.

Drancourt M and Raoult D (2002). Molecular insights into the history of plague. *Microbes and Infection*, **4**, 105–9.

Francis T, Napier IA, Voight RB, *et al.* (1955). Evaluation of the 1954 field trials of poliomyelitis vaccine. *American Journal of Public Health*, **45**(Suppl.), 1–63.

Fung YW, Lau LT, and Yu AC (2004). The necessity of molecular diagnostics for avian flu. *Nature Biotechnology*, **22**, 267.

Halstead SB (1992).The XXth century dengue pandemic: need for surveillance and research. *World Health Statistics Quarterly*, **45**, 292–8.

Halstead SB, Tugwell P, and Bennett K (1991).The International Clinical Epidemiology Network (INCLEN): a progress report. *Journal of Clinical Epidemiology*, **44**, 579–89.

IEA (1977). History of the International Epidemiological Association 1954–77. *International Journal of Epidemiology*, **6**, 309–24.

IEA (1984). The history of the International Epidemiological Association brought up to date. *International Journal of Epidemiology*, **13**, 139–41.

Keawcharoen J, Oraveerakul K, Kuiken T, *et al.* (2004). Avian influenza H5N1 in tigers and leopards. *Emerging Infectious Diseases*, **10**, 2189–91.

Krieger, N (1992). The making of public health data: paradigms, politics and policy. *Journal of Public Health Policy*, **13**, 412–17.

Krieger N (1994). Epidemiology and the web of causation: has anyone seen the spider? *Social Science and Medicine*, **39**, 887–903.

Mao SB (1989). Development and mission of parasitology. *Chinese Journal of Parasitic Diseases*, **2**, 150–4.

Macfarlane SB, Evans TG, Muli-Musiime FM, Prawl OL, and So AD (1999). Global health research and INCLEN. International Clinical Epidemiology Network. *Lancet*, **353**, 503.

Microbiology @ Leicester. *Online notes: malaria.* www-micro.msb.le.ac.uk/224/Malaria.html

Mannion R and Davies HT (2002). Reporting health care performance: learning from the past, prospects for the future. Journal of Evaluation in Clinical Practice, **8**, 215–28.

Ministry of Public Health (2003). *TB and STDS.* Bureau of AIDS. Department of Disease Control, Ministry of Public Health, Nonthaburi.

Morris JN, Kagan A, Pattison DC, *et al.* (1966). Incidence and prediction of ischemic heart disease in London businessmen. *Lancet*, **10**, 553–9.

Mustaffa BE (1985). Diabetes mellitus in peninsular Malaysia: ethnic differences in prevalence and complications. *Ann Acad Med Singapore*, **14**(2), 272–6.

Payanandana V, Bamrungtrakul T, Sareebutra W, and Na Songkla S (1992). Present situation of tuberculosis. *Thai Journal of Tuberculosis and Lung Disease*, **13**, 49–57.

Payanandana V, Kladphuang B, Somsong W, Jittimanee S. (1999). Battle against TB: National Tuberculosis Programme Thailand. Tuberculosis Division, Department of Communicable Disease Control, Ministry of Public Health, Bangkok, Thailand. p. 28.

Pearce N (2004). The globalization of epidemiology: introductory remarks. *International Journal of Epidemiology*, **33**, 1127–31.

Punpanich W, Ungchusak K, and Detels R. Thailand's response to the HIV epidemic: yesterday, today, and tomorrow. *AIDS Education and Prevention*, **16**(Suppl. A), 119–36.

Ramsay S (2001). Ethical implications of research on the human genome. *Lancet*, **357**, 535.

Sitthi-amorn C, Pongpanich S, Somgrongthong R, Likitkirirat T, and Likitkirirat P (2002). The Asian voice in building equity in health for development—from the Asian Forum for Health Research, Manila, February 2000. *Health Policy and Planning*, **17**, 213–17.

Sriyabhaya N, Payanandana V, Bamrungtrakul T, and Konjanart S (1993). Status of tuberculosis control in Thailand. *South Asian Journal of Tropical Medicine and Public Health*, **24**, 410–19.

Tarwater PM, Mellors J, Core ME, *et al.* (2001). Methods to assess population effectiveness of therapies in human immunodeficiency virus incident and prevalent cohorts. *American Journal of Epidemiology*, **154**, 675–81.

Timasarn K (1997). The history of malaria control in Thailand. *Malaria Journal*, **32**, 178–81.

Truong DH, Hedemark LL, Mickman JK, Mosher LB, Dietrich SE, and Lowry PW (1997). Tuberculosis among Tibetan immigrants from India and Nepal in Minnesota, 1992–1995. *Journal of the American Medical Association*, **277**, 735–8.

Ungchusak K, Auewarakul P, Dowell SF, *et al.* (2005). Probable person-to-person transmission of avian influenza (H5N1). *New England Journal of Medicine*, **352**, 323–4.

United Nations Development Programme (2004). *Thailand's response to HIV/AIDS: progress and challenges: thematic MDG report*. United Nations Development Programme, Bangkok.

Ward NA, Milstein JB, Hull HF, and Kim-Farley RJ (1993). The WHO EPI Initiative for the global eradication of polomyelitis. *Biologicals*, **21**, 327–33.

White K (1991). *Healing the schism: epidemiology, medicine and public health*. Springer-Verlag, New York.

White ME, McDonnell SM, Werker DH, Cardenas VM, and Thacker SB (2001). Partnerships in international applied epidemiology training and service, 1975–2001. American Journal of Epidemiology, **154**, 993–9.

World Health Organization (2002). *Global tuberculosis control: surveillance, planning, financing*, WHO Report WHO/CDS/TB/2002.295. WHO, Geneva.

World Health Organization (2005). Responding to the avian influenza pandemic threat: recommended strategic actions. WHO/CDS/CSR?GIP/2005.8.

Wu GL (2002). Emergence and development of parasitology and parasitic diseases. In *Modern issue of parasitic diseases* (ed. X Chen, GL Wu, X Sun, *et al.*), pp. 1–5. People's Press of Military Medicine, Beijing.

Wu GL (2005). Medical parasitology in China: a historical perspective. *Chinese Medical Journal*, **118**(9), 759–61.

Xu ZJ (2000). Human parasitology. In General history of medicine in China (ed. TT Deng and ZF Chen), pp. 377–81. People's Health Press, Beijing.

31

Epidemiological methods: a view from north Asia/Japan

Kunio Aoki and Itsuzo Shigematsu

Personal experiences

Kunio Aoki: I graduated from Nagoya University School of Medicine in 1952. In 1953–54 I had post-graduate education in clinical tuberculosis at the Department of Internal Medicine, Nagoya University Hospital, and also learned modern anatomy of the lung, pathogenesis of tuberculosis and the reading of chest X-rays of the TB patients at the Research Institute of the Anti-Tuberculosis Association in Tokyo. Then I engaged in examining patients at the TB dispensary affiliated to the Nagoya University Hospital. At the same time I studied the clinico-epidemiological characteristics of TB patients and evaluated modern TB treatments on the patients who registered in more than 10 hospitals and dispensaries. I was also interested in analysing TB mortality statistics nationally and internationally. In 1959, I started an epidemiological study in the Department of Preventive Medicine, Nagoya University School of Medicine as a research assistant, although I expected to return to the Department of Internal Medicine. In 1963, I had a chance to study epidemiology at the Department of Preventive Medicine and Public Health, University of Pennsylvania, Philadelphia, USA for 18 months, obtaining grants from the Rockefeller Foundation and others. I discovered a higher risk of lung cancer among the chronic active TB patients registered in the city of Philadelphia since 1955. The finding was against the common idea that TB and cancer are antagonistic. But a similar association was observed in other countries. In order to resolve this problem, I continued to study the causal mechanism in Japan for a long time, although I had similar results in the epidemiological studies and the autopsy series. My colleagues clarified causal mechanisms between chronic inflammation and cancer from molecular biological studies in 1980s. As a result, epidemiology became my life's work.

Itsuzo Shigematsu: After graduation from the Faculty of Medicine, University of Tokyo in 1941, I started my medical career as an assistant in the Department of Internal Medicine at the above Tokyo University Hospital. However, my interest shifted from clinical medicine for individuals to preventive medicine for groups during my military service of about four years in the Second World War. When I returned from overseas in 1946, various infectious diseases were rampant in Japan due to the post-war chaos, so I engaged in the prevention of epidemic disease at a quarantine station for about a year. This became my direct motivation for specializing in epidemiology, and in 1947 I was appointed as a member of the research staff at the Department of Epidemiology, National Institute of Public Health, which was, at that time, the only epidemiological institution in Japan. I held the position of director of the department from 1966–81 and since 1981 I served for 16 years as chairman of the Radiation Effects Research Foundation, a cooperative Japan–United States research organization, in Hiroshima and Nagasaki; this is well known as a long-term (more than 50 years) cohort study of the atomic bomb survivors.

A century of epidemiology in Japan is briefly described in four stages: the period of birth extending to the early 1940s, the period of growth from 1945 to 1970, the period of development from 1971 to 1990, and the period of expansion from 1991.

Period of birth to the early 1940s

The concept of epidemiology for infectious diseases was introduced to Japan in the 1880s and medical researchers came to understand epidemiology as a methodology for studying typical features of diseases and detecting causal mechanisms leading to prevention. Studies on cholera, typhoid fever, dysentery, smallpox, plague, typhus, tuberculosis, and others were conducted using classical epidemiological methods in the early twentieth century. These studies were conducted by physicians, bacteriologists, staff of medical school hygiene department, government officers, and others. A worldwide epidemic of influenza was the subject of study around 1920. An experimental study on a typhoid fever epidemic among mouse colonies was carried out in Japan, based on Müsendorf's study (Aoki 1996; Shigematsu 1988, 2000a).

Besides infectious diseases, causal factors for non-infectious diseases such as beriberi in the navy and rickets in rural districts were studied, with fruitful results. A group of pathologists tried to detect the causative factors of malignant neoplasms related to dietary habits, quality of drinking water, alcohol consumption, income, labour conditions, natural environmental factors, and so on, comparing those in areas with high and low mortality from malignant neoplasms in 12 prefectures from 1905 to 1936; they found several risk and protective factors for cancer similar to our recent findings (Aoki 2001). In the 1930s, a preliminary study on cerebrovascular diseases among inhabitants of the Tohoku district (the northern part of the main island of Honshu) was conducted by a hygienist.

The University of Tokyo established a department of hygiene in its Faculty of Medicine in 1885. The Laboratory of Epidemiology was, however, set up in 1930 at the Institute of Infectious Diseases, University of Tokyo, and the laboratory was elevated into the Department of Epidemiology in 1938, at the time of the founding of the National Institute of Public Health. Keizo Nobechi, who graduated from the Harvard University School of Public Health, was the first Chief of the Laboratory of Epidemiology, where he initiated research and education in epidemiology. The Second World War, however, disturbed his efforts to develop the field (Shigematsu 1988, 2000a).

The paradigm of statistics had already been introduced to Japan around 1860 and the Meiji Government, which took office in 1868, set up the Bureau of Statistics in the Ministry of Home Affairs. Starting in 1882 the Bureau of Statistics published annual population statistics, including vital statistics. Population census efforts have been carried out based on the Koseki (family registration) system since 1872. Economists and specialists other than those in medicine were placed in charge of the Bureau of Statistics (Hayashi 1957). Population censuses based on international rules were initiated in 1920 and then conducted quinquennially.

Period of growth from 1945 to 1970

In 1944–45, towards the end of the Second World War, Japan was devastated by air raids and the living conditions of the Japanese people in 1946–47 were miserable. However, epidemiological studies on infectious diseases resumed immediately after the end of the war, with the aim of controlling epidemics of infectious disease. It is surprising that 51 research papers on infectious diseases and 30 papers on personal and environmental hygiene were presented at the first scientific meeting of the Japanese Society for Public Health, which had just been formed in 1947. Mortality from acute infectious diseases and other infections such as gastroenteritis, bronchitis/pneumonia, and parasitic diseases was rapidly reduced by the efforts of not only government workers but also volunteers under the preventive laws newly enacted (Table 31.1) (Aoki 1996; Shigematsu 1988, 2000a). It should be noted that the Occupied Japan Allied Forces General Head Quarters (AFGHQ), which had adequately advised on control programmes for infectious diseases, greatly

Table 31.1 Brief chronology of enactment and promulgation of the laws for disease

1897 Promulgation of the Communicable Disease Prevention Law (eight diseases)
1898 Enactment of the Marine Port Quarantine Law
1907 Enactment of Leprosy Prevention Law
1909 Enactment of the Smallpox Vaccination Law
1919 Enactment of the Trachoma Prevention Law, and Tuberculosis Prevention Law
1927 Enactment of the Venereal Diseases Prevention Law
1931 Enactment of the Parasitosis Prevention Law (four diseases)
1937 Enactment of Law of Public Health Centre
1947–48 Enactment of the Food Sanitation Law, Revision of Public Health Centre Law, Promulgation of the Preventive Vaccination Law (12 diseases), and the Venereal Disease Prevention Law (four diseases)
1950–51 Enactment of the Daily Life Security Law and the Mental health Law, Enactment of the Tuberculosis Prevention Law, Promulgation of the Quarantine Law (four diseases)
1953 Enactment of the Leprosy Prevention Law
1954–59 Revision of the Communicable Diseases Law, Designation of acute poliomyelitis as a specially designated communicable disease
1961 Enactment of the Universal Health Insurance Law
1967 Enactment of the Basic Law for Environmental Pollution Control
1972 Enactment of the Industrial Safety and Health Law
1980 Deletion of smallpox vaccination from routine vaccination
1981 Start of the infectious diseases surveillance system
1982 Enactment of the Health and Medical Service Law for the Aged
1987 Enactment of the Law on the Health and Welfare of the Mentally Handicapped, National AIDS Control Programme
1994 Revision of Preventive Vaccination Law, Repeal of Parasitosis Prevention Law
1996 Repeal of Leprosy Prevention Law

Most laws were renewed in 1945–51.

contributed to this effort, donating abundant pesticides, precious drugs and chemicals, and offering food and other requirements. The organization also sponsored Japanese students to study in the USA. AFGHQ staff believed that strengthening the field of public health was urgent for Japan, and ordered the establishment of departments of public health, besides departments of hygiene, in all medical schools, and the promotion of public health activities in all 675 public health centres throughout Japan (Japanese Association of Public Health 1967). These policies resulted in increases in the government budget for such efforts as well as the number of staff and officials working in public health.

The population census resumed in 1950, and vital statistics have been published annually since 1947. Other surveys, such as patient surveys, surveys of living conditions of people on welfare, hospital reports, public health administration reports, and others were initiated between 1946 and 1948 and thereafter reports were published annually. The National Nutritional Survey was initiated in 1945, even under such difficult living conditions, and has been conducted each year thereafter (Aoki 1996).

After a decline in deaths from infectious diseases, Japan was found to have a serious situation with respect to tuberculosis (TB). The renewed TB Prevention Law was enacted in 1951, and a TB registration system was established. Under this law, the medical costs of registered patients were covered, and primary and secondary prevention programmes for those under 30 years of age were intensively executed. In 1953, after independence from occupation, the Japanese government carried out the National TB Prevalence Survey, in which areas throughout Japan were stratified and randomly selected using modern sampling methods. Based on the estimated 2.93 million patients from this survey, modified TB programmes were developed. Various epidemiological studies on TB in local areas were followed up by public health workers and physicians with the aim of obtaining more detailed information in each district (Aoki 1996; Sasaki and Aoki 1992).

With declining mortality from tuberculosis, the leading cause of death shifted to cerebrovascular diseases, followed by cancer. The epidemiological study on cerebrovascular diseases was resumed in the towns and villages of the Tohoku district in the 1950s by Naosuke Sasaki and colleagues (Sasaki *et al.* 1962). Using traditional survey methods, confirmation of living conditions, physical examinations, including blood pressure, urinalysis, and others, they reported a high incidence of stroke associated with poor nutrition and high salt intake, which confirmed his predecessor's work. In response to the increased number of deaths from apoplexy, epidemiologists in many districts tried to survey the current features of stroke and hypertension in small communities. Screening methods in the early stages were similar to those used in the previous study. ECG and thickness of subcutaneous fat were added later around 1965. The papers from the Framingham Study and the scheme of the Seven Country Study in the USA greatly stimulated Japanese epidemiologists (Komachi 1987; Sasaki and Aoki 1992; Ohno 1996).

In 1961 and 1962, the government conducted nationwide surveys on 'adult diseases' for estimating their exact prevalence and incidence, based on which the National Programme for Preventing Apoplexy was issued. The term 'adult diseases', which comprises cerebrovascular diseases, cardiac diseases, hypertension, cancer, and others, became popular from that time. Local governments of cities and towns concentrated on reducing the incidence of adult diseases through education and screening programmes, in addition to medical treatment. International collaborative studies on circulatory diseases started to draw comparisons utilizing these data (Komachi 1987). Participation by Japanese epidemiologists generated new concepts and tools for study. The Japanese Society of Administration for Circulatory Diseases was organized in 1962 and consisted of clinicians, epidemiologists, and others engaged in this field of study.

Japan's cancer death rate was not high in 1950, and a hospital cancer patient survey was conducted by pathologists in 1953 (Japanese Cancer Association and Japanese Foundation for Cancer Research 1957). Mitsuo Segi, the researcher responsible for the epidemiological study in the above survey, carried out a case–control study to detect the factors causing cancer. Segi worked to establish a cancer registry in the Miyagi prefecture in 1957, after surveying all cancer patients in the Miyagi prefecture from 1951 to 1953. Hiroshima was the first city to set up a cancer registry in 1957, and Nagasaki followed in 1958, in order to pursue the health status of the atomic bomb survivors (Aoki and Kurihara 1994). Segi also published a paper on age-adjusted mortality rates of cancer by site in 24 countries, using the 1950 world population as a standard. This study achieved worldwide recognition (Segi 1960).

In response to the trend of increasing cancer deaths, the Japanese Government conducted the Nationwide Cancer Patient Survey in 1958, and similar surveys in 1959 and 1963. Confirming the increasing trend, the government issued its strategy for controlling cancer in Japan: (1) public education on cancer; (2) cancer screening programmes; (3) the establishment of medical institutes for cancer; (4) training of specialists; and (5) the promotion of cancer research.

The National Cancer Centre was established in 1962 in Tokyo, and the Osaka Adult Disease Centre and the Aichi Cancer Centre followed within 2 years. These three cancer centres all have a department or division of epidemiology.

Mass screening programme for cervical, uterine, and stomach cancers were begun by physicians and spread throughout Japan in the 1960s in response to public demand. Epidemiologists did not participate in such programmes in the early stages, so the efficacy of the screening was not planned (Aoki 1996).

In 1965, a large-scale cohort study on smoking and cancer, including of 265,000 inhabitants of Japan, was launched in 1964 by a research team (under the chairmanship of T. Hirayama) based on a government grant, to confirm the Surgeon General's Report on Smoking and Health (Hirayama 1990). This was the first large-scale cohort study on cancer to be conducted in Japan.

The high rate of economic growth in Japan since 1960 produced various industrial products and pollutants that became closely related to specific diseases and/or health hazards, such as chronic bronchitis/Yokkaichi asthma (due to air pollution) (Imai *et al.* 1967), Minamata disease (due to methyl mercury) (Tsubaki and Takahashi 1986), itai-itai (ouch-ouch) disease (related to cadmium) (Shigematsu 1973), yusho (due to poisoning with polychlorinated biphenyls (PCBs)) (Kuratsune 1996), and so on, all of which are shown in Table 31.2. Kawasaki disease, a new infantile syndrome like scarlet fever, appeared in this period, although its relation with pollution is not clear (Yanagawa *et al.* 2004).

Multidisciplinary study teams including epidemiologists started to scrutinize the causes and causal mechanisms of such diseases, and each study team successfully elucidated the causal mechanisms.

Table 31.2 Brief chronology of disease outbreaks and countermeasures related to development of epidemiological study in Japan after 1945

1946–50 Epidemics of cholera, smallpox, typhus, typhoid fever, dysentery, Izumi fever (scarlet fever-like disease), viral enteritis/hepatitis and parasitosis. Tuberculosis (leading cause of death). Establishment of Atomic Bomb Causality Commission (ABCC)
1951 Cerebrovascular diseases occupied the leading cause of deaths
1953 Outbreak of Minamata disease in Kumamoto prefecture
1955–56 Outbreak of Arsenic milk poisoning. The first report of itai-itai (ouch-ouch) disease
1955–56 Thalidomide babies
1955–56 Yokkaichi asthma (due to air-pollution)
1962 Epidemic of Asian influenza
1963–68 Strategy for controlling cancer by the Ministry of Health and Welfare. Clustering of SMON patients in concentrated small areas throughout country. The second outbreak of Minamata disease in Niigata prefecture. Outbereak of Yusho (due to PCBs)
1969–70 Cerebral apoplexy prevention measures by the government. Photochemical smog (due to air-pollution). Research Committee on Kawasaki disease
1971 Establishment of the Environmental Agency. Research committees on intractable diseases determined by the Ministry of Health and Welfare
1981–85 Cancer became the leading cause of death. Excess risk of lung cancer among asbestos workers in Osaka. 10-year strategy for cancer control by the government. Karoushi (sudden death due to overwork) recognized by the WHO
1991 CIOMS: International Guidelines for Ethical Review of Epidemiological Studies.
1993 The second 10-year strategy for cancer control

Ironically, the term 'epidemiology' became widely known through the mass media because epidemiological outcomes were recognized as important evidence of such health hazards in the legal system.(Aoki and Kurihara 1994) On the other hand, epidemiological studies with less rigorous design and conducted by inexperienced researchers were severely criticized. The Japanese Society of Epidemiology provided a focus to which criticism of epidemiological studies could be directed (Shigematsu 1988, 2000b).

The long-term health effects of ionizing radiation from the atomic bombings were for many years carefully and intensively studied by the Atomic Bomb Casualty Commission (ABCC) in Hiroshima and Nagasaki, starting in 1947. Excess incidence of leukaemia was first reported by this organization (Yokoro 1991).

As for infectious diseases, clinicians and bacteriologists faced problems of increased drug-resistant strains of major infections. Worldwide epidemics of influenza, viral hepatitis, and El Tor cholera, among others, caused problems for epidemiologists and public health workers, although mortality from such infectious diseases approached negligible levels.

It can be said that during this period the field of epidemiology was steadily climbing the ranks of the medical sciences.

Period of development from 1971 to 1990

The period of the 1970s was characterized by the pervasiveness of information technologies in all scientific fields, including epidemiology, and by the demand for more positive involvement of epidemiology in the area of medicine, for which evaluation of studies of various interventions was based on monitoring, surveillance, and disease control systems.

At the same time, epidemiology began to study newly recognized and intractable diseases of unknown aetiology. The first such disease was subacute myelo-optico-neuropathy (SMON). SMON appeared around 1955 in Osaka–Kobe and surrounding areas but soon spread. In 1965, the epidemic-like spread of SMON reappeared in many areas throughout Japan with seasonal variation. The government organized an interdisciplinary study team consisting of clinicians, pathologists, neurologists, microbiologists, chemists, pharmacologists, epidemiologists, and others. Fortunately, the study team was able to determine within a year that clioquinol, a drug for treatment of diarrhoea and gastroenteral disorders, was the cause of SMON. A subsequent ban of clioquinol soon eliminated SMON. Epidemiologists participated in a study of the situation a bit later, and thereby contributed to the clarification of clinical features, mode of transmission, and causal mechanisms in the human population.(Gent and Shigematsu 1978) The role of epidemiology was now well understood not only by clinicians and researchers but also by the government.

There were many diseases with unknown aetiology and without effective treatments, which were difficult for small groups of researchers to study due to their low incidence. From the SMON study, the government expected that the well-organized interdisciplinary study team might clarify the causal mechanisms of such diseases leading to treatment and prevention. In 1972, the government launched a new project dubbed 'Specified diseases as intractable', determined by the Ministry of Health and Welfare. The diseases targeted by the project included multiple sclerosis, myasthenia gravis, Behçet's disease, systemic lupus erythematosus, aplastic anaemia, SMON, and sarcoidosis. These diseases were chronic, of low incidence, of unknown aetiology, without effective treatment, and accompanied by severe sequelae and tremendous social and psychological burdens. The patients were scattered throughout the country. In order to save laborious work and cost, epidemiologists who were involved in a total of eight interdisciplinary study teams planned to coordinate their work by nationwide surveys of eight diseases to obtain clinico-epidemiological disease characteristics as basic data and to detect causal factors. The surveys obtained very useful results not only for the researchers in each study team but also for the government officers to make future plans. Epidemiologists gained valuable experience conducting the surveys with clinicians and other researchers from different study fields. An increase in the number of young epidemiologists was another benefit gained from the studies.(Yanagawa *et al.* 1992)

A large-scale cohort study on smoking by Dr Hirayama confirmed a causal relation with lung cancer and cancer of other sites. Hirayama then revealed the effect of passive smoking on lung cancer, which contributed greatly to the worldwide anti-smoking movement (Hirayama 1990).

The increased number of cancer deaths stimulated researchers and epidemiologists to start epidemiological research on cancers of the stomach, cervix/uteri, lung, oesophagus, liver, breast, bladder, and other sites successively in the 1970s, but their efforts were hampered by the small size of government grants. The Society of Cancer Epidemiology, consisting of around 50 members and established by Suketami Tominaga and others in 1977, held annual scientific meetings. Cancer registries were conducted in two cities and 15 prefectures at that time. The Research Group for Population-based Cancer Registration in Japan was organized by Isaburo Fujimoto in 1975 for collaborative study of cancer incidence (Aoki 1996).

In 1984, the 10-Year Strategy of Cancer Control supported by more substantial governmental funding was initiated in Japan. In relation to this strategy, a new project, the Monbusho Overseas Scientific Investigation (later Scientific Research)—Special Cancer Study, was started with the aim of detecting causal factors of cancer based on comparisons of the different features of outcomes between two areas, Japan and another country, with the expectation that the results would be different from those generated in Japan alone. Epidemiologists requested that they be allowed to plan and execute the study by organizing multidisciplinary research teams. This programme continued for more than 20 years, as the outcomes in the early stages were very encouraging (Sasaki and Aoki 1990).

The ABCC in Hiroshima and Nagasaki was reorganized into the Radiation Effects Research Foundation (RERF) in 1975, and this new organization actively engaged in basic and clinico-epidemiological studies. RERF's research results circulated throughout Japan and the high-quality papers contributed worldwide not only to the understanding of cancer but also lifestyle-related diseases. RERF provided its support to the Chernobyl accident and made great efforts in research and prevention (Yokoro K 1991; Shigematsu 2000b). It is noteworthy that Dr Shigematsu, a former RERF chairman, stated in a lecture that most RERF efforts are devoted to dose estimation, especially individual dose, and referred to the comprehensive evaluation and limitations of radiation effects on the atomic bomb survivors based upon review of the results of 50 years of follow-up (Shigematsu 2000b).

Studies on environmental pollution leading to illnesses such as itai-itai disease, Minamata disease, and chronic respiratory diseases were continued through longitudinal study of such diseases with various aftereffects.

Few research facilities conducted epidemiological research in name, except for the Department of Epidemiology of the National Institute of Public Health. In this period, however, a department of epidemiology was established at the School of Health Sciences, University of Tokyo, followed by the founding of several schools of medicine and related research institutes. A short course of epidemiology was initiated at the National Institute of Public Health. The Society of Theoretical Epidemiology was organized by Kazuya Horiuchi and Kunihiro Sakamoto in Japan's Kinki district. Thus, the chance for epidemiologists to meet was gradually increased.

For occupational hazards, epidemiological studies have increased in place of toxicology studies, reflecting lower dose exposures. Of course, longer observation is needed for asbestosis and other diseases involving exposure to high doses of toxic material. Karoushi (unexpected sudden death due to overwork), mental disorders, vibration disorders, and other problems related to recent working conditions have been studied. Many screening programmes for workers have been planned and conducted (Aoki 1996).

In 1983, the Health and Medical Services Law for the Aged was implemented. The law includes guidance on health education, counselling, health examination, functional training, and in-home visits. Physical examinations consisted of basic health check-ups and cancer screening (stomach, uterus, lung, breast, and colon). This project was evaluated from an epidemiological point of view – the compliance rate was about 30% for the basic examinations and less than 15% for the cancer screening. Numerous epidemiological studies on disorders related to aging are under way (Sasaki and Aoki 1992; Aoki 1996; Ohno 1996). The increase in life expectancy since 1985 is 2.12 years for males and 3.51 years for females. The effects of such programmes are partly reflected in these figures.

Data accumulated over more than 50 years in the National Nutrition Survey were good indicators of the nutritional status and lifestyle of the Japanese people and the data were indispensable not only for research but also for policy-making (Aoki 1996).

Surveillance systems of various infectious diseases were computerized in 1987 and have been used effectively for a number of purposes, and no major epidemic happened in the meantime.

In the 1980s, however, the worldwide outbreaks of AIDS greatly changed the conventional strategy for dealing with infections. In relation to AIDS, the human rights of the patient became irrelevant. Both epidemiologists and the public should understand the meaning of weak infectivity and human rights. The traditional countermeasures for the increasing number of infectious diseases, including evolving and recurrent infectious diseases such as TB, needed to be changed (Aoki 1996). Adult T-cell leukaemia/lymphoma, a disease specific to Japan, is a disease that has been present for a long time but which began to be newly studied. Basic research revealed the cause and causal mechanisms and epidemiology greatly contributed to prevention (Sasaki and Aoki 1992). As for hepatitis B and C infections, many efforts continue, and the problem of hepatitis B is mostly resolved.

An increasing number of epidemiologists requested the establishment of an association where discussions could be conducted freely and mutual assistance enhanced. After 2 years of talks, the Japanese Epidemiological Association (JEA) was founded in 1990 and the relevant societies replaced by the association were discontinued. About 300 members initially registered, consisting of epidemiologists, biostatisticians, clinicians, pathologists, microbiologists, public health workers, psychologists, sociologists, health nurses, engineers, technicians, and others, and the number of members has continuously increased.

Period of expansion from 1991

The field of epidemiology is now growing in various ways. All health information systems described above were computerized to send timely information throughout the country. Detailed information can be obtained with the permission of the national government. Health promotion activities aimed at controlling smoking, alcohol consumption, dietary habits/nutrition, exercise, and mental stress have attracted attention. A study on health risk appraisal showed effective results in Japan, although further study is necessary based on more evidence from epidemiology (Aoki 1996).

Ischaemic heart disease has become a major item in the study of circulatory diseases, and cancer continues to be the leading cause of death, even though the pattern of cancer by site has changed.

Two large-scale cohort studies on cancer and circulatory diseases consisting of more than 100,000 subjects were started around 1990 (Aoki 1996). In parallel with the above cohort studies, several small-scale cohort studies were initiated in local areas, from which detailed prevention data specifically geared for such locales are expected. In this way, intervention studies on cancer and ischaemic heart diseases based on the control of risk factors have increased.

One new finding was that chronic infection with *Helicobacter pylori* is a causative factor in stomach cancer. At the same time, close associations between chronic infections of *Salmonella typhi* and biliary cancer, *Chlamydia trachomata* and cervical cancer, chronic active TB and lung cancers, among others, were also uncovered (Aoki 1993; Maeda and Akaike 1998). These study results suggest that controlling chronic inflammation may be a new way of preventing cancer.

In the 1990s, epidemiological evaluations of the cancer screening programme in Japan were conducted and reported the efforts to be effective for all except lung cancer. However, effectiveness was not as high as physicians expected (Aoki 1996).

The incidence of diabetes mellitus (DM) has been increasing for decades, and according to a nationwide survey in 1997 the estimated number of DM patients was 6.9 million with 6.8 million more borderline cases. Multidisciplinary studies, including epidemiology, of DM are ongoing.

It is notable that case–control studies of specific intractable diseases have detected risk or protective factors in their aetiology, including smoking and dietary factors (Yanagawa and Sasaki 1992).

The aged population has increased so rapidly that those aged over 65 years made up 17.4% of the total Japanese population in 2000, rising to 19% in 2003. In 1990 the government issued a so-called 'golden plan' for promoting the health and welfare of the aged and included subsidies in the plan. Epidemiologists and gerontologists have joined in partnership to work on this difficult problem. Besides diseases related to aging, studies on diminished functional capacities and behavioural changes among the aged are under way, which could prove important for maintaining good health among the elderly.

A computerized surveillance system compiling reports from 3000 designated clinics and hospitals operates smoothly for 27 communicable diseases including TB. In addition, a predictive surveillance system of communicable diseases is in place, checking antibody levels and isolating causal agents. And laborious efforts continue to be made with respect to AIDS, HTL, sexually transmitted diseases, and other viral diseases.

The contribution of epidemiology to the study of occupational hazards has been growing and the field of epidemiology has become more and more commonly utilized in the workplace.

The very first scientific meeting of the JEA (Chairman Yoshio Komachi) was held in 1991, at which 45 papers were presented, followed by 90 papers presented at the second meeting in Fukuoka (Chairman Tomio Hirohata) in 1992. The first IEA Regional Scientific Meeting in the Asia-Pacific region (Chairman Kunio Aoki) was held in Nagoya and 300 participants from 12 countries attended. In August 1996, the 14th International Scientific Meeting of the International Epidemiological Association (IEA) was held in Nagoya, Japan (Honorary Chairman Itsuzo Shigematsu, Chairman Kunio Aoki), and about 900 participants from 52 countries attended. Several satellite meetings on such topics as molecular epidemiology, and diet/nutrition and cancer were successfully held, in addition to the WHO Environment and Health meeting, the WHO GEEnet meeting, and the meetings on epidemiology of leprosy and smoking and health. Epidemiological researches in Japan in the past and present were introduced by specially issued monographs and panel exhibitions. The meetings indicated that the level of epidemiology in Japan seemed to be approaching the level of epidemiology internationally. It was a good chance for young Japanese epidemiologists to come into contact with established epidemiologists of global standing.

The Japanese government has issued a strategy on health promotion in the twenty-first century dubbed 'Health Nippon 21', which aimed at good health by improving dietary habits, exercise, rest, psychological care, and dental hygiene. Anti-smoking and anti-alcohol movements, and screenings for DM, cancer, and circulatory diseases were strongly recommended. The strategy based on attainment of certain targets will now be evaluated.

Molecular epidemiology is a new wave in the general field of epidemiology, anticipating clearer understanding of causal mechanisms at the cell or tissue level, and many papers have resulted. However, gene polymorphisms and limited DNA information related to disease may prove to be obstacles. Mendelian randomization is now common as a study topic, and other new study designs seem to be required.

With respect to epidemiology including genetic studies, however, medical ethics protecting human rights are a standard feature of human studies. Ethics is the basic condition for the conduct of any studies in medicine. Increased attention to ethics has been paid to the field of epidemiology in Japan since the 1980s and has intensified since 2003. In 2004, the government legislated to protect human rights in any scientific study. The government's aim in so doing was to better promote research, by insisting on careful study planning considering human rights implications.

Epilogue

In the first half of the twentieth century epidemiology seemed to be rooted in the soil of Japanese medicine, as researchers and physicians used epidemiology as a methodology within medicine. A laboratory of epidemiology was established at the National Institute of Public Health in 1938, but its activities were limited by the Second World War.

Although the term epidemiology was still used only for infectious diseases, after 1945, occupied Japan's AFGHQ strongly emphasized the importance of public health, in which epidemiology served as a methodology to provide evidence supporting public health activities.

However, experiences of epidemiological studies on chronic non-infectious diseases and new information abroad prompted the wide use of modern epidemiology. And thus, since 1965, the paradigm of epidemiology was clearly described in Japanese textbooks.

Government officials have planned and conducted nationwide surveys since 1953 on tuberculosis and other health hazards using modern epidemiological methods and supported by a few epidemiologists or statisticians.

When epidemics or clustering of diseases or health hazards of public concern occurred, government officers organized adequate study teams including epidemiologists. Such participation did not require a great many epidemiologists and the true role that epidemiology played was not apparent to the public.

Increasing deaths from cerebrovascular diseases and cancer demanded the study of epidemiological features of the diseases and causative factors for prevention. It was at that time that epidemiological studies of such diseases were initiated in small communities and special populations throughout Japan. The studies required many epidemiologists, and public health workers and physicians interested in epidemiology participated in the studies, ultimately becoming involved in the field of epidemiology. As mentioned before, it was a good time for epidemiologists when epidemiology was regarded as part of the studies on specified diseases supported by the Ministry of Health and Welfare, as epidemiologists throughout Japan could participate in the studies and gather valuable experience in research and gain information about relevant methodologies etc. The numbers of epidemiologists gradually increased. Before 1965, there were few official epidemiology positions, but the positions started to increase in the 1970s, beginning in medical schools, as stated before. This proved to be another fortunate trend for the emerging field.

In 1990 the Japanese Epidemiological Association (IEA) was established, and epidemiological activities have since developed rapidly. The quality of the papers published gradually improved, and papers originally written in English started to increase from the end of the twentieth century. This advance is a reflection of the increased grants made available for epidemiology.

International contributions in the field, such as training of epidemiologists, technology transfers, and the like are continuously being realized.

Epidemiology in Japan developed through studies on diseases and health hazards, although studies on health started later. However, epidemiology in Japan was not positively involved in the evaluation of governmental polices on medicine, such as the long-term effects of Japan's universal health-insurance system established in 1961, the medical security system, the medical system of facilities, personnel and services, or the safety of medicines, including costs and benefits. Neither was epidemiology engaged in recent study topics of globalization, inequality and health, the low birth rate, women's rights, and health and social impacts, and so on. This may have been due to the lack of epidemiologists over a long period, but it is possible that the scope of such studies was narrow compared with those conducted in Western countries.

Methodologically speaking, epidemiology in Japan is still immature, not only in terms of infrastructure, but also with respect to design and tools for study. Co-working with biostatisticians should be strengthened. Consideration of patients and participants is apparently insufficient, and the feedback system for study outcomes is often incomplete. There is little discussion regarding what patients or lay people think about and expect with regard to epidemiology, or what expectations are held by politicians, economists, and social psychologists. With great expectations placed on the field, epidemiology in Japan still has many tasks to resolve.

References

Aoki K (1993). Excess incidence of lung cancer among pulmonary tuberculosis patients. *Japanese Journal of Clinical Oncology*, **23**, 205–20.

Aoki K (ed.) (1996) Epidemiological research in Japan; historical perspectives and selected major studies. *Journal of Epidemiology*, **6**(Suppl.).

Aoki K (2001). Contribution to cancer prevention of non-governmental organizations 2. The dawn of cancer control activities: Comparison of Japan and the US. *Asian Pacific Journal of Cancer Prevention*, **12**, 15–26.

Aoki K and Kurihara M (1994). The history of cancer registration in Japan: contribution of Dr. Mitsuo Segi cancer surveys. *Trends in Cancer Incidence and Mortality*, **19**, 563–70.

Gent M and Shigematsu I. (ed.) (1978). *Epidemiological issues in reported drug-induced diseases—SMON and other examples*. McMaster University Library Press, Hamilton, Canada.

Hayashi F (1957). Study on history of statistics in Japan. Mori Rintaro's view on statistics. *Waseda Shogaku*, **127**, 811–36 (in Japanese).

Hirayama T (ed.) (1990). *Lifestyle and mortality; a large-scale census-based cohort study in Japan*. Karger, Basel.

Imai M, Oshima H, Takatsuka Y, *et al*. (1967). On Yokkaichi asthma. *Japanese Journal of Hygiene*, **22**, 323–35 (in Japanese).

Japanese Association of Public Health (ed.) (1967). *Development of public health 1967*. Japanese Association of Public Health, Tokyo (in Japanese).

Japanese Cancer Association and Japanese Foundation for Cancer Research (1957). An epidemiological study on cancer in Japan. The report of the committee for epidemiological study on cancer, sponsored by the Ministry of Welfare and Public Health. *Japanese Journal of Cancer Research*, **48**, S1–S63.

Komachi Y (ed.) (1987). *Changing features of circulatory diseases in relation to nutrition and living environment*. HokenDojinSha, Tokyo (in Japanese).

Kuratsune M, Yoshimura H, Hori Y, Okumura M, and Masuda Y (1996). *Yusho, a human disaster caused by PCBs and related compounds*. Kyushu University Press, Fukuoka.

Maeda H and Akaike T (1998). Nitric oxide and oxygen radicals in infection, inflammation, and cancer. *Biochemistry (Moscow)*, **63**, 854–65.

Ohno Y (ed.) (1996). Epidemiology for global health in a changing environment. *Journal of Epidemiology*, **6**(Suppl.)

Sasaki N (1962). High blood pressure and salt intake of the Japanese. *Japanese Heart Journal*, **3**, 313–24.

Sasaki R and Aoki K (ed.) (1990). *Epidemiology and prevention of cancer*. University of Nagoya Press, Nagoya.

Sasaki R and Aoki K (ed.) (1992). Recent progress in research on epidemiology, Japan and other countries. *Journal of Epidemiology*, **2**(Suppl.)

Segi M (1960). *Cancer mortality for selected sites in 24 countries (1950–1957)*. Department of Public Health, Tohoku University School of Medicine, Sendai.

Shigematsu I (1973). Itai-itai (ouch-ouch) disease and cadmium pollution. *Society of Occupational Medicine*, **2**, 1–6.

Shigematsu I (1988). Epidemiology in Japan and future problems. *Asian Medical Journal*, **31**, 620–7.

Shigematsu I (2000a). Looking back at epidemiology in Japan during the twentieth century. *Journal of the National Institute of Public Health*, **49**, 354–62 (in Japanese).

Shigematsu I (2000b). The 2000 Silvert Lecture—lessons from atomic bomb survivors in Hiroshima and Nagasaki. *Health Physics*, **79**, 17–24.

The 1st Scientific Meeting of the Japanese Association of Public Health (1947). *Journal of Public Health*, **3**(Special Issue) (in Japanese).

Tsubaki T and Takahashi H (ed.) (1986). *Minamata disease studies—methylmercury poisoning in Minamata and Niigata/Japan*. Kodansha Ltd, Tokyo.

Yanagawa H, Sasaki R, Nagai M, *et al.* (ed.) (1992). *Recent progress of epidemiologic study of intractable diseases in Japan*. The Epidemiology of Intractable Diseases Research Committee, Ministry of Health and Welfare of Japan, Tokyo .

Yanagawa H, Nakamura Y, Yashiro M, and Kawasaki T (ed.) (2004). *Epidemiology of Kawasaki disease— a 30-year achievement*. Shindan-to-Chiryosha, Tokyo (in Japanese).

Yokoro K (ed.) (1991). A review of forty-five years of study of Hiroshima and Nagasaki atomic bomb survivors. *Journal of Radiation Research*, **32**(Suppl.).

32

Health transitions in Mexico and Central America: implications for health policy

Julio Frenk, Rafael Lozano, and
Octavio Gómez-Dantes

In the past half century Mexico and the Central American countries have experienced a profound transformation in their health conditions. These changes are having important impacts on the organization of health and other social services. The most salient features of these transitions are an increase in life expectancy, a decline in infant mortality, and an increasing complexity in the pattern of causes of death. Communicable diseases, malnutrition, and reproductive health problems have lost their previous predominance at the expense of non-communicable ailments and injuries.

In this chapter the interaction of epidemiological and health systems analysis in Mexico and Central America (Costa Rica, El Salvador, Guatemala, Honduras, Nicaragua, and Panama) is discussed. Emphasis is given to the specificities of health transitions in the region and what has been called the double burden of disease, and their influence on health policies. Mexico is used as a case study to illustrate the use of population health and health services assessment in the design, implementation, and evaluation of health policies.

Information sources

The information on populations, mortality, and fertility used in this chapter was derived from estimates generated by the Latin American and Caribbean Demographic Centre (CELADE in Spanish). Information on deaths and resources was generated by the World Health Organization (WHO). Important differences on national data were detected. Table 32.1 presents an assessment of the availability and quality of data on causes of death using criteria developed by Mathers *et al.* (2005), which include variables such as coverage and ill-defined conditions. Coverage was calculated by dividing the total number of deaths reported by country–year by the total numbers of death estimated by the WHO. The last column presents an evaluation of the quality of death registries. Usually the data on these registries only include those deaths coded under Chapter XVIII of the International Classification of Diseases (ICD) (10th R00–R99). However, these authors were stricter and also added those deaths with codes defined as 'useless'. These 'garbage codes' deaths include deaths from injuries where the intent is not determined (ICD-9 codes E980–E989 and ICD-10 codes Y10–Y34 and Y872); cardiovascular disease categories lacking diagnostic meaning, such as cardiac arrest and heart failure; and cancer deaths in unspecified sites.

Using the most recent year for which the cause of death data were available for each member state, the WHO computed the proportion of deaths coded to each of these four groups of ill-defined codes. This provides one set of indicators of the quality of the coding of causes of death. If we

Table 32.1 Quality assessment of the causes of death registries in North-Central America

Country	Years available	ICD rev.	Coverage	Ill-defined[a]	Quality
Costa Rica	1961–2002	10th	79	6	Medium
El Salvador	1950–1999	10th	73	19	Medium
Guatemala	1963–1999	9th	86	14	Medium
Honduras	1968–1983	9th	–	–	–
Mexico	1955–2003	10th	96	5	High
Nicaragua	1961–2002	10th	55	9	Low
Panama	1955–2002	10th	86	12	Medium

Source: Mathers et al. (2005).

[a]Includes 'garbage codes'.

take into account other factors, such as the type of coding for causes, the completeness of death registries, and the status of the latest available data, it is possible to broadly categorize the overall quality of mortality data.

The annexes of the World Health Reports and the Pan American Health Organization (PAHO) Health of the Americas and country profiles for Mexico and Central America were also consulted.

Since CELADE did not provide data for Belize, and considering the lack of information on causes of death in Honduras, the former was excluded from all the analyses that follow and the latter was excluded from most of them.

Health transitions

The health systems of Mexico and Central America have been confronting what has been called a double burden of disease. On the one hand they have been addressing the unfinished agenda of those diseases traditionally identified with the 'health backlog' (common infectious diseases, malnutrition, and reproductive health problems), that affect mostly the lower income groups, particularly children under 5 and women of reproductive age. On the other hand, as these societies age they have to confront an increasing demand for health services for non-communicable diseases which affect both high- and low-income groups. These diseases require on-going, complex, and expensive care. This changing situation can be analysed through the discussion of child and adult mortality, life expectancy, pattern of main causes of death, and general situation of health expenditure and resources.

Child and adult mortality

Important gains were achieved in the area of child survival in the second half of the twentieth century worldwide. The mortality rate of under 5s declined from 159.3 per 1000 live births in 1955 to 70.4 in 1999 (Ahmad *et al.* 2000). Similarly, in Mexico and Central America large reductions in child mortality were observed between 1950 and 2000. According to CELADE, mortality rates in this age group decreased from 224 to 33 per 1000 live births, a reduction of around 85%. In Costa Rica the decline in this period reached 92%. The decline in the region as a whole was pronounced in the 1970s and 1980s, and slowed down during the 1990s.

Considerable country differences in the rate of progress in reduction of infant mortality were observed. In the 1950s infant mortality rates in Honduras were two times higher than in

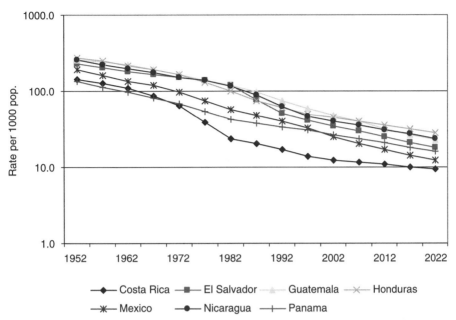

Fig. 32.1 Child mortality in North-Central America, 1950–2025. (Source: CELADE (2004) Latin America. Life table 1950–2025. *Demographic Bulletin*, **XXXIV**, 74.)

Costa Rica. By the year 2000 the gap had increased to four times. Likewise, Costa Rica reached an infant mortality rate of 21 per 1000 live births in 1987, and it took Mexico 20 more years to reach that level. Guatemala and Nicaragua will reach this level around 2025 and Honduras will probably reach it after 2030 (Fig. 32.1).

Adult mortality rates also fell by half between 1950 and 2000 worldwide. In Mexico and Central America adult mortality dropped 53% in males and 68% in females. Progress in the reduction of male mortality was lower in those countries that experienced periods of war during the 1970s and 1980s (Guatemala, El Salvador, and Nicaragua).

If differences among countries in the reduction of child mortality in the region in the last 50 years were important, in adult mortality they were huge. According to CELADE estimates, Mexico and Panama will take probably 30 years to reach the present levels of Costa Rica's adult mortality. The other countries in the region will probably take more than 50 years (Fig. 32.2).

The WHO has used a combination of both infant and adult mortality to create a mortality stratification of the world. Mexico and Central American countries can be situated in three strata. Mexico and Panama could be included in the group of countries with low infant and adult mortality. El Salvador, Guatemala, Honduras, and Nicaragua could join the group of nations with high infant and low adult mortality. Finally, Costa Rica could probably join those countries with very low infant and adult mortality (Table 32.2).

Life expectancy

The trends in mortality rates discussed above translate directly into changes in life expectancy at different ages. Just as there has been a steady decline in overall mortality rates since 1950, life expectancy has also risen in all the countries of the region, albeit at different rates. Table 32.3 shows the dynamics of life expectancy at birth for the seven countries of the region between 1950 and 2025 as estimated by CELADE (2004). Life expectancy in the region increased steadily

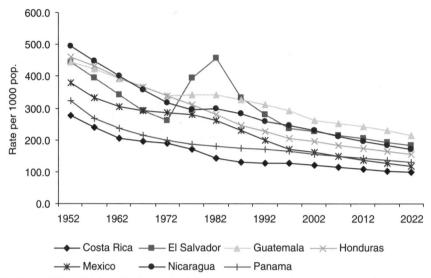

Fig. 32.2 Probability of dying of adult males in North-Central America, 1950–2025. (Source: CELADE (2004) Latin America. Life table 1950–2025. *Demographic Bulletin*, **XXXIV**, 74.)

Table 32.2 Child and adult mortality in Mexico and Central America, 2003

Country	Probability of dying in children under 5 years per 1000 births	Probability of dying in adults aged 15–60 per 1000 population		WHO region
		Males	Females	
Costa Rica	10	129	76	Low IM–low AM
El Salvador	36	248	181	High IM–low AM
Guatemala	47	289	165	High IM–low AM
Honduras	41	248	181	High IM–low AM
Mexico	28	166	95	Low IM–low AM
Nicaragua	38	209	138	High IM–low AM
Panama	24	146	84	Low IM–low AM

IM, infant mortality; AM, adult mortality.

Source: World Health Organization (2005). *World Health Report 2005. Make every mother and child count*. WHO, Geneva.

between 1950 and 2000, but the rate of progress declined after the year 2000, reflecting the large gains achieved earlier in the last century and the likely existence of some kind of natural upper limit to the length of life. One can think of the production of life expectancy as exhibiting increasing marginal costs, so that additional improvements can only be reached by incurring ever larger costs.

Dynamics of the demographic and epidemiological transitions

A framework used to analyse epidemiological transitions published in 1996 (Frenk *et al*. 1991) recognizes fertility as important for health policy because it is the main determinant of the

Table 32.3 Life expectancy at birth in Mexico and Central America, 1950–2025

Country	1950–1955		2000–2005		2020–2025	
	Males	**Females**	**Males**	**Females**	**Males**	**Females**
Costa Rica	56.0	58.6	75.8	80.6	78.0	82.9
El Salvador	44.1	46.5	67.7	73.7	71.8	78.1
Guatemala	41.8	42.3	65.5	72.5	70.1	77.2
Honduras	40.5	43.2	68.6	73.4	72.5	77.5
Mexico	48.9	52.5	72.4	77.4	76.6	81.3
Nicaragua	40.9	43.7	67.2	71.9	72.1	77.1
Panama	54.4	56.2	72.3	77.4	75.0	80.6

Source: CELADE (2004). Latin America. Life table 1950–2025. *Demographic Bulletin*, **XXXIV**, 74.

population's age composition. Measures of fertility relate the number of births to the female population of reproductive age, providing a useful measure of reproductive performance.

As shown in Table 32.4, between 1950 and 1970 fertility rates declined. All countries in the region showed high fertility rates during the baby-boom period. This rate started to decline in the 1950s but at a very low rate, with the exception of Costa Rica. In the 1980s and 1990s the declining rate increased considerably from 5.5 to 2.7 child per women of reproductive age in the region as a whole. CELADE estimates that in the period 2025–30 four countries will reach the substitution rate.

Table 32.4 also shows that total fertility rates in Mexico and Central America varied among countries and across time. In the 1950s there were no differences in fertility rates between Guatemala and Costa Rica. In the 1960s and 1970s a gap was created, and this gap has remained in the last 30 years.

From the point of view of the epidemiological transition, the major effect of fertility decline is the resulting change in age structure. The growing proportion of adults and elderly raises the relative importance of non-communicable diseases and injuries. Table 32.5 shows changes in the age structure in two countries of Central America in the period 1950–2025. It is better not to present a regional average because the size of Mexico's population biases the final result.

Table 32.4 Total fertility rates in Mexico and Central America, 1950–2030

Country	1950–55	1975–80	2000–05	2025–30
Guatemala	7.0	6.2	4.6	2.6
Honduras	7.5	6.6	3.7	2.2
El Salvador	6.5	5.6	2.9	2.2
Nicaragua	7.3	6.4	3.3	2.1
Panama	5.7	4.1	2.7	2.1
Mexico	6.9	5.4	2.4	1.9
Costa Rica	6.7	3.8	2.3	1.9
Region	6.9	5.5	2.7	2.0

Source: CELADE (2004). Latin America. Life table 1950–2025. *Demographic Bulletin*, **XXXIV**, 74.

Table 32.5 Population age structure of Guatemala and Costa Rica, 1950 and 2025

	Guatemala 1950		Costa Rica 1950		Guatemala 2025		Costa Rica 2025	
	Population (million)	%	Population (million)	%	Population (million)	%	Population (million)	%
Young people, 0–14 years	1.4	44.6	0.4	38.5	7	34.4	1.2	20.9
Adults, 15–59 years	1.6	51.2	0.5	53.9	12	58.4	3.5	63.3
Elderly 60+ years	0.1	4.2	0.1	7.6	1	7.2	0.9	15.8
Total	3.1		1.0		20		5.6	

Source: CELADE (2004). Latin America. Life table 1950–2025. *Demographic Bulletin*, **XXXIV**, 74.

Individuals in lower age groups have decreased their contribution to the population structure in all countries of the region. For instance, in Costa Rica and Guatemala the percentage of children under 15 will decline in a very different way in the period 1950–2025. The starting point in Costa Rica was 38.5%. By the year 2025 it will reach 20.9%. The decline in Guatemala will be from 44.6 to 34.4%, which means that in 2025 one-third of the population will be under 15. On the other hand, the proportion of the elderly is increasing in all countries of the region. According to the CELADE projections, the elderly in Costa Rica and Guatemala will grow in this period from 8 and 4% to 16 and 7%, respectively. In both countries the increase in the elderly in absolute and relative terms is important. However, Guatemala will not reach the Costa Rican figure for 1950 until the year 2025.

Attributes of the epidemiological transition

There are three attributes of the epidemiological transition that need to be discussed in order to understand the differences among countries: the changes in the age structure of mortality; the changes in the predominant causes of death; and the duration and timing of these changes.

Changes in the age structure of mortality

At the onset of the epidemiological transition, most deaths occur in children under 15 years old. During the transition the burden of death shifts into older groups. This process is due to multiple factors; one is that children are mainly affected by communicable diseases and malnutrition problems. With the control of infectious diseases, survival of children increases more rapidly than survival of adults and the elderly.

The age structure of mortality has changed in Mexico and Central American countries over the past 50 years. Since the 1950s almost one out of two deaths occurred before the fifth birthday. At the beginning of the twenty-first century they occur in only one in ten or less in Panama, Mexico, El Salvador, and Costa Rica. That is not the case for Nicaragua, where the contribution of infant deaths is still considerable. The worst scenario that of Guatemala, where more than four out of each ten deaths occur in children under 5. On the other extreme, in the middle of the last century deaths in the elderly accounted for around 20% of deaths. In the year 2000 more than half of the deaths occur in adults over 60 with the exception of Guatemala (Table 32.6). These change in the age structure of death influence the profile of the predominant causes of death.

Table 32.6 Percentage of deaths by age groups, Mexico and Central America,1955 and 2000

Country	1955–60		2000–03	
	<5 years (%)	60+ years (%)	<5 years (%)	60+ years (%)
Costa Rica	52.0	27.0	6.0	64.0
El Salvador	52.0	8.0	8.0	52.0
Guatemala	52.0	16.0	28.0	36.0
Mexico	50.0	21.0	9.0	60.0
Nicaragua	51.0	21.0	18.0	46.0
Panama	44.0	27.0	10.0	61.0

Source: CELADE (2004). Latin America. Life table 1950–2025. *Demographic Bulletin*, **XXXIV**, 74.

Table 32.7 Deaths attributed to non-communicable and communicable diseases in Mexico and Central America, 1950–60 and 2000–2003

Country	1950–60				2000–03			
	Commun.	Non-commun.	Injuries	Ill-def.	Commun.	Non-commun.	Injuries	Ill-def.
Costa Rica	43.8	36.1	5.1	15.0	8.5	76.5	12.3	2.6
Mexico	61.8	22.1	6.2	9.9	13.8	73.0	11.1	2.1
Panama	41.4	33.6	5.1	19.9	15.6	65.5	11.5	7.4
El Salvador	52.8	14.3	5.5	27.4	16.7	53.2	18.1	12.0
Nicaragua	52.3	20.1	6.1	21.6	20.0	63.4	13.3	3.3
Guatemala	70.0	11.5	2.8	15.7	38.7	40.0	12.1	9.2

Source: World Health Organization (2005). *Mortality database. Causes of death statistics.*

Changes in the predominant causes of death

The decline in mortality that accompanies the initial phases of the transition is concentrated on communicable diseases, which tend to be displaced by non-communicable diseases. Table 32.7 shows the contribution of deaths related to communicable diseases, malnutrition, and reproductive diseases in Mexico and Central America. Fifty years ago, almost five out of every ten deaths in the region were due to these causes. In the twenty-first century, with the exception of Guatemala, fewer than two in ten are related to infectious diseases, malnutrition, and reproductive ailments.

Health expenditures and resources

Even with some countries spending a relatively large proportions of their GDP on health care (9.3 and 8.9% of GDP in Costa Rica and Panama, respectively), Mexico and the Central American nations invest small amounts of their resources in health, as shown by the small per capita expenditure on health (Table 32.8). At one extreme we have Costa Rica, Mexico, and Panama, spending close to US$400 per capita on health care in 2002. In contrast, Honduras and Nicaragua spend only US$60 per capita on health. The insufficiency of health expenditure is particularly relevant to the fact that, given the epidemiological transition in the region, health systems

Table 32.8 National expenditure indicators for Mexico and Central America, 1998–2000

Country	Total expenditure on health as % of GDP					General government expenditure in health as % of total expenditure on health					Private expenditure on health as % of total expenditure on health				
	1998	1999	2000	2001	2002	1998	1999	2000	2001	2002	1998	1999	2000	2001	2002
Costa Rica	8.1	7.9	8.3	8.8	9.3	69.3	68.1	66.7	65.2	65.4	30.7	31.9	33.3	34.8	34.6
El Salvador	8.2	8	8	7.7	8	42.5	43.5	45.1	42.4	44.7	57.5	56.5	54.9	57.6	55.3
Guatemala	4.4	4.7	4.8	4.8	4.8	47.4	48.3	48.6	48.3	47.5	52.6	51.7	51.4	51.7	52.5
Honduras	5.6	5.7	5.9	6.2	6.2	51.9	50.8	52.5	52.1	51.2	48.1	49.2	47.5	47.9	48.8
Mexico	5.4	5.6	5.6	6	6.1	46	47.8	46.6	44.8	44.9	54	52.2	53.4	55.2	55.1
Nicaragua	7.3	6.9	7.6	7.6	7.9	49.3	45.8	49.3	49.2	49.1	50.7	54.2	50.7	50.8	50.9
Panama	9	7.7	9	8.6	8.9	73.5	69.4	71.9	71.4	71.7	26.5	30.6	28.1	28.6	28.3

have to provide increasing care for non-communicable diseases and injuries, which are more expensive to treat than common infections and reproductive problems.

In addition to the problem of amount of health expenditure, the health systems of Mexico and Central America face a problem concerning origin of health expenditure. With the exception of Costa Rica and Panama, a large proportion of the total health expenditure in these countries is private, and most of it is out-of-pocket. Since there is always an element of uncertainty in health, out-of-pocket expenditure poses a risk for households incurring catastrophic illnesses, possibly impoverishing them. The risk of incurring such expenses increases when the health problem to be confronted requires complex and expensive care. In fact, catastrophic health expenditures are increasing in the region and it was only recently that most countries started documenting this problem, very probably as a consequence of the publication of the fair financing figures for 191 national health systems published by WHO in the year 2000 (World Health Organization 2000).

As a consequence of the low investment in health care, health resources are also scarce, as shown in Table 32.9. Again, at one extreme we have Costa Rica and Mexico, with ratios of physicians and hospital beds per 10,000 population above 12 and 1, respectively, and, on the other extreme, Guatemala with ratios below 10 and 0.6, respectively.

Health and health system assessment for health policy: the Mexican case

Since the late 1980s the transition in health conditions in Mexico has been thoroughly researched (Frenk *et al.* 1989, 1993). Work in this field has been complemented by various assessments of the national burden of disease that made use of several national health surveys carried out in the 1990s (Frenk *et al.* 1994). These studies showed that Mexico was involved in a clear aging process. Life expectancy at birth had risen from 40 years in 1943 to more than 70 in 2000 and fertility rates had declined from 6 in 1976 to less than 2.5 in 2000. By the year 2050 an estimated one out of every four Mexicans will be over the age of 60 (Consejo Nacional de Población 2002).

Research results also showed that Mexico was going through a profound, protracted, and polarized epidemiological transition. As shown in the previous section of this chapter, the burden of disease had shifted dramatically. Between 1950 and 2000, the proportion of deaths attributable to non-communicable diseases increased from 44 to 73% and the proportion attributable to

Out-of-pocket expenditure on health as % of total expenditure on health					Private prepaid plans as % of private expenditure on health					Per capita total expenditure on health at average exchange rate				
1998	1999	2000	2001	2002	1998	1999	2000	2001	2002	1998	1999	2000	2001	2002
98.4	98.7	98.8	98.9	99	1.6	1.3	1.2	1.1	1	304	324	339	358	383
94	90.2	95.6	93.6	93.9						165	163	170	169	178
93.2	85.6	86.2	85.7	86.2	4.5	5.4	5.2	5.3	5.2	78	78	81	86	93
85.5	85.6	85.4	85.4	85.4	7.2	7.2	7.3	7.2	7.3	48	49	56	60	60
95.9	95.9	95.3	95	94.6	4.1	4.1	4.7	5	5.4	232	271	321	367	379
98.1	95.6	92.9	92.9	96	1.9	4.4	7.1	7.1	4	54	52	59	59	60
83.5	82.4	81.5	84.5	81.8	16.5	17.6	18.5	15.5	18.2	345	307	353	336	355

accidents from 6 to 13% (Secretaría de Salud 2001). At the same time, the poorer states and population groups were suffering from an epidemiological backlog and continued to face burdens associated with common infections, malnutrition, and reproductive health. This posed an extremely complex challenge to the health system which has to battle simultaneously the diseases of underdevelopment and the higher-cost, chronic illnesses associated with urbanization and an aging population.

In the 1990s the Mexican Health Foundation, in collaboration with several academic groups and international organizations and making use of National Households Income and Expenditure Survey, also developed a system of national health accounts which showed that Mexico was investing a relatively small proportion of its GDP in health (5.3%). This proportion was below the Latin American average and was also not enough to meet the demands of the epidemiological transition. In addition more than half of that expenditure was out-of-pocket, which increased the risk of incurring catastrophic spending leading impoverishment. This proved to be a direct result of the fact that approximately half of the country's population

Table 32.9 Resources for health care in Mexico and Central America, 1998–2004

	Physicians ratio (per 10,000 population)	Last year available	Hospital beds ratio (per 10,000 population)	Last year available
Costa Rica	11.5	2000	1.4	2003
El Salvador	12.6	2002	0.7	2004
Guatemala	9.5	2003	0.5	2003
Honduras	8.7	1999	1.0	2002
Mexico	12.1[a]	2004	1.2[a]	2004
Nicaragua	16.4	2004	0.9	2004
Panama	13.8	2003	1.8	2004

Source: Pan American Health Organization (PAHO), 2004.

[a]Source: Secretaría de Salud, 2004

(around 50 million) lacked health insurance. These findings were unexpected as it was generally believed that the Mexican health system was financed predominantly with public resources.

As a direct result of its high levels of out-of-pocket spending, Mexico performed very poorly on the international comparative analysis of fair financing developed as part of the health system performance assessment by WHO in 2000 (World Health Organization 2000). This poor result spurred a detailed country-level analysis in 2001 that showed that impoverishing health expenditures were concentrated among poor and uninsured households. The analysis was undertaken jointly by the Ministry of Health of Mexico, the WHO, and the Mexican Health Foundation.

The findings of the burden of disease, the national health accounts, and the fair financing assessments showed that Mexico was experiencing a mismatch between its health needs and its health system. The need for comprehensive health reforms seemed obvious.

These same findings were used as an advocacy tool to promote major legislative reform establishing a system of social protection in health which was approved in April 2003 by a large majority of the Congress. The Popular Health Insurance (PHI) is the operational programme of the new system.

This system will reorganize and increase public funding over 7 years in order to provide universal health insurance, including the 50 million Mexicans, most of them poor, who have been excluded until now from formal social insurance schemes. The affiliation process runs from 2004 to 2010, so that 14.3% of the approximately 11 million families that make up the uninsured population will be included each year. Preference must be given to families from the lowest deciles.

Affiliation to the PHI guarantees access to an essential package of services that include ambulatory care at the primary level and outpatient consultations and hospitalization for the basic specialties at the secondary level. This package is covered by funds administered at the state level, because these services are associated with low-risk, high-probability health events. The number of covered interventions is being gradually expanded as funding increases, going from 91 interventions and 168 medications to 154 and 172 (Knaul and Frenk 2005).

The PHI also provides access to a package of services covered by the Fund for Protection against Catastrophic Expenditures that is being updated annually. This package is now offering funding for cancer in children, cervical cancer, HIV/AIDS, and neonatal intensive care. The criteria for selecting specific conditions and interventions are based on burden of disease, cost effectiveness, and resource availability (Frenk *et al*, 2004).

The System for Social Protection in Health will mobilize enough resources to solve the health backlog that mostly affects the rural poor. It will also allow the country to start meeting in a rational way the increasing demand for services for non-communicable conditions (diabetes, cancer, and cardiovascular diseases) which are now the main causes of death and disability. Thirdly, given that this system is basically a public insurance, it will help reduce catastrophic and impoverishing health spending that mostly affect the poor and uninsured, and will increase the financial fairness of the health system as a whole.

Finally, it is important to acknowledge that those same analytical tools—burden of disease, national health accounts, and system performance assessment—that provided the evidence to develop a solid diagnosis, design the reform, and politically support its approval and implementation, are also being applied at the state and national levels in Mexico to benchmark health system performance and mark progress toward implementation of the reform initiative.

Conclusions

The interaction of epidemiological and health services analysis has been key to the development of rational health policies. However, political circumstances do not always allow for the necessary use of evidence in the design, discussion, implementation, and evaluation of health initiatives, programmes, and policies. It is necessary to create arrangements that promote evidence-based health policies.

The analysis of the demographic and epidemiological transition that is taking place in Mexico and Central America is generating evidence that will be central to address, in some cases, and anticipate, in others, the challenges being confronted by national health systems in the region. Without careful in-depth national epidemiological and health services studies, countries in the region will not be able to meet in a rational way either the needs of those suffering from common infections, malnutrition problems, and reproductive health problems or the demands of an increasing proportion of the population for health interventions against non-communicable diseases and injuries.

The Mexican case is particularly useful for two main reasons. On the one hand, it has had success with the use of evidence for policy formulation. On the other hand, Mexico is going through a process of transition that anticipates what may happen elsewhere, and is offering solutions that can be useful for the health systems of other developing countries.

References

Ahmad O, López A, and Inov M (2000). The decline in child mortality: a reappraisal. *Bulletin of the World Health Organization*, **78**, 1175–91.

Behm H and Robles A (1990). Costa Rica: El descenso reciente de la mortalidad en la infancia por grupos socioeconómicos. In *Factores sociales de riesgo de muerte en la infancia*. CELADE, Santiago de Chile.

CELADE (2004). Latin America. Life table 1950–2025. *Demographic Bulletin*, **XXXIV**, 74.

CELADE (2005). Latin America: estimates and population projections 1950–2025. *Demographic Bulletin*, **XXXIV**, 73.

Consejo Nacional de Población (2002). *Envejecimiento demográfico en México: retos y perspectivas*. CONAPO, Mexico City.

Frenk J, Bobadilla JL, Sepúlveda J, *et al.* (1989). Health transition in middle-income countries. New challenges for health care. *Health Policy and Planning*, **4**, 29–39.

Frenk J, Bobadilla JL, Stern C, Frejka T, and Lozano R (1991). Elements for a theory of transition in health. *Health Transitition Review*, **1**, 21–38.

Frenk J, Bobadilla JL, Lozano R, and Stern C (1993). The epidemiological transition and health priorities. In *Disease control priorities in developing countries* (ed. DT Jamison, WH Mosley, AR Measham, and JL Bobadilla). Oxford Medical Publications, New York, pp. 51–63.

Frenk J, Lozano R, González-Block MA, *et al.* (1994). *Economía y salud. Propuestas para el avance del sistema de salud en México*. FUNSALUD, Mexico City.

Frenk J, Knaul F, Gómez-Dantés O, *et al.* (2004). *Fair financing and universal social protection: The structural reform of the Mexican health system*. Secretaría de Salud, Mexico City.

Jamison D and Mosley H (1991). Disease control priorities in developing countries. Health policy responses to epidemiological change. *American Journal of Public Health*, **81**, 15–22.

Knaul F and Frenk J (2005). Health insurance in Mexico: achieving universal coverage through structural reform. *Health Affairs*, **24**, 1467–76.

Mathers CD, Ma Fat D, Inoue M, Rao C, and Lopez AD (2005). Counting the dead and what they died from: an assessment of the global status of cause of death data. *Bulletin of the World Health Organization*, **83**(3), 171–7.

Olshansky SJ and Auldt BA (1986). The fourth stage of the epidemiological transition: the age of delayed degenerative disease. *Milbank Memorial Fund Quarterly*, **64**, 355–91.

Omran AR (1983). The epidemiologic transition: a theory of the epidemiology of population change. *Milbank Memorial Fund Quarterly*, **49**, 509–38.

Pan American Health Organization (2002). *Health in the Americas*. PAHO, Washington, DC.

Pan American Health Organization/World Health Organization (2003). *Health situation in the Americas. Basic indicators 2002*. PAHO, Washington, DC.

Secretaría de Salud (2001). *Programa Nacional de Salud. La democratización de la salud. Hacia un sistema universal de salud*. Secretaría de Salud, Mexico City.

Secretaría de Salud (2005). *Salud: México 2004*. Secretaría de Salud, Mexico City

World Health Organization (2000). *World Health Report 2000. Improving health system performance*. WHO, Geneva.

World Health Organization (2005a). *Mortality database. Causes of death statistics* (www.who.int/whosis/en).

World Health Organization (2005b). *World Health Report 2005. Make every mother and child count*. WHO, Geneva.

33

The development of epidemiology: the United States of America

Warren Winkelstein Jr and Elizabeth Barrett-Connor

Personal experiences

Warren Winkelstein Jr: I was born into it. On the day of my birth, 1 July 1922, Simon Flexner, Director of the Rockefeller Institute for Medical Research published an article entitled 'Experimental epidemiology' in the *Journal of Experimental Medicine* [1922; **xxxvi**, 9–14]. The first sentence of that article tells it all, namely 'Ever since Hippocrates and especially since Sydenham, the study of epidemics of disease with a view to penetrating their hidden meaning has engaged the attention of occasional men ....

Oh, there have been a few contributing factors along the way, for example socially concerned parents, a 'progressive' secondary education, a liberal higher education, early commitment to a career in public health, training in an innovative health department with wonderful mentors, and exciting and challenging field experiences.

Elizabeth Barrett-Connor: I began my post-medical school career in infectious disease. I now realize that what I liked best about infections was the possibility of making a bedside diagnosis based on epidemiological questions—who, when, and where—and on the recognition of common source outbreaks. In communicable disease, the transition from patients to populations and from treatment to prevention was obvious. I was doing epidemiology daily, but I did not know it.

My graduate education in epidemiology included a year studying tropical medicine (including public health and statistics) at the London School of Hygiene and Tropical Medicine, and an advanced summer seminar at the University of Minnesota (where my small-group mentors included Milt Terris, Abe Lillienfeld, and Al Evans).

When I decided to stay in academic medicine, I was offered a faculty position if I agreed to teach an unpopular epidemiology course to medical students. Just one step (at best) ahead of them at every lecture, I loved the teaching first, and later, through generous mentors and fortunate circumstances, contributed to the science as well.

Introduction

While some epidemiological studies were recorded in the United States during the nineteenth century, substantial developments occurred only during the last decades of the century, after the introduction into the USA of microbiology developed in France and Germany. With the resultant rapid growth of laboratory science came a concurrent development of epidemiology. By the end of the second decade of the twentieth century, the accomplishments of epidemiological science were substantial. By the early 1920s, formal instruction was being introduced into academic schools of public health, professional organizations were being formed, and the field was increasingly recognized as central to the implementation of public health policy and administration. During its formative period, American epidemiology was largely concerned with the elucidation of the aetiology, transmission, and natural history of acute infectious diseases. However, after the Second World War, attention was extended to chronic (presumably non-infectious) diseases, and emphasis was directed toward the identification of predisposing risk factors. As the focus broadened, epidemiologists considered a wide range of environmental, social, behavioural, and genetic factors as they strove to explain factors responsible for chronic diseases. New advances in biostatistics, computer science, and later, molecular biology, gave epidemiologists increased ability to address diverse scientific questions as the twenty-first century began.

Nineteenth-century antecedents

Three nineteenth-century events provided an impetus for the development of epidemiology in the United States. First, in 1843, 31-year-old Austin Flint, destined to become the second leading American medical man of the century, superseded only by William Osler, investigated an outbreak of typhoid fever in a small hamlet southwest of Buffalo in New York State. In a population of 43, 28 developed the disease and 10 died. Flint got it half right when his investigation concluded that the epidemic was spread by contagion, not miasma, then still the dominant theory explaining epidemic phenomena. Flint's paper describing this typhoid fever epidemic was published in a major journal in 1845 (Flint 1845). To his credit, almost 30 years later, then internationally recognized, he re-examined the data and, at the first meeting of the American Public Health Association in 1873, reported that the epidemic had been propagated by drinking water from a contaminated well (Flint 1873). So, in the end, he got it wholly right. But, additionally, he lent his prestige to the infant public health movement and revealed the power of an epidemiological strategy to explain the dynamics of an epidemic.

Second, in 1850, the Sanitary Commissioners of Massachusetts, led by Lemuel Shattuck, founder and first president of the American Statistical Association, issued its report (known as the 'Shattuck report'). The report was divided into four major areas of concern: a review of health conditions in Europe, a corresponding review of health conditions in Massachusetts, recommendations for remediation, and appendices. The commissioners (probably solely Lemuel Shattuck) presented tables on mortality classified by age, sex, year of death, season, occupation, geographical location, marital status, and socio-economic status! Based primarily on these data, 50 recommendations were presented to include such diverse issues as the composition of boards of health, planning of communities, training of health professionals, and the need for personal hygiene. Finally, the appendices contain discussions of the reasons for adopting the recommendations, predictions of the arguments that will be presented in opposition to the recommendations, and, most importantly, a model public health law. This model, largely unmodified, was enacted into law in Massachusetts in 1868 and by many states thereafter. The Commission's recommendations and model law can be considered a good example of epidemiological 'evidence-based' public health policy.

Third in 1887, the Marine Hospital Service, forerunner of the US Public Health Service, established a bacteriology laboratory at its Staten Island Hospital in New York Harbor and put Joseph J. Kinyoun in charge. Kinyoun had trained in the laboratories of both Koch and Pasteur. Besides studies of water and air pollution and the introduction of immune serum technology, Kinyoun trained a number of laboratory directors who were destined to establish bacteriology laboratories throughout the country. It was a combination of the development of technology at the Hygienic Laboratory, the name given to the laboratory, and its wide dispersion that contributed substantially to the development of epidemiology in the United States.

Early twentieth-century developments

In 1899, Milton Rosenau succeeded Kinyoun as director of the Hygienic Laboratory, where he conducted epidemiological research, recruiting a cadre of brilliant and innovative investigators, including Wade Hampton Frost and Joseph Goldberger. Frost's studies of the epidemiology of poliomyelitis, published in the *Hygienic Laboratory Bulletin* No 90, elucidated the comprehensive epidemiology of the disease including the recognition of healthy carriers and subclinical cases as the source of transmission prior to the isolation of the causal agent. Goldberger's studies with Edgar Sydenstricker of pellagra in southern institutions for the mentally retarded and in South Carolina mill villages revealed the nutritional deficiency that caused the disease. These studies are considered classics of US epidemiology.

In 1918, the Johns Hopkins School of Hygiene and Public Health was established—the first school of public health in the United States. Wade Hampton Frost left the Hygienic Laboratory to become the first professor of epidemiology there. At Johns Hopkins he continued his research, making major contributions to the epidemiology of tuberculosis, introducing cohort analysis, and pioneering prospective methodology. In addition, Frost contributed to the development of epidemiology by his approach to instruction and the cadre of epidemiologists he trained. Drawing primarily on his own experience, he developed a case-study teaching style that continues to form the basis of modern instruction in the field.

Epidemiological organizations

Between 1923 and 1928, three epidemiological professional organizations were created: the Biggs Club, a small social club; out of the Biggs Club grew the American Epidemiological Society (AES), an elite organization with limited membership; and the Epidemiology Section of the American Public Health Association (APHA), which was for many years the principal venue for the presentation of epidemiological research.

In early 1941, with war imminent, the US Army created an advisory board made up of civilian and military experts to advise the army's surgeon general on matters related to preventive medicine, to provide assistance in the investigation of infectious disease outbreaks, and to conduct research on diseases of concern to the army. The board implemented its mandate through the development of a series of commissions each concerned with a specific problem. In 1949 the advisory board was extended to all military services and it became known as the 'Armed Forces Epidemiological Board'. The board continues to function and its many commissions have contributed significantly to the understanding, control, and prevention of a broad range of medical conditions.

Because older and more established investigators dominated the available venues for the presentation and consideration of epidemiological research and issues, in 1968 the Society for Epidemiologic Research (SER) was established, primarily as a vehicle for the presentation of research by younger epidemiologists. As time passed, the SER replaced the APHA to become a major venue. In recent years a number of additional organizations have been created to address specific diseases.

In 1979, the American College of Epidemiology was established, primarily to establish criteria to define the field. This organization is active in addressing professional concerns, sponsoring scientific meetings and educational activities, and promoting the development of policy statements.

Federal agencies

Two federal agencies have had a major role in the development of American epidemiology. They are the National Institutes of Health, an outgrowth of the Hygienic Laboratory, and the Centers for Disease Control and Prevention.

National Institutes of Health (NIH)

In 1930, the Hygienic Laboratory became the National Institutes of Health (NIH) and greatly expanded its role. It rapidly became the principal funding resource as well as a major centre for the development of biomedical science, including epidemiology, in the USA, carrying out these functions through a series of issue-centred institutes, for example the National Heart and Lung Institute and the National Institute of Allergy and Infectious Diseases. By 2005, there were 26 institutes in the NIH. Each institute provided for extra-mural research support as well as intra-mural research. All of the institutes created disciplinary divisions, and most have included a division of epidemiology.

Centers for Disease Control (CDC)

The Centers for Disease Control and Prevention has played an enormous role in setting standards for public health, epidemiology, and surveillance in the USA as well as in the training of legions of state and territorial epidemiologists.

This organization began in the 1940s as a unit of the US Public Health Service called Malaria Control in War Areas; it was established in Atlanta to fight malaria in the southeastern USA and thereby create safe training sites for the military during the Second World War. In 1946, its name changed to the Communicable Disease Center, reflecting a broader mission to detect and contain all tropical diseases. Under the leadership of Joseph W. Mountin, the centre developed an excellent laboratory and a distinguished reputation. In the 1960s the CDC expanded beyond communicable disease, and offered epidemic investigation services to the states and even began to evaluate epidemics overseas.

When concern about germ warfare was raised at the beginning of the Korean War, the CDC used this as an opportunity. Mountin observed that the nation needed 'epidemiologic intelligence' as an early warning system against man-made epidemics. The resulting Epidemiologic Intelligence Service (EIS) made public health surveillance an essential component of public health practice in the USA, and similar programmes have developed around the world, not only for surveillance and evaluation of epidemics, but also as training centres for generations of epidemiologists.

Over the years, the CDC has been home to many investigators. For example, Alexander D. Langmuir was an associate professor at Johns Hopkins when he was invited to take a leadership role at the CDC in 1949. Two years later he initiated the Epidemic Intelligence Service (EIS). When polio rates increased in the 1950s, Langmuir argued that state health officials should be included in a national programme to control polio, led by the CDC. During a major polio epidemic the CDC collected detailed polio data from more than 40 states and about 90% of the US population. These data were compared with past experience in the USA. The CDC also organized a prospective study of polio patients carried out by physical therapists, which provided the first standardized description of residual paralysis. During the first field trial of the new Salk vaccine, conducted in 1954 by Thomas Francis, the CDC provided 20 EIS officers and statisticians. Later Langmuir used the limited supply of polio vaccine as an opportunity for evaluation studies. EIS officers were involved in the collection of data from 8.5 million children, vaccinated and unvaccinated. The results showed 75% protection (Etheridge 1992).

Langmuir was an enthusiastic supporter of the *Morbidity and Mortality Weekly Report* (MMWR) when it was transferred to a reluctant CDC from the Washington DC National Office of Vital Statistics. He recognized that the agency charged with controlling and preventing disease should also collect and distribute data. The MMWR was able to report epidemics recently evaluated by the CDC. Publication began in January 1961 and never missed an issue. Langmuir himself supervised MMWR for many years; most of the staff were EIS officers. In 1961 circulation was 6000; 20 years later it exceeded 80,000.

Epidemiological epitomes

As indicated earlier, after the Second World War, US epidemiology substantially expanded its subject matter and methodology. To accommodate its output a number of new journals were created. Furthermore, epidemiology has been widely used for the development of public policy, programme planning and evaluation, coping with disasters, and many other functions. Thus, it would be impossible in this brief overview to chronicle the accomplishments of US epidemiology since the mid-twentieth century. We have, therefore, chosen to encapsulate these accomplishments with nine brief epitomes.

Smallpox—the sleeping scourge

Edward Jenner's first treatise on smallpox vaccination, in 1798, demonstrated the protective effect of natural infection by the causal agent of cowpox and described the protection provided by artificial infection. This work is one of the great documents of science (Jenner 1798). In an 1801 sequel to the original publication, Jenner predicted '... the annihilation of Small Pox ... must be the final result of this practice' (Jenner 1801). His prediction was realized in 1978 when the World Health Organization (WHO) declared smallpox to be eradicated worldwide.

Ten years earlier, in 1968, the WHO had estimated 10 to 15 million cases and 2 million deaths from smallpox in 30 countries worldwide. The consequent human suffering and financial expense were immense. In 1958 the Soviet Union proposed a worldwide eradication effort, and when the United States backed the proposal in 1966, the WHO launched the international 'Intensified Smallpox Eradication Programme' under the direction of US CDC epidemiologist Donald A. Henderson.

There were biological and technical reasons why eradication was feasible. The biological reasons were: no subclinical cases, infectivity accompanies the rash, no recurrent cases, only one serotype, and no animal reservoir. These characteristics made the epidemiological strategy of mass vaccination augmented by surveillance and containment vaccination effective. This latter strategy, introduced by William Foege of the CDC during a pilot project in Nigeria, was a key factor in the final worldwide eradication. The principal technical reason enabling eradication was the availability of an effective, stable (freeze-dried) vaccine.

After eradication was certified, many nations pushed for the destruction of all stocks of smallpox virus. Two repositories were designated—the Vaccine Institute in Moscow and the Centers for Disease Control and Prevention in Atlanta. In 1996 the World Health Assembly voted to have the remaining stocks of virus destroyed but the resolution has never been implemented.

When former deputy director of the Soviet Union's bioweapons programme Dr Ken Alibek defected to the United States in 1993, he brought the information that the Soviet Union had large stocks of weaponized smallpox virus. To what extent this technology has been disseminated outside of Russia is unknown. What is known is that smallpox virus remains a serious potential biological weapon.

Goldberger: public health activist

Joseph Goldberger's remarkable career in public health began in 1899, when, after a few years as a general practitioner, he joined the US Marine Hospital Service—probably as much for financial security as for a deliberate career choice. His first epidemic investigation was a typhoid outbreak in Washington. Between 1902 and 1914 Goldberger investigated epidemics of cholera, yellow fever, typhoid, dengue, and typhus, and was himself infected with at least three of these.

In 1912 he was appointed to supervise the Federal government's pellagra investigation, and so began the classic investigations that consumed the rest of his life (Kraut 2003). At this time most physicians thought that pellagra, and most other diseases, were caused by infection. Within a very short time Goldberger concluded that the cause could not be communicable, based on the absence of pellagra in staff caring for patients. He then confirmed non-transmissibility by the failure to induce pellagra after inoculating himself, his wife, and his staff with blood, urine, stool, or skin scales from pellagra patients. He quickly hypothesized that pellagra was due to a deficient diet, and later confirmed this thesis based on a series of eating experiments (conducted in orphans, mental patients, and prisoners without their consent). These trials led to his suggestion that meat and milk could cure a protein deficiency, but he later recognized the superior preventive and therapeutic benefit of brewer's yeast.

Although Goldberger did not identify the essential protein (tryptophan), or its role as a precursor for the essential nutrient in yeast (niacin), and was unable to put the biochemistry together, he identified effective inexpensive nutrients for prevention and cure of pellagra. And he correctly attributed seasonal pellagra epidemics in the rural south to poverty and to sharecropping, which discouraged growing diversified crops.

When neither politicians nor physicians endorsed his conclusions or recommendations, Goldberger became a public health activist, advocating small gardens and shared ownership of a cow to prevent further pellagra epidemics. In 1928 he sent a cautiously written recommendation to the Surgeon General. The political will was lacking, however, and Goldberger died in early 1929 without seeing vitamin-fortified foods or the disappearance of pellagra. Nor was he ever awarded the Nobel prize, although he was nominated three times.

Before his death, Goldberger's wife Mary had been an active advocate for a Federally funded institute for the study of all human diseases, a proposal sponsored by Louisiana Senator Joseph Ransdell. In May 1930, only a few months after Goldberger' death, President Herbert Hoover signed the Ransdell Act into law, converting the Hygienic Laboratory into the National Institutes of Health. (Ironically the Ransdell Act specifically prohibited the award of its fellowships to commissioned officers in the US Public Health Service.)

Salk vaccine trials set the 'gold standard' for vaccine field trials

At the turn of the twentieth century, poliomyelitis was an 'emerging infection'. Sporadic outbreaks had been reported, first from northern Europe and subsequently from countries worldwide. In the USA the first major epidemic occurred in 1905 followed by the most serious recorded epidemic in 1916—29,000 cases and 6000 deaths. The epidemiology of poliomyelitis had been worked out before identification of the causal agent in observational studies between 1910 and 1912 by Wade Hampton Frost, one of the brilliant investigators assembled in the Hygienic Laboratory of the US Public Health Service. The only gap was Frost's inability to recognize the existence of antigenically distinct substrains of the virus. Frost's recognition that most infections were immunogenic and subclinical and that these 'passive carriers' (his term) were responsible for dissemination of infection indicated that control could not be accomplished by isolation or quarantine (Frost 1913). The alternative control strategy was vaccination. When Bodian demonstrated the existence of three distinct antigenic serotypes of poliovirus in1948 and Enders and colleagues propagated the virus in tissue culture (earning them a Nobel prize) in 1949, the stage was set for the development of a vaccine.

By 1953, Jonas Salk and colleagues at the University of Pittsburgh had developed a formalin-inactivated trivalent poliovirus vaccine and had tested it for immunogenicity and safety on family members, laboratory staff, and student volunteers (Salk 1953). After controversy over the study design, i.e. whether to conduct an observed controlled trial or a double-blind placebo controlled trial (the more rigorous design), both strategies were implemented. In 1954 the National Foundation for Infantile Paralysis sponsored and organized an evaluation of the vaccine under the direction of eminent virologist and epidemiologist Thomas Francis of the University of Michigan. Because of the low incidence of clinical poliomyelitis, the trials required large numbers of study subjects, over a million in the observed controlled communities and 400,000 in the placebo-controlled communities. Despite the large number of participants, a total of only 726 cases were recorded in the trials, 451 in the observed controlled communities and 275 in the placebo-controlled areas. The results, similar for both study designs, showed the vaccine to be effective against all three serotypes.

Although an attenuated live virus vaccine, adopted without a double-blinded placebo controlled trial, supplanted the 'Salk vaccine' in the USA, the double-blinded placebo-controlled component of the 1954 field trial provided the template for most subsequent vaccine evaluations in the USA. By 1995 poliomyelitis was eliminated from North America.

Fluoride and dental caries: epidemiology drives public health practice

In 1916, McKay and Black, practicing dentists in Colorado Springs, Colorado, reported a condition known as mottled enamel (an unsightly, irregular thickening of dental enamel) (McKay and Black 1916). Subsequently, mottled enamel was shown to be caused by the fluoride ion in drinking water and renamed 'fluorosis'. It was also shown to be inversely associated with dental caries. The consequences of dental caries being substantial and serious and the prospect that the cause of fluorosis had been identified led to the establishment of a Dental Hygiene Unit at the National Institutes of Health under the direction of H. Trendley Dean, a dental epidemiologist. Dean had conducted a series of surveys to document the prevalence of fluorosis nationwide and its association with dental caries. These surveys confirmed and quantified the inverse association between fluorosis and dental caries and established a standard of 1.0 parts per million (ppm) as a lower limit for mild fluorosis and maximum caries prevention.

To test the hypothesis that adjusting the fluoride content of community water supplies to 1.0 ppm would result in reductions of caries among children, a major field trial was carried out by the New York State Health Department between 1945 and 1955. Two cities, Newburgh and Kingston—of similar size, socio-economic status, and industrialization located near each other in the Hudson River Valley and without detectable fluoride in their water supplies—were studied. The fluoride content of the water supply of one, Newburgh, was adjusted to 1.0 ppm, and the dental health of children in the two cities was observed prospectively for 10 years. A reduction of 58% in decayed, missing, and filled teeth among 6- to 9-year-old children in Newburgh compared with Kingston was observed. Lesser, though substantial, effectiveness was observed among older age groups (Ast *et al.* 1956). Intensive paediatric studies demonstrated the safety and lack of side-effects of low-level fluoride exposure.

Despite the objections of many individuals and organized groups, adjustment of fluoride content of public water supplies to 0.08–1.2 ppm became widespread in the USA after 1945. By 2000, 66%, or 162 million Americans, received optimally fluoridated water from municipal supplies. According to the latest National Health Examination Survey (NHANES III, 1996), 55% of children aged 5–17 were caries free, representing a 5% reduction from the previous NHANES survey completed in 1987.

The lessons of Framingham

The community-based cohort approach to epidemiological investigation of chronic disease in the USA began in 1948 with the Framingham Heart Study, under the leadership of T. R. Dawber and the long-term productive guidance of William B. Kannel. In its first 40 years, the results of the Framingham Study almost completely changed the clinical perception of the causes and consequences of cardiovascular disease. Before Framingham, physicians thought that it was meddlesome to label, alarm, and treat persons with asymptomatic conditions such as hypertension or hypercholesterolaemia; further, the definition of these asymptomatic conditions was based on average or usual levels, without appreciating that these levels were not optimal; and accepted teachings were based on case studies and clinical impressions. The Framingham Study introduced the term 'risk factors' to clinicians.

Framingham taught us that neither increasing blood pressure nor left ventricular hypertrophy were healthy compensatory changes of aging, and that their adverse consequences were not primarily caused by diastolic hypertension. Before Framingham, physical exercise was thought to be dangerous for heart patients, and dietary cholesterol and a fatty diet were of debatable concern. Even cigarette smoking was not accepted by the American Heart Association as a risk factor for heart disease until data from Framingham and the Albany Cardiovascular Health prospective study on smoking and the incidence of coronary heart disease were combined and a three-fold excess risk in heavy smokers was published in 1962 (Doyle *et al.* 1962).

The importance of treating risk factors and not waiting to treat disease was dramatically illustrated by the Framingham observation that about one-third of patients with a heart attack presented with sudden death. Before Framingham, the disabling and lethal nature of congestive heart failure was not appreciated, and atrial fibrillation not associated with clinical heart disease was thought to be a benign arrhythmia. Framingham studies showed that risk factors clustered, and that the risk of heart disease increased with the number of risk factors and increasing levels of risk factors; these observations were later applied to the Framingham risk score—the first method designed to help clinicians predict the individual risk of their patients based on age, sex, and number and level of risk factors. The risk score concept of 5- and 10-year risk has been adopted by most Western countries to help patients and their doctors decide about therapy.

Smoking and health—establishing the link to lung cancer

By 1950 it became apparent in Europe and America that lung cancer was assuming epidemic proportions and had become the leading cancer cause of death for men. Also, in 1950, two case–control studies were published establishing an association between cigarette smoking and lung cancer (Levin *et al.* 1950; Wynder and Graham 1950). Subsequently, a plethora of case–control and cohort studies were carried out worldwide. (By 1964, 29 case–control studies, 11 of which included women, had been published. All but one confirmed the association. Also, by 1964, the results of seven cohort studies had become available. Crude mortality ratios in these studies ranged from 8.2 to 46.3. Six of the seven provided data indicating a dose–response relationship between amount smoked and lung cancer mortality.)

In 1957 the Surgeon General of the US Public Health Service had issued a warning that cigarette smoking was a probable cause of lung cancer, and 2 years later the warning was repeated more explicitly in a major article in the *Journal of the American Medical Association*. Nevertheless, many influential organizations and public health leaders considered these warnings insufficient. In 1961, urged by the executive officers of five major health agencies, the Surgeon General, with the explicit approval of President Kennedy, appointed a 10-member 'blue ribbon' Advisory Committee to comprehensively evaluate the consequences of tobacco use. Its report is a classic (Report of the Advisory Committee to the Surgeon General of the Public Health Service 1964). Of particular interest to epidemiologists is Chapter 3, entitled 'Criteria for judgment'. Therein the committee indicated that epidemiological evidence played a major role in the conclusion that cigarette smoking was '… causally related to lung cancer…'. The Committee also commented, 'The causal significance of an association is a matter of judgment which goes beyond any statement of statistical probability'. They then proceeded to advance specific criteria that might be helpful in making a judgment of a causal association: (1) consistency, (2) strength, (3) specificity, (4) temporality, and (5) coherence. (These 'criteria' were published a year before the address to the Royal Society of Medicine in which Sir Austin Bradford Hill laid out a similar set of guidelines for assessing the causal validity of an association.)

The report was a turning point in the acceptance by the public and by public health and medical agencies of the harmful effects of smoking. Perhaps the reason for its influence was partly its comprehensiveness (it was a model of evidence-based conclusions) but, more importantly, it had the credibility of the independence and authority of the expertise of its members.

HIV/AIDS—a modern scourge

On 5 June 1981, the CDC reported the occurrence of five cases of a rare opportunistic infection, *Pneumocystis carinii* pneumonia, in three Los Angeles hospitals (MMWR 1981). All five cases occurred in homosexual men. Shortly after publication of these five cases, the CDC established a task force to monitor and study this new epidemic. At a workshop convened during the following several months, the pathophysiology and rudimentary epidemiology were identified. Nationwide surveillance was initiated. By the end of 1982 additional 'at risk' groups had been identified and the syndrome had been named 'acquired immune deficiency syndrome' (AIDS). Most cases were in gay men; much less common risk groups were identified as: heterosexual contacts of AIDS cases, drug abusers sharing needles, recipients of blood transfusions, haemophiliacs treated with Factor VIII, and children born to women with AIDS. In 1983, a causal agent, a retrovirus, was identified and named Human Immunodeficiency Virus (HIV). By the end of 2002, more than 880,000 cases and 500,000 deaths from AIDS had been recorded in the USA.

Two major cohort studies were funded by the National Institutes of Health for epidemiological studies of HIV/AIDS in the USA. The Multi-Center AIDS Cohort Study (Chmiel *et al.* 1987) studied convenience samples in four urban areas: Los Angeles, Chicago, Pittsburgh, and Baltimore/Washington/Wilmington. The San Francisco Men's Health Study (SFMHS) (Winkelstein *et al.* 1987) was based on a probability sample of single men aged 25 to 55 years living in 19 census tracts of San Francisco, where the AIDS epidemic had been most intense. These studies revealed the mechanism of transmission of infection among gay men, the infectivity of the virus, various immunological markers of progression, behavioural factors influencing infection and progression, the immunological profile of long-term survivors, and the time trend of incidence in the study populations. This information was used in developing epidemic control strategies, but success was constrained by issues related to confidentiality and stigma.

Because HIV/AIDS seemed to be occurring almost exclusively in gay men, neither the US Government nor the WHO saw much reason for concern. An epidemic of disease in homosexuals was thought to have limited potential for transmission to the majority of society. Soon thereafter investigators from the CDC and elsewhere discovered that AIDS was widespread in Africa— where it was transmitted mainly by heterosexual contact. Few wanted to believe that this almost uniformly fatal disease could be spread by heterosexual transmission. A 1983 paper describing the epidemiology of HIV/AIDS and evidence for its heterosexual transmission was rejected for publication by at least 10 major journals before it was finally published in *The Lancet* in 1984 (Piot *et al.* 1984) nearly a year later. When the senior author of this paper and Bill Foege, then the Director of the CDC, called the assistant secretary of the Department of Health and Human Services to alert him to the overwhelming epidemiological evidence for heterosexual spread and its implied potential for a global epidemic, the reaction was denial. (In retrospect, at the time of this failed warning, 40,000 had already died and 1 million HIV infections had accrued worldwide (Behrman, 2004).) Two consecutive US presidents said little and did almost nothing. Not until

1987 did President Reagan, speaking at the American College of Physicians, call HIV-AIDs 'public enemy number one'. Reagan called for abstinence. In 2004 the appropriations bill for the US plan to combat HIV/AIDS stipulated that one-third of the education and prevention programme be spent on an abstinence-promoting programme. At this writing the US Government is still opposed to condom use.

The pandemic continues to grow. The official death toll of 1.3 million in 1995 rose to at least 26 million in 2004. The death toll does not include the unmeasured number of children orphaned, or the economic implications of the loss of working-age adults while children and elders remain. According to the US Census Bureau, 40 nations will have declining life expectancy by 2010; AIDS will be the primary cause in 35 of these countries. The story of the HIV/AIDS epidemic, the greatest epidemic of the twentieth century, recapitulates on a grand scale what happened to the public health in the Goldberger era, when prejudice and politics denied epidemiological evidence and delayed resources.

Cervical cancer: an infectious disease

Cancer of the uterine cervix (cervical cancer), is the second most common cancer of women worldwide. As early as the mid-nineteenth century, clinical observations indicated that cancer of the uterine cervix was common in prostitutes and rare in Jewish women. In 1962, an American case–control study showed associations with low economic status, early age of first coitus (later confirmed by observations that coitus after maturation of the cervical mucosa at around age 21 was less of a risk factor), and multiple sexual partners (Rotkin, 1962). The story of multiple sexual partners was strongly suggestive of a transmissible causal agent and the search for such an agent was intensive. By the 1980s, human papilloma viruses (HPVs) had been demonstrated to be the principal cause of cervical cancer. More than 100 distinct serotypes of HPV have been identified, of which at least 30 are associated with an increased risk of developing cervical cancer (Bosch *et al.* 1995).

Studies of cervical cancer worldwide have consistently shown infection with high-risk serotypes among women with cervical cancer in over 90% of cases. However, it should be noted that many infections are transient and many infected women do not develop cervical cancer. Additionally, the International Agency for Research on Cancer (IARC) classified cigarette smoking as an independent risk factor in 2002. A recent case–control study limiting cases and controls to HPV-infected women showed a more than two-fold increase of risk of high-grade squamous intraepithelial lesions among smokers (Plummer *et al.* 2003).

Clearly, a vaccine to prevent infection by HPV high-risk serotypes would have important public health consequences. Vaccines immunizing against HPV-16 and -18, high-risk serotypes, have been tested in double-blind placebo-controlled trails and found to safely prevent cervical intraepithelial neoplasis (Harper *et al.* 2006).

Prophylactic HPV vaccines are now being licensed for commercial use. Their actual public health effect will depend on duration of protection, degree of cross-protection against non-vaccine types of virus, and availability of vaccine to economically disadvantaged women.

Hormones and heart disease in women

In every country, whether heart disease rates or risk factors are high or low, women between the ages of 45 and 64 are at lower risk of fatal coronary heart disease (CHD) than men. This sex difference is universal despite diverse lifestyles, diets, and work patterns. Heart disease is uncommon in women before the menopause, and is more common in women who have a premature surgical menopause. Heart disease is less common in post-menopausal women who use hormone therapy. A meta-analysis of 25 observational studies published through mid-1997 showed an overall 30% reduced relative risk for heart disease among women who had ever used HT, compared with never users. Taken together, these observations support the hypothesis that female cardioprotection is due to an intrinsic factor, probably oestrogen. Laboratory studies show a favourable effect of oestrogen on high-density lipoprotein and low-density lipoprotein cholesterol, homocysteine, and vasoreactivity.

These consistent and biologically plausible results led several professional and volunteer organizations to conclude that post-menopausal hormone therapy (HT) cardioprotection was proven, that clinical trials were not only unnecessary but also unethical, and that HT should be offered to every post-menopausal woman. Others pointed out that no mass pharmacological therapy to prevent disease had been recommended in modern times in the absence of clinical trial evidence of benefit (Barrett-Connor *et al.* 2005).

And so, after 50 years of HT use in the USA, three large placebo-controlled randomized clinical trials were finally conducted: the Heart and Estrogen/Progestin Replacement Study (HERS) published in 1998, the Women's Health Initiative (WHI) Estrogen plus Progestin trial published in 2002, and the WHI Estrogen Only trial, published in 2005. All showed no cardioprotective effect of HT. In HERS and the WHI Estrogen plus Progestin trials, there was actually an increased risk of CHD during the first year. Both WHI trials showed an increased risk of stroke first apparent after 1–2 years.

The most plausible explanations for the trials' failure to demonstrate the cardioprotection reported in observational studies is that women prescribed oestrogen in observational studies were healthier and wealthier to begin with, and hormones took the credit for benefit. Since WHI, sales of post-menopausal hormones have decreased dramatically—and thousands of asymptomatic menopausal women were spared medication for an unproven indication. One other positive result of these trials has been the increasing attention paid to heart disease in women, a disease previously studied and treated mainly in men.

Conclusion

From its birth in the USA in 1843, epidemiology has played a critical role in elucidating the aetiology and natural history of many diseases, and in developing and providing its methodology. Although American epidemiology was originally concerned primarily with the investigation and control of epidemics, its functions and content have progressively expanded, providing the data for programme planning and evaluation and formulation of health policy.

Introduced into the curriculum of the first American school of public health at Johns Hopkins University in 1919, epidemiology is now a core component of curricula in all 37 accredited schools of public health. Further, all 125 accredited schools of medicine are required to include 'preventive medicine' in their curricula, of which epidemiology is usually a prominent component.

References

Ast DB, Smith DJ, Wachs B, and Cantwell BA (1956). Newburgh-Kinston caries-fluorine study, final report: combined clinical and roentgenographic dental findings after ten years of fluorine experience. *Journal of the American Dental Association*, **52**, 290–325.

Barrett-Connor E, Grady D, and Stefanick ML (2005). The rise and fall of menopausal hormone therapy. *Annual Review of Public Health*, **26**,115–14.

Behrman G (2004). *The invisible people. How the U.S. has slept through the global AIDS pandemic, the greatest humanitarian catastrophe of our time*, pp. 10–29. Free Press, New York.

Bosch FX, Manos MM, Munoz N, *et al.* (1995). Prevalence of human papilloma virus in DNA in cervical cancer: a worldwide perspective. *Journal of the National Cancer Institute*, **87**, 796–802.

Chmiel JS, Detels R, Kaslow RA, *et al.* (1987). Factors associated with prevalent human immunodeficiency virus (HIV) infection in the Multicenter AIDS Cohort Study. *American Journal of Epidemiology*, **126**, 568–77.

Doyle JT, Dauber TR, Kannel WB, *et al.* (1962). Cigarette smoking and coronary heart disease: combined experience of the Albany and Framingham studies. *New England Journal of Medicine*, **266**, 796–801.

Etheridge, EW (1992). *Sentinel for health: a history of the Centers for Disease Control*. University of California Press, Berkley, CA.

Flint A (1845). Account of an epidemic fever which occurred in North Boston, Erie County, New York, during the months of October and November, 1843. *American Journal of Medical Science New Series*, **10**, 21–35.

Flint A (1873). *Relations of water to the propagation of fever. Reports and papers presented at the meeting of the American Public Health Association*, pp. 164–72. Hurd and Houghton, New York.

Frost WH (1913). Epidemiologic studies of acute anterior poliomyelitis. *Hygienic Laboratory Bulletin*, No 90.

Harper DM, Franco El, Wheeler CM, *et al.*, on behalf of the HPV Vaccine Study group (2006). Sustained efficacy up to 4.5 years of a bivalent L1 virus-like particle vaccine against human papillomavirus types 16 and 18: follow-up from a randomised control trail. *Lancet*, **367**, 1247–55.

Jenner E (1798). *An inquiry into the causes and effects of the Variolae Vaccinae, a disease discovered in some of the western counties in England, particularly Gloucestershire, and known by the name of the Cow Pox*. Sampson Low, London.

Jenner E (1801). *The origin of the vaccine inoculation*. D. N. Shury, London.

Kannel WB (1995). Clinical misconceptions dispelled by epidemiological research. *Circulation*, **92**, 3350–60.

Kraut AM (2003). *Goldberger's war, the life and work of a public health crusader*. Hill & Wang (Farrar Straus and Giroux), New York.

Levin ML, Goldstein H, and Gerhardt PR (1950). Cancer and tobacco smoking. A preliminary report. *Journal of the American Medical Association*, **143**, 336–8.

McKay FS and Black CV (1916). An investigation of mottled teeth: an endemic developmental imperfection of the enamel of the teeth, heretofore unknown. *Dental Cosmos*, **5**, 477–84.

MMWR (1981). Pneumocystis pneumonia – Los Angeles. *Morbidity and Mortality Weekly Report*, **30**, 250–1.

Piot P, Quinn TC, Taelman H, *et al.* (1984). Acquired immunodeficiency syndrome in a heterosexual population in Zaire. *Lancet*, **2**, 65–9.

Plummer M, Herraro R, Franceschi S, *et al.* (2003). Smoking and cervical cancer: pooled analysis of the IARC multi-centric case-control study. *Cancer Causes and Control*, **14**, 805–14.

Report of the Advisory Committee to the Surgeon General of the Public Health Service (1964). *Smoking and health*. US Department of Health, Education and Welfare, Public Health Service, Washington, DC.

Rotkin ID (1962). Relation of adolescent coitus to cervical cancer risk. *Journal of the American Medical Association*, **179**, 486–91.

Salk JE (1953). Studies in human subjects on active immunization against poliomyelitis: preliminary report of experiments in progress. *Journal of the American Medical Association*, **151**, 1081–98.

Winkelstein W, Lyman DM, Padian N, *et al.* (1987). Sexual practices and the risk of infection by the Human Immunodeficiency Virus: the San Francisco Men's Health Study. *Journal of the American Medical Association*, **257**, 321–5.

Wynder EL and Graham EA (1950). Tobacco smoking as a possible etiologic factor in bronchiogenic carcinoma. A study of six hundred eighty-four proved cases. *Journal of the American Medical Association*, **143**, 329–36.

34

Poland

I: Development of the epidemiology of non-communicable diseases in Poland

Miroslaw J. Wysocki and Jan E. Zejda

II: Epidemiology, prevention, and control of infectious diseases in Poland in the twentieth century

Wieslaw Magdzik

Personal experiences

Miroslaw J. Wysocki: When in 1964 I completed medical studies in Warsaw, I started to look for a good place for my obligatory 2 year clinical internship. It soon became apparent that I would have to wait long months for an assignment in Warsaw, but the organization of a health care (public health) specialization fellowship enabled me to spend 2 years working in a very good clinical departments and the third year of this fellowship included courses in various areas of public health including epidemiology taught then by Dr Marek Sanecki who told me the fascinating story about new challenges for epidemiology in the area of non-communicable diseases (NCDs).

Later I met Jan Kostrzewski, the founder of modern epidemiology in Poland and Feliks Sawicki, who encouraged me to join the Department of Epidemiology of the National Institute of Hygiene and work in the team running the epidemiological study of chronic obstructive pulmonary diseases (COPDs) in Cracow. I did this between 1968 and 1971 and was heavily involved in the field study and in analysis of Cracow data on symptoms and spirometry which led me to my doctoral thesis (1971). Around this time Jan Kostrzewski asked me whether I would like to go to UK for 1 year's training in epidemiology and social medicine, because there was a possibility of getting a World Health Organization (WHO) research grant. In September 1971 I found myself in London in the Department of Clinical Epidemiology and Social Medicine of St Thomas's Hospital (under Walter W. Holland).

The 11 months I spent there were great and I learned a lot, attending various courses, taking part in the Harrow study and other work of the department, and working and discussing with Walter, Charles Florey, Doug Altman, Mike Adler, Mike Clarke, Ron Corkhill, Tony Swan, and many others including Philip Wood from the Medical Research Council then in Manchester. These nice and friendly people really knew what modern epidemiology, health statistics, and public health were. I also met Archie Cochrane and later translated into Polish his book *Effectiveness and efficiency*. It was a very important time in my professional life. The last month of my fellowship was spent at Erasmus in Rotterdam working in the epidemiology department of Hans Valkenburg, one of most brilliant people and epidemiologists I ever met. In September 1972 I returned to Poland, fully converted to modern epidemiology and with lots of knowledge and many new ideas.

Since then I have worked primarily as an epidemiologist in the NIH in Warsaw and the WHO Regional Office of Southeast Asia, planned and coordinated a number of national and international epidemiological studies of NCDs and published quite a few papers. Now, in 2005, as the deputy director of NIH, professor of epidemiology and chairman of the National Sanitary-Epidemiological Council I sometimes try to think about the turning point in my professional life. What really made me, who wanted to be a brilliant clinician, become an epidemiologist. There were a few such moments and the first of them—taking up the public health post-graduate specialization curriculum—was rather accidental. Later I met in Poland Marek Sanecki, Jan Kostrzewski, and Feliks Sawicki who were able to show me what epidemiological work is and to convince me that to be an epidemiologist may be equally as interesting as being a clinician. And finally, working with Walter Holland and his people at St Thomas's and with Hans Valkenburg at Erasmus made me almost a professional in epidemiological work and opened prospects for international cooperation which was extremely important in Poland at this time.

On the other hand, with the reluctant blessing of Jan Kostrzewski, I continued for many years in part time clinical work, having patients, completing specialization curricula, and finding it very useful in my epidemiological work which also required clinical knowledge and good cooperation with clinicians.

Jan E. Zejda: Having completed medical education in 1978 I joined the staff of the Clinical Department of Occupational Medicine (Institute of Occupational Medicine, Sosnowiec, Poland) and in addition to the regular duties of a house physician (internal and occupational medicine) I engaged in field studies on the health effects of various occupational exposures. My early interest in clinical and physiological aspects of occupational lung diseases resulted in a research stay at the Respiratory and Exercise Laboratory in the Department of Occupational Health, University of Newcastle upon Tyne, UK. Discussions with the centre's head Dr John E. Cotes brought to my attention the importance of good epidemiological practice. Following his advice I focused on that issue; however, scarce opportunities for standard epidemiology training in Poland at that time hampered the goal. Thanks to the Romer Foundation Scholarship, in 1989 at the Respiratory Epidemiology Laboratory (Department of Epidemiology and Biostatistics, McGill University, Montreal, Canada; Dr Margaret R. Becklake) I worked on diagnostic and epidemiological aspects of mineral dust-related respiratory disorders. At the same time, I completed a university course leading to the Diploma in Epidemiology and Biostatistics, in 1990. This was a turning point in my professional career. Further experience in occupational medicine led to a post-doctoral fellowship at the Centre for Agricultural Medicine in 1990, Department of Medicine, University of Saskatchewan, Canada (Dr James A. Dosman). In 1992 I returned to Poland and organized the Department of Epidemiology at the Institute of Occupational Medicine and Environmental Health in Sosnowiec, Poland. I helped to organize a team of young colleagues who received proper training, both 'hands on' and via formal training opportunities in Europe and the USA. In 2000 I accepted a position as the head of the Department Epidemiology at the Medical University of Silesia (Katowice, Poland) which gave me a much needed opportunity to reshape the training of medical students in epidemiology and biostatistics. The impact of eminent British and Canadian mentors was instrumental in my engagement in organization and management of the Faculty of Public Health in 2002 (Medical University of Silesia). That step was possible due to the emerging role of public health, including epidemiology, in the region and completed a preparation for a spectrum of formal education in epidemiology both at the undergraduate (medical and non-medical students) and post-graduate (physicians and other health professionals) levels.

Part I: Development of the epidemiology of non-communicable diseases in Poland

Introduction

In October 1964, during the 3rd National Congress of the Polish Association of Epidemiologists and Infectionists, J. K. Kostrzewski and K. Lachowicz presented a lecture entitled 'Tasks and perspectives of epidemiology in Poland' (Naruszewicz-Lesiuk and Magdzik 2005). The authors expressed the strong view that the burden, determinants, and prevention of socially important NCDs should become a new challenge for epidemiologists in Poland. Therefore October 1964 is often considered to be the date which marked the beginning of the study of the epidemiology of non-infectious diseases in Poland.

But even before October 1964 a number of studies on the frequency and determinants of cardiovascular diseases, cancer, diabetes, rheumatic diseases, mental impairment, and other groups of diseases had been carried out, often on representative population samples in different regions of the country. We must stress that because of restrictions on space only selected epidemiological studies are discussed.

The real beginning—Cracow study of COPDs

In 1965 the team of the Department of Epidemiology of the National Institute of Hygiene in Warsaw in cooperation with the Department of Epidemiology of the Medical Academy in Cracow initiated an epidemiological, prospective study of COPDs in Cracow, in part supported by a research grant from the National Centre for Health Statistics, Washington, DC and in later phases by research grant from the National Heart, Lung and Blood Institute, Bethesda, Maryland. The leader of the study team was Feliks Sawicki. After his sudden death in 1978, Miroslaw J. Wysocki took over; both were from the National Institute of Hygiene in Warsaw. (Field surveys in Cracow were coordinated by Wieslaw Jedrychowski.)

Results were extensively published and quoted in the Polish and foreign medical literature. This was the first large-scale epidemiological study of NCDs in Poland, and for many years served other epidemiologists as a model for planning, execution of field work, and the way in which the methodology and results were described and interpreted. The original objective of the study was to determine the previously unknown prevalence of COPDs in an urban population and its relation to various environmental factors as well as to develop methods for studies on the epidemiology of NCDs (Sawicki 1972). Selected methodological issues and results of this study are presented below.

After the preparatory phase, which included *inter alia* sampling design, preparation of measurement tools, training of interviewers and other staff as well as a pilot study, the cross-sectional survey was carried out in 1968. A random sample of 4355 (93.6% of the original sample) people aged 19–70 years was examined. From each subject information was collected by a questionnaire based on that developed by the UK Medical Research Council (MRC). All respondents were invited to a clinical examination which included spirometric tests made with the use of a Vitalograph spirometer. The spirometric measurements were performed in 3047 subjects. Chronic bronchitis, according to the MRC criteria, was found in 15.6% of interviewed males and 5.0% of females. It was also found that COPDs was more frequent in smokers and inhabitants of areas with high levels of air pollution. A synergistic effect of smoking and level of air pollution on the symptoms of COPD was observed (Sawicki 1972).

In 1981, 13 years after the original study, the next survey was conducted. An attempt was made to contact all those interviewed in 1968; 70.8% responded and were interviewed again. The remaining 11.2% were not interviewed but it was confirmed that they were still alive and 6% were lost from follow-up. Death had occurred in 523 cases (12%) of those interviewed in 1968. Deaths were confirmed by examination of death certificates which provided the underlying cause of death and its date. The relation of mortality to ventilatory function and some respiratory symptoms has been studied in 3047 men and women with spirometric tests performed in 1968 and followed-up for 13 years (Krzyzanowski and Wysocki 1986). The analysis was performed for all natural causes of death (327 deaths) and separately for deaths due to circulatory diseases and neoplasms.

The results confirmed the strong predictive power of ventilatory impairment for overall and circulatory mortality, even after adjustment for age, cigarette smoking, and other factors in logistic regression models. The risk of cancer death in men increased with decrease of FEV1. However, chronic cough, mucous hypersecretion, or asthmatic syndrome were not related to subsequent mortality. A strong predictor of overall and circulatory disease mortality in men was self-assessed health status. This was independent of other factors. The significance of the level of air pollution in chronic respiratory symptoms was also analysed (Wojtyniak *et al.* 1984) and epidemiological evidence on the relationship of air quality to health in children and adults was described and summarized in the light of Cracow and other epidemiological studies (Jedrychowski *et al.* 2002).

The longitudinal trends in lung function in a study population were presented in a number of publications including comparisons of FEV1 longitudinal annual changes with cross-sectional estimates (Jedrychowski *et al.* 1986) and comparison of the results of Cracow and Tucson studies (Krzyzanowski *et al.* 1990).

The end of the twentieth century—epidemiological studies of environmental factors and children's health in Upper Silesia

Political changes in Poland at the beginning of the last decade of the twentieth century, gave an impetus to investigations into the adverse health effects of environmental pollution. The topic received well-justified attention in the Upper Silesian Industrial Zone (Voivodship of Katowice). This densely populated region (containing 10% of Poland's population) affected by a legacy of the decades of extensive coal mining, metallurgical, and chemical industries was one of the most contaminated Eastern European environmental 'hot spots', suffering from 50 years of increasing environmental degradation. These important large-scale population-based environmental epidemiology studies were originated within the programme of the WHO Collaborating Centre for Environmental Pollution/Health Impact Assessment and Training in Environmental Health established in 1993 at the Institute of Occupational Medicine and Environmental Health in Sosnowiec. Based on the evidence provided by the assessment of environmental health risk, the focus of the studies was on children's health in relation to ambient air pollution and heavy metal exposures (Fitzgerald *et al.* 1988).

Projects on ambient air pollution and health included an array of studies. The panel studies showed an effect in terms of symptom occurrence, lung function, and respiratory morbidity. In particular, the findings confirmed statistically significant associations between concentration of particulate matter and sulphur dioxide and incidence of acute respiratory diseases. It was estimated that during the days of 'high' air pollution levels (in the mid-1990s) the incidence of common respiratory illnesses could increase by 50% (Biesiada *et al.* 2000). The impact of gaseous and particulate air pollution on paediatric respiratory health was also seen in large cross-sectional studies evaluating symptom occurrence and lung function.

Subsequent confirmatory evidence came from a multicentre Eastern European CESAR-PHARE Project. The CESAR Project was a far reaching initiative resulting in an apparent upgrade of skills and competence in all aspects of good epidemiological practice, risk assessment, and risk communication, and it introduced some specific techniques. The consistent finding, also seen in a 2-year time series analysis of daily mortality, was the predominant effect of exposure to sulphur dioxide, the leading harmful ambient air pollutant due to coal combustion. The results triggered a series of descriptive studies targeting the prevalence of childhood asthma in the region. A number of child populations throughout the region participated in questionnaire surveys that revealed a 6–8% prevalence of asthma.

Childhood asthma was the subject of a series of studies at the Medical University of Silesia. A cohort approach allowed the examination of risk factors. The cumulative incidence of asthma appeared to relate to using coal for cooking/heating and parental smoking, in addition to the known effects of parental asthma, history of atopic eczema, or allergic conjunctivitis (Zejda and Kowalska 2003). The role of indoor exposure to tobacco smoke was also confirmed by another project on chronic respiratory symptoms. The studies addressing various indoor exposures were reviewed by a 1997 Joint Symposium on the Indoor Environment and Respiratory Illness, Including Allergy, performed in the region under the auspices of International Programme on Chemical Safety.

The second major activity, the health effects of exposure to heavy metals, focused on exposure to lead. These projects involved biomonitoring and questionnaire-based assessment of pre-school and early primary school children and were performed in a wide range of populations. The results identified 'hot spots' and led to the estimation of the risk of environmental lead intoxication from the principal environmental causes. Furthermore the studies revealed that the principal risk factors of increased blood lead levels was place of residence, time spent playing outdoors, and socio-economic standing of the family (Osman *et al.* 1998).

Other topics addressed by the environmental epidemiological studies in the region included occupational exposures, biomonitoring of chemicals, and health effects of hazardous wastes. Increasing activity in the field of environmental epidemiology stimulated a number of doctoral theses, resulted in *ad hoc* courses, and was essential in the development of a comprehensive curriculum in epidemiology and biostatistics, a separate track within undergraduate teaching of public health students at the Medical University of Silesia. These environmental epidemiology programmes prepared the ground for preventive measures in two priority areas: the environmental lead exposure project led to a population-based programme composed of education, screening, and medical assessment of exposed children and recognition of the magni-tude of childhood asthma in the region triggered a population-based asthma screening programme.

Epidemiological studies of cardiovascular diseases

The first epidemiological cross-sectional field studies on the frequency of ischaemic heart disease and arterial hypertension were carried out in different areas of Poland in the 1950s and 1960s. In the late 1960s and in the 1970s the WHO epidemiological study of the registered incidence from acute myocardial infarction (AMI) and the pre-hospital and annual fatality were carried out in three districts of Warsaw and in Lublin—a town in southeast Poland (Askanas *et al.* 1975). In Warsaw the annual registered incidence in males aged over 20 was 311 and in females 169 per 100,000 inhabitants and in Lublin it was two times higher among males and four times higher among females. The annual fatality was 45%, and did not depend on gender or age. It should be stressed that pre-hospital fatality was 27% in males and 22% in females.

In 1984 the WHO international epidemiological programme MONICA started in Poland (Pol-MONICA) with the objectives of monitoring the incidence, fatality, and mortality due to CVDs (including acute myocardial infarction (AMI) and stroke) as well as the levels of factors recognized as their determinants. The study covered some 240,000 inhabitants aged 25–64 years of two districts of Warsaw, and over 280,000 inhabitants of the whole of the Tarnobrzeg province (southeastern Poland) in the same age group. The registered incidence and mortality from AMI significantly increased in Warsaw between 1984 and 1990 in males and females and then declined in between 1990 and 1994 in both sexes (Broda *et al.* 1996). Similar trends in registered incidence and mortality from AMI were observed among males in Tarnobrzeg province (Pajak *et al.* 1996). It should be mentioned that the WHO MONICA studies were also carried out in the areas of the present Czech Republic, the former East Germany, Lithuania, the present Russia, and former Yugoslavia (Tunstall-Pedoe 2003).

The analysis of the transformation of the health situation in Poland and in other countries of central Europe, especially the mortality from cardiovascular diseases before and after 1988, based on routinely collected mortality data and results of number of epidemiological and sociological studies was published in 1996 (Zatonski and Boyle 1996). The authors of this paper showed a significant increase in overall mortality rates among middle-aged Polish males (aged 45–64) and a stagnation of death rates in middle-aged females which occurred between 1965 and 1988 was primarily caused by constant rise of mortality rates from cardiovascular diseases. Mortality rates from cancer and sudden death from external causes also increased in men but remained stable in women during this period. In the years 1989–91, another significant increase in overall mortality rates occurred in Poland. It lasted for 3 years and took place mainly in men aged 15–64. This increase was due primarily to higher mortality from sudden death and to a lesser extent to higher mortality from cardiovascular diseases. Unexpectedly, from 1992 to 1994, there was an appreciable fall in mortality rates in both sexes which continued in later years and resulted mainly from a decline in cardiovascular deaths. Zatonski and Boyle argued that this positive mortality trend reflected the lifestyles changes of the Polish population which started to happen in 1980s and the beginning of 1990s and included a decline of the number of smokers, changes in drinking habits (from vodka to wine and beer), and a decline of alcohol consumption per capita as well as dramatic changes to a 'healthy' diet. From the beginning of the 1990s the average daily food energy intake began to drop, animal fat was largely replaced by vegetable fats, and there was increased consumption of local and exotic vegetables and fruits. The changes in the health situation occurring in Poland, although similar to those in other countries of Central Europe (the Czech Republic, Slovakia, and the former East Germany), have been greater and more striking.

The further (1995–2002) significant and continuous decline of mortality from coronary heart disease in Poland, especially among men and women aged 45–64, has been analysed and attributed primarily to a fall in the consumption of saturated fats and a rise of the consumption of polyunsaturated fats and to lesser a extent to the fall of the prevalence of smoking among males (Zatonski and Willet 2005).

Epidemiological studies of malignant neoplasms

The establishment of the Polish Cancer Registry in 1952 by Professor Tadeusz Koszarowski set up the basic conditions for long-term and obligatory collection of uniform and internationally comparable clinical and epidemiological data on malignant neoplasms in the whole of Poland. The experience gained during the first decade of the registry's activities showed the need for an additional registry of selected areas, which would offer better completeness and quality of data. Such registries were founded in 1963 in Warsaw, Cracow, and Katowice provinces (voivodships) covering some 6 million people, i.e. 20% of the Polish population.

The organization of this register was made possible with the assistance of the National Cancer Institute in Bethesda, USA, and especially with the personal help and advice of Professor William Haenszel (Wronkowski and Bielska-Lasota 1990). Professor Haenszel also helped to initiate the training of Polish oncologists in epidemiology at leading US centres and to carry out important international studies (Haenszel and Staszewski 1990).

A comprehensive description and analysis of mortality trends as well as geographical differences in malignant neoplasms in Poland was published in 1988 (Zatonski and Becker 1988) and mortality data in the countries of Central Europe in 1996 (Zatonski *et al.* 1996). The research team headed by W. Zatonski from the Maria Sklodowska-Curie Memorial Cancer Centre and Institute of Oncology, Warsaw, took part in a number of international epidemiological studies of neoplasms of the larynx, breast, pancreas, stomach, and gallbladder. The risk factors for gastrointestinal cancer in Poland were also studied in the 1980s and 1990s by W. Jedrychowski (2004).

The results of a number of epidemiological studies on malignant neoplasms carried out in Poland suggested that the main cause of the rise in cancer incidence in Poland after the Second World War was the constant and linear increase in the prevalence of cigarette smoking which lasted until the beginning of 1980s (Zatonski 2004). The well-coordinated long-term anti-smoking and health promotion campaign run by W. Zatonski with the help of mass media eventually led to a significant decline in smoking, especially among males. Comprehensive anti-smoking legislation was passed by the Polish Parliament in 1996.

Epidemiological studies of diabetes

In the 1950s and 1960s various groups of researchers in different areas of Poland carried out cross-sectional studies of diabetes. For example A. Czyzyk and T. Kasperska examined representative groups of the population of Warsaw over 14 years of age ($n = 4100$) and inhabitants of country areas ($n = 3456$) and found a prevalence of diabetes of about 0.8% and 0.5%, respectively.

In the early 1970s the Medical Academy and National Institute of Hygiene in Warsaw began a prospective study of the natural history of diabetes and its vascular complications among diabetic patients registered in the diabetic outpatient clinics of Warsaw who were born between 1905 and 1956 and had diabetes diagnosed after 1 January 1963. There were 5666 (2684 males and 2982 females) patients meeting these criteria, and of this group 2120 (79%) males and 2518 (84.4%) females took part in the initial study in 1973–74 (Czyzyk *et al.* 1975). The initial study included a standard questionnaire interview, biochemical and anthropometric tests, as well as measurement of blood pressure and an ECG.

In the period 1973/74 to 1995 a prospective mortality study covered 1990 males and 2430 females with type 2 diabetes. In the 22 years nearly 80% of the initial cohort died. The overall risk of death was two times higher, the death risk from cardiovascular diseases three times higher, and from coronary heart disease five times higher in diabetics than in the general population observed in the same time period. The overall and cardiovascular ratio of death were the same for women and men but was selectively higher for females than males for coronary heart disease and cerebrovascular diseases. Diabetics, especially women, also died more frequently from cancer than the general population (Janeczko *et al.* 1998). Out of 105 males and 66 females aged 18–30 with type 1 diabetes followed up during the same period of time 31.6% died (32.4% males and 30.3% females). The relative overall mortality risk was five times higher than in the general population (3.5 for men and 7.5 for women). Almost 30% of deaths were caused by renal disease and 17% by coronary heart disease.

Risk factors of the incidence of late micro- and macrovascular complications of diabetes were also analysed in the same study among 1329 type 2 diabetics followed for 17 years (Kopczynski *et al.* 1998). For new cases of proteinuria, hyperglycaemia was the common predictor (with diastolic hypertension, smoking, and overweight); hyperglycaemia and glycosuria were among significant predictors for leg vascular disease (with duration of diabetes, smoking, male gender, diastolic hypertension, and proteinuria). On the other hand, systolic hypertension and male gender prevailed among factors predicting both ischaemic heart disease (with high cholesterol and overweight), and stroke.

In the 1980s an incidence study of type 1 diabetes mellitus (IDDM) in children (0–14 years) and young adults (15–29 years) was carried out in Warsaw between 1 July 1983 and 30 June 1988 (Wysocki *et al.* 1992). This was possible because a distinctive feature of the health-care system in Poland is that virtually all newly diagnosed IDDM patients are referred to a specialized diabetic outpatient clinics for lifelong care. The overall number of new IDDM aged 0–29 registered in Warsaw during more than 5 years was 165, and the completeness of the registries of diabetic outpatient clinics was ascertained. The average incidence rates in the age groups 0–14 and 15–29 were respectively 5.2 and 6.5 per 100,000 population in males and 4.5 and 4.4 in females. The highest incidence was observed in the age groups 25–29, 10–14, and 15–19 in males and 5–9 and 25–29 in females. More patients reported the onset of their first symptoms in autumn and winter than in spring and summer. The incidence rates of IDDM in Warsaw appeared to be lower than those in some other countries (including the former East Germany) for which data at ages 0–29 were available.

The Polish Multicentre Study on Diabetes Epidemiology was financed by the Ministry of Health and was carried out from 1998 to 2000 on a representative randomized population sample of people over 35 years age inhabiting urban and rural areas of Krakow, Lublin, and Lodz provinces. The prevalence rates of type 2 diabetes (NIDDM) in this age group were respectively 10.8%, 15.6%, and 15.8%. It was estimated that the overall prevalence of type 2 diabetes in the Polish population is about 5.4% which accounts for over 2 million subjects, with around 50% of them representing 'unknown' diabetes. The major risk factors of newly diagnosed NIDDM were identified as fasting hyperinsulinaemia over 9.7 mIU/ml, body mass index over 30.0, and age over 65. Evaluation of the annual incidence rates of IDDM in 10 selected urban and rural areas revealed rates from 8.4 to 14.7/100,000 population in the age group 0–14 and from 4.4 to 11.2/100,000 in the age group 15–29 (Szybinski 2001). The prevalence and incidence rates found in this survey were much higher then rates found in previous epidemiological studies carried out in the 1980s or earlier. It was recommended that a research-based national programme to prevent NIDDM, which is a major public health issue, should be worked out and widely implemented. The coordinators also recommended that treatment of IDDM should be centralized in specialized centres to optimize the standard of care, and that the education of diabetic patients is an essential part of the management of diabetes.

Epidemiological studies of other selected groups of diseases

Until recently, the mental health of the Polish population was generally evaluated on the basis of such indirect indicators as the incidence of suicide or admissions to psychiatric outpatient clinics and hospitals. In 1996 the National Health Interview Survey, based on WHO recommendations, was carried out by the Central Statistical Office in collaboration with Polish and Dutch experts. The study was a representative survey of the entire non-institutionalized Polish population by means of a randomized, stratified (urban and rural census tracks) two-stage method. The response rate was very high (88%)—39,449 inhabitants aged 15 and over took part in the survey. The prevalence of psychiatric morbidity was based on GHQ-12 and the assessment of sleep-related problems was based on a six-item questionnaire.

Psychiatric morbidity was noted in almost one-quarter of women and one-fifth of men in Poland, with small differences between urban and rural populations. Every tenth woman reported such a complaint at up to 25 years and every second above 75 years of age. A higher prevalence of psychiatric morbidity was noted in unemployed and especially in disabled persons. The higher the level of education, the lower the frequency of psychiatric morbidity (Kiejna et al. 2004a).

Nearly one-quarter of the Polish population suffers from insomnia. The percentage is significantly higher among women (28.1%) than among men (18.1%). The prevalence of insomnia increases with age and is highest in divorced respondents. Respondents of both sexes with higher education suffer from insomnia less often than subjects with a lower level of education. The problem of insomnia affects similarly inhabitants of rural and urban regions. About 5% of people experienced recent deterioration of sleep related to some trouble. It is positively associated with age, female gender, and lower education. About 20% of the population get up tired in the morning—significantly more women than men and urban residents than rural ones (Kiejna et al. 2004b).

Almost one-tenth of Polish inhabitants usually sleep badly or very badly and this problem is more common among women than men. The quality of sleep decreases with aging and this process is more rapid in women than in men over 40 years of age. Highly educated respondents have the highest quality of sleep. The mean duration of sleep was 7.7 hours, without a gender difference. Usage of over-the-counter (OTC) medications is significantly lower than those prescribed by the physician (5% versus 16%). Women use OTC drugs twice as often as men.

The evaluation of the prevalence and natural history of rheumatic diseases including rheumatoid arthritis, other diseases of the musculoskeletal system, and rheumatic complaints has been the subject of a number of epidemiological population studies in urban and rural areas of Poland. In 1979 the Standing Committee of Epidemiology of the European League Against Rheumatism (EULAR) met in Stockholm to examine and analyse the situation, to recommend methods of improvement, and to suggest areas for epidemiological research. The burden of disease issues and epidemiological criteria were also reviewed (Allander *et al.* 1982). The outcome of this meeting appeared to be very helpful to epidemiologists in many European countries, including Poland. A critical summary of the epidemiological studies carried out in Poland in the second half of twentieth century was published in 1994 (Moskalewicz 1994). One of the important findings was that among males aged 30 to 60 years some 10% had serious rheumatic complaints according to Cobb's criteria modified by Adler and Abramson. Among females this percentage was about 25. It was also estimated, taking into account the results of a number of epidemiological studies, that in 1993 some 220,000 females and 80,000 males suffered from rheumatoid arthritis. The burden of arthrosis was also estimated. The author concluded that some 2 million of the 38 million inhabitants of Poland had, in 1993, symptoms and signs of this disorder.

To complete the picture of the development of epidemiology of NCDs in Poland in the twentieth century it should be mentioned that a number of molecular epidemiology studies were initiated in the 1990s (Jedrychowski *et al.* 2003) and a handbook of clinical epidemiology was published in 1997 (Brzezinski and Szamotulska 1997). This was the first book in Polish on this subject and included chapters on basic aspects of clinical trials, evaluation of diagnostic tests, clinical decision analysis, economic analysis, evaluation of the quality of medical care, meta-analysis, and evidence-based medicine. There is also a useful and clear Polish handbook on epidemiology used by medical students and professionals interested in the epidemiological approach and methodology (Jedrychowski 1999).

Part II: Epidemiology and prevention and control of infectious diseases in Poland in the twentieth century

Personal experiences

Wieslaw Magdzik: I studied in the medical faculty at the Medical Academy in Warsaw from 1950–55, during which time I chose to specialize in the epidemiology of infections and hygiene. Thus together with a diploma of Bachelor of Medicine I received the first degree of specialization in epidemiology (at that time in Poland there were two degrees of specialization). So I came into epidemiology before graduation.

During my course of medical study I was employed at the Department of Epidemiology of the National Institute of Hygiene as technical and laboratory worker.

After graduation I worked as an epidemiologist in the army and at the Ministry of Health where I was a chief of the operational group for the control of epidemics and later a chief of the Sanitary–Epidemiological Department. I received the second degree of specialization in epidemiology and the first degree of specialization in infectious diseases. Further training in epidemiology and other public health problems took place as a fellow of the World Health Organization in the UK and in Denmark in 1965. I received the scientific degree of doctor in 1965, habilitated doctor in 1971, and became a professor in 1982. In 1979 I returned to the National Institute of Hygiene where I was appointed the chief of the Epidemiological Department (1979–2002) and director of the Institute (1981–90). I retired in 2002.

Table 34.1 Infectious diseases in Poland, 1975–2004

Disease	1975	1976	1977	1978	1979	1980	1981	1982	1983	1984	1985	1986	1987	1988
Number of cases														
Typhoid fever	276	181	132	94	103	80	98	79	74	79	45	41	41	
Shigellosis	9220	3220	3524	2961	6988	2194	2863	1337	5789	8243	2649	5480	8217	11,321
Tetanus	111	112	115	105	104	89	91	122	116	87	86	76	71	67
Diphtheria	0	3	0	I	0	0	I	0	I	0	0	0	1	i
Pertussis	1156	512	1068	633	508	232	281	452	185	326	304	122	295	174
Measles	146,664	125,168	44,949	84,073	30,653	24,882	35,283	7620	11,271	54,403	35,680	6806	1286	1005
Rubella	519,56	127,650	68,678	49,575	52,318	143,120	207,029	14,036	18,602	24,456	74,705	462,593	19,120	15,529
Hepatitis (total)	74,559	73,392	76,516	65,283	52,004	48,245	47,164	50,028	61,729	52,287	42,610	28,880	22,363	21,827
Hepatitis A														
Hepatitis B					15,345	16,089	15,371	15,276	15,372	16,285	16,763	14,571	14,346	14,161
Hepatitis C														
Mumps	138,118	82,493	97,847	170,519	105,072	116,851	115,362	56,220	146,511	214,516	98,350	156,683	113,795	67,427
Incidence per 100,000														
Typhoid fever	0.811	0.527	0.380	0.269	0.292	0.225	0.273	0.218	0.202	0.214	0.121	0.109	0.109	0.074
Shigellosis	27.10	9.37	10.16	8.48	19.82	6.17	7.97	3.69	15.83	22.33	7.12	14.63	21.82	29.90
Tetanus	0.33	0.33	0.33	0.30	0.29	0.25	0.25	0.34	0.32	0.24	0.23	0.20	0.19	0.18
Diphtheria	0	0.009	0	0.003	0	0	0.003	0	0.003	0	0	0	0.003	0.003
Pertussis	3.40	1.49	3.08	1.8	1.44	0.65	0.78	1.25	0.51	0.88	0.82	0.33	0.78	0.46
Measles	431.08	364.26	129.55	240.71	86.94	69.94	98.28	21.03	30.82	147.38	95.91	18.17	3.41	2.65
Rubella	152.7	371.5	197.9	141.9	148.4	402.3	576.7	38.7	50.9	66.3	200.8	1235.0	50.8	41.0
Hepatitis (total)	219.1	213.6	220.5	186.9	147.5	135.6	131.4	138.1	168.8	141.6	114.5	77.1	59.4	57.6
Hepatitis A														
Hepatitis B					43.5	45.2	42.8	42.2	42.0	44.1	45.1	38.9	38.1	37.4
Hepatitis C														
Mumps	406.0	240.1	282.0	488.2	298.0	328.4	321.3	155.2	400.6	581.1	264.4	418.3	302.1	178.1

Introduction

The history of sanitary–epidemiological services in Poland, providing prevention and control of infectious diseases, in the twentieth century began in 1918. In that year, as a result of the First World War, Poland gained independence and Polish territories were reunited after 124 years of occupation by Austria, Germany, and Russia.

The first step to establish the services was bringing together in one institution experts in diagnosis, prevention, and control of infectious diseases. Relatively quickly several people were designated

1989	1990	1991	1992	1993	1994	1995	1996	1997	1998	1999	2000	2001	2002	2003	2004
23	25	13	21	14	14	12	9	7	2	6	13	6	5	0	3
8578	10,052	3608	1894	1290	3210	815	530	439	555	292	121	128	220	75	74
59	65	58	52	51	54	44	46	37	22	21	14	21	20	30	25
0	0	0	I	10	2	2	9	0	0	0	I	0	0	0	0
107	292	302	590	314	697	549	330	2092	2871	876	2269	2411	1788	2034	2955
7225	56,471	2419	3695	1410	864	752	639	338	2255	99	77	133	34	48	11
20,663	17,396	59,425	398,704	64,043	52,703	57,351	79,286	138,782	43,239	30,958	46,181	84,419	40,518	10,588	4857
25,078	29,906	36,728	40,531	41,778	37,360	30,276	18,456	10,715	8106	6729	5360	5183	4449	4228	3834
								4045	2011	1024	262	738	338	150	95
15,308	15,116	13,603	13,237	13,296	10,924	9034	6435	4896	4074	3508	2825	2394	2021	1812	1568
								1064	1710	1988	2086	1953	1978	2255	2152
81,212	140,156	54,370	42,202	I15,300	219,516	82,337	39,596	83,588	217,452	90,214	17,548	16,724	39,978	87,336	135,050
0.061	0.066	0.034	0.055	0.036	0.036	0.031	0.023	0.018	0.005	0.016	0.034	0.016	0.013	0	0.008
22.60	26.37	9.43	4.94	3.35	8.33	2.11	1.37	1.14	1.44	0.76	0.31	0.33	0.58	0.20	0.19
0.16	0.17	0.15	0.14	0.13	0.14	0.11	0.12	0.10	0.06	0.05	0.04	0.05	0.05	0.08	0.07
0	0	0	0.003	0.026	0.005	0.005	0.023	0	0	0	0.003	0	0	0	C
0.28	0.77	0.79	1.54	0.82	1.81	1.42	0.85	5.41	7.43	2.27	5.87	6.24	4.68	5.33	7.74
19.03	148.14	6.33	9.63	3.67	2.24	1.95	1.65	0.87	5.83	0.26	0.20	0.34	0.09	0.13	0.03
54.4	45.6	155.4	1039.2	166.5	136.7	148.6	205.3	359.1	111.8	80.1	119.5	218.5	106.0	27.7	12.7
66.1	78.5	96.0	105.6	108.6	96.9	78.5	47.8	27.7	21.0	17.4	13.9	13.4	11.6	11.1	10.0
								10.5	5.2	2.6	0.7	1.9	0.9	0.4	0.2
40.3	39.7	35.6	34.5	34.6	28.3	23.4	16.7	12.7	10.5	9.1	7.3	6.2	5.3	4.7	4.1
								2.75	4.42	5.14	5.40	5.05	5.17	5.90	5.64
213.9	367.7	142.2	110.0	299.8	569.5	213.4	102.5	216.3	562.4	233.4	45.4	43.3	104.6	228.7	353.

to take over these tasks, among others Professor Ludwik Serkowski from Warsaw University, Dr Feliks Przesmycki from the military health service, Dr Ludwik Rajchman from London and Dr Ludwik Hirszfeld from Zurich. They began working in 1918. In 1919 the State Central Institute of Epidemiology was founded, which in 1923 was renamed as the National Institute of Hygiene (NIH) (its present name)—in Polish 'Panstwowy Zaklad Higieny (PZH)'. The Central Institute in Warsaw supervised local branches, at first 6 and then 13, in the voivoidship (provincial) capital cities. These branches collaborated with local authorities to implement effective prevention and control of infectious diseases and served as a base for microbiological and serological diagnosis.

Before the Second World War PZH and its branches constituted the core of Polish sanitary–epidemiological services. The structure of these services in Poland, as well as in other Central European countries, resembled the structure of services in Western European countries.

After a big epidemic of typhus in 1919 an Emergency Committee to Control Typhus was established by the Minister of Public Health. Parliament passed an act to establish the 'Office of Chief Extraordinary Commissary to Fight Epidemics'.

In 1919 three Acts were passed: the Basic Sanitary Act, the Act on Infectious Diseases Control, and the Act on Compulsory Smallpox Vaccination. Further legislative work was carried out as needed, and additional acts for the control of communicable diseases were passed in 1935, 1963, and 2001.

Beside the public health laboratory, educational activities, and field interventions, there was an increasing interest in public health research. In the beginning, the major research projects were initiated at the National Institute of Hygiene by Professor Ludwik Hirszfeld. The Rockefeller Foundation also supported the creation of the School of Hygiene in the PZH to train public health specialists, with a focus on the prevention and control of infectious diseases.

In 1920 the PZH started to issue a scientific journal *Przeglad Epidemiologoczny* [Epidemiological Review], in which research carried out in the PZH as well as in other Polish institutes was published. In 1923 the journal was renamed *Medycyna Doświadczalna i Spoleczna* [Experimental and Social Medicine]. The original title was restored in 1947. One part of this journal, '*Kronika Epidemiologiczna* [Epidemiological Chronicle], a major source of information on the occurrence of infectious diseases in Poland, is still being published annually.

During the Second World War from 1939–1945, the PZH branches located in the so-called General-Government areas in Warsaw, Cracow, Lublin, and Kielce continued infectious disease control and prevention activities. After the war the PZH temporarily moved to Lodz until the Warsaw building was rebuilt. PZH branches were set up in all but three voivodship capital cities.

On 24 November 1944, in response to the alarming infectious disease situation in Poland (the threat of epidemics related to the fighting and deportation of large numbers of people), the Office of the Chief Extraordinary Commissary to Fight Epidemics was re-established on the territories captured by the Soviet Army. This office was discontinued in April 1947.

Until 1952, as before the war, local health departments were in charge of control and prevention of infectious disease in collaboration with the local PZH branches, which provided reference laboratory diagnosis. In 1952, a network of sanitary–epidemiological stations was organized with the voivodship stations, based on the PZH branches, and poviat-level stations including poviat, town, district, and port stations, based on the sanitary–epidemiological organizations and the poviat physician offices.[1] This network served as a foundation for the State Sanitary Inspection

---

[1] Voivodships and poviats are administrative units in Poland. Up to 1975 Poland was divided in to 17 voivodships and five cities. Voivodships were divided into 392 poviats and cities were divided into 33 city districts. The total Polish population 32,909,000. The average population of one unit was 1,496,000—the highest 3,701,000 (Katowice) and the lowest 472,000 (Poznań city). The average number of poviats or city districts in one voivodship or city was 19.3; the highest was 35 (voivodship of Poznań) and the lowest 4 (Kraków, city). Between 1975 and 1998 Poland was divided into 49 voivodships In this period there were no poviats in Poland. In 1998 the population of Poland was 38,666,145. The average population of a voivodship was 789,105; the highest being 3,903,276 (Katowickie) and the lowest 249,238 (Chelmskie). Since 1999 Poland has been divided into 16 voivodships. Voivodships are divided into 379 poviats. In 2004 the population of Poland was 38,180,249. The average population of one voivodship is 2,386,265; the highest being 5,139,545 (Mazowieckie) and the lowest 1,009,177 (Lubuskie). The average number of poviats is 23.7; the highest being 42 (Mazowieckie) and the lowest 14 (Lubuskie and Świętokrzyskie).

required by the Decree of 14 August 1954. The division of production of sera and vaccines in PZH was restructured into three serum and vaccine facilities in Warsaw, Krakow, and Lublin.

In the early 1950s the sanitary–epidemiological services in Poland were reorganized in a similar way to that in the Soviet Union and its satellite countries Czechoslovakia, Romania, Bulgaria, East Germany, and Hungary. Compared to the situation prior to the 1952 reform, the major change was the setting up of a technical supervisory body of the sanitary–epidemiological service within the Ministry of Health. This took over the supervising functions from PZH. PZH assumed a consultative role and concentrated on research.

Beginning in 1954, the sanitary–epidemiological services were gradually transformed into the State Sanitary Inspection, i.e. an institution authorized to initiate public health interventions and use administrative sanctions. This institution included the public health agency of the Ministry of Health and the sanitary–epidemiological stations.

Research institutes collaborating with the sanitary–epidemiological stations provided technical and professional support. The network of stations and institutes formed a highly specialized unit dealing with specific and general prophylactics and health promotion. The structure described here functioned with minor changes, which had no impact on the prevention and control of infectious diseases, throughout the beginning of the twenty-first century.

The history of the control and prevention of infectious diseases in the Polish territories (and to some extent other countries in Central Europe) in the twentieth century can be divided into six periods:

1. The period before the First World War (1900–14).

2. The First World War, the Polish–Russian war and several years afterwards (1914–22).

3. The interwar period (1922–39).

4. The Second World War and the period of deportations after the war (1939–49).

5. The period of enthusiasm related to achievements in the control and prevention of infectious disease (1949–90).

6. The end-of-the-century period (1990–present).

During the first period the Polish territories were under the partition of Austria, Germany, and Russia and were therefore administered differently, with different legislation, different sanitary situation, and different public awareness of health issues. The conditions for the spread of infectious diseases were least favourable in Germany, moderately favourable in Austria, and very favourable in Russia, where the sanitary state of the cities was poor, public awareness, especially in villages was low, and the general living conditions very poor. Pediculosis was very common, as were the louse-borne diseases, including typhus. The food-borne diseases, most importantly typhoid fever and shigellosis, but also other diseases such as smallpox, tuberculosis, syphilis, and malaria, all represented great problems. After gaining independence in 1918 there were almost no cases of smallpox in the territories previously under the German partition, a few dozen of cases in the ex-Austrian partition, and a few thousand cases on the territories of Russian partition.

In the second period, from 1914 to 1922, comprising military operations during the First World War, the situation regarding infectious diseases worsened noticeably. During the First World War the majority of the military fighting on the Eastern Front took place on the territories of Poland. Due to the fighting, movement of armies, confiscation of goods, and disintegration of both industry and agriculture, the population became impoverished. As a consequence, a significant increase was observed in the incidence of tuberculosis, louse-borne diseases (mostly typhus), diseases affecting the military, e.g. trench fever (also known as Wolhynia fever), and food-borne diseases, including cases of cholera.

During the third, interwar period (1922–39) efforts were undertaken with the aim of improving the control and prevention of infectious diseases. The sanitary conditions and public awareness at this time had not yet attained a satisfactory level, but were getting better. Mass smallpox immunization campaigns were implemented and the first groups of children were vaccinated against diphtheria, tetanus, typhoid fever, and tuberculosis. Furthermore, research on bacteriological diagnostics and immunization of populations was initiated.

Due to mass vaccinations, the last death attributed to indigenous smallpox was registered in 1933, and the last indigenous case was notified in 1937. The overall epidemiological situation was considered severe, but it was gradually improving. Infectious diseases, however, were the principal cause of death and approximately every fifth Polish citizen during that time died of an infectious disease.

The fourth period extended over the years 1939–49, during the Second World War and several following years. This was a period of intensive military operations and mass deportations of the civilian population, first initiated by the Germans during the occupation of Poland, from Western territories to the Central regions, from the region of Zamosc to different parts of Poland, and after the war from the former Eastern territories of Poland taken over by the Soviet Union to the Northern and Western territories annexed from Germany after the Second World War as a result of the Yalta agreements. The health and sanitary infrastructure was destroyed to a great extent. The socio-economic situation worsened in the general population and the living conditions were extremely bad in Nazi camps and prisons, including concentration camps located in several places in Poland. All these factors contributed to a very difficult epidemiological situation with increasing incidence of tuberculosis, typhus, typhoid fever, dysentery, diphtheria, scarlet fever, malaria, and sexually transmitted diseases (STDs) (Chomiczewski *et al.* 2001, 2002).

The fifth period could be defined to begin in 1949, and end between the years 1981 and 1996, depending on the selected criteria, and was arbitrarily set to extend over to 1990. During this period, multiple effective approaches of prevention and treatment of infectious diseases were introduced, leading to improvement of the epidemiological situation for several diseases, as well as eradication of single disease entities.

Among the most effective measures were the following:

+ introduction of effective insecticides;
+ improvement of sanitary conditions, particularly the supply of uninfected and good quality water and food, and effective waste disposal;
+ improvement in the living conditions of citizens;
+ effective mass active immunization (vaccination) against many infectious diseases, and to a lesser degree passive or passive–active immunization;
+ improvement of the quality and coverage of medical treatment.

The efficacy of these measures was higher because they were often used in an organized manner in mass prophylactic actions, for example the tuberculosis prophylactic programme or STD prevention action (Action W). The implementation of preventive measures, which combined effectiveness and safety (for example, vaccination programmes and implementation of antibiotic treatment) required the design and realization of numerous scientific projects. Two studies deserve to be mentioned here:

+ A study of the efficacy and effectiveness of vaccinations against typhoid fever carried out in 1960–63 using the controlled field trials methodology in 25 districts in Poland, involving approximately 700,000 vaccinated subjects. The study was performed under the auspices of the WHO in Poland, the Soviet Union, Yugoslavia, and British Guyana.
+ A study comparing the efficacy and safety of measles vaccines based on the Leningrad 16 and Edmonston strains.

The most spectacular effects were achieved as a result of implementation of the national immunization programme. They included substantial improvement in the epidemiological situation of such infectious diseases as tetanus, pertussis, diphtheria (which was eliminated), measles, congenital rubella syndrome, and eradication of smallpox and poliomyelitis.

During the fifth period, in 1949–1990, three outbreaks of smallpox imported from India occurred. In 1953 an epidemic in Gdansk involved 13 cases and 3 deaths. In 1962 in the seaport of Gdansk 29 imported cases were reported, and in 1963 a countrywide outbreak occurred, involving 99 cases and 7 deaths in Wroclaw, Opole, Wieruszow, and Gdansk.

In the 1970s Polish epidemiologists contributed to the implementation of the smallpox eradication programme worldwide, especially in India. Professor Jan K. Kostrzewski and Dr A. Oles played a special role in this programme. In 1980 the worldwide eradication of smallpox was announced. In 1988, the poliomyelitis eradication programme was implemented. The last cases of poliomyelitis in Poland caused by the wild poliovirus were notified in 1982 and 1984.

The occurrence of diphtheria also decreased considerably and is now limited to imported cases. During the diphtheria epidemic in the countries located to the east of Poland, 24 cases were imported, but only 1 person contracted the disease in Poland.

In the second part of the twentieth century the situation concerning hepatitis A and B initially became more severe and then improved partly as a result of anti-epidemic measures. For hepatitis type A and B, in particular, evaluation of the effectiveness of the preventive and control measures undertaken merits a detailed commentary. Improvement in the sanitary situation and living conditions of the population and, to a lesser degree, implementation of vaccinations, led to a reduction in the case numbers of hepatitis A. Before 1978, the number of hepatitis A cases exceeded 50,000 or even 60,000 cases per year (an incidence of over 150 per 100,000 population). After 1978, the number of cases was decreasing with periodic fluctuations. Since 2000, the annual number of cases went down to several hundred, and in 2004, declined below 100. Before 1978 the endemicity of hepatitis A was classified as high, from 1978 to 1997 as intermediate, between 1997 and 2002 as low, and, finally, following the year 2002 as very low. These changes influenced both the epidemiological and clinical characteristics of the disease, and the population immunity against hepatitis A.

Before 1993, the situation for hepatitis B was highly unfavourable, compared with most European countries. The number of cases exceeded 16,000 per year, and the incidence reached 45 per 100,000 population. Beginning in 1993, a comprehensive programme of prevention and control of hepatitis B was implemented, combining the elimination of sources of infection, breaking the transmission routes, universal vaccination of infants and adolescents, and vaccination of persons from high-risk groups. These activities contributed to a decrease in the number of hepatitis B cases to below 2000 in 2004 (incidence approximately 4). This was a 90% decrease compared to 1993.

During the fifth period (1949–90), the incidence of infectious diseases with high case-fatality rate was decreasing. Therefore, the proportion of mortality attributable to infectious diseases dropped below 1% (usually 0.7–0.8%), compared to over 20% in the third period (1922–39). The mean lifespan systematically increased, from 58.6 years in 1952 to 66.5 years in 1990 for men, and from 64.2 to 75.5 years for women.

At the end of the fifth period, euphoria and enthusiasm associated with the belief that the problem of infectious diseases would be eliminated in short order were very common. In some regions of Poland health-care units necessary for the proper diagnosis and treatment of infectious diseases were closed down, and in some instances rigorous monitoring of diseases was disrupted. This was the case for diseases spread parenterally, especially hepatitis B, food-borne infections, and intoxications as typhoid fever, dysentery, hepatitis A, certain types of meningitis, tick-borne encephalitis, nosocomial infections, and infections in immunocompromised persons.

The Charles Nicolle theory of the birth, life, and death of infectious diseases was generally neglected.

The emergence of AIDS and identification of the HIV virus in 1981 were astonishing and caused consternation among the policy-makers. On the wave of a world epidemic, the first AIDS case was diagnosed in Poland in 1985. A thorough analysis of the new situation led to the development in 1992 of a new concept of emerging and re-emerging diseases. This problem was further studied and recognized by the WHO in a special report in 1996.

Furthermore, an increase in hepatitis C cases was observed. Registration of hepatitis C cases began in Poland in 1997. Despite significant under-reporting of cases, the number of newly diagnosed cases increased during the last 10 years, exceeding 2000 per year in 2004. The lack of effective measures for prevention and control of hepatitis C implies the possibility of a continuous increase in hepatitis C incidence in the forthcoming years.

During the same period, the improvement in the epidemiological situation for tuberculosis slowed down, and in some years an increase in incidence and mortality was observed. Furthermore the problem of antimicrobial resistance became more important. Recently recognized epidemiological threats comprise the nosocomial infections caused by commensal bacterial flora, imported cases of tropical diseases, and possible bioterrorist attacks. Particular concerns are related to the threat of a terrorist attack using the smallpox virus or its genetically modified derivative, *Bacillus anthracis*, *Yersinia pestis*, or agents of viral haemorrhagic fevers.

Based on these phenomena, the sixth period of infectious disease epidemiology in the twentieth century was defined as the era of emerging and re-emerging diseases. This started during the 1980s and 1990s and continues today.

To summarize the twentieth century, some infectious diseases constituted a serious problem throughout the whole century (tuberculosis, influenza), some had a serious health impact mainly in the first half of the century (malaria, typhus, typhoid fever, diphtheria, pertussis, measles), and some emerged in the second half of the century and continue to influence the present epidemiological situation (viral hepatitis, AIDS) (Table 34.1).

Major epidemiological research in infectious disease

Epidemiological research on infectious diseases was performed by the Department of Epidemiology at National Institute of Hygiene in cooperation with sanitary epidemiological stations. Professor Jan Kostrzewski was the chief of the department up to 1978 and I succeeded him for the period 1979–2002. Professor Andrzej Zielinski is the present chief.

In the 1960s a large programme evaluating vaccination against typhoid fever and the efficacy of typhoid fever vaccines was performed in 25 poviats in 5 voivodships in Poland as a controlled field trial, and five typhoid fever vaccines were evaluated in comparison with the placebo group as control. Formol-phenol and acetone vaccines were found to be the most effective. As a result of this trial the typhoid vaccine used routinely in Poland was changed for formol-phenol vaccine.

Epidemiological evaluation of the sequelae of hepatitis was performed. This was the first such study connected with hepatitis as a infectious disease with chronic consequences. This was followed by a programme for the control of hepatitis B, which caused a 10-fold reduction in hepatitis B cases.

The next controlled field trial was an evaluation of measles vaccines, especially comparing the efficacy of the Russian vaccines with the vaccines produced in Western countries. No significant differences were found.

Epidemiological evaluation of the side effects connected to vaccination, especially those performed as universal vaccinations, were evaluated in the whole country. The findings of this study were implemented by the routine notification of the side-effects of vaccination.

An important piece of research was on food infections and food poisoning. Trials were started when the problem of diseases caused by *Salmonella enteritidis* transmitted by chicken products increased considerably. The results of this research were included in the routine public health activities in the country, especially in the field of surveillance of these diseases and their control.

References

Allander E, Behrend T, Henrard JC, *et al.* (1982). Rheumatology in perspective, the epidemiological view. *Scandinavian Journal of Rheumatology*, Suppl. 48.

Askanas Z, Kedra M, and Rywik S (1975). Registration of myocardial infarction in Warsaw and Lublin. Data on incidence. *Polski Tygodnik Lekarski*, **30**, 192–6 (in Polish).

Biesiada M, Zejda JE, and Skiba M (2000). Air pollution and acute respiratory diseases in children: regression analysis of morbidity data. *International Journal of Occupational Medicine and Environmental Health*, **13**, 113–20.

Broda G, Rywik S, and Kuriata P (1996). Hospital care of patient with myocardial infarction between 1986 and 1992—program Pol-MONICA, Warsaw. *Kardiologia Polska*, **44**, 482–91 (in Polish).

Brzezinski ZJ and Szamotulska K (1997). *Epidemiologia kliniczna (Clinical epidemiology)*. Wydawnictwo Lekarskie PZWL, Warszawa (in Polish).

Chomiczewski K, Gall W, and Grzybowski J (2001). *Epidemiology of war and catastrophes*. Alfa-medica Press, Bielsko-Biala.

Chomiczewski K, Kocik J, and Szkoda M (2002). *Bioterrorism*. PZWL Medical Publishing, Warsaw.

Czyzyk A, Brzezinski ZJ, Krolewski AS, Janeczko D, Wysocki M, and Puncewicz B (1975). Fate of diabetic patient. I. Plan of the study, methods and study group. *Przeglad Epidemiologoczny*, **29**, 449–59 (in Polish).

Fitzgerald EF, Schell LM, Marshall E, Carpenter DO, Suk WA, and Zejda JE (1988). Environmental pollution and child health in Central and Eastern Europe. *Environmental Health Perspectives*, **106**, 307–11.

Haenszel WM and Staszewski J (1990). Cancer among migrant Poles. In *Cancer prevention, vital statistics to intervention* (ed. W Zatonski, P Boyle, and J Tyczynski). The Maria Sklodowska-Curie Memorial Cancer Centre and Institute of Oncology, PA Interpress, Warsaw. pp. 25–8.

Janeczko D, Kopczynski J, Czyzyk A, Janeczko-Sosnowska E, Tuszynska A, and Lewandowski Z (1998). Mortality of diabetic patients in Warsaw – 22-years follow-up (1973/74–1995). Part I. Mortality of diabetic patients in type2 (NIDD). *Polskie Archiwum Medycyny Wewnetrznej*, **100**, 153–64 (in Polish).

Jedrychowski W (1999). *Epidemiologia, wprowadzenie i podstawy* [Epidemiology, introduction and basics], 4th edn. PZWL, Warsaw (in Polish).

Jedrychowski WA, Perera FP, Maugeri U. (2003). *Molecular epidemiology in preventive medicine*. International Center for Studies and Research in Biomedicine in Luxembourg, Luxembourg.

Jedrychowski W (2004). *Gastrointestinal cancer in Poland. Nutritional epidemiologic study*. Jagiellonian University Press, Cracow.

Jedrychowski W, Krzyzanowski M, and Wysocki M (1986). Changes in lung function determined longitudinally compared with decline assessed cross-sectionally. The Cracow study. *European Journal of Epidemiology*, **2**, 134–8.

Jedrychowski W, Maugeri U, and Jedrychowska-Bianchi I (2002). *In search for epidemiologic evidence on air quality and health in children and adults*. Center for Research and Studies in Biomedicine in Luxembourg, Luxembourg.

Kiejna A, Wojtyniak B, and Rymaszewska J (2004a). Prevalence of psychiatric morbidity in Poland – National Health Interview Survey. *Acta Neuropsychiatria*, **16**, 295–300.

Kiejna A, Rymaszewska J, Wojtyniak B, and Stokwiszewski J (2004b). Characteristics of sleep disturbances in Poland – results of the National Health Interview Survey. *Acta Neuropsychiatria*, **16**, 124–9.

Kopczynski J, Janeczko D, Lewandowski Z, Janeczko-Sosnowska E, Tuszynska A, and Czyzyk A (1998). Risk factors of the incidence of late vascular complications of diabetes. *Polskie Archiwum Medycyny Wewn Trznej*, **100**, 236–44 (in Polish).

Kostrzewski J (ed.) (1964). *Infectious diseases in Poland – epidemiology and control in 1919–1962*. PZWL Medical Publishing, Warsaw (in Polish).

Kostrzewski J (ed.) (1973). *Infectious diseases in Poland – epidemiology and control in 1961–1970*. PZWL Medical Publishing, Warsaw (in Polish).

Kostrzewski J (ed.) (1984). *Infectious diseases in Poland – epidemiology and control in 1970–1979*. PAN Publishing, Wroclaw (in Polish).

Kostrzewski J (1994). *75 years of sanitary-epidemiological services in Poland*. Lecture on 10 October 1994 during the Jubilee Celebration in Tarnow. Published in the Proceedings of Tarnow Conference, Tarnow, 1–6 (in Polish).

Kostrzewski J, Magdzik W, and Naruszewicz-Lesiuk D (ed.) (2001). *Infectious diseases in Poland – epidemiology and control in the twentieth century*. PZWL Medical Publishing, Warsaw (in Polish).

Krzyzanowski M and Wysocki M (1986). The relation of thirteen-year mortality to ventilatory impairment and other respiratory symptoms. The Cracow Study. *International Journal of Epidemiology*, **15**, 56–64.

Krzyżanowski M, Camilli AT, and Lebowitz MD (1990). Relationships between pulmonary function and changes in chronic respiratory symptoms – comparison of Tucson and Cracow longitudinal studies. *Chest*, **98**, 62–70.

Magdzik W (1988). *Epidemiological threats*. Lecture on the Annual Congress of the Polish Association of Epidemiologists and Infectiologists, Published in Proceedings of Annual Congress, Pulawy 8–15 (In Polish).

Magdzik W (2004). Achievements of sanitary-epidemiological services in Poland during 85 years of activity and perspectives for the future. *Przeglad Epidemiologiczny*, **58**, 569–81.

Magdzik W, Naruszewicz-Lesiuk D, and Zielinski A. (ed.) (2005). *Vaccinology*. Alfa-medica Press, Bielsko-Biala (in Polish).

Moskalewicz B (1994). Rheumatic complaints and diseases in Poland – epidemiological and social evaluation. *New European Rheumatology*, **2**, S1–S4 (in Polish).

Naruszewicz-Lesiuk D and Magdzik W (2005). *Jan Karol Kostrzewski, 1915–2005*. Panstwowy Zaklad Higieny (National Institute of Hygiene), Warsaw (in Polish).

Osman K, Zejda JE, Schutz A, Mielzynska D, Elinder CG, and Vahter M (1998). Exposure to lead and other metals in children from Katowice district, Poland. *International Archives of Occupational and Environmental Health*, **71**, 180–6.

Pajak A, Jamrozik K, Kawalec E, *et al.* (1996). Myocardial infarction – threats and medical care. Longitudinal observational study in 280 000 women and men – POL-MONICA Krakow Project. Part III: Epidemiology and treatment of myocardial infarction. *Przeglad Lekarski*, **53**, 767–78 (in Polish).

Sawicki F (1972). Chronic nonspecific respiratory diseases in Cracow. *Epidemiological Review*, **26**, 230–49.

Szybinski Z (2001). Polish Multicenter Study on Diabetes Epidemiology (PMSDE) – 1998–2000. *Polskie Archiwum Medycyny Wewn Trznej*, **106**, 751–8 (in Polish).

Tunstall-Pedoe H (ed.) (2003). *MONICA. World largest study of heart disease, stroke, risk factors, and population trends, 1979–2002*. WHO, Geneva.

Wojtczak A (1992). Sources of social medicine and public health. *Zdrowie Publiczne*, **103**, 117–31 (in Polish).

Wojtyniak B, Krzyzanowski M, and Jedrychowski W (1984). Importance of urban air pollution in chronic respiratory problems. *Zeitschrift fur Erkrankungen Der Atmungs Organen*, **163**, 274–84.

World Health Organization (1996). *The World Health Report 1996. Fighting disease. Fostering development*. WHO, Geneva.

Wronkowski Z and Bielska-Lasota M (1990). Vital statistics in Poland. In *Cancer prevention, vital statistics to intervention* (ed. W Zatonski, P Boyle, and J Tyczynski). The Maria Sklodowska-Curie Memorial Cancer Centre and Institute of Oncology, Pa Interpress, Warsaw, pp. 18–24.

Wysocki MJ, Chanska M, Bak M, and Czyzyk AS (1992). Incidence of insulin-dependent diabetes in Warsaw, Poland, in children and young adults, 1983–1988. *World Health Statistics Quarterly*, **45**, 315–20.

Zatonski W (2004). Tobacco smoking in central European countries: Poland. In *Tobacco, science, policy and public health* (ed. P Boyle, N Gray, J Henningford, J Seffrin, and W Ztonski). Oxford University Press, London, pp. 235–52.

Zatonski W and Boyle P (1996). Commentary; Health transformations in Poland after 1988. *Journal of Epidemiology and Biostatistics*, **1**, 183–97.

Zatonski W and Willet W (2005). Changes in dietary fat and declining coronary heart disease in Poland: population based study. *British Medical Journal*, **331**, 187–8.

Zatonski W and Becker N (in collaboration with Gottesman K, Mykowiecka A, and Tyczynski J) (1988). *Atlas of cancer mortality in Poland, 1975–1979*. Springer Verlag, Heidelberg.

Zatonski W, Smans M, Tyczynski J, and Boyle P (1996). *Atlas of cancer mortality in Central Europe*, IARC Scientific Publication No 134. International Agency for Research on Cancer, Lyon.

Zejda JE and Kowalska M (2003). Risk factors for asthma in school children – results of seven-year follow-up. *Central European Journal of Public Health*, **11**, 154–9.

Przesmycki F. *The role of National Institute of Hygiene in formation of the health care system*. Lecture at the meeting of the Scientific Council of National Institute of Hygiene (PZH) celebrating the 45th Anniversary of the foundation of PZH.

35

Epidemiology and public health in Finland and Scandinavia: development and current state

Arpo Aromaa

Personal experiences

I was born in 1942 and graduated in medicine (Helsinki, 1966) and in social medicine (Edinburgh, 1968). In 1981 I obtained a MScD with a dissertation on hypertension as a public health problem. Between 1971 and 1995 I was the Medical Director and Director of the Social Insurance Institution's research unit. Since 1995 I have been a Research Professor in the National Public Health Institute and Head of the Department of Health and Functional Capacity. I have also been the Vice-president of the International Federation of Medical Students Associations 1966–67, a Member of the Council of the International Epidemiological Association (IEA) from 1984 to 1993 and its Secretary from 1987 to 1993.

Chance played a large role in my career, as always. However, there was obviously a relevant background. Chairmanships of associations of medical students and doctors, comprising also the International Federation of Medical Students' Associations, provided the view and personal contacts leading me toward a career in epidemiology. Also, I had become interested in macro level thinking and influencing policies. Professionally, a decisive moment was a 2-year grant given to me by a Finnish foundation. Their selection was based on activities in student and professional organizations. Personal contacts led me to the above-mentioned post-graduate course just set up in Edinburgh.

From then on the next steps were quite natural, from appointments in the health services, university public health departments, the Social Insurance Institutions Research Department, and now the National Public Health Institute. Chance led me to the IEA. An acquaintance from the British Medical Students Association, Michael Garraway, was Secretary of the IEA when the association was looking for a place to hold its meeting in 1987. He consulted with Leo Kaprio, the WHO Regional Director. Then I was contacted and after discussion with colleagues we found the place in Helsinki.

Introduction

Since the 1960s the Nordic countries and in particular Finland have been known for their high standards of public health policy and epidemiological research. Finnish health policy had probably the closest ties to the World Health Organization's (WHO) 'Health For All' policy. After the year 2000 Swedish health policy was reformed and is currently based on modifying the determinants of health whereas its previous emphasis was on provision of health care, particularly hospital care. In Finland during the latter half of the twentieth century epidemiology and health services research were in direct response to the high cardiovascular disease mortality and efforts to improve provision and access to health-care services.

In this description I will mainly deal with Finland, but brief overviews about epidemiology in the other Nordic countries are presented in the incorporated boxes. Regardless of the effects of international trends on Nordic health policy and epidemiology it is remarkable that public health policy, epidemiology, and health services research have been strengthening now for six decades in Finland. The following account is an effort to explain the development in Finland and why it is both similar and different from that in the other Nordic countries.

The four Nordic countries and their health care

Today the larger Nordic countries, Finland, Sweden, Denmark, and Norway, jointly have about 24 million inhabitants. Historically the countries have had close ties by belonging to the same kingdoms. Early developments in Sweden and Finland were similar, as Finland was part of the Swedish kingdom for many centuries until it was surrendered to the Russian Empire in 1809. Despite their common roots the situation of the Nordic countries in Europe is quite different today. All of them vouch for the welfare state model, but its implementation is different. The four countries share a high standard of living with GNPs close to each other and among the highest in the world. Much of the prosperity is derived from high-technology production and extensive services financed in whole or in part by taxation. In Norway oil production is the main source of income from natural resources and in Sweden and Finland a comparable source of wealth is the paper and pulp industry based in part on the availability of wood from their extensive forests; in the last decade mobile phone production has become a significant source of income. Denmark's wealth is derived from a mix of high-technology production, agricultural production, and services. In all the Nordic countries social welfare is of a high standard and one of the indicators of health—life expectancy—is among the highest in the world.

In the 1800s much of public health care was provided by provincial or municipal doctors employed by the state or the local communities. The ensuing expansion has led to administratively quite divergent systems. Whereas the basic structure in all countries comprises publicly employed primary-care doctors and several levels of publicly funded specialized hospitals, all of them have organized and financed these services differently. Recently the main types of solutions have been coverage of costs of the hospital system by local communities and their federations (Finland), by counties (Sweden), and by the State (Norway).

In Finland, primary-care doctors are mainly employed by local municipalities in health centres. In addition there are doctors working part-time or full-time in the private sector, where fees are reimbursed in part by the sickness insurance scheme. There is a long tradition of midwives and public health nurses taking care of maternity and child welfare and also health education at large. The hospital system comprises regional hospitals run by federations of municipalities. In Sweden primary-care doctors are mainly employed by the local authority or county, but a large proportion are private. In Denmark primary care is provided by British style general practitioners remunerated by local communities. In Norway the majority of primary-care providers are also remunerated from public funds.

In the early years of hygiene, public health, and epidemiology these disciplines had much impact on the provision and organization of preventive and curative care. This can be understood on the basis of the immediate impact of infectious diseases and poor hygiene on public health, such as maternal and infant mortality as well as mortality from common infectious diseases. In the current situation the acceptance of epidemiology may be more difficult to understand. Whereas epidemiology and public health have certainly contributed to the developments of preventive and curative care there have been other major influences. There are examples of basic epidemiological findings influencing policy and content decisions in prevention. However, health services research and its findings are often too close to politics to be able to overcome other considerations. Therefore, in the organization of health care the gap between what is known and what is done remains large.

Origins of epidemiology and public health

In all Nordic countries, just as elsewhere in Europe, the beginning of today's public health is in the prevention of infectious diseases and of premature mortality due to them. Early in the twentieth century Pasteur Institutes were set up in many countries with the task of diagnosis and prevention of communicable diseases. These state institutes were the backbone for controlling infections endangering public health. Lacking specialized public health doctors, the local and provincial health personnel were the representatives of these institutes in the whole country. Local community doctors had realized late in the 19th century and early on in the twentieth century that it was important to understand the occurrence and causes of malnutrition and infectious and chronic diseases and their variation in the community. In the late 1800s and the early 1900s disciplines like hygiene also emerged in the medical curricula in order to enable doctors to prevent communicable diseases not only by vaccinations but also by advising on nutrition and environmental issues, such as clean food and water.

A still earlier development leading to one of the basics of epidemiology, demography, was the censuses and population statistics originally meant to help the Crown in raising taxes and men (and horses) for war. In Sweden–Finland these were supplemented by registers of births and deaths kept by parish priests. To their task was added also the recording of causes of death. During recent decades these books have been a rich source for genetics and genetic epidemiology in the reconstruction of family trees.

Since the early 1900s prevention and treatment of tuberculosis understandably preoccupied a large number of doctors interested in controlling major public health problems. Following the containment of infectious diseases by vaccinations and hygienic measures the next preventable health problems, i.e. maternal and perinatal mortality, gained ground in the 1930s and 1940s. In the post-Second World War period the scientific community's attention was drawn to the toll of non-communicable diseases, and this era continues. In terms of scientific disciplines public health after the 1940s and 1950s covers a much broader field than before. In the Nordic countries, as elsewhere, its current foundations comprise disciplines such as epidemiology, health services research, hygiene, microbiology and virology, molecular medicine, the social sciences, and biometrics. Epidemiology is subdivided into communicable disease epidemiology and non-communicable disease epidemiology.

Finland

Developments in Finland are an excellent demonstration of all the above. The mortality statistics (tables) prepared by priests had since about 1748 to record one of 30 causes of death.

But it took a long time before the system was modernized. Since 1936 the causes of death were recorded on the basis of death certificates issued by doctors. In Finland, the first reported survey of the population's health was carried out by a local municipal doctor (Relander 1892) but church population registers (parish registers) go back to the sixteenth century. The Pasteur Institute today is KTL (www.ktl.fi), a comprehensive public health institute, many of the previous health threats have been contained, and comprehensive monitoring of population health has become systematic.

Combating tuberculosis

Tuberculosis prevention was initiated early in the 1900s with BCG vaccination. A systematic public health approach resulted from the combination of vaccinations, early detection by tuberculin tests and mass chest X-rays, and treatment by a network of tuberculosis sanatoriums built in the supposedly healthy environments of pine forests. This comprehensive scheme was employed from the 1920s to the 1970s, and in terms of the near eradication of tuberculosis results have been excellent. Over the years a multitude of scientific reports have dealt with the incidence and prevalence of tuberculosis infections, with their prognosis, and with the efficacy of drug treatment. These were applications of epidemiology with the data coming from the comprehensive tuberculosis detection and treatment scheme. The findings were also compiled into detailed articles in the Finnish Tuberculosis Association's yearbook. Some of the key personalities were Risto and Jorma Pätiälä and A. Sakari Härö. The Finnish Tuberculosis Association also took initiatives in many other fields of public health.

Laying the foundation for good child health

Surveillance and health promotion for infants was initiated by Arvo Ylppö, who developed his ideas whilst studying in the Charité in Berlin in the 1920s. Upon his initiative a network of child welfare clinics was set up throughout the whole country. All children were followed up regularly, they were vaccinated, and their mothers received advice on feeding, diet, and other matters. This practice continues until today and covers practically all infants. It is also the basis for the comprehensive vaccination programme. The visits to child welfare clinics resulted in millions of records held manually and containing a description of health and growth from birth through to school entry. For many decades Finnish infant mortality has been among the very lowest in Europe. However, it is well known that the work in child welfare needs to be reformed to correspond to present needs. One can only hope that the invisible organizational hurdles to this can be overcome. A recent initiative is the establishment of a Department of Child and Youth Health in the National Public Health Institute, KTL.

Besides being a first-class paediatrician and prime promoter of child welfare, Arvo Ylppö is an example of a multitalented person promoting health and public health in such diverse areas as building a large children's hospital for which he raised the funds and founding the major pharmaceutical company in Finland.

Due to their public health orientation many paediatricians have also been active in epidemiology and health services research. In the 1950s they initiated the first follow-up surveys of children's health and growth, resulting in an understanding of healthy growth and in the growth curves similar to those still used today in the welfare clinics. Others carried out surveys of the child population in their region to make sure that needs were met. However, the boom of epidemiology in child health began in the 1970s and continues (see below).

Epidemiology and health services research

Cancer epidemiology

Immediately after the Second World War Erkki Saxén, Professor of Pathology in the University of Helsinki, initiated a country wide cancer registry, which has been functioning since 1951 (Saxén and Teppo 1978). The registry's strength is its comprehensive high-quality data covering all incident cancers and its epidemiological expertise. Early years were largely devoted to producing tabulations of cancer occurrence and to descriptive epidemiology. The registry continues to publish a yearbook with complete tabulations of cancer incidence and participates in compiling comparable Nordic publications. It also has direct links with cancer screening and screening trials and evaluates their efficacy. Since the 1970s the opportunities have been used to their fullest. Often this has required linking cancer data to those from various population studies. The latter were initially designed for cardiovascular or other chronic disease epidemiology, but large stores of frozen serum samples and linkage of records to the cancer registry and other registers has been an excellent opportunity for cancer epidemiology. Key people in the cancer registry from the 1960s have been Lyly Teppo, Matti Hakama, and Timo Hakulinen, who is the present director.

To name just some important topics of applied research, reports have dealt with modelling prognosis in breast cancer, assessing socio-economic differences in cancer and survival in cancer, estimating the impact of cervical screening, and recently of prostate-specific antigen (PSA)—screening for prostate cancer and assessing future cancer trends. Causal research based on longitudinal population studies has concerned possible determinants such as serum antioxidants and vitamins, dietary fatty acids, and infections.

Cardiovascular diseases and other chronic conditions

The beginnings of modern epidemiology and public health in Finland can be traced back to the early 1950s when in parallel with the establishment of the cancer registry the nationwide fight against cardiovascular diseases was initiated by surveys of coronary heart disease and its risk factors. The first surveys were linked to the beginnings of Ancel Keys' Seven Country Study (Karvonen *et al.* 1967) and one of the key Finnish workers was Martti Karvonen. The need to do something about the main killer of middle-aged men, coronary heart disease, was a strong motivation for research. Around 1960 coronary heart disease mortality of middle-aged men was higher than anywhere else in Europe. At the same time also the ratio of male mortality to female mortality was much higher than elsewhere.

The introduction of the sickness insurance scheme in 1964 was also a milestone for epidemiology. The law stipulated that 2% of its revenue should be used for prevention, rehabilitation, and relevant research. One of the preventive measures was to set up in the mid-1960s the Social Insurance Institution's Mobile Clinic Unit (Heinonen 1966). Its initial purpose was to screen for chronic diseases and their risk factors. Later its task was transformed and it was to investigate the occurrence of chronic diseases, their treatment situation, and their risk factors in the population. This transition from screening to epidemiology was due to the insight that the latter would be more important for the health of the population. Field work involved close to 100,000 persons. During field work the key figures were Olli P. Heinonen, and Jouni Maatela, and during data analysis Arpo Aromaa. In collaboration with the University of Helsinki a large dietary history interview survey of more than 10,000 subjects was carried out. The subjects have been followed-up with registers and this work continues out. The epidemiological studies have resulted in a very large number of epidemiological observations.

Furthermore, to evaluate and develop sickness insurance a series of nationwide health interview surveys (Purola *et al.* 1968) was initiated, the first one was in 1964 and the most recent so far in 1995/6. The Social Insurance Institution also set up a research unit for analysing and reporting on their findings. Several current senior epidemiologists were trained in their work in the Social Insurance Institution. However, as part of a streamlining process, by the late 1990s epidemiological research (or as it was called social medicine) was transferred to KTL, the National Public Health Institute.

A remarkable development in the early 1970s was the initiation of the North Karelia Project (Puska *et al.* 1981), an effort to reduce the burden of cardiovascular diseases in the community by methods now defined as promotion, prevention, and information dissemination. Key persons initially were Pekka Puska and the late Kai Sievers, and one of the important promoters was Martti Karvonen. Up to that time it was one of the largest community-level intervention projects based on epidemiological findings.

The North Karelia project started to carry out yearly postal surveys of health behaviour and 5-yearly risk factor surveys, and set up myocardial infarction registers. The project was also closely tied to the WHO Monica Project, in fact its disease registers and surveys were the Finnish Monica surveys. Amongst the numerous key people involved in the multicountry project Kari Kuulasmaa of KTL played a key role, being responsible for the databases and much of the analysis. The various surveys continue to this day and provide valuable information on health behaviour, risk factors, and dietary habits. In the 1980s the central staff of the North Karelia Project was attached to the National Public Health Laboratory, KTL.

The activity of the mobile clinic unit requires a few more words. First, several large epidemiological field investigations were carried out. In 1973–76 there was a follow-up study of 20,000 people previously investigated and in 1978–80 the Mini-Finland Health Examination Survey (Aromaa *et al.* 1989), the first of its kind in Europe, was carried out. The survey was broader than the well-known US National Health Examination Surveys. It was based on a broad view of health and covered all the major chronic conditions, their determinants, and functional limitations. The study was led by Arpo Aromaa. The Mini-Finland survey comprised a thorough home interview and a health examination of 8000 people aged 30 or over and representing the country's population. Remarkably, its participation rate was 95%. Its main emphasis was on the major chronic conditions, cardiovascular diseases, respiratory diseases, musculoskeletal diseases, mental health problems, oral health, and functional limitations. The study was a forerunner, in Europe at least, in regard to the epidemiology of musculoskeletal diseases, mental health problems, oral health, and functional limitations. All the people examined were followed up with record linkage to central Finnish registers (see below). An additional benefit was that several clinicians were trained in the epidemiology of their respective field. Numerous articles from the above studies cover a vast array of descriptive epidemiology and causal research ranging from the occurrence of chronic conditions to their impact on mortality, from the occurrence of risk factors to their impact on disease occurrence and death, to the study of possible determinants such as physical and mental strain, physical activity, serum antioxidants, vitamins and infections, or intake of various items from food.

A recent equally large joint effort is the nationwide Health 2000 Survey (Aromaa and Koskinen 2004) which is a modernized version of the Mini-Finland survey comprising a home health interview and a comprehensive health examination of a two-stage sample of 10,000 adults aged 18 and over. A subsample of people who originally participated in the Mini-Finland survey was also examined. Comparability with the previous survey was a first priority. Thus, Finland now has a set of interview and examination data describing not only a population cross-section but also enabling the estimation of 20-year trends and a longitudinal data set.

Epidemiology in children and young people

The first long-term multipurpose follow-up study was initiated by Paula Rantakallio in the 1960s when all newborns in North Finland were registered. Their follow-up with intermediate field surveys and register-based data has lasted over 40 years and is continuing now by KTL. As a logical follow-up to the cardiovascular disease studies in adults, two other studies in children were initiated in the early 1980s with initiatives also from the Academy of Finland. One (atherosclerosis risk factors in children) comprised several urban and rural cohorts of children aged 0, 1, 3, 6, 9 and 12 years from various parts of the country and it was led by Hans Åkerblom, Jorma Viikari, and Matti Uhari with support from several experienced epidemiologists. The children have also been followed up by repeated surveys. The other (Strip) is a follow-up and experiment in newborns with dietary intervention directed by Olli Simell. In addition to themes relating to tracking of risk factors and causes these studies have shown that considerable reduction of levels of low-density lipoprotein (LDL) cholesterol levels by dietary means is feasible and safe in children. Both of these studies have been carried out in collaboration with the SII, and are now proceeding with collaboration with the Department of Health and Functional Capacity of KTL.

The impact of child health, particularly undernutrition (Barker's hypothesis), on adult health has been studied utilizing the records of maternity and child welfare clinics and hospitals. These studies have been carried out in collaboration between Johan Eriksson and David Barker.

Repeated postal surveys have concentrated on school-age children. One of them is the Health Habits Survey of Arja Rimpelä, providing three-decade-long time series of a random sample of Finnish children. The other is the School Health Survey led by Matti Rimpelä based on total school classes. The third one is the Finnish arm of the WHO School Health survey.

Health services research

The Sickness Insurance Act of 1964 also meant the beginnings of large-scale health services research in Finland. The first phase was a nationwide household survey in 1964 and the aim of the second phase in 1967 was to evaluate the initial effects of sickness insurance.

These surveys were led by the social policy specialist Tapani Purola, who became the first director of the Research Institute for Social Security of the Social Insurance Institution of Finland. Today there are 60 employees in the research department of SII. After Tapani Purola it was led by Esko Kalimo, Arpo Aromaa, and Mikael Forss.

Later, the SII repeated its health surveys in 1976, 1987, and 1995. As mentioned above, its other research activity was epidemiological research based on the mobile clinic surveys and the Mini-Finland survey. Other large-scale studies carried out were on the causes of sickness absence in Finland, the development of occupational health care for farmers, and the family doctor experiment (Aromaa *et al.* 1998). Occupational health care for farmers resulted in a model for health care adopted by the National Board of Health. The family doctor experiment demonstrated clear benefits of the experimental model but none of its elements have so far been adopted.

Demographic research

Demographics is taught at the Department of Sociology of the University of Helsinki. A forerunner in the field was the Actuary of Statistics Finland Väinö Kannisto, who already by the late 1940s prepared population forecasts and demonstrated the effect of diseases. In the 1960s Tapani Valkonen joined forces with Statistics Finland and created a long-term research programme on socio-economic differences in mortality (Valkonen *et al.* 1993). Several of the scientists from that programme have in the meantime joined the Department of Health and Functional Capacity at KTL.

Intervention studies and experiments

The largest epidemiological intervention studies have been the North Karelia Project and the ATBP Study. The ATBP Study was led by Jussi Huttunen and Olli P. Heinonen and it was a randomized intervention to evaluate the effect of certain vitamins on health. It was carried out in collaboration with US National Cancer Institute.

The quasi-experimental family doctor study mentioned above was carried out in four large cities over 9 years. A combination of a personal doctor, reduced costs, and a simple possibility to consult private sector specialists improved satisfaction with primary care in all population groups.

The tradition of evaluation research

The foundation for modern evaluation research was laid with the repeated SII National Household Health surveys carried out in 1964 and 1967 with the aim of assessing the impact of the sickness insurance scheme on use, met need, and costs of health-care services. Many criticisms could be raised about the before–after design, but nevertheless the findings proved extremely important. Large regional differences were observed in the use of health care. Sickness insurance enhanced use and reduced costs but could, of course, not correct the lack of service provision. These observations were important when the Public Health Act of 1972 was directed at enhancing provision of municipal primary care in all parts of the country.

Another imbedded series of findings were those concerning dental care, clearly demonstrating the inadequate provision despite abundant availability of trained personnel. It also became clear that the out of pocket costs of dental care prevented use according to need. After these observations were widely known in the late 1970s it still required a national clinical dental survey (Mini-Finland Survey) and many committee memoranda before the whole adult population was covered by reduced-price services in the early 2000s. The evaluation tradition was continued by the second national survey of dental health in conjunction with the Health 2000 survey and a four-phase postal survey, repeated so far three times, with the specific task of assessing the impact of the new legislation on dental care.

The family doctor study lasting 9 years not only continued the tradition but also introduced into real settings an experimental design based on intervention and control groups in four cities. As a research project it was unusual, since primary care services for 40,000 people were funded by the Social Insurance Institution for 9 years. The findings mentioned above were very promising, but none of the recommendations has so far been taken on board in the Finnish health-care system.

Surveillance and health monitoring

The communicable disease notification scheme and register of KTL is the foundation for communicable disease surveillance. One of the early schemes involved notification of tuberculosis. Outbreak investigation is also part of traditional surveillance at KTL. In recent years surveillance has mainly been used to establish the causes of water- and food-borne infections.

Health monitoring is deeply rooted in the tradition of the national health interview and health examination surveys. It has also always been combined with research interests, making it more attractive to researchers. In addition to the survey data, indicators from various registers (see below) are used. The population survey system today comprises yearly postal questionnaires to a sample of the adult population, postal questionnaires to young people at 2-year intervals, FinRisk surveys at 5-year intervals and comprehensive surveys similar to Health 2000 surveys at 10–15-year interval. The FinRisk surveys are a continuation of the North Karelia Project and FinMonica Project surveys and they comprise a moderate risk factor survey. The Health 2000 type surveys comprise a thorough health interview and a comprehensive health examination. At present, efforts are on-going to add the health monitoring of children to the system. It is intended that in future Finnish health policy will be based on a comprehensive view of health and health-care needs, their past development, and their future (Data Reform 2004 Report). The information is interpreted and disseminated in books entitled *Health in Finland*, with the latest English-language version published in 2006 (Koskinen *et al.* 2006).

Organizational basis

Registers of health and health care

One of the prerequisites of epidemiological research in Finland is the capacity to link national register-based data on health and its determinants to population surveys. Record linkage is straightforward due to the national person identification number (PIN) which was introduced in the early 1960s together with sickness insurance. In many countries record linkage is still seen as a threat to privacy. According to Finnish legislation on personal data and medical research, processing and linking of personal data for research purposes is explicitly allowed, provided that the required precautions are taken (Aromaa *et al.* 2006). The Information 2005 Report contains a description both of health surveys and of registers (Data and Information Reform 2004).

Important national registers comprise those on causes of deaths, causes of disability pensions, hospital discharges, cancer, occupational diseases, as well as specially reimbursed and other medicines. It is customary to link these with each other or with population survey data using the PIN. Much of epidemiological research has been carried out utilizing these data sources. In order to enhance the use of registers several institutes have together funded a support centre for register based research (Retki). Typical approaches have been to follow up examinees by several of the registers, use their health data as end-points, and assess the impact of suspected determinants on those outcomes.

Public research institutes

The four state-financed research institutes in the sector of the Ministry of Social Affairs and Health are the Finnish Institute of Occupational Health (FIOH, Työterveyslaitos; www.ttl.fi), the National Public Health Institute (KTL, Kansanterveyslaitos; www.ktl.fi), the National Research and Development Centre for Welfare (STAKES, Sosiaali-ja terveysalan tutkimus-ja kehittämiskeskus; www.stakes.fi), and the Institute for Radiation Protection (STUK, Säteilyturvakeskus; www.stuk.fi). Other important state institutes are the Social Insurance Institution's (Kela; www.kela.fi) Research Department and Statistics Finland (Tilastokeskus; www.stat.fi). Universities also play a role, but perhaps are not as important as in some other countries.

The FIOH stems from the 1950s when Leo Noro was able to persuade Finnish and American stakeholders, including the Finnish labour organizations, of the need for an institute to improve occupational health. His successor Jorma Rantanen managed to further strengthen the institute. The general manager now is Harri Vainio, previously at IARC. The institute has over 650 employees. In more than six decades it has researched and developed the working conditions in the whole country. Its backbone is the obligatory occupational health-care system with several thousands of nurses and doctors trained by the institute. Its methods range from molecular biology and toxicology to epidemiology and biometrics.

The National Public Health Institute (KTL) was founded in the early 1900s as the State Serum Institute to prevent infectious diseases and to produce vaccines. After the Second World War it was led by Eero Uroma. Major changes resulting in its present structure began after Jussi Huttunen was appointed its Director General in 1980. On the basis of the work of a State Committee KTL was developed to become a central research institute for chronic communicable diseases, communicable diseases, and environmental health. Currently, KTL is headed by Pekka Puska, the leader of the North Karelia Project, and KTL's activities range from infectious diseases and environmental health to health promotion and chronic communicable diseases, molecular biology, and genetics. At present KTL has about 900 employees, of whom 250 are in the two general epidemiology units. The first boost to general epidemiology in KTL was the affiliation of the key persons of the North Karelia Project to KTL, leading to the establishment of the Department for Epidemiology and Health Promotion led today by Erkki Vartiainen. The second was the affiliation of the SII medical research group in 1995, leading to the foundation of the Department of Health and Functional Capacity led by Arpo Aromaa. The latter department was strengthened by a further

40 people from the SII in 2004. Two other major changes had occurred in the mid-1980s when the Department for Mental Health was established to investigate suicides and their prevention under the leadership of Jouko Lönnqvist. In the late 1990s the research department of the Finnish alcohol monopoly (ALKO) was transferred half and half to KTL and to STAKES, and the department in KTL was renamed the Department for Mental Health and Alcohol Research. One of KTL's strengths is genetic epidemiology directed by Leena Palotie. It is currently involved in researching genetic determinants of common chronic conditions. Its more traditional approaches have led to the identification of a large number of inherited conditions grouped under the title 'The Finnish Disease Inheritance'.

The third Institute (STAKES) is a result of transforming parts of the previous central administration (National Board of Social Welfare, National Board of Health) into a research institute. Since its establishment in the early 1990s it has been headed by Vappu Taipale, a psychiatrist and a former Minister of Health. STAKES received some of the alcohol research from ALKO, as mentioned above. STAKES is the central organization for health-care and social services registers and statistics and a research institute for welfare and health-care research. It has also done some work in the field of epidemiology.

The Institute for Radiation Protection (STUK) is mainly responsible for radiation safety and surveillance of environmental radiation but it has also been involved in epidemiological research on the effects of both high and low levels of radiation. Recently a large programme has been related to researching the possible relationship of radio wavelength radiation from cellular phones to intracranial cancers.

The Social Insurance Institution (SII, Kela) has since the 1960s had a research department, originally called the Research Institute for Social Security. It currently has 60 staff members. A process of reorientation has been ongoing for many years and it seems finally to have a more stable future. The major research areas are expected to be social science, economics, social security in general, pension policy, health and safety care, rehabilitation, and sickness insurance. In addition to its own research the SII has a major impact on research, first due to holding large numbers of data on the population and its health, and second by granting research funding available on the basis of the current rehabilitation law, 24% of the income of sickness insurance.

Statistics Finland (Tilastokeskus) is the central agency for statistics. It hosts the mortality and causes of death register and carries out numerous household interview surveys. In earlier years its Level of Living surveys provided important data on health. In recent years its interviewers have been employed to carry out health interviews in the SII Health Survey 1995/6 and the KTL Coordinated Health 2000 Survey in 2000 and 2001.

Until recently the state research institutes have been growing, but much of the growth has been due to outside grants. From 2005 there have been strong pressures mainly from the Ministry of Exchequer to transfer some of their resources to other activities and also to reduce their staff. The outcome of these ongoing disputes is not yet known.

The Academy of Sciences of Finland

The Academy of Sciences has played a major role, particularly in the 1970s and 1980s. During those years part of the grants were given to target-oriented research. Many groups with relatively little experience in chronic disease epidemiology were financed. Although criticized at the time those grants were probably the seed money needed for many epidemiological careers.

In later years the competition for funding between real science, i.e. basic research, and applied research, such as epidemiology and health services research, has been quite fierce. Those with an applied orientation have often felt that they are losing the battle.

European Union research and public health

Since Finland joined EU in 1995 Finnish researchers have been involved in both the EU Public Health Programme and the Research Programme. The Research Programme has been an important source of funds and European collaboration. Recently, in the Public Health Programme, the position of Finnish researchers has become much stronger with new important R&D projects. KTL is currently leading two EU-wide projects: the ECHIM (European Community Health Indicators and Monitoring) Project intending to implement health indicators in all member states and the FEHES (Feasibility of Health Examinations in Europe) Project. The background for both is the expertise, experience, and the well-developed health-care and research structures in Finland.

It is essential to mention the other international sources of funding. Two US bodies, the National Institutes of Health and the National Cancer Institute, have funded major Finnish projects. To a large part this has been due to the excellent population study materials, the ability to implement successful population-level experiments, and the exceptionally high participation rates. It is fair to say that Finnish researchers have been welcomed as collaborators in many US-led and funded projects.

But international funding schemes share a problem, and a great deal of trouble is caused due to their unnecessary attention to budgeting detail. Many researchers are likely to share the view that it is fine to make sure that the research to be carried out is of the highest class but that it is not sensible to try to make pre-project calculations accurate to very small amounts.

Public health as a speciality, universities and training

In Finland, public health is a medical speciality although there are no designated public health doctors employed by the health-care system. Instead, their natural duties are traditionally being taken care of by municipally employed doctors and by physicians in administrative positions in hospital districts and large municipalities. Nevertheless, with support of university departments of public health and the Public Health Doctors' Association formal training and specialist examinations have been kept up. As has been planned, many of the post-graduates have been employed in public health and administrative positions.

After the era of hygiene, universities have not been particularly strong in public health. However, with the increasing number of young doctors in training, university research is also getting a boost. Another strategy has been their alliance with the State research institutes. The third has been the close tie with the two main associations in the field, the Society for Social Medicine and the Finnish Public Health Doctor's Association. It is fair to say that many of the international contacts and opportunities have arrived at the universities via key persons in these associations. Certainly the rebuilding of the medical speciality is almost entirely due to the work of people active in the Public Health Doctor's Association.

Its most recent chairmen are Kimmo Koskenvuo, Arpo Aromaa, and since 2006, Taina Mäntyranta.

However, universities have also been involved in some important epidemiological projects, often together with State research institutes. Examples are both the child health surveys mentioned above, the East–West Diabetes Survey and several of the SII and KTL national surveys, which have drawn on universities to provide special knowledge in fields such as mental health, oral health, or cognitive testing. Doctors in post-graduate training have been proposed themes for their theses and they have often been a major addition to the workforce for reporting on the surveys.

Training abroad and other international contacts

'Early birds' in public health and epidemiology after the Second World War were several physicians who went for training abroad, first particularly to public health schools in the USA and later to the UK. Examples from the 1950s are Leo Kaprio, previously Regional Director WHO Europe and A. S. Härö, Chief of Planning of the National Board of Health. In the early 1960s Olli Miettinen went to Boston to concentrate on epidemiology and biometrics. He came back every year to hold 3-week epidemiology courses in Helsinki. Most current Finnish public health specialists attended those. The last years of the 1960s saw Olli P. Heinonen, later Professor of Public Health in Helsinki, go to Harvard to work in the Boston Collaborative Drug Surveillance Program and to work on his thesis. In the 1960s and 1970s Arpo Aromaa, Professor at KTL, and Kimmo Leppo Chief Medical Officer at the Ministry of Health attended training in UK. Other persons attending London courses were Jarkko Eskola, Chief Medical Officer, Timo Klaukka, Director of Health Research, and Seppo Koskinen, Chief Physician in my department at KTL. Several post-graduates went to Harvard University or other US schools of public health. To name just a few Timo Sahi, who became Chief Medical Officer of the Armed Forces, and Matti Rajala, who until recently was Chief of Unit in EU Sanco (Directorate for Consumer Affairs and Health).

The International Society of Cardiology, at the time chaired by J. Stamler, organized 10-day summer schools in different parts of the world. In the 1970s those were attended by many of those who were to become key figures in Finnish cardiovascular disease studies such as the Mobile Clinic Health Examination survey and the North Karelia Project.

However, public health was not alone in this trend since many later leading physicians went for periods of post-graduate training in the early years after the Second World War, first to the UK, for example to the Hammersmith Hospital or the Hospital for Sick Children, and later mainly to the USA. During the era after 1980 practically all research-inclined post-graduates spent at least a year in one of the US centres.

In the 1970s a private foundation (the Yrjö Jahnsson Foundation) giving grants for both economics and medicine decided to fill the gap in a related speciality, health economics. It created a grant scheme for training in health economics and over the years practically all Finnish health economists have completed their PhD studies in York, UK. The first was Harri Sintonen, Professor in the Department of Public Health Science in the University of Helsinki.

Additional advantages of these training periods have been the networks created. Some of the outcomes have been close contacts with international research groups and societies such as the International Epidemiological Association and the European Public Health Association.

Conclusion: why is epidemiology strong in Finland?

Taking into account the above description and other less formal information it is first of all fair to say that epidemiology and health services research are both more developed and used more in Finland than in many other European countries. Although attracting young graduates to public health and epidemiology is quite difficult, partly due to the lack of career prospects, interest among the younger generation is alive. People interested in health policy and health-care administration find the discipline attractive. Judged on the basis of numbers of researchers and senior experts in the field the resources devoted to the disciplines are considerable, and probably larger than in many other countries. However, future prospects may be more ambiguous.

The current relative strength is probably mainly related to quite a few factors. First, a systematic approach to disease control had been adopted early to control tuberculosis. Second, since the 1940s visionary paediatricians were able to push for the creation of a nationwide network of child welfare clinics. Third, after the Second World War the whole of Finnish society expressed an urge for international contacts. This led amongst other things to post-graduate public health training in the USA and the UK. Those early and later contacts were highly valued during post-war reconstruction. At the same time the expertise gained abroad served to improve both scientific and public health activities. Fourth, a critical mass was probably created by the 1970s when it started to perpetuate actions in both research and public health. The activities of the speciality associations should not be underestimated.

However, the above arguments alone cannot explain why epidemiology has been successful. There must be an underlying cause. It may well be that the Finn's positive approach to life has

---

Denmark

- In the 1880s the first epidemiological survey on measles was carried out by Panum in the Faeroe Islands.
- The first national health interview survey was carried out soon after the Second World War.
- A mortality and causes of death register as well as a cancer register were established in 1943.
- The predecessor of the National Public Health Institute (www.niph.dk) was the Danish Tuberculosis Index founded in 1954. From 1972 to 1999 it was called the Danish Institute of Clinical Epidemiology. The institute has about 90 employees.
- Communicable disease surveillance and prevention is placed in another national institute (Statens Seruminstitut, serum@ssi.dk) founded in 1902.
- The well-known epidemiological cardiovascular disease survey began in Glostrup in the 1950s.
- National Health Interview surveys have been carried out since 1987 and record linkage has also been used. The setting up of the surveys was preceded by a period of Nordic experts working together with Danish colleagues.

Norway

- In the 1950s and 1960s epidemiological studies were a strength of Norway. Large surveys provided excellent data on obesity and hypertension (Bjerkedal 1957).

- In the 1960s and 1970s remarkable regional cardiovascular disease studies were carried out. Later the infrastructure of the chest X-ray screening system was used.

- Compared to the other Nordic countries Norway was late in establishing a comprehensive national public health institute.

- The National Public Health Institute in Oslo (Folkehelseinstituttet; www.fui.no) has about 800 employees working in communicable and non-communicable diseases and environment and health.

- Norway has a large number of national health-related registers (Cappelen and Lyshol 2004), which comprise, for example, mortality, cancer, births, communicable diseases, tuberculosis, vaccination, treatment quality.

Sweden

- Due to the common history the description of Finland covers most of the developments in Sweden until the early 1900s.

- Early chronic disease epidemiology beginning in the 1960s was centred in Gothenburg (study of men born in 1913, Tibblin 1967).

- The Värmland Study (Socialstyrelsen 1968) was initiated and inspired by the progress of laboratory automation. Large numbers of individuals were subjected to multiphasic screening.

- In 1970 a population follow-up survey of 70-year-olds had been initiated in Gothenburg by Alvar Svanborg.

- In the 1970s and 1980s experimental health centres were set up to examine ways to improve health-care provision. These centres became hallmarks of health services research.

- Some county-wide health surveys have been carried out, but the only national survey is the Level of Living Survey (ULF) by Statistics Sweden. This interview also comprises health data.

- The Swedish National Public Health Institute (SNIPH) was established in 1992 and has some 160 staff. It has played a major role in formulating the new public health policy. The approach is based on policies and programmes to modify risk factors and other determinants.

- Sweden has well-developed health and health-care registers. Their data and information have been organized in an exemplary fashion by the Epidemiological Center of the National Board of Welfare and Health (Socialstyrelsen). Data such as mortality, cancer incidence, and hospital use can be viewed over the Internet using a straightforward user interface. The centre has about 60 employees. The Epidemiological Centre (www.sos.se/epc) publishes numerous reports, specifically a regular National Health Report (latest, Folkhalsorapport 2005).

favoured looking for explanations and evaluating reforms on the basis of empirical research. In health and health care this translates into epidemiology and health services research.

References

Aromaa A and Koskinen S (ed.) (2004). *Health and functional capacity in Finland. Baseline results of the Health 2000 health examination survey*, National Public Health Institute B 12/2004. National Public Health Institute, Helsinki (available at www.ktl.fi/health2000).

Aromaa A, Heliövaara M, Impivaara O, et al. (1989). *Terveys, toimintakyky ja hoidontarve Suomessa* [Health, functional capacity and need for care in Finland], Social Insurance Institution AL:32. Social Insurance Institution, Helsinki and Turku.

Aromaa A, Linnala A, Maljanen T, and Mattila K (1998). *Yksityislääkärit omalääkäreinä* [Private doctors as family doctors], Social Insurance Institution of Finland 39. Social Insurance Institution, Helsinki.

Aromaa A, Huovinen P, Leena M, et al. (2006). Good research practice in the National Public Health Institute Handbook. Publications of the National Public health Institute B4 (www.ktl.fi/publications).

Bjerkedal T (1957). Overweight and hypertension. *Acta Med Scandinavica*, **159**, 13–26.

Cappelen I and Lyshol H (2004). Oversikt over helseregistre I Norge [An overview of health registers in Norway]. *Norsk Epidemiologi*, **14**, 33–8.

Data and Information reform — Working Group report, English summary (2004). Ministry of Social Affairs and Health Working Groups Memorandums, **12**, Helsinki.

Folkhälsorapport (2005). Health in Sweden. The National Public Health Report. *Scandinavian Journal of Public Health*, Suppl. 67.

Heinonen OP (1966). Autoklinikka [The mobile clinic]. *Duodecim*, **82**, 1161–4.

Karvonen MJ, Blomqvist G, Kallio V, et al. (1967). Men in rural east and west Finland. In Epidemiological studies related to coronary heart disease: characteristics of men aged 40–59 in seven countries. *Acta Medica Scandinavica*, Suppl. 460.

Koskinen S, Aromaa A, Huttunen J, and Teperi J (2006). *Health in Finland*. National Public Health Institute, National Center for Research on Welfare and Health, Ministry of Social Affairs and Health, Helsinki.

Purola T, Kalimo E, Sievers K, and Nyman K (1968). *The utilization of the medical services and its relationship to morbidity, health resources and social factors*, National Pensions Institute of Finland, Series A:3. National Pensions Institute of Finland, Helsinki.

Puska P, Tuomilehto J, Salonen J, et al. (1981). *Community control of cardiovascular diseases in North Karela, Finland 1972–1977*. WHO, Copenhagen.

Relander K (1892). *Terveyshoidollisia tutkimuksia Haapajärven piirilääkäripiirissä I. Kuopio*. [Health studies in the district doctor area of Haapajärvi, near Kuopio].

Saxén E and Teppo L (1978). *Finnish Cancer Registry 1952–1977. Twenty-five years of a nation wide cancer registry*. Finnish Cancer Registry, Helsinki.

Socialstyrelsen (1968). *Hälsoundersökningen i Värmland 1962–1965*. Socialstyrelsen, Stockholm.

Statens Seruminstitut, Denmark (www.ssi.dk).

Tibblin G (1967). High blood pressure in men aged 50. *Acta Medica Scandinavica*, **470**, S1–S84.

Valkonen T, Martelin T, Rimpelä A, Notkola V, and Savela S (1993). Socioeconomic mortality differences in Finland 1981–1990. *Statistics Finland, Population*, **1**.

36

History of modern epidemiology: Italy

Rodolfo Saracci, Benedetto Terracini,
and Franco Merletti

From 25 April 1945, the end of the Second World War in the country, Italy was confronted with the major task of reorganizing, and often of reconstructing, all branches of collective life, from political to economic, from industry to the health services. Modern epidemiology, which was taking its first steps in UK and USA, was initially weak in Italy, and its beginnings took a long time, some 30 years. This was followed from the mid-1970s to about 1990 by a period of rapid and sustained development and differentiation into a variety of areas of investigation. The mature phase of the most recent years has seen epidemiology being consolidated as a complex permanently evolving and expanding research field.

Slow beginnings: 1945–75

The first post-war census (in 1951) enumerated a population of 47.5 million. Crude death rates per 100,000 (both sexes combined) had been falling from around 1352 in the last pre-war year (1939) to 1028 by 1949, essentially due to advances in the control of infectious and respiratory causes, mainly tuberculosis: cancers and cardiovascular diseases already ranked as the leading causes of death, although rates were substantially lower than in the UK or USA, for instance. A vigorous economic expansion took off and lasted for three decades, with a real (corrected for inflation) rate of increase of GDP close to 4.5% per year. Marked health improvements occurred during this period, the life expectancy at birth increasing between the early 1950s and the early 1970s from 63.7 to 69 years for males and from 67.2 to 74.9 years for females. Infant mortality was more than halved from 29.9 per 1000 to 14.2 for males and from 24.6 to 10.6 for females. Expenditure for health services as a proportion of GDP was less than 2% in the early 1950s but had increased to around 5% in the early 1970s, while the corresponding figures for research (all sectors) were less than 0.5% and about 0.8%.

Within this context it was only in the second half of the 1945–75 period, during the 1960s, that recognizable signs of modern epidemiology appeared in Italy, the preceding years having elapsed as an 'incubation period', in which both interest in epidemiology and the need for it increased.

Inputs to the early development came from four main sources: the academic institutes of hygiene, a number of hospital and academic medical departments, academic institutes concerned with genetics and medical statistics, and the social movement of the late 1960s and early 1970s.

The academic departments of hygiene

Research, teaching, and, more generally, matters of health of the population were the province of the university institutes of hygiene as Italy had not—and does not have even today—schools of public health outside the medical schools. While remaining informed of the results of modern epidemiological studies these institutes were, with some exceptions (Checcacci *et al.* 1965), slow in absorbing research, adopting research as a priority, and spreading its messages. Two likely and important reasons were the wide range of tasks that these institutes had to attend to and the political choices that shaped the organization of the Italian health services. Regarding the first reason, a partial table of contents of a standard manual of hygiene for medical students would list subjects as heterogeneous as health legislation, health services organization, health statistics, methods of prevention and control of infectious diseases, description and prophylaxis of individual infectious diseases, sewage systems, thermal regulation systems, and drinking water assessment methods. Besides posing an obvious burden at the teaching and consulting level, several of these subjects could each represent an entire field for research; it is therefore not surprising that, for instance, the developing field of laboratory virus research became a higher priority than epidemiology for personnel who mostly had a bacteriological background. One may also conjecture that epidemiological methods, particularly the new ones, would of necessity have become a higher priority if the health services had been reorganized along the lines proposed in September 1945 by the Health Committee of the Veneto region. With remarkable foresight the committee, led by A. Giovanardi, the hygiene professor at Padua University, proposed the institution of a national health service, uniform throughout the country but decentralized in its technical and economic operations. It was to be operated at the level of municipal districts under the coordinating responsibility of the local regional governments, in turn nationally guided by a Ministry of Health: to be functional this structure would have demanded an extensive use of epidemiology. Unfortunately the proposal was dismissed and conservative political choices prevailed, favouring the continuation, with adaptations, of the fragmented mixture of different health insurance schemes existing during the fascist era (Delogu 1967). The advent of a national health service had to wait more than 30 years before starting in December 1978 and a main potential stimulus for developing epidemiology was lost.

The hospital and academic medical departments

A different kind of intellectual stimulus was pervading the post-Second World War medicine. On one hand the advent of drugs like antibiotics and corticoids clearly showed that efficacious agents could indeed be discovered and developed, raising the issue of how to test them in humans. On the other hand the very efficacy of antibiotics made many of the common and serious infectious diseases treatable, shifting the research interests of clinicians and pathologists towards 'degenerative' diseases, like cancers and atherosclerotic disease, still largely obscure in aetiology. Both stimuli promoted the use of epidemiological methods. In 1961 a periodical was first published in Milan (*Quaderni della Sperimentazione Clinica Controllata* [Controlled Clinical Trials Notes]) at the initiative of a small group of industrial clinical pharmacologists, later linked to the Institute of Medical Statistics of the local university. It contributed for more than a decade to familiarization of clinicians and pathologists with the quantitative approach and statistics in medicine, with particular attention to clinical trials methodology. An early development in aetiological investigations, marking a distinctive and continuing (to present day) contribution to modern epidemiology, has been the Italian component of the now classic Seven Countries prospective study of coronary heart disease (Puddu and Menotti 1969). It was only at the beginning of the 1970s that a mortality study (actually published in 1976; Rubino *et al.* 1976) of talc workers in a Piedmont valley showed for the first time the feasibility of a historical cohort investigation in an Italian context, contributing to dispel the prejudice that epidemiological studies feasible elsewhere would meet insurmountable practical obstacles in Italy.

The academic institutes of genetics and medical statistics

The key impulse to the development of modern epidemiology, however, came from quite a different quarter. Applied human genetics had been instrumental over many decades in the rise of racism, culminating in the mass exterminations by the Nazis, allies of Italian fascism. But genetics was also developing as a fundamental science, strongly research based, rapidly advancing on the experimental side using relatively simple materials such as bacteria and insects, and—alone among the biological sciences—inherently quantitative and probabilistic. In post-Second World War Italy it was new as an academic discipline. The Institute of Genetics of the University of Pavia was directed by A. Buzzati-Traverso (1913–83), an outstanding scientist combining creativity in research, managerial skills, and a progressive cultural and international outlook. He rapidly made his institute the focal point of the discipline in the country: in the 1950s it became the cradle of young geneticists destined for international repute and acted as a magnet for scientists in biology and medicine. R. Fisher lectured at the Pavia Institute and G. A. Maccacaro (1924–77) gave courses in microbial genetics, his field of research which brought him to a Chair in Microbiology in 1964. A full mastering of quantitative methods in biology joined with an acute intelligence of biology and medicine, a vast cultural knowledge, and a deep social concern prompted Maccacaro's decision to abandon microbiology and establish in 1966 the first Italian Institute of Medical Statistics and Biometry at the University of Milan. He saw medical statistics as a conceptual and technical tool to innovate and reform medicine and public health from the interior. From the outset the institute became the national reference in methodological matters: although initially these concerned mostly biological and clinical studies, room was soon more specifically made for modern epidemiology, as witnessed by studies on human growth (Marubini and Barghini 1969) and health services (Saracci 1969), the publication of the first Italian monograph on epidemiological methods (Saracci 1967), and the translation of the epidemiologically based monograph by Richard Doll on cancer prevention (Doll 1968). The institute also became a focal point for methodological development (Marubini *et al.* 1971) and training, including the organization of the 3-week courses on statistics applied to biology and medicine started in the late 1950s by the Biometric Society. A regular teacher at these courses was G. Barbensi (1875–74), a numerate general practitioner from Florence and an honorary life member of the International Biometric Society, whose books had been, from the 1930s until the early 1960s (Barbensi 1962), the only work in Italian on mathematics and modern inferential methods of statistics available to biomedical researchers.

The social movement of the late 1960s and early 1970s

At the end of the 1960s a major wave of social unrest shook Italy. In essence it arose from the blatant discrepancy between a society which had progressed markedly in economic terms while being blocked in several respects, from workers rights to school organization, from legislation on marriages to research structures. Medical research and practices also underwent sharp attacks, the Milan Institute of Medical Statistics standing as an active centre in many of these debates. The modern epidemiological approach was raised, amid great expectations, to the level of the main tool for critical analysis of health conditions at work and of the many dysfunctionalities in the health area (the disappointing discovery was soon made that epidemiology *per se* is no panacea for society's ills, including ill-health, and that political activism counts more for producing change). By being propelled to the forefront of public attention modern epidemiology gained on two counts: it became widely if superficially known, and by involvement in the social movement epidemiologists learned to better appreciate the strengths and limitations of their discipline; this applied particularly in the area occupational epidemiology where, for instance, a neglected element, the exposed subjects' assessments of their working environment, became recognized as a valuable tool for a comprehensive evaluation of exposures (Bertazzi 1975).

The emergence of modern epidemiology

As a net result of all these inputs, fairly often in competition, by the early 1970s epidemiology had become by a visible and evolving subject. A dozen or more essentially self-trained, or trained on the job abroad, epidemiologists were at work and some collaborations had developed between researchers with separate backgrounds and traditions as epidemiologists, clinicians, medical statisticians, and hygienists (Rose *et al.* 1968; Bianchi *et al.* 1972; Rolli *et al.* 1974). The first population-based cancer registry started in Piedmont, and began to report its initial epidemiological work (Terracini *et al.* 1974). But epidemiology remained by and large fragmented into initiatives by dispersed individuals or small units. Perhaps the clearest illustration of the shortcomings of this situation came when in 1973 an outbreak of cholera occurred in the three southern regions of Campania (Naples), Puglia, and Sardinia. To identify and control the responsible vectors (contaminated seafood) the 'Istituto Superiore di Sanita' in Rome, where a nucleus of competent infectious disease epidemiologists was active, sought the supporting expertise of other specialists: after careful pondering they decided to ask for collaboration from the USA Centers for Disease Control (CDC) rather than from some of the potentially antagonistic Italian experts (Baine *et al.* 1974).

The need for more communication, coordination, and more convergent efforts to upgrade epidemiological resources to create groups with critical mass, prompted the foundation in Pisa of the Associazione Epidemiologica Italiana (AEI) in April 1975 (Meeting News 1975). It arose in response to a request from the newly established 'Panel of Epidemiology and Social Medicine in the European Community', grouping the national scientific societies of the relevant disciplines, and assembled a number of clinicians, pathologists, occupational physicians, statisticians, and epidemiologists, several of whom had in 1974 participated in the first Italian IEA-sponsored course in modern epidemiological methods in Pisa. Soon afterwards the 'Societa' Italiana di Epidemiologia' was founded in Milan, assembling mostly hygienists, public health officers, statisticians, and epidemiologists. Members of the Milan Institute of Medical Statistics were present in both societies. It became immediately clear that the existence of two societies could only be counterproductive, and discussions about their unification started; in 1977 they merged into the AIE (Associazione Italiana di Epidemiologia).

The growth of epidemiology: 1975–90

The creation of the Italian Association of Epidemiology, the foundation by G. A. Maccacaro of *Epidemiologia e Prevenzione*, which later became—and still is—the official journal of the association, and the introduction of new methods of investigation in occupational medicine were not the only landmarks in the development of the discipline during the 1970s. The perception of the need for epidemiological skills was catalysed by several events taking place during those years, some of which are outlined below. However, the rationale of the 1978 health reform, which created a national health service along the lines of the 1948 British model, relied much more on a general quest for social justice and equity than on estimates of loss of health brought about by the existing system.

The presence of Italian epidemiological studies in the international scientific literature expanded progressively and significantly since 1975. Early studies related to the areas of cancer and occupational studies, other applications of epidemiological methods being added later.

The academic milieu had a minor role in the expansion of epidemiological investigations in Italy. Indeed, until the early 1990s medical schools were not particularly sensitive to the increasing need that the country had for epidemiological skills. In the 1970s, in a country of some 50 million, there were a handful of chairs of medical statistics, in addition to a position of non-tenured Professor of Cancer Epidemiology in the University of Turin. Post-graduate courses in medical statistics were offered in the universities of Milan—at the leading institute created by Maccacaro—Rome, and Pavia. The epidemiology of non-infectious diseases was not a focus of interest of departments of hygiene in Italian universities (until recently modern Italian epidemiology almost exclusively evolved outside the universities, i.e. within the laboratories of the National Research Council, the private research institute 'Mario Negri' in Milan, a handful of National Cancer Institutes and the National Health Service, including the central Istituto Superiore di Sanita' in Rome and several regional observatories or agencies). Research articles started to appear in international journals (Buiatti *et al.* 1978; La Vecchia *et al.* 1982; Forastiere *et al.* 1986; Costa and Segnan 1987; Merletti *et al.* 1987), including in the 1980s the report of a nationwide randomized trial which had considerable impact on the practice of cardiology (GISSI 1987). The work of all key investigators was regularly documented by papers in *Epidemiologia e Prevenzione*, indexed in Medline. Rather than systematically review (at the risk of partiality) this material it is of interest to briefly comment on some significant stimuli to the sustained growth of epidemiology in the period 1975–90: the occurrence of several environmental disasters, the opportunities offered by the new International Agency for Research on Cancer (IARC) in Lyon, with which strong links were developed from its inception, the judicial recourse to epidemiological expertise, and, last but not least, the mounting and inescapable need to assembling and analyse informative health databases.

Environmental disasters

Icmesa was a chemical company associated with Hoffman La Roche located in Seveso, near Milan. On 10 July 1976 a reactor used for the production of trichlorophenol exploded and released in the general environment a cloud containing at least 200 g of 2,3,7,8-tetrachlorodibenzodioxin (TCDD). The episode made the public, politicians, and epidemiologists aware of the lack of preparedness of the country in the face of an environmental accident. One of the four branches of the special office set up by the regional government of Lombardy in order to manage post-disaster programmes was concerned with epidemiological and health activities. However, in the early phases there was a total inability to plan and conduct valid epidemiological investigations. Several teams were called to the scene, but they were unable to cooperate and coordinate their activities. The interpretation of many early studies was impaired by the insufficient size of the samples, the lack of proper control groups, the unknown validity of existing records, and the incomplete standardization of ascertainment and measurements methods (World Health Organization 1997). For instance, the local impact of TCDD on spontaneous abortions in the first months after the accident, if any, has never been clarified. Adequate long-term studies investigating cancer incidence and mortality were launched only at a later stage, when the epidemiological skills of the Clinica del Lavoro of Milan were brought to bear (Bertazzi *et al.* 1989).

All over the peninsula, other episodes of health concern consequent to the release of industrial chemicals into the general environment occurred in the same period, but they also started to be the object of proper epidemiological studies only at a much later stage. After the Seveso episode, and in the light of the growing concern of the public about environmental issues, the Italian Ministry of Health created in 1978 the National Advisory Committee for Toxicology, a multidisciplinary body one of whose tasks was unravelling the health consequences of environmental problems in Italy. It operated for over 20 years with modern (for the country) procedural rules, such as interdisciplinarity, transparency, and circulation of the opinions which were expressed (Mucci *et al.* 1998). It was dismantled in 2000.

In 1986, law 348 recognized a number of areas 'at high risk of environmental crisis' requiring decontamination (which in fact has proceeded much more slowly than expected) as well as an evaluation of the environment–health associations at local level. The task has been undertaken by the Rome branch of the European Office of the WHO (Martuzzi *et al.* 2002). These studies have taken advantage of the availability of mortality statistics for each of the approximately 10,000 municipalities as well as of the development of skills within the country for the application of sophisticated methods to geographical analysis.

Support from the International Agency for Research on Cancer (IARC)

The rationale of General De Gaulle and his collaborators in the early 1960s for promoting the creation of the IARC, namely the need to investigate the cause of diseases and primary prevention, was not too different from the principles of the Italian 1978 health service reform. Since its inception, the IARC fellowship programme seemed to be tailored for Italian needs in terms of training epidemiologists. Among the current leading Italian epidemiologists more than a dozen were trained in epidemiology in those years, in the UK, in the USA, or at IARC itself thanks to IARC fellowships. However, the impact of IARC's support was something more than the provision of fellowships. For Italian groups which had just started, taking part in multicentric IARC case–control studies was a unique opportunity to learn the tools of analytical epidemiology. The first opportunity to be offered was the case–control study on cancer of the larynx in Mediterranean countries coordinated by the late A. Tuyns (1921–2001) (Tuyns *et al.* 1988). In 1977 he created GRELL ('Groupe pour la recherche épidémiologique dans les pays de langue latine') also known as the 'Groupe de l'Ascension', from the date of the religious spring festival on which epidemiologists from countries speaking Latin languages have established the habit of meeting for almost 30 years. Tuyns was correctly convinced that in order to develop modern epidemiology (and cancer registries) southern European countries had to face cultural, legal, and technical obstacles different from those which had been successfully met in Scandinavian and other northern countries. He also stressed the importance of cancer risk factors which had peculiar patterns in southern Europe, such as tobacco colour (black or blond) and type of alcoholic drink. There was hardly any Italian cancer registry active in the 1980s that missed the privilege of working with A. Tuyns.

Epidemiology in court

The first outbreak of occupational cancer to attract public attention (and reach the Italian courts) occurred at the Industria Piemontese Coloranti Anilina (IPCA), a relatively small dye factory in the outskirts of Torino, where working conditions were very poor and hazardous aromatic amines had been produced for years in spite of evidence of carcinogenicity. Although the outbreak had been reported by occupational doctors in an Italian medical journal (with no mention of the name of the factory), the case exploded in the early 1970s because of the perception of some of the victims that so many bladder cancers in young men who had worked in the same factory was unusual. In 1977, the court in Torino deemed the owner, the director, and the physician of the factory guilty of negligent homicide on the basis of more than 20 claimants who had bladder cancer (where less than one would be expected), and the sentence was confirmed in 1979 by the Italian Supreme Court.

Other outbreaks of occupational bladder cancer were brought to court in the late 1970s, but most episodes in which cases of occupational cancer reached the court concerned the consequences of asbestos exposure (at present, a cautious estimate is that at least 750 asbestos-related mesotheliomas and as many lung cancers occur annually in Italy). As a consequence of much interaction between epidemiologists and magistrates with regard to occupational cancer, the Supreme Court stressed in 1990 'the need for an epidemiological investigation…on those sectors of the population who have been and those who have not been exposed … so that a significant opinion can be formed about the possible excess of the former over the latter rate' (Guariniello 2005). Other courts, however, even in recent times, have justified acquittal with the impossibility of diagnosing the aetiology of polycausal tumours at the individual level.

The availability of health statistics

Mortality statistics in Italy were computerized in 1969, but only some years later was access allowed (with some restrictions, in order to ensure confidentiality) to data broken down by age, sex, and municipalities (approximately 10,000 municipalities all over the country). In earlier years the only available data were the absolute numbers of deaths by cause by province (around 100 provinces all over the country). The indirect standardization method was used to produce the first statistical atlas on Italian cancer mortality which covered the years 1970–72 (Cislaghi *et al.* 1987). Albeit limited, the information provided by the atlas put into proper perspective the geographical differences in the occurrence of cancer and focused attention on the protective factors which in those days were typical of southern Italy. It also led to subsequent analyses of the large populations which had migrated within Italy during the 1950s and 1960s.

Morbidity statistics had started initially for cancer registration (Bianchi *et al.* 1972) with data from an Italian registry (Varese province, founded in 1976) included for the first time in the IARC reference publication *Cancer incidence in five continents* in its fifth edition (Muir *et al.* 1987). Registration of birth defects started much later on a regional basis (Bianchi *et al.* 1997), while quality-controlled statistics on hospital discharge became available only in the late 1990s.

Epidemiology, a mature activity: 1990 to the present

The sustained development of epidemiology in Italy during the period 1975–90 had brought the discipline on a par with other European countries, so that the history of epidemiology in Italy during the last 15 years largely reflects the general trends of epidemiology in economically developed countries, compounded with the chronic structural and underfunding problems which affects all research in Italy (Saracci 2004). Some other country-specific features likely to persist in time, and hence of potential historical relevance, are also worth mentioning.

At the middle of the 1980s no summer schools of epidemiology were available in Europe, and it was customary for students from European countries to cross the Atlantic to attend such schools in North America. In 1988, at the initiative of the Panel of Epidemiology and Social Medicine in the European Community (regrouping a number of national scientific societies), the first 3-week European summer school of epidemiology started in Florence—the 'European Educational Programme in Epidemiology' (EEPE). By 2005, the yearly summer courses of the programme, taught in English by lecturers from Europe and supported by Italian (regional) health authorities, have been attended by more than 1500 students from both European and non-European countries.

A second significant initiative was taken in the mid-1990s: in contrast to research, education and training remained clearly inadequate in volume and quality with respect to the demand growing within scientific and health services institutions under the stimulus of research. The Italian Association of Epidemiology decided, after extensive consultation of its membership, to start a Master of Epidemiology programme, with countrywide recruitment of both teachers/tutors and students and, in the initial and experimental phase, no formal academic attachment. The programme began in 1997. Students attended every month from January to May of the 2 years of the programme one full-time week of methodological lectures and practical computer-based sessions, for a total of 10 weeks: this proved particularly suitable for participants who already had a job, for instance within the health services, which would have prevented long absences. In addition students had to prepare a short dissertation at the end of the first year and a thesis at the end of the second year, these two tasks requiring—under the supervision of one or two tutors—several months of work. The programme developed successfully, setting a standard in the country, and became recognized and incorporated as an academic activity at the University of Turin, enrolling an average of 15 students every 2 years. Most of the final theses produced publishable articles, about a third already being close to the form required of papers for international journals in English. Lately the programme has entered a circuit of European Masters of Epidemiology, with some modules taught in English.

A sustained didactic programme, particularly through courses in applied and field epidemiology, was also developed by the Istituto Superiore di Sanita', which had been active in epidemiology since the early days. Its engagement in research amplified over the years leading to the constitution of a National Centre for Epidemiology, Health Surveillance and Promotion, with 12 sections ranging from clinical epidemiology to pharmaco-epidemiology, to bioethics.

Cancer registries, which have been important in epidemiology since its beginning, have also multiplied in number. Of the 22 population registries (19 general and 4 specialized) only four (three general and one specialized, i.e. some 18% of the total) are in the south of the country and islands (Sicily and Sardinia) an area which includes more than a third of the country's population. This imbalance closely follows a similar imbalance in epidemiological activities in general, a reflection of the more pervasive and persistent phenomenon of a socio-economic lag affecting the southern regions.

At the turn of the century epidemiology in Italy showed all the signs of a mature sector of research, teaching, and applications. Which of the many activities will leave a historical mark is obviously impossible to say today. In virtually every specialized area of epidemiology one can find at least a few experts with an active record of publications in the international peer-reviewed literature. Epidemiological methods appear in the curricula of all 33 medical schools, although the quality of the teaching is highly variable, as there are no explicit quality standards or links to research projects. Epidemiology also appears as a topic in the curricula of the recently reformed schools of nursing and of a large number of medical specialities. The Italian Association of Epidemiology holds an annual general meeting, the number of participants ranging from 200 to 400; occasionally a second smaller meeting may be held on special issues, for instance in environmental epidemiology or health services research. Epidemiology is well represented not only within the central Istituto Superiore di Sanita' but also in the public health structures of the 20 regions. Several of these the regional health agencies or observatories carry substantial amounts of epidemiological research focused on issues of local relevance which often have national or European ramifications. This expansion has been favoured, on the whole, by the successive reforms that the national health service has undergone after its establishment in 1978. The 1992 reform (regarded by some as a 'counter-reform' of the 1978 bill) was oriented to management and competition between health-care providers. The 1999 reform went in a different direction, re-establishing the priority of actual health objectives to be attained, and the year 2000 legislation on regional 'federalism' made the regions autonomously responsible (with a relatively minor compensation system between higher and lower income regions) both for income and expenditure for health. Although divergent in their orientations all these laws accentuated—for different reasons—the need for epidemiological data collection and analysis at all levels, from national aggregates to local hospitals. Notwithstanding the increasing regionalization of the health services, or maybe just because of it, a notable and positive trend is the generally good level of cooperation between different groups of epidemiologists—as well as of the public services carrying out environmental measurements—which often join forces outside the restricted limits of their region in nation-wide studies such as those on air pollution (Biggeri *et al.* 2004).

References

Baine WB, Mazzotti M, Greco D, *et al.* (1974). Epidemiology of cholera in Italy in 1973. *Lancet*, **2**, 1370–4.

Barbensi G (1962). *Metodologia statistica applicata alle scienze biologiche*. Valsalva editrice, Firenze.

Bertazzi PA (1975). Homogeneous groups of workers in an epidemiologic study in industrial medicine. *La Medicina del Lavoro*, **66**, 119–26.

Bertazzi PA, Zocchetti C, Pesatori AC, Guercilena S, Sanarico M, and Radice L (1989). Ten-year mortality study of the population involved in the Seveso incident in 1976. *American Journal of Epidemiology*, **129**, 1187–200.

Bianchi F, Cianciulli D, Pierini A, and Seniori-Costantini A (1997). Congenital malformations and maternal occupation;: a registry based case-control study. *Journal of Occupational and Environmental Medicine*, **54**, 223–8.

Bianchi P, Porro CB, Coltorti M, *et al.* (1972). Occurrence of Australia antigen in chronic hepatitis in Italy. *Gastroenterology*, **63**, 482–5.

Biggeri A, Bellini P, and Terracini B (2004). Meta-analysis of the Italian studies on short-term effects of air pollution 1996–2002. *Epidemiologia e Prevenzione*, **28**, S1–S98.

Buiatti E, Cecchini S, Ronchi O, Dolara P, and Bulgarelli G (1978). Relationship between clinical and electromyographic findings and exposure to solvents, in shoe and leather workers. *British Journal of Industrial Medicine*, **35**, 168–73.

Checcacci L, Meloni C, and Romero E (1965). Prevalence of ischemic cardiopathies in municipal personnel employed in sedentary work. *Annali della Sanita Pubblica*, **26**, 787–93.

Cislaghi C, Decarli A, Morosini P, and Puntoni R (1987). *Atlante della mortalita' per tumori in Italia 1970–72*. Lega Italiana per la lotta contro i tumori, Milan.

Costa G and Segnan N (1987). Unemployment and mortality. *British Medical Journal (Clinical Research Education)*, **294**, 1550–1.

Delogu S (1967). *Sanita' pubblica, sicurezza sociale e programmazione economica*. Giulio Einaudi, Torino.

Doll R (1968). *Le basi epidemiologiche della prevenzione del cancro*. Centro G. Zambon, Milan.

Forastiere F, Lagorio S, Michelozzi P, *et al.* (1986). Silica, silicosis and lung cancer among ceramic workers: a case-referent study. *American Journal of Industrial Medicine*, **10**, 363–70.

GISSI (1987). Long-term effects of intravenous thrombolysis in acute myocardial infarction: final report of the GISSI study. Gruppo Italiano per lo Studio della Streptochinasi nell'infarto miocardico (GISSI). *Lancet*, **2**, 871–4.

Guariniello R (2005). Epidemiology in the Italian courts: the experience of a magistrate. *International Journal of Occupational and Environmental Health*, **11**, 47–52.

La Vecchia C, Franceschi S, Gallus G, *et al.* (1982). Prognostic features of endometrial cancer in estrogen users and obese women. *American Journal of Obstetrics and Gynaecology*, **144**, 387–90.

Martuzzi M, Mitis F, Biggeri A, Terracini B, and Bertollini R (2002). Environment and health status in the population of the areas at high risk of environmental crisis in Italy. *Epidemiologia e Prevenzione*, **26**, S1–S56.

Marubini E and Barghini G. Research on the average age at puberty in school girls in Carrara. *Minerva Pediatrica*, **21**, 281–5.

Marubini E, Resele LF, and Barghini G (1971). Comparative fitting of the Gompertz and logistic functions to longitudinal height data during adolescence in girls. *Human Biology*, **43**, 237–52.

Meeting News (1975). *International Journal of Epidemiology*, **2**, 151.

Merletti F, Rosso S, Terracini B, and Cappa AP (1987). Cancer of the breast in women born in southern Italy and who migrated to the city of Torino. *Tumori*, **73**, 229–32.

Mucci N, Terracini B, and Camoni I (1998). Evaluation of carcinogenicity of chemical and productive processes by the National Advisory Toxicology Committee. *La Medicina del Lavoro*, **89**, 78–83.

Muir C, Waterhouse J, Mack T, Powell J, and Whelan S (1987). *Cancer incidence in five continents*, 5th edn. International Agency for Research on Cancer, Lyon.

Puddu V and Menotti A (1969).An Italian study of ischemic heart disease. *Acta Cardiologica*, **24**, 558–78.

Rolli GP, Tenconi MT, and Marinoni A (1974). Prevalence of ischaemic heart disease in the residents of the Republic of San Marino. *Giornale Italiano di Cardiologia*, **4**, 261–9.

Rose GA, Ahmeteli M, Checcacci L, *et al.* (1968). Ischaemic heart disease in middle-aged men. Prevalence comparisons in Europe. *Bulletin of the World Health Organization*, **38**, 885–95.

Rubino GF, Scansetti G, Piolatto G, and Romano CA (1976). Mortality study of talc miners and millers. *Journal of Occupational Medicine*, **18**, 187–93.

Saracci R (1967). *Metodi statistici elementari per l'epidemiologia clinica*. Centro G. Zambon, Milan.

Saracci R (1969). Factors affecting accuracy and precision in clinical chemistry: a survey of 404 Italian laboratories. *American Journal of Clinical Pathology*, **52**, 161–6.

Saracci R (2004). La ricerca scientifica in Italia: come prima, peggio di prima. *Epidemiologia e Prevenzione*, **28**, 69–70.

Terracini B, Anglesio E, Cappa AP, Coverlizza S, Panero M, and Pastore G (1974). High incidence of laryngeal cancer in the province of Torino (Italy). *Tumori*, **60**, 143–56.

Tuyns AJ, Esteve J, Raymond L, *et al.* (1988). Cancer of the larynx/hypopharynx, tobacco and alcohol. The IARC case control study in Turin and Varese (Italy), Zaragoza and Navarra (Spain), Geneva (Switzerland) and Calvados (France). *International Journal of Cancer*, **1**, 483–91.

World Health Organization (1997). *Assessing the health consequences of major chemical incidents— epidemiological approaches*, WHO Regional Publications, European Series No 79. WHO, Copenhagen.

37

The development of epidemiology: Spain

Francisco Bolúmar

The aim of this chapter is to describe the development of epidemiology in Spain, with special emphasis on the period from the mid-1970s to the present day. After a brief historical introduction, I shall first present the major factors which influenced me to start in epidemiology and the options available at that time for training. I shall follow this with a description of the major obstacles encountered by people of my generation in the practice of epidemiology, including the restricted availability and use of data sources. I shall continue by highlighting the relationship with and the influence of epidemiology on some public health policies. Finally, I shall discuss the future perspectives for epidemiology in Spain.

Brief historical introduction

Possibly the first book in the world in which the word epidemiology appeared in the title was published in Spain in the sixteenth century by Tito Angelerio and described a plague epidemic. Later, the word epidemiology was used in Spain in 1802 by Joaquín Villalba in his book *Epidemiología Española* (1803), a compilation of the epidemics registered in Spain since the fifth century BC.

However, in spite of the pioneering work developed in the eighteenth century in Asturias by Gaspar Casal (1762), who associated pellagra with a poor diet, in Valencia by Cavanilles (1797), who studied the relation between malaria and rice growing, and in the nineteenth century in Catalonia by Monlau (1841;1856), who related living conditions in the inner cities with disease, there were no further studies in Spain that explored the association between poor living conditions or lifestyle and the incidence of certain diseases, since epidemiologists had neither the competence nor the interest to do this during the first half of the twentieth century.

The generalized movement in Europe, at the end of the nineteenth century, to the use of vital statistics for public health policies was reflected in Spain with significant contributions by Hauser (1913). However, and in spite of an early systematic collection of vital data at the end of the nineteenth century, it was nonetheless peripheral to the development of public health at the beginning of the twentieth century.

Life expectancy in Spain was roughly 40 years at the beginning of the twentieth century, with a mortality rate of 28 per 1000 inhabitants, and a high infectious disease mortality (standardized rate of 1588 per 100,000) mainly due to diseases of faecal–oral and air transmission. Thus, it was activities related to the control of transmissible diseases that guided the development of epidemiology, both institutional and scientific, in accordance with the transmissible pattern predominant in morbidity and mortality.

In this context, the development of epidemiology in Spain occurred mainly within the framework of the health administration, and the contribution of the universities was negligible. This probably explains to a large extent the absence of Spanish theoretical or methodological contributions to the development of epidemiology in Europe.

The twentieth century represents a sustained effort to update public health in Spain and, consequently, epidemiology. This effort became more evident during the second half of the 1920s, when the nation began to reap the fruits of the programme set up jointly by the Spanish Government and the Rockefeller Foundation for the training of public health personnel. The programme (Curso de Oficial Sanitario) was established with the aim of setting up a corps of sanitary personnel at the service of the health administration. In charge of their training was the National School of Public Health (Escuela Nacional de Sanidad), created in 1924 and directed by Pittaluga (1930), that completed the training programme in Spain with a stay in the USA for the best students, financed by the Rockefeller Foundation (Bernabeu Mestre 1994; Rodríguez Ocaña 1994; 2000).

This training programme, which ran from 1923 to 1930, had a major impact on the practice of epidemiology in Spain, and may be illustrated by the work of two of the students (Ortiz de Landázuri and Marcelino Pascua) who spent 1 or 2 years at Johns Hopkins University. On his return to Spain, Ortiz de Landázuri published an important paper (Ortiz de Landázuri 1929) that should be considered as the first attempt to organize a modern epidemiology unit in the country. He clearly established the difference between the traditional and modern practice of epidemiology, and his work greatly contributed to shape the new epidemiological services (Martinez Navarro 1994).

Pascua, General Director of Health from 1931 to 1933, made a systematic study of vital statistics and contributed significantly to the organization of the first Spanish surveillance system of transmissible diseases (Pascua 1934). He taught statistical methods in the Curso de Oficial Sanitario, and his book *Bioestadistica* became a classic teaching book even up to the 1960s (Rodríguez Ocaña 1988; 1992; Benavides 2000).

This training programme and the process of incorporation of competent post-graduate students into key posts of the public health services was drastically interrupted by the Spanish Civil War. A substantial number of academics and notable public health physicians loyal to the Republic (among them Pittaluga, Ortiz de Landazuri, Marcelino Pascua, etc.) went into exile during and after the Civil War. This dramatic drain, that enriched the academic staff of many universities in America, resulted in an impoverishment of the academic life and in the practice of public health in Spain, and had long-term consequences for the development of epidemiology and public health in the country, and some of these consequences were already evident when I arrived at university to study medicine.

The teaching of epidemiology and public health (a personal digression)

In the 1970s a substantial proportion of students at Spanish universities were involved in Agitprop activities within the frame of the fight against Franco's dictatorship. Leftwing ideology had even permeated the ranks of upper-middle-class students. This ideology matched well with what we thought, as students, was the mission of public health. But our views clashed with reality. With the only exception of Associate Professor Martinez Navarro, competent in epidemiology and who was later instrumental in the development of the Spanish Epidemiological Corps, the rest of the staff in charge of the teaching of public health still had a microbiological view of the subject, were unaware of the new epidemiological methods, and lacked any sort of social consciousness. Fortunately, our interest was strengthened by López Piñero, at the time Professor of the History of Medicine, who was the most progressive and influential professor at the Valencia School of Medicine and who had a particular interest in the history of public health.

My internship in his department was crucial to my future orientation, since it not only allowed me to understand the evolution of medicine up to then but introduced me to a series of books such as *World health* by Fraser Brockington, *Sociology of medicine* by Rodney McCoe, and Thomas McKeown's *Introduction to social medicine*, that enlarged in a definitive way my view of medicine which up until then had too narrowly focused on the clinical perspective. George Rosen's *A history of public health*, which I read and discussed thoroughly with colleagues, was essential to comprehend the population perspective of disease. In the end, it was this realization of the population perspective of disease that led me to epidemiology. Thus, I and other colleagues in Valencia came into epidemiology through public health, and to public health through the history of medicine.

When I qualified in medicine in the mid-1970s, post-graduate courses in epidemiology or public health were not available and field work was too narrow to be instructive. Therefore, people from my generation were forced to go abroad in order to have formal training in these subjects. At the beginning, those of us who were relatively fluent in English went to the UK (mostly to the London School of Hygiene and Tropical Medicine), and later on, in the mid-1980s, the younger generation also set off for the USA (Johns Hopkins, Harvard) taking up again what was a tradition in Spain during the 1920s and was interrupted by the Spanish Civil War. The Cuban National School of Public Health was the favourite destination for Spanish-only speakers and the Université Libre de Bruxelles for French speakers.

After this personal and generational account of the vicissitudes encountered in our training I shall continue by describing the difficulties of carrying out epidemiological research in Spain in the 1970s, that were fairly similar to those experienced in other areas of scientific research.

Major obstacles to epidemiological research

The major obstacles to epidemiological research in Spain in the mid-1970s came from the absence of good public health practice and of competent public health practitioners, together with the lack of visibility of epidemiology as a scientific discipline. At that time, the immense majority of practising Spanish physicians would have been unable to give a reasonable description of the contents of the discipline.

The absence of a research tradition in public health administration was another drawback. The epidemiology practised in the public health services was conceptually backward and focused on routine activities of epidemiological surveillance. In this context, there was no room for research.

Unskilled personnel was another important obstacle. The National School of Public Health had been training physicians and nurses in public health matters since its creation in 1925. The 1-year course of Official Sanitario taught at the school was highly prestigious at the beginning but by the 1960s was totally outdated and was discontinued a few years later. Thus, the unavailability of formal training in modern epidemiology in Spain had the consequence that those physicians joining the public health services in the 1970s had a lack of expertise in modern epidemiological methods. This made them unable to conduct rigorous epidemiological studies.

The situation in the university departments was no better. Restricted access and nepotism in the appointment of junior staff made the groups uncompetitive. Team working culture was absent, with the result of a concentration in small groups without a critical mass for conducting good epidemiological research.

Given the shortage of money available for field epidemiological studies, the use of secondary data could have helped to develop epidemiology in the country. Unfortunately, the status of health information systems was relatively poor at the time, and was thus another major drawback to epidemiological research. Mortality data appeared with a delay that limited its usefulness. Hospital morbidity data were based on the diagnosis at entry, and only by the end of the 1970s was the coding of the diagnosis at discharge firmly established as practice. By the mid-1970s there were only two cancer registries in operation, limited to the provinces of Zaragoza and Navarra, which covered only a small proportion of the Spanish population. Finally, systematic data from surveys was not available; the first National Health Survey was only carried out in 1987 (with the precedent of the Barcelona Health Survey done in 1983).

Financing was another major problem. In the mid-1970s the possibilities of obtaining funding for epidemiological studies were scant, and funds came mainly from town councils and provincial councils interested in specific studies.

The principal funding body at the time was the Fondo del Descuento Complementario of the pharmaceutical industry, devoted entirely to clinical research in hospitals of the National Health Service and with absolute disregard for epidemiology. Private financing for epidemiology, either from the industry or other non-governmental bodies, was, obviously, non-existent.

This catalogue of obstacles to epidemiological research began to change gradually during the 1980s, following the path of economic growth occurring in the country, that was consolidated with Spain's entry into the European Union. The new situation favoured the introduction of some public policies whose repercussions in the improvement of public health was notable.

Public policies and the development of epidemiology

The changing epidemiological pattern was making evident the need to introduce changes in the public health services. With this aim, the State Epidemiological Corps was given a new impetus in 1978 by calling for, under the direct supervision of the Directorate General of Health, a public competition for posts that had been blocked for many years.

A group of the first 45 members that joined the Corps in 1978 founded, in the same year, the Spanish Epidemiological Association (SEE). The association came into being as a response to the attempt by the Ministry of Health to concentrate most of the jobs offered at the central level which clashed with the ideas and interests of the professionals. Thus, at the beginning, the association had strictly a professional orientation, but soon also became a scientific society.

In 1981, a progressive multisystem disease, later called toxic oil syndrome, broke out in epidemic proportions in Spain, affecting thousands of people. Toxic oil syndrome resulted from the consumption of rapeseed oil that had been denatured with 2% aniline for industrial use. Until then, the epidemiological surveillance system had proved adequate since it was mainly concerned with cholera, and the possibility of a massive outbreak of the disease was minimal given the degree of economic development in Spain during the 1980s. However, the eruption of a huge and previously unknown public health problem, such as toxic oil syndrome, highlighted the shortcomings of the Spanish public health services, bringing into question the role played by the epidemiologists, chemists, and veterinarians of Sanidad Nacional. It was clear that food control, public health inspection, and epidemiological surveillance services required a thorough reorganization and strengthening. As part of the strategy aimed at improving the epidemiological services, the new entrants to the Epidemiological Corps were deployed all over the country.

The crisis triggered by the toxic oil syndrome had also shown the need to develop a new normative framework for public health matters that made effective the coordination between local, regional, and central services. Therefore, the Ley General de Sanidad [General Health Law] was enacted in 1986 in an attempt to match the health structures to the health needs of its time, and to articulate mechanisms for cooperation between the Ministry of Health (set up in 1978) and the health services of the autonomous regions. A key actor in the preparation of the General Health Law was Enrique Nájera, at the time Professor of Hygiene and Social Medicine at the University of Seville. The law, in the sixth article, established that the actions of the health administration would be aimed at the promotion of health and prevention of illness, two of the main strategies of public health. More specifically, in its eighth article, the General Health Law considers as a fundamental activity of the health system the carrying out of epidemiological studies required in order to address with higher efficacy both the prevention of health risks and health planning and evaluation, based upon an organized health information system. In addition, the law had a mandate by which each autonomous region should prepare a health plan addressing all necessary health actions in order to achieve the objectives set by their respective health services. Several regions worked out their health plans with a strong component of preventive activities that required the cooperation of epidemiologists, and with the intention of allocating human resources in an equitable manner into the different health districts of their respective regions.

With regard to public health, the development of this law, by both the Ministry of Health and the health services of the autonomous regions, involved the need to increase substantially the number of epidemiologists and to improve their training. At the time, the supply of epidemiologists fell short of demand. With no possibility of substantially increasing their output, due to limitations imposed by the fixed number of graduate students entering the medical training programme, and by the reduced number of hospital preventive medicine services offering such training, the regional health authorities of several autonomous regions took the decision to design methods to train the epidemiologists they required. Thus, four new schools of public health, which greatly contributed to the training in epidemiology of the new generations of health professionals, were set up in Barcelona, Granada, Madrid, and Valencia. On the whole, these schools, that were short of human resources and overwhelmed by their teaching burden, paid little attention to research activities. In the long run it worked against them, and at present, with Madrid and Barcelona closed and Valencia languishing, only Granada and the National School of Public Health continue their training programmes.

The future for epidemiology

Looking to the future, epidemiology is nowadays more included and far better understood than it was three decades ago when I started.

The rise of clinical epidemiology has brought epidemiological methods into the mainstream of clinical research. A substantial number of clinicians, mainly cardiologists, oncologists, and GPs, have followed courses on basic epidemiology in Spain and are willing to cooperate with epidemiologists. Thus, epidemiology is now a respected discipline among Spanish clinicians and is recognized as a core scientific method for clinical research. A growing number of research units in the main hospitals carry out collaborative studies in clinical epidemiology, and the prospects for the future are good. In this respect, the Fondo de Investigaciones Sanitarias FIS [Medical Research Fund] has been crucial in the development of epidemiology in general and of clinical epidemiology in particular. The FIS, an evolution of the Fondo del Descuento Complementario, has shown since its inception a good understanding of and great commitment to epidemiology, financing numerous epidemiological studies carried out at the universities and hospitals. Its policy of supporting new and inexperienced epidemiological groups that could hardly obtain any financing from other sources has greatly contributed to the improvement of the scale and scientific level of epidemiological studies in Spain. The constant growth in the budget section devoted to epidemiology experienced over these years augurs well for the future.

In recent years there has been a growing appraisal in Spain of the relation between epidemiology and policy. New tools for conducting epidemiological research, together with the increasing capacity to manage and analyse large databases, have increased the usefulness of epidemiological evidence for answering policy-makers' questions.

The relevance of epidemiological evidence for policy-making has slowly gained momentum in Spain. This has occurred with a combination of better technical facilities for Spanish epidemiologists, both in the universities and in the public health services, and the need to respond to social demands by decision-makers based on the best evidence. In addition, there has been an increasing awareness by individual researchers of their responsibility to the public and a greater commitment to public health intervention, leading them to take active steps to disseminate the results of their studies. As a result, there has been a growing presence of epidemiologists in the media. In this respect, the case of smoking is paradigmatic. The implication that epidemiologists in the public debate have presented incontrovertible data has represented a turning point. Through both direct and indirect action epidemiologists have made the control of smoking a cross-party issue in the political debate, putting it into the agenda of all political parties which have in this way assumed a stronger commitment to prevention. This represents a clear success for epidemiology and public health, and a considerable change with respect to the previous situation. This change in attitude by all parties is a guarantee for future interaction based on a new and promising climate of trust and cooperation.

The Spanish epidemiological society, SEE, has been growing ever since its foundation in 1978, and now with its nearly 900 members is one of the largest and most active epidemiological societies in Europe. The society is multidisciplinary, and apart from physicians, who make up the majority, there are also sociologists, statisticians, nurses, psychologists, chemists, etc. In many respects the SEE has been crucial in the development and consolidation of modern epidemiology in Spain. Over the years, 23 annual meetings have been held at which, under themes as diverse as the impact of epidemiology on public health programmes, ethics, environment and communication, or the epidemiological evaluation of the 'Health For All' strategy, the progress made in the descriptive, analytical, and methodological aspects of epidemiology has been presented. From the outset, all the abstracts submitted have gone through a rigorous peer review process that has definitely contributed to improving the quality of the works presented.

The SEE, together with the Spanish Public Health Society (SESPAS), publishes *Gaceta Sanitaria* which is the journal that has the highest impact among all journals published in Spanish in the area of epidemiology and public health. It is worth highlighting that the SEE has paved the way for the interaction between academic epidemiologists and those working in the public health services, with mutual benefit.

It is largely acknowledged that epidemiologists need to work more effectively with those who communicate with the public, and in particular with the media. The Spanish Epidemiological Society has played, and continues to play, a very active role in the diffusion of the results of epidemiological studies, and its implications for public health policies. Finally, the SEE has played an active role in consultancy, particularly with the Ministry of Health, in an attempt to translate research results into practice.

Parallel to the expansion of the SEE, most academic departments of public health in Spain have experienced a profound transformation in the last 15 years, affecting both the contents of the discipline and the personnel. As older professors have progressively retired, the microbiological tradition to which they belonged has lost ground and the inclusion in the teaching programmes of areas such as health promotion, social determinants of health, etc., to the detriment of the infectious diseases, reflect the conceptual shift in the subject. In addition, epidemiology has now been incorporated as a main subject in the undergraduate teaching programmes of all schools of medicine in the country, and as an optional in other health-related sciences. As regards personnel, the vacancies left by retirement have progressively been filled by professors with a formal training in epidemiology, some of them trained abroad, and with a large experience in epidemiological research. Their incorporation has notably revitalized the academic departments of public health.

Until quite recently the training of epidemiologists and other public health specialists has occurred separately from the university departments. In fact, with the exception of the schools of public health that offered a series of Masters courses with a variable content in epidemiology, no other formal training has been available for non-physicians. Due to the aforementioned changes in the academic departments, they now have the capacity to offer post-graduate training programmes. Nowadays, PhD programmes in public health run by some universities, with a strong epidemiological component, attract students from health-related areas, as well as foreign students, mostly from Latin American countries.

The National Commission for the Medical Speciality of Preventive Medicine and Public Health has played a key role in the transformation of the training programme for medical residents (Gómez and Benavides 2004), shifting from a hospital-based conception of the speciality, with special emphasis on the control of nosocomial infections, to a community perspective in which epidemiology becomes essential. Nowadays, all medical residents in the speciality have to take a 1-year Masters course with a strong component of epidemiological methods. Afterwards they spend only 1 year in a hospital and then go on to public health centres. In addition, the new training programme has established five routes for the speciality (epidemiology, preventive medicine, health promotion, occupational and environmental health, and health administration and management) one of which will have to be chosen by the residents according to their future interests. Thus, epidemiology will have the consideration of a subspeciality in the training of medical specialists in public health. The Masters course must be done at the National School of Public Health (ENS) or at one of the three academic departments in Alicante, Barcelona, or Granada accredited by the National Commission. The National School, after years of hesitation and pressed by the Bolonia requirements for a European Space for Higher Education (Benavides *et al.* 2006), is now undergoing a process of transformation that affects its administrative structure and the configuration of the teaching programmes. These changes introduced by the National Commission have only been possible thanks to the enormous improvement in the professional qualifications of epidemiologists that has taken place both at the universities and at the public health centres. As regards the future, the document issued by the National Commission, following the Bolonia process, leaves the door open for specialization in epidemiology by non-medics.

The admission of Spain into the European Union favoured the incorporation of Spanish groups into ongoing or new epidemiological research projects of a much larger scale than they were used to. Working on these projects allowed some of the groups to enhance their methodological skills and undertake new and more ambitious research projects. At the same time, the groups were able to recruit young staff and grow since the policy of the Medical Research Fund was to finance all research projects that were part of a larger European project. At present, several groups play an active role in various European projects and it is expected that their contribution will increase in the future.

As elsewhere, the perception of confronting a change in paradigm, both in the process of the production of knowledge and its organization and management, has prompted the establishment of research networks in Spain; a phenomenon to which has included epidemiology. In 2002, a research network on epidemiology and public health (RCESP) was set up by the Ministry of Health through the Carlos III Institute. The network, made up of 11 research centres from different institutions belonging to six autonomous regions, brings together 40 groups and nearly 300 researchers who share common research objectives. The centres cover a wide range of experience in research and development: from centres of excellence in aetiological research to public health agencies and regional departments of health.

The objectives of the RCESP are to coordinate and to supplement the ongoing research projects of the centres that make up the net and to set up new collaborative research projects between them, to provide an adequate framework for the training of young researchers in epidemiology, and to define strategies in order to promote a greater interaction of public health research with the Spanish health services. In this respect, it is hoped that the coexistence and collaboration within the RCESP network of research groups from centres of excellence and groups from the departments of health can be seen as an asset, which might facilitate the translation of knowledge from research into public health practice, and in turn promote evidence-based public health.

The RCESP network has taken advantage of the previous existence of cohorts (such as EPIC) as a platform to expand the scientific reach of their studies. However, largely due to financial restrictions, the network has not been sufficiently proactive in capitalizing on the resources offered by the different databases built and supplied by the research groups integrated into the network.

At present, the Carlos III Institute of the Ministry of Health has gone a step further in the configuration of research networks and has decided to establish seven national biomedical research centres (CIBER), with a network structure and virtual character. The CIBER on epidemiology and public health will be among this seven, and will constitute an essential tool for the future of epidemiology in Spain.

Epidemiology is nowadays in a good position to face the future, but new cross-cutting issues such as road accidents, working conditions, migration, etc. will try the capacity of epidemiologists to work with other social scientists in order to answer all those problems.

Acknowledgements

I am grateful to Dr F Martinez Navarro, Dr FG Benavides, Dr I Hernández, and Dr A Segura for their comments on the manuscript.

References

Benavides FG (2000). Epílogo para después de un paseo con don Marcelino de Pascua. Revista. *Española de Salud Pública*, **74**, 95–8.

Benavides FG, Bolúmar F, and Gómez López L (2006). El Espacio Europeo de Educación Superior, una gran oportunidad para la salud pública. *Gaceta Sanitaria*, **20**, 89–90.

Bernabeu Mestre J (1994). El papel de la Escuela Nacional de Sanidad en el desarrollo de la salud pública en España, 1924–1934. *Revista de Sanidad e Higiene Publica*, **68**, 65–90.

Casal G (1762). De affectione, que Vulgò in hac Regione mal de la Rosa nuncupatu. In Historia Natural *y Médica del Principado de Asturias*. Oficina de Manuel Martín, Madrid.

Cavanilles AJ (1797). *Observaciones sobre la Historia Natural, Geografía, Agricultura, población y frutos del Reyno de Valencia*. Imprenta Real, Madrid.

Gómez L and Benavides FG (2004). El nuevo programa de la especialidad en medicina preventiva y salud pública, una apuesta por mejorar la práctica profesional. *Gaceta Sanitaria*, **18**, 79–80.

Hauser PH (1913). *La geografía médica de la península ibérica*. Imprenta Eduardo Arias, Madrid.

Martinez Navarro JF (1994). Salud publica y desarrollo de la epidemiología en la España del siglo xx. *Revista de Sanidad e Higiene Publica*, **68**, 29–43.

Monlau PF (1841). *Abajo las murallas!! Memoria sobre las ventajas que reportaría Barcelona y especialmente su industria, de la demolición de las murallas que circuyen la ciudad*. Imprenta del Constitucional, Barcelona.

Monlau PF (1856). *Qué medidas puede dictar el gobierno a favor de las clases obreras?* Gorcho, Barcelona.

Ortiz de Landázuri A (1929). La función epidemiológica moderna. *Revista de Sanidad e Higiene Publica.*

Pascua M (1934). *La mortalidad infantil en España.* Dirección General de Sanidad, Madrid.

Pittaluga G (1930). *La constitución de la Escuela Nacional de Sanidad de Madrid (España),* Publicaciones de la Escuela Nacional de Sanidad Núm. 11. Escuela Nacional de Sanidad, Madrid.

Rodríguez Ocaña E (1988). *La constitución de la Medicina Social como disciplina en España (1882–1923).* Ministerio de Sanidad y Consumo, Madrid.

Rodríguez Ocaña E (1992). La estadística en la administración sanitaria española del siglo veinte. In *Las estadísticas demográfico-sanitarias. Primer Encuentro Marcelino Pascua,* pp. 35–60. Instituto de Salud Carlos III, Madrid.

Rodríguez Ocaña E (1994). La salud pública en España en el contexto europeo, 1890–1925. *Revista de Sanidad e Higiene Publica,* **68**, 11–28.

Rodríguez Ocaña E (2000). La intervención de la Fundación Rockefeller en la creación de la sanidad contemporánea en España. *Revista Española de Salud Pública,* **74**. 27–34.

Villalba J (1803). *Epidemiología española o historia cronológica de las pestes, contagios, epidemias y epizootias que han acaecido en España desde la venida de los cartagineses hasta el año 1801.* Villalpando, Madrid.

Name index

Subject index